Trim Healthy Mama

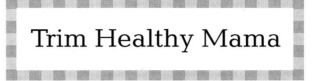

Trim Healthy Mama

Serene Allison & Pearl Barrett

Cover Design:
Jami Saunders
imadairyqueen@gmail.com

Interior design and typesetting:
PerfecType, Nashville, TN

Illustrations:
Monique Campbell (Serene and Pearl's sister-in-law)
smoochymctwain@att.net

Publisher:
Welby Street Press
www.welbystreetpress.com

ISBN: 978-0-9887751-1-4

Unless otherwise noted, all Scriptures are taken from the King James Bible.

Serene and Pearl are also recording artists. To order their music, go to *Book & Music Store* at www.aboverubies.org

CONTENTS

Part I: Gain the Knowledge

Part II: Practice the Knowledge

Part III: Join Us in the Kitchen (the Recipes)

Part IV: Our Past and Present

Part V: More Than Food

FOREWORD

by Charlie Barrett

March 20, 1994. The first day of spring. The first day of the new year on the Solar Calendar. The first day of the rest of my life—the day I married Pearl Priscilla Campbell.

Little did I know that the sweetest girl I had ever met in my 38 years was "The Food Dictator!" Now, I'm not complaining (well, maybe I did once in a while), but I should probably give a little background to my eating habits.

I am a true country boy. I love meat and potatoes—and junk food. I don't cook, and I always ate out. Not one to be bothered with breakfast, my first meal of the day was usually mini doughnuts, chocolate-dipped granola bars (they're healthy, right?), or cookies. Whichever I chose, it was accompanied by a diet soda. After all, one good choice counteracts a bad one, doesn't it?

Lunch was usually a burger and fries (large size), with a diet soda or unsweetened tea. Or, maybe a five piece fried chicken meal with potato salad, biscuits, and green beans or macaroni and cheese. Or, a foot long sub with a bag of potato chips.

Supper was usually one of the above that I didn't have for lunch. Sometimes I would treat myself to a restaurant meal of steak, salad, one of the potato choices, and dessert. Often, I would end up at home watching TV and eating a bag of potato chips with dip, a hunk of cheese, and of course, a diet soda. There were also plenty of sandwich choices—peanut butter and jelly, bologna and cheese, deli meat with cheese, peanut butter and banana, peanut butter and butter. You get the picture.

A couple of times a day between meals, I ate a candy bar and diet soda. Or, I had about a pint of ice cream. I have a terrible sweet tooth. I love Pecan Pie, Chess Pie, No Bake Cookies—the sweeter, the better.

When I met Pearl and Serene, they were on their vegetarian kick. Pearl recognized her biggest challenge and project in me. I wasn't in bad shape at first. Still pretty active and not quite middle aged, my body was holding up okay. I am six feet tall, large frame, and despite eating all that junk, weighed about 210 pounds when we met. However, marriage does strange things to a man's body. It didn't take long to hit 220 pounds. Pearl didn't push the issue of health too much at first; we were newlyweds. She cooked healthy meals at night but I didn't change my morning and daily eating habits. I still ate my cookies or ice cream after her supper.

Ten pounds or so later, the "Food Dictator" took charge. We went through several "fad" diets trying to find one I could accept. First, with Serene's help, she put me on a strict vegetarian diet. That was okay for a while. I could eat all the potato salad I wanted, which I really love. I could still eat most desserts, although I ate more than I should, especially when she wasn't watching! I lost weight for a while. I still had lots of potato and corn chips with dips (dairy wasn't out) and the vegetarian sandwiches with chips or potato salad (or both) for lunch didn't keep the pounds off for long. Pearl was still challenged, but not defeated.

She decided to put me on the Atkins Diet. That sounded good to me. Finally, a diet I could sink my teeth into! Any man would be happy eating all the meat, cheese, and eggs he wanted. It worked great for a while, but I started missing potato salad, cornbread, beans, and desserts. I was pretty frustrated and found ways to cheat on my diet as often as I could.

When I turned 50, I weighed over 235 pounds and was starting to feel "my age." I told everyone that life was all downhill after 50. My joints ached, I didn't have any energy, and I was depressed a lot of the time. Pearl's biggest challenge yet, but she wouldn't be defeated!

Pearl studied with the intensity of a postgraduate college student. She spent hour upon hour reading books and scouring the internet. The plan you are about to learn is the result of her and Serene's intense study, their love for health, and their wisdom gained from trial and error. I have a brother/sister relationship with Serene. I tease her a lot, I'm kind of a "mean" big brother. Once a year, usually at Christmas, I say something nice to her to make up for all the teasing. I never thought I would call her wise, but I guess I just did. Will that cover the next 10 or 15 Christmases?

I'm now 56 years old and weigh less than 200 pounds. I feel better than I have in more than 20 years and I love my diet and have little desire to "cheat." The hormones and supplements Pearl encourages me to take are a true miracle. She pushed hard for some of Serene's exercise programs, but I'm a little, I mean very stubborn. Finally, we settled on a steady regimen of push-ups every other day.

It's been over four years since being on "the plan" and I don't complain. I don't even feel like a reformed junk food eater. I no longer feel I am missing out as I get to eat so many treat foods. What? No potato salad! The *Cauliflower Potato Salad* is a surprisingly good replacement.

Pearl doesn't mind when I cheat now and then because my body has adapted so well. We have popcorn at the movies. I eat non-approved desserts once in a while (and even some real potato salad now and then). But, for the most part, I submit completely to my "**Former** Food Dictator" and am very happy to do so.

You will too, I know. I am Pearl's personal guinea pig. I am one stubborn junk food lover, her greatest challenge, and (so far), Pearl and Serene's greatest success story.

After reading my Foreword, Pearl reminded me that Serene and her have helped many people lose even more weight than I have. However, I still think I was the most stubborn challenge they had. That's my story and I'm sticking to it—the plan, that is!

FOREWORD

by Samuel Allison

She's incredible, she's a Christian, she can sing, she's absolutely beautiful, but the only problem is she's a vegan."

These were the words my father said to me when he first told me about my future wife. He met her before I did!

I have watched my beautiful wife come from veganism and then a raw lifestyle to a balanced view of diet and nutrition. She has built her current solid foundation one fact at a time.

The first discussion I had on the subject of health after Serene and I met was with Pearl, surprisingly enough, about the evils and dangers of dairy. I thought it was ludicrous, but took it with a grain of salt. Even though Serene was a vegan at the time and in complete agreement with Pearl, she decided to marry me anyway. "To meat do us part" was thankfully not in our marriage vows.

Like most people, the idea of health didn't enter my daily thoughts until I had a health crisis myself (battling cancer) and I realized the importance of eating and exercising properly. We have now been married 15 years and have nine children (two adopted), and although I have not always been 100 percent on board at all times, the wealth of knowledge I have gained and the benefits I have received to my overall health and body are immense.

Through it all, whether the veganism or the raw food craze, Serene has always created the type of cuisine in our home that you would find in world class restaurants. Now, however, Serene and Pearl's nutrition knowledge has reached beyond the fads and pit stops where so many get stuck. Their delicious meal creations and their intense research have taken the whole concept of nutrition to the next level.

When our daughter, Chalice was young and trying to drink her green spirulina smoothie, we found her playing finger puppets with her fingers.

"It don't look very good," one hand said to the other. "But, it good for you," replied the other hand. This is the stereotypical reaction to healthy food that you have to force it down to reap the benefits.

However, for me, it's not about the things I can't eat. The world of things I can eat in my home that not only taste good, but are good for me, never ends.

Open your mind to a world where healthy eating and good habits are something to look forward to, not something from which you have to run away.

INTRODUCTION

Almost daily, we hear from women who have arrived at a place called "done." They want to put their hands over their ears to drown out all the conflicting and confusing noise about what to eat. What are they "done" with? All the dietary nonsense.

"Ten ways to drop ten pounds in ten days."

Ridiculous!

They no longer have time for this sort of craziness. They no longer have the fight. Diet headlines continue to scream ludicrous promises, diet gurus inflict rigid rules, and diet trends constantly rise and fall. It's no wonder more and more women want to tune it all out.

Yes, these women want to have trimmer figures and healthier bodies but they don't want to do it with the answers they've already been given. Day after day, we hear from mothers who are right at this point. They are massively pressed for time and are discouraged with how difficult and time-consuming it is to eat "right." They are almost resigned to live with their extra pounds.

They are not willing to accept anything less than a sane approach to tackling their problems, something that's actually doable in their busy lives. Even then they're still skeptical. Any answers offered that are less than pure common sense, a common sense that resonates deep in their gut, and their eyes glaze over. They have heard it all before.

They no longer want to be told to eat less, eat healthier, or strip more fat from their diet. They've tried it all and it led them right to where they are right now—fed up!

But the danger with being "done" is that it is stagnant. It's like a vehicle stopped on the side of the highway. It will only rust and deteriorate if it doesn't get back on the road. The previous direction may have been wrong, but skidding to a halt and remaining in one precarious place is not going to fix anything. Stopping has to be the initiation of a new direction, the beginning of a turnaround.

Are you one of these mamas? You don't have to raise your hand, but are you happy with your weight? Would buttons be popping if you tried on your wedding dress? But, all this constant changing information about how to trim down puts you off trying again? Maybe you haven't had major weight changes, but how are your energy, skin, hormonal balance, and libido? Is depression creeping up on you?

Most of us mamas have been in at least one of these sinking boats. But, the life lines thrown to us do not pull us to any better place.

How about . . . count every calorie. *No thanks!*

Okay then . . . at least count your fat grams. *Double no, been there!*

Hey, I've got it . . . pull all meat from your diet and replace it with tofu! *Great, just what my husband wants for dinner!*

All right then . . . get a gym membership and workout for at least one—no, two hours at the Y. *You think I have the time for that? And why on earth would I want to work out with 50 other people watching me? Last thing I want to do, thanks.*

You'd better stop eating desserts then. *If you tell me to give up chocolate I might hit you!*

Hmm . . . here's a good one. Don't fully clean your plate. Leave one third of your meal uneaten and watch the pounds drop. *Sure, being constantly hungry will really put me in a good mood. Might as well padlock the fridge because I am getting hungry just thinking about having to stay hungry.*

Try this as a last resort. Eat bland foods. You'll be less likely to overeat that way. Don't eat sweet, savory, or fatty tasting foods as they cause you to want bigger helpings. Cut back on salt. Only steam your foods and you'll find yourself eating smaller portions. *In other words . . . just be miserable and get no enjoyment out of anything I eat?*

You'd better take some Prozac. You sound depressed. *Been considering it and all these suggestions only make me feel like I need a high dose!*

Well, at least you'd better get on birth control for your "female conditions," your adult acne, and mood swings. *I thought you were trying to help me lose weight. I gained ten pounds by taking the pill. Just stop, I can't hear anymore!*

All these rescues are more disasters in disguise. Roads to nowhere. No big surprise that many women are idling in the place called "done."

The Juggling Act

Recently, at a women's conference where we were invited to speak on nutrition, we asked for a show of hands for those who felt they were able to juggle a healthy weight along with feeding a whole family. Maybe two hands went up. "Who finds it all too hard and overwhelming?" we asked. Hands rose all over the building.

Women look skeptical when we first tell them it doesn't have to be so difficult. That's because they've been constantly bogged down with the "no pain, no gain" approach to eating. While it's true we all need a certain amount of self control, God wants you to enjoy life. He wants you to enjoy food. What a notion! Punishing yourself to get to a healthy weight only robs joy and peace from your life, your marriage, and your entire family.

We're not saying you can pop a pill and be slim. This is not a "drink an infomercial diet shake for dinner, but you can still eat all the pizza you want" way of life. However, there is an ease and a peace that comes when dietary truth and common sense shines through. Mamas who are standing up and saying No to the risks of ruining their metabolism, becoming hormonally imbalanced, depressed, and aging faster to fit into a size six are a growing multitude. They're wise to perceive the dead ends ahead.

But, here's the beauty. You can keep a great shape, or find a great shape again if you have lost it, yet you don't have to be denied a love relationship with food. You can happily eat hearty food, cooked food, tasty food, sweet food, comfort food, or even fried food for that matter, and you can have all these in satisfying portions.

We want to offer you food sanity. Finally, an ease of eating that flows without having to muster up a lot of self-denial or by making the kitchen a concentration camp. Your kitchen should waft delicious aromas that draw your family and guests. If the kitchen has been your war zone, the place where you fight your demons, we want to help you change. Come on out of the trenches, and we'll show you how the kitchen can be your place of peace.

Can you almost taste the freedom? You want to hope, but it all sounds too good to be true?

We live this life. We are busy moms with lots of children, tight budgets, and yes, both of us have husbands who can be picky when it comes to food. We know your challenges because we face them daily. Yet, we embrace a way of eating that is male friendly. Steaks and chicken wings—bring them on! Your husband can be satisfied with hearty meals without growing a big belly. In our world, female cravings are not denied, but encouraged. Chocolate? Absolutely! If you love baking, great! Bake on, because homemade treats are not frowned upon when they are prepared smartly. All of this is possible to enjoy even while losing weight at a sensible pace. We repeat—sensible. We're not saying weight loss must be painfully slow, but we go against the grain, and say it shouldn't be too fast, either.

Four Letter Word

All of us are sick of the word d-i-e-t. Yet, diet really means "the way you eat." Even if you never have a thought about what you put into your mouth, it is still a diet. It is the "I Don't Care Diet." All sorts of diets and food programs are pushed on us from every corner. Lately, due to the dislike and overuse of the word, many of these diets pretend they are not diets at all, but they do not fool anybody. The problem with them is not that they are disguised as non-diets, but they don't make sense for real life. Sure, maybe if you're rich, maybe if you have oodles of will power, maybe if you have too much time on your hands, maybe if you are a single person with not much else to do but focus on yourself, maybe you might achieve some sort of success on these programs. But, they are simply not going to work for busy mothers with the important responsibility of feeding their families.

It makes no nutritional or budgeting sense to spend good money purchasing your own prepackaged diet meals while the rest of your family eats boxed lasagna from the frozen foods section of your grocery store. At the other extreme, you shouldn't have to spend all day juicing fruits and vegetables and dehydrating food to drop pounds and be healthy. We'll show you how to merge your needs with the rest of your family, because if something is not easy and achievable, it can never be sustained long term, no matter how much will-power you can summon at first. We had to figure that out the long and hard way.

You'll notice that most of the recipes and ideas for breakfast and lunch contained in this book take no longer than five to ten minutes. The evening meal recipes should generally take no more than half an hour or so of preparation. We have large families, so if your family is smaller, our evening meal recipes can be prepared in the quantities suggested, divided, and then frozen for lots of "no thought required" suppers.

There is an easier way than switching from the "I Don't Care Diet" to an "I am now going to Suffer Diet." Results occur while you eat the best you ever have in your life. It wasn't our Creator's plan for it to be almost impossible to have a nice figure after the age of 25 and a few pregnancies under your belt. It just takes some understanding.

New Power Tool

Knowledge will be your new power. Knowledge about how to make each meal burn one primary fuel source will change the way you shape your meals. Armed with this new understanding, your new savvy food choices will have absolutely nothing in common with deprivation, but excess pounds will naturally melt away.

We want to equip you with a bigger dietary picture. Our greatest hope is that we can help install in your mind true understanding about how your body reacts to food. There are so many half truths about nutrition that are constantly flung around. Learning how to be a *Trim Healthy Mama* will enable you to see the whole "diet" subject with new eyes. Once the shackles of confusion fall to the ground, true dietary freedom can begin.

We should be able to enjoy the aroma of a delicious hearty meal that's gently cooking as evening falls without a sense of guilt about how many pounds it will add. We should look forward to a satisfying main meal, but also be kind enough to ourselves to enjoy dessert, if desired. And, above all, we should have the assurance that this meal will nourish the whole family while also being friendly to our waistline. This ideal is not too good to be true but it cannot happen accidentally. Greater understanding enables this state of food peace in your home.

If you have thrown up your arms and thrown your "I might fit back into these clothes one day" into boxes, don't drop them off at Goodwill yet. Give us some baby-step belief here.

Dare to Toddle

Think about a baby learning to walk. They take a lot of hard knocks, always falling on their behinds. Sometimes they get mad, frustrated, and have a good cry. But give up? Not when there's tag to play, balls to chase, and the thrill of running in the wind. They instinctively know all the joy that is ahead of them if they can only master the challenge.

Maybe you've fallen on your behind again for what seems like the zillionth time. You're mad, sad, and feel like screaming for your pacifier. To continue the metaphor, that would be a donut or a bowl of Häagen-Dazs, right? But, there is still that dream of feeling vibrant, slim and healthy and more able to celebrate your life, marriage, children, and all your meals.

Therefore, what are you going to do? Stay down on the floor, or find a better way to learn to toddle?

We want to hold your hand while you take your first steps, then laugh with joy right along with you once you're running in the wind. We are not going to inspire you like so many diet books do and then leave you alone to figure out the hard reality. We are going to lead you through the particulars, the struggles, and all the questions.

Our Own Bumpy Ride

We didn't arrive at this place of dietary peace without our own share of bumps and knocks on the journey. It's been a long path of learning for us. We have spent the last two decades on this quest to find an optimum diet that still allows for a happy life. It was no easy task to sift through all the half-truths and confusion. Countless hours studying our passion at night after the children were in bed taught us one thing—diet books contradict one another. The same applies to the internet. You can find scientific evidence for a certain way of eating then find a different article saying the complete opposite, each with its own evidence.

We had to keep digging. Surely, finding a way to eat that promotes health and manages weight without causing misery wasn't too much to ask. Being mothers on a budget, it had to fit a penny-pinching lifestyle and could not take all the hours in a day to implement. Did such a thing exist?

We want to be honest about the pitfalls we fell into so you don't have to repeat them. We were crazy enough to use ourselves as guinea pigs. And unfortunately, we wore the experimental side effects. If there was a new diet, we tried it, (except for maybe the Hollywood Brownie Diet or some other crazy notion). We didn't explore the different styles of eating because we had excessive weight to lose, but we were bound and determined to find the best way of eating to prevent us from sliding into the middle-age spread.

During all these years of searching, we swung the gambit by going too high in carbohydrates, then too low. In the early nineties, many vegetarian diet gurus placed little emphasis on protein and touted vegetarianism as the ultimate human experience. We rode precariously on their bandwagon for a good while.

At times, we believed dietary fat was the enemy, even though we still craved it. We then learned of its many benefits, brought it back into our diet, but still didn't understand how to use it to our advantage without gaining weight.

Raw foods have an important place in this plan, but we've gone too far down that path for too long. For years, we juiced vegetables and fruits until we were blue in the face. Or, should we say, orange from all the carrots? There could even have been a tint of green, too! We eventually discovered juicing carrots and apples was like drinking soda all day as far as our blood sugar was concerned. Glucose tests showed extremely high numbers after these juicing concoctions. We digested thousands of vegetable-only salads, convincing ourselves they were complete meals while the dehydrator droned continually all day. But, who can last at this while trying to raise a family, keep a husband happy, and stay sane?

Scriptures to the Rescue

Like the Hebrew children of Israel wandering around in the wilderness, we ran around in circles looking for answers. Finally, a very drawn out "finally," the biblical approach hit us in the face and everything swung into place. The Bible clearly outlines what we should eat. Science and historical context infallibly back up the Scriptures. Why were we blind to biblical simplicity, spending our time frantically searching for the next "guru" to give us wisdom on what to eat, when God had already told us the truth in simple terms?

God has given us all the food groups and He wants each one to be enjoyed in a balanced way. Every gift God gives is good. Why would we shun any of his gifts? Why would we dismiss their value with a "we know best" attitude? As we came to this understanding, the pieces of the missing puzzle came together. Even little nuggets of truth extracted from all the conflicting diet books we had read lined up in agreement. We noticed recurrent themes that finally fit together. We could now take the good from all the extreme dietary journeys we had traveled and shed the nonsense. Balance at last! And what happened to our weight? All the constant angst and effort we'd previously poured into staying in our skinny jeans was no longer needed. Trim naturally happened. Health naturally flourished.

Essence of Womanhood

This is not only a book about nutritional healing, although that will follow. This is a book about keeping a youthful figure, a youthful zest for life, and love (yes, we mean the love that happens between the sheets). Coming from two conservative Christian women this could sound like needless vanity and frivolity, but this *Trim Healthy Mama* way of life is about embracing the most practical basics of being a woman. The Bible talks about food groups. It talks about sex, and concerning many of the heroines of the Bible, it mentions the beauty of their physical form. God put a lot of thought and design into molding the female body. We honor Him by looking after it. Rachel and Esther were both described as being beautiful of both form and face (Genesis 29:17 and Esther 2:7). If that didn't matter at all, it wouldn't be mentioned in the Bible. Queen Esther's mission from God involved preparing her body, and not just her spirit, to save a nation.

Of course, becoming a *Trim Healthy Mama* is not about trying to be a Barbie doll or becoming consumed with outward looks. It's being the best "us" we can be. Esther's approach to beautifying her body was not for prideful reasons. It wasn't out of conceit. Her obedience reached far beyond her own benefits. As married women, and mothers, our body is not only our own. You are your husband's investment and your children's role model. Attaining a healthy weight and learning the art of maintaining that weight is not only a gift to yourself, but it is one you keep giving to your husband and children throughout the years.

We are not saying a perfect figure makes a marriage, but learning to keep your body in a pleasant form is a way of esteeming and respecting your husband as well as yourself. Your husband is worth it. Maybe he'll see you doing so well and join you for the ride. And, let's be honest, when we look and feel healthy and trim, it's easier to be a happier mama in the home.

Two Basic Essentials

What do you need to start performing your own transformation? The two ingredients are an open mind and a willingness to shed bad habits. This is very attainable when you replace bad habits with new ones that are fun and easy. Once the results show up, those old "weigh you down" ways will be a thing of the past. The new you will shine and you'll be equipped with tools for a lifetime of healthy eating. We are interested in nothing less than a lifelong healthy body weight for you. You will not find us insisting you set six week or six month goals. Short term weight loss goals often result in long term defeat. You are going to baby step your way to forever trim.

You don't need to wait until your circumstances are perfect before you start this new lifestyle. Your husband won't need a raise. These foods are affordable. Since we both live on tight budgets, we understand if you have to go to three different grocery stores to find the cheapest prices on items like cheese and produce. It won't be necessary to belong to a co-op or live next door to a Whole Foods Market. You'll find a good majority of the foods you need at your local supermarket (or three, if you care about the best values).

You won't have to join a gym or buy expensive workout equipment. Of course, we believe in exercise. But, let's make it quick and efficient so we can get it over with. Best of all, you won't even have to possess a lot of self control. You'll never come away from a meal hungry. We adamantly discourage that. Neither will you have to constantly count calories and fat grams or weigh food. Crazy! These practices are far too dull, and in our opinion, lead to obsession. Also, low-fat diets make you fat and depressed. You'll find out why. Bland foods that don't satisfy should have a "BANNED" sign on them!

One Size Does Not Fit All

This *Trim Healthy Mama* approach is fluid. It moulds easily to all personalities. It's not only for women who are able to resist junk food and naturally have a lot of will power. You don't have to be a scratch cook or a granola mom. In fact, if food is your weakness, that's okay. If you're the indulgent type, it's a good thing, because many of the meals we want you to eat are designed to be just that—indulgent.

We want to help you customize your own way of eating that works for you and your family. We don't agree with stringent food programs you can never vary. As sisters, we have very different personalities. Our households run differently, and while our core eating philosophy is the same, we're not identical twins when it comes to food. We both share a passion for nutrition

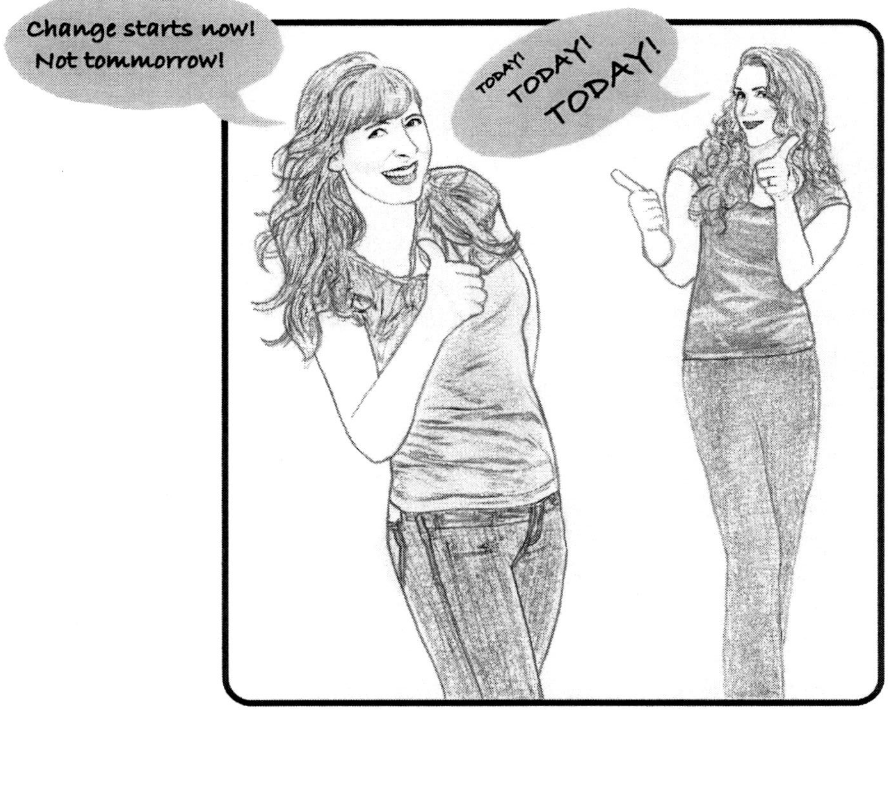

and talk daily about our latest ideas. We admit it. Sometimes we engage in sisterly argument—you'll get a taste of this in chapters to come. But, this tends to help us keep a balanced point of view.

Serene is much more of a food purist and always comes from the angle of what produces optimum health and nutrition. She, and her family, like spicy exotic foods and take an unconventional approach to eating. Pearl likes to figure out shortcuts, is only interested in what is easy and practical, using sneaky little tools to make everyday American-style food without their usual negative effects on health. Our vastly different approaches will show you that you don't have to be a "certain type" to attain health and a sleek waistline. We will offer you our varying opinions and choices on menu ideas so you can implement them to fit your own lifestyle.

We also think specific diets for each individual in the family, such as blood type diets, are neither practical nor scientifically sound. You can't cook four separate meals at supper time to keep everybody in the family happy. Remember, the food groups God created are good for all of us. Tangents are outta here! Obviously, some folk have real allergies to certain foods, but you'll still have plenty to eat. Gluten intolerant people will find plenty of wheat alternatives in our recipes.

First Page to Last

This book has been a drawn out four year project, now trickling into the fifth year . . . agghhh! We could not keep up with all the emails and calls as our sanity style approach of feeding mamas and families trickled out and passed on by word of mouth. Things took on a life of their own and we knew a book was necessary. We wanted to write the majority of it together, but the busyness of life and family commitments did not always allow time to make that to happen. Since we both homeschool, we had to rely on summer breaks to get the bulk of this book completed.

Whenever we did manage to get together at the computer, it also meant our combined 13 children were with us. If you picture a house full of children bouncing off the walls and generally creating an atmosphere not conducive to academic thought, you'd be right. Our brain space was more like, "Must wipe baby poop off living room floor, must run and get sharp stick off five-year-old who's now jumping on trampoline with six year old cousin—Uh oh, also with stick, must stop toddler from feeding baby marbles, and must pull two wrestling boys apart before bleeding noses occur!" Get the picture? If there is even one grammatically correct sentence, we'll count it a miracle. Some of you have been waiting years for this book. Thank you for your patience.

Forget formality. We figured attempting to pass ourselves off as professionals would drive us crazy and you, too. We are what we are, stay at home moms who are passionate about doing our best for our own health and the health of our families. We have no PhDs or any other impressive credentials on our walls. We are chatting to you as if you are in our living room with us. Welcome to the inner circle of our lives—chaos and all.

We can bet your living room is probably a lot like ours most days, and we doubt you're living a life of leisure either. Let's sit down together, forget pretention, and talk, even with crazy stuff happening all around! Keeping it real has been the only way for us to write and maintain our sanity. This book is our way of passing along ideas that actually work, even amidst hectic lifestyles. If we have found a way to implement these truths into our busy and often chaotic lives, you can too.

Yes, it's a big book, but please don't let that overwhelm you—a large chunk of it is recipes. We share them in a more unconventional recipe style. We want to include all the nitty gritty details about our recipes that make them really work and chat about ways to tweak them. That's the way we share recipes between ourselves. Don't neglect to read Part V of the book, *More Than Food*. It's tacked on the end, but we've written life-changing goodies there for you, too.

Don't Say We didn't Warn You

Come on in and enjoy our frank (sometimes overly frank) sisterly discussions. Sisters, you know, can get pretty blunt. Let's just say, although we attempted good behavior, we didn't always manage to stay perfectly polite. Forgive us for that in advance. We started out with our best manners, but things sort of went downhill the longer we were together and sisterhood silliness got the better of us.

You can do this with us! You *can* naturally find your trim, and then keep your trim. We are going to walk you through it all and have a little fun on the way. That's what we do when we're together.

Scriptures that talk about the woman's body:

Genesis 12:11, 14; 24:16; 26:7; 29:17; 1 Samuel 25:3; 2 Samuel 11:2; 14:25-27; 1 Kings 1:4; Esther 1:11; 2:7; Job 42:13-15; Song of Solomon (throughout the whole book).

Part I

Gain the Knowledge

Let's clear away the clouds of confusion
and bring on the blue skies
of dietary freedom and truth.

Chapter One

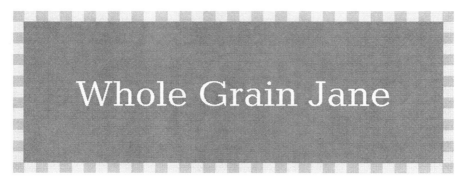

Whole Grain Jane

We'd like to introduce you to four different women. Which one are you? Maybe you'll see yourself in a couple of these women. Or, like us, you've been on similar paths to almost all of them at one time or another.

Let's meet Jane.

Jane is a homeschooling mother of five. She is interested in health and knows quite a bit about nutrition. She grinds her own wheat and bakes bread for her family. Her diet leans heavily on organic whole grains as her nutritional studies have taught her these are best for optimum health. Brown rice, oats, and whole wheat pasta are staples on her meal table. She's even studied the benefits of ancient grains, using spelt and kamut in her baking.

She eats her salads every day, but even more plentiful than greens in her diet is fruit. She chooses fruit for snacks over refined or heavy foods. Jane loves to make banana based smoothies and has an array of dried fruits always at hand.

Her husband loves potatoes and since they are a fat free, higher fiber vegetable, they are a popular side dish on the family's plate, including Jane's. She forgoes butter and sour cream, instead garnishing her baked potato with a little dribble of olive oil and salt free Mrs. Dash seasoning.

Are her Treats Healthy?

Like many homeschooling mothers, Jane likes to bake healthy treats with her older girls. They make whole grain muffins, cookies, and granola bars with honey, organic unrefined cane juice crystals, or even agave syrup instead of table sugar. She has learned to cut back on oils in her baking by replacing them with apple sauce. Jane regularly indulges in these treats as she is certain every ingredient is healthy. No trans fats or preservatives for this woman!

She freely pours pure, Grade A maple syrup on her homemade whole grain pancakes on Saturday morning, but she does not allow that same freedom with fats. She is especially fearful of saturated fats like red meat, butter, or too many egg yolks. Although she would not call herself a vegetarian, Jane has become creative in substituting some meat meals for more vegetable based proteins like legumes and soy. She tries to get the whole family on board with her "Meatless Mondays and Fridays" idea. They're still complaining about it, however.

When she does cook meat, Jane makes sure to use lean cuts only. She has also managed to cut back on cheese and often uses soy replacements on her whole grain sandwiches and in cooking. That took some getting used to, but she figures her family's health is worth it. Soy and rice milk have replaced regular milk on her organic raisin bran in the morning. Jane feels proud, that like the National food guidelines recommend, her diet is higher in fiber, whole grains, fruits and vegetables and lower in fat.

While Jane is careful not to eat refined foods, she will admit to a couple of weaknesses. One being corn chips, the blue organic kind, of course. Well, at least they're whole grain and they make a great taco salad with beans and crumbled soy burger. She also allows herself one naughty treat a couple of nights a week when all the children are finally in bed and she has a moment's peace. Pepperidge Farm chocolate chip cookies are a delicious indulgence, but only a couple.

Jane's Dilemma

For many years this type of diet worked well for Jane. She was able to maintain her figure after her first three babies, but lately, her size 10 clothes no longer fit. She cannot figure out why she is always bloated! Her diet is sufficiently high in fiber and constipation is not the problem.

Grains and Fruit . . . Toot, Toot, Toot!

No other way to put it delicately, it's the gas! All this gas is becoming an embarrassing problem. Lately, this windy, and often painful, gastric issue has become so distressing that Jane is considering doing an expensive colon cleanse.

If she gets pregnant again there will be a reason for the pooch around her middle, but right now, a pinch test tells her it's more than a bloated tummy. There's a new thickness also.

Why, when doing your Best?

This is so frustrating for Jane. She has used a lot of self control and expertise for this sort of diet. She's been very careful to keep it low in fat and high in complex carbohydrates as most current nutritionists advise. Why does her body feel like it's wearing down? Her skin is drying out and showing other signs of aging. Where is the energy she once enjoyed? In her recent physical checkup, she was surprised to find that her cholesterol was too high, including the dreaded LDL cholesterol. Her triglycerides were dangerously close to the top of the limit. She wonders how this is possible when she is very careful to avoid cholesterol laden foods.

Recently, she even cut out her Pepperidge Farm cookies to see if that would make a difference to her struggling weight gain. The scales hardly budged. Disappointed, Jane sought comfort by adding a third cookie to her ritual. After all, they obviously weren't the problem.

Her cravings for sweets are often alarmingly strong. Of course, knowing Jane, candy will not pass her lips, but she can finish off a few handfuls of dates or raisin trail mix and still crave for more. She's taken to making carob balls with dried fruit to help satisfy these cravings, but is left wondering whether she will ever be a size 8-10 again.

Don't worry, Jane, help is on the way. We've been you. We understand the cravings since we spent several years eating that way. Yes, it did some damage, but God also gave food for our healing. Many of the problems you have now can be eliminated.

Sugar is the Culprit! Huh . . . What Sugar?

Jane would be surprised how her unrefined, whole grain diet easily escalates into more carbohydrates than her body can handle. It's simple enough. Carbohydrates raise blood sugar or what is commonly known as glucose. You don't have to eat sugar to accumulate too much sugar in your blood. All forms of starchy carbohydrates result in a raised blood sugar level. It's true that some forms of carbs, like whole grains, take a little longer for the rise to occur than with refined grains, but it will happen. And while all whole grains contain more nutrients and fiber than their refined counterparts, some of them like whole grain pasta are not any gentler on levels of blood sugar. If Jane took a blood sugar test after any one of her meals, she may be shocked at the high number and the damage it is doing to her body.

Now please don't put this book down thinking we're pushing another Atkins type diet. Constant low-carb diets like that go to extremes, and many who try them end up lowering their metabolism and overdoing certain food groups while eliminating others. They also often end up calorie counting since our bodies always learn to get efficient at metabolizing the same food groups over and over. Who wants to end up counting calories as well as carbs? No thanks!

However, much can be learned from Dr. Atkins' research. His science was mostly accurate. Severely restricting carbs does result in shedding pounds and his diet is certainly healthier than the Standard American Diet. But, carbohydrates are essential for well-rounded health. The trick is to eat the right ones in the right amounts. We'll show you how to do it soon.

We have to give Jane credence for the things she's doing right. Whole grains are certainly full of more nutrients than white or refined grains and a diet that is liberal in vegetables and fruits must be given its dues. Kudos to Jane for this! She is not loading her body with chemicals and toxins from processed foods and she avoids harmful trans fats. Another cheer!

Basic Physiology 101

Jane's problem lies in her imbalance. In the end, it is not only the quality of the foods that you eat, but the quantity. In high amounts, whole grains, even with their higher fiber levels can be deceivingly destructive to a slim waistline and a healthy mind and body.

It's all about proportions. To make up for the lack of fat and satisfying protein in her diet, Jane steers her diet in the complete opposite direction and relies too heavily on carbohydrates. They make up the bulk of her meals. Even though she may choose the healthiest of carbs like organic whole grains, when she indulges too heartily (and she will need to in order to feel satisfied), they raise her blood sugar to the point where it is as detrimental as eating plain old junky white bread. Jane's blood is constantly overloaded with glucose, meal after meal. This is stored as fat, first as extra padding around the mid section.

All that so-called "whole grain goodness" is the reason for the thickness she can now easily pinch around her middle. Who woulda thought it? Not Jane, but now she's going to get the download.

Basic Physiology 101: Any extra padding around the waistline is related to an excess of carbs, creating a problem with the hormone insulin.

Insulin—Your Friendly Neighborhood Delivery Truck

Jane would be surprised to learn that eating fat doesn't make you fat. Yes, you read correctly! You can eat lots of fat in a meal and not gain a pound. You can actually lose some of your own body fat if your fat filled meal is not eaten with sugars or starches which convert to glucose in the blood stream.

Your knowledge to freedom—EXCESS INSULIN MAKES YOU FAT! Insulin is your storing hormone. It promotes the storage of nutrients in your body, which is good and necessary. But, when insulin is over secreted, it becomes a fat storing monster, and that's why it is notoriously known as the fat-promoting hormone of your body. Constantly creating excess insulin in your body meal after meal is the perfect way to get fat.

But, God didn't design your insulin hormone to fatten you up. It was designed to transport glucose, proteins, and fats out of your blood stream and into your cells so your body can use them. Without insulin, the amino acids that protein contains would not be driven into your muscle cells where they are needed to make repairs. Fatty acids would not have a way out of the blood stream to nourish your skin, brain, and nervous system. Glucose would stay locked in the blood stream and could eventually lead to coma and death. The key is to ensure insulin works for your good, the way God intended, not to your detriment.

How do you get excess insulin? By eating excess carbs. Carbohydrates are the main food group that will stimulate a large insulin surge. The reason is that carbohydrates are converted to blood glucose much more quickly than fat and protein. That, in turn, causes rapid, large rises of insulin. Dietary fat has very little effect on insulin, but protein causes small to medium rises.

The important difference between the way protein and carbs stimulate insulin is that protein also causes the body to release glucagon, a hormone that helps counteract the more hazardous sides of insulin. Glucagon helps to halt insulin's stimulation of fat synthesis. Animals in a laboratory setting that are given injections of pure glucagon fail to gain weight and reduce their food consumption. This is why protein is so important in every meal. We will drill this protein precept into you as the book continues. A carb heavy meal with little protein will cause insulin to surge ahead without the buffering effects of glucagon.

Insulin's most important job is the task of clearing elevated sugar from your blood. Your body prefers your blood sugar to stay in a safe zone of about 80-100 (measured by a glucose monitor). Once your blood sugar bumps up above this threshold, insulin must go to work to bring it down again. It is like the truck that carries the sugar out of your blood stream and delivers it elsewhere. It cleans up and delivers after every meal you eat. Insulin has to do this because too high blood sugar for too long is fatal. Therefore, if your diet is very carb heavy, your pancreas will have no choice but to over-react and send out large amounts of insulin to take care of the big mess of excess sugar in your blood. It's only doing this to keep you alive!

Jane's Average Lunch

Let's say Jane eats a peanut butter and honey sandwich for lunch made from her whole wheat bread, maybe pretzels on the side, and a little fruit flavored, honey sweetened, low-fat yogurt for dessert. This meal doesn't look so bad at first glance, but it contains lots of starch and some sugar. It's highly possible that Jane's post meal sugar levels will spike well into the 150's, maybe even higher.

Out surges Jane's insulin to the rescue. It loads up all the blood sugar it can manage, takes it out of the blood stream and offers it to her muscle cells for energy. Job well done.

But, red alert! Insulin cannot rest yet. Jane's body just signaled that her blood sugar is still in the 130's. Not low enough yet, says her body. Uh, oh. The pancreas has no choice but to release more insulin to get that blood sugar down below 100. Therefore, insulin has to haul off another load of blood sugar. Back to the muscle cells it goes with a second delivery. But, now

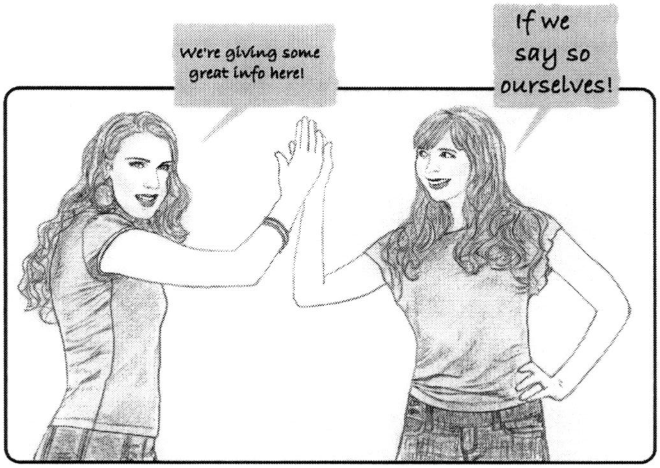
We're giving some great info here!
If we say so ourselves!

there's a problem. Her muscle cells are full. They cannot accept any more glucose. Poor insulin has no choice but to drive over to the fat cells and load off the excess glucose to them. Fat cells don't say "No thanks" to glucose.

It doesn't matter that a food may start its life as a carb. Once blood sugar is stored in a fat cell, it is no longer distinguishable as a carb. Abracadabra, it is now fat. This is how insulin makes you fat.

Insulin doesn't make you fat because it is inherently evil, gleefully plumping you up to cackle at your suffering. It is forced to fatten you up due to the content of your meals. And, it doesn't work in a vacuum. It affects other hormones that when thrown off kilter make you fatter still. Highly elevated insulin, or what is known as hyperinsulinemia, goes hand in hand with a condition called hyperleptinemia. Together, they are a double whammy on your weight.

Leptin is a very important hormone that tells your brain when you are full. Once leptin is thrown out of whack, you no longer know when to stop eating. This hormone gets elevated in the blood stream just like insulin, but is unable to be received by the leptin receptors in your brain. Therefore, you feel compelled to keep on eating. Not good, right?

What goes up must come down. Remember a sugar low always follows a sugar high. This cycle constantly repeats itself in Jane's body. That is why she feels tired in the afternoon and craves a banana muffin. Insulin had to work overtime. It had to make too many deliveries to finally get its job completed and clear Jane's blood stream of the abundant sugar her grain-based diet causes. However, the extra surges of insulin required for the task cleared things too well. Jane now suffers from a sugar low. Her blood sugar level is now significantly below the healthy 80-100 range. Sugar lows are not great for the body either. Now Jane feels lethargic, slightly shaky, and quite grouchy. She often feels like she needs a "pick-me-up" banana based smoothie, sweetened with more honey, or a bowl of granola and vanilla flavored soy milk.

Is the picture becoming clearer? It is not only Pepsi and Snicker bars which create sugar highs and then lows. Even "so-called" healthy carbohydrates can be damaging if they take up too large a space in the diet. They must find their optimum place if long term health and weight management is to be achieved.

When Jane eats her generous bowls of whole grain cereals, brown rice and beans, dried fruit snacks, or her three or four slices of home baked, whole wheat bread, she is unknowingly eating herself out of her size 10's. Whole grains are necessary. It would not be the right approach to throw them out and miss out on a whole food group that God made for our health, but Jane will have to learn to scale them back and let them work in harmony with other foods which she will learn to increase.

Aging Cells Reject Sugar Delivery Truck

Jane is approaching 40. She's noticing the extra weight, because as we get older, we become more "insulin resistant." We're sure you've heard that term before. The idea of insulin resistance can easily confuse people, especially if they already have the knowledge that insulin is our fat storing hormone. They wonder, "Why on earth do we get fatter in an insulin resistant state when insulin is supposed to be making us fat. Shouldn't resisting insulin be a good thing?" More confusion!

To clear this up, all you need to know is that it is only our muscle cells that become resistant to insulin. If muscle cells stayed receptive to insulin, that would be fantastic as muscles burn glucose rather than store it as fat. But once they begin to resist insulin, fat cells have to take up the slack and receive the loads of blood sugar that our muscle cells used to be able to handle, but don't want anymore. Insulin resistance essentially means less glucose burning, more glucose storing. Two words: fat gain.

It is rare for fat cells to ever develop this resistance issue, but some very skinny people do have fat cells that are more resistant to insulin than their muscle cells. Folk with this condition have the opposite problem to most of us and have trouble putting on enough weight.

Generally, most people have fat cells that stay highly insulin receptive and greedily gobble anything insulin has to offer them. Fat cells keep gobbling, getting larger since they don't burn fuel like muscles cells do. Unfortunately, as we age, it is only our muscle cells that become a lot fussier. High-carb intake over the years only makes this worse. Dr. Diana Schwarzbein, author of *The Schwarzbein Principle*, says on page 13: "By the time you are thirty years old, your cells do not utilize sugar as well as they did when you were younger; this is cellular aging. What you have eaten and how you have lived your life will determine the actual age of your cells and therefore the health of your metabolism at any given time."

When we are young, our muscle cells are open and ready to welcome the insulin truck with its load of blood sugar. Think of young cells like hungry baby birds in a nest with their mouths wide open to accept any food they can scarf down. As we age, these cells become less ready to accept the glucose that insulin offers us for energy. They are simply not as hungry for it. You can use a similar visual image of the nest of birds to picture insulin resistant cells. These baby birdies would have mouths half open in a lackluster way, listless, and disinterested in wolfing down anything insulin has to offer.

Jane is simply not able to use the amount of blood sugar that she could in her youth. She is left with more and more leftover glucose in her bloodstream. This has to be removed. It's insulin to the rescue again. However, since all her muscle cells are already full from her last carb laden meal, it has only one place to go. Guess where? You got it. It is stored as fat! Insulin enables carbs and sugars to magically turn into fat more easily as her cells age and become more insulin resistant.

The kicker is that this state of insulin resistance causes the body to make even more insulin, which means the body will also consequently make more fat. It's a vicious cycle. It's a worse state than having to store excess glucose as fat after a high-carb meal. The same kind of carb rich meal can cause an insulin resistant person to store twice the fat because the muscles refuse to receive as much of the glucose.

The truck arrives at Jane's cell loading zones, beeps, and gets ready to tip its sugar load. It yells out to the muscle cells, "Are you ready?"

"No thanks," her cells respond. "We couldn't handle a mouthful more. We're not as interested anymore."

Insulin replies, "Fine, I will store, store, store in your fat cells. They're not so picky and always accept anything I have to offer."

This scenario is the reason Jane's waist is expanding. We may have over explained, but it is imperative that you "get" this fundamental point.

Watch for Phytates

Grains contain phytates that bind with minerals in Jane's body and leech them out in her urine. Many people on high grain diets become mineral deficient. This shows up as dull, lifeless hair and skin and lack of energy—the regular blahs. Excess carbs increase the depletion of B vitamins causing lack of energy, shorter temper, and bloating. Some of Jane's belly bloat is not only due to the overgrowth of yeast and sugar in her digestive system from excess grain, but also from the difficulty she has in digesting the un-soaked grains.

We're not saying you have to soak every grain or bean you eat. You do not need to worry about lentils and millet as they are lower in phytates. Oats are one of the highest in phytates, so we do suggest soaking them. But, don't beat yourself up. We're all busy women. It's unrealistic to always remember to soak grains. Poor Jane would need pots and pans of soaking grain covering all her kitchen counters to eradicate the phytates that are robbing her of her vitality and energy. When grains are reduced to a health promoting portion of the diet, this problem is no longer overwhelming. We'll be honest. Serene soaks. Pearl usually forgets, or doesn't bother about it.

Soy, Goodie or Baddie?

Soy is not doing Jane any favors either. All the soy in Jane's diet which she believes to be so health promoting could be a problem. A little tofu here and there doesn't hurt too much, but soy beans have some of the highest phytate levels. Her daily soy milk on her cereal is not only too high in sugars, because it has been pre-sweetened, but because it is full of phytates, which cause a large mineral leech for Jane's body. Soy's effect on estrogen levels in the body is not completely understood, but it has been shown to be a powerful aromatase stimulator. That means it is an enzyme that converts testosterone into estrogen. Dr. Russell Blaylock, a neuroscientist and widely read author, says in an interview in the book *Knockout* by Suzanne Somers: "We know that breast cancers produce a lot of aromatase and things that stimulate a breast cancer also stimulate aromatase . . . Soy massively increases aromatase, so that's a reason not to consume soy."

Dr. Blaylock goes on to explain that soy has very high concentrations of fluoride, manganese, and glutamate. He says, "We know that manganese, fluoride, and glutamate are terrible brain toxins and in my neuroscience journal, it shows that giving soy formula to children is associated with Parkinson's because of the manganese. Women have been lulled into thinking that eating and drinking all this soy is good for them, but it is loaded with manganese, which is a powerful brain toxin and has been shown to cause brain atrophy."

Dr. Blaylock points out that most soy is genetically modified. There is increased evidence that GMO foods induce sterility. He cautions that young women who consume a lot of soy may find that they have trouble getting pregnant.

In order to keep a well functioning metabolism, Jane should worry less about fat in her food and consider her thyroid. There are serious questions about soy's impact on thyroid.

A 1991 Japanese study found that soy consumption can suppress thyroid function and cause goiters in healthy people, especially in elderly subjects. European researchers found in one study that even a week of consuming unprocessed boiled natural soybeans caused changes to thyroid levels.

Czech researchers, in a 2006 study that examined thyroid hormones and thyroid antibodies, found that even small differences in soy phytoestrogen intake can influence thyroid function, especially in those who are deficient in iodine. In 2004, researchers carried out a study at the *Department of Pediatrics at Northwestern University Medical School.* The study, published in *Arch Dis Child*, found that babies fed soy formula had a long lasting increase in their TSH (Thyroid Stimulating Hormone) levels. An increase means the thyroid is becoming hypo or less efficient. In a 1997 study published in the journal of *Biochemical Pharmacology* researchers concluded, "It was observed that an extract of soybeans contains compounds that inhibit thyroid peroxidase catalyzed reactions essential to thyroid hormone synthesis."

It's not our aim to march around holding "We Hate Soy" banners. Our approach to food hopes to avoid all extremes and that would include suggesting that someone never put soy in their mouths again. Soy is a controversial subject and while we have brought to your attention studies that show its negative effects, there are some studies that show the opposite. Jane could still comfortably use small amounts of naturally fermented soy in her diet, as fermented soy is lower in harmful phytates as the fermentation process breaks them down. Jane could also eat a little tofu now and then or some soy beans.

It is the constant barrage of soy in Jane's diet that poses risks for the balance of her hormones. Like grains, soy enjoys too prominent a place in her diet. Jane has simply gone too far using soy crumbles to replace meat, soy milk to replace dairy, soy slices to replace cheeses on her sandwiches, and tofu to replace meat protein. It comes down to common sense again. Soy cheese looks processed and fake, smells processed and fake, and tastes processed and fake. It's sad that Jane has come to believe it is a better choice for her than the real thing, simply because it has less fat, is considered cholesterol free, and is not an animal product.

Try This on for Size

You don't often hear this, but the truth is that Jane would be better off adding more fat to her diet, including saturated fats!

Retrial for Fat

Americans have only gotten fatter since the low-fat, high-complex carb diet was recommended in the seventies and eighties. Saturated fat intakes have dropped substantially while bellies have grown bigger. Kind of makes you go, "Hmmmm."

We know there is much debate on this subject, and conventional doctrine says that eating saturated fat causes high cholesterol and makes you susceptible to heart attacks. However, science now reveals that high insulin levels generated from more high-carb and lower saturated fat diets causes plaque to be deposited in the arteries.

A diet that is too high in carbs results in smaller cholesterol particles, rather than bigger. This is a problem, because bigger, fluffy, cholesterol particles are safer. They are less likely to slip through blood vessel walls and form dangerous plaque deposits. Bigger particles, nice healthy ones, form when a diet is tipped higher toward fat and lower towards carbs. Fats help lower glucose levels, which, in turn, result in lesser need for insulin, and these lower insulin levels have a more balancing effect on the cholesterol profile.

It sounds crazy, but triglyceride levels can rise by simply eating too much fruit! Triglycerides are circulating forms of fat found in the blood stream. Most of us would think that a higher fat diet would raise triglyceride levels and a lower fat diet like Jane's would lower them. Not so. A 2004 study in *The Journal of Nutrition* shows that reduced carb consumption consistently decreases triglycerides in the fasting state and in response to meals. Other studies continue to back this one up. Fats, (including saturated fats) actually lower "trigs," while carbs raise them. This information is seldom heard because there is so much noise about how low-fat diets are the requirement for a healthy lipid profile.

Poor Jane is stumped since she was told by her doctor that her triglycerides were close to 200 on her recent blood test during a full physical. High triglycerides are a key warning sign of declining cardio vascular health and often precipitate both strokes and heart attacks. Any time triglycerides are over 150 the first suspect that needs to be seriously checked out is a high-carb diet.

Fat deprivation in diet causes many imbalances in the body, including loss of lean muscle mass and more fat gain around the middle. Jane is now experiencing this for the first time. Eliminating fat can actually cause a halt in hormone production, and this can cause cell abnormalities. Also, believe it or not, fiber is not the only important requirement for preventing constipation. Fat is necessary to stimulate bile flow which allows bowel action. Fat also helps to prevent heavy mood swings, is essential for brain function, and keeps skin soft and less lined. Real fats like butter, saturated oils, cream, and yes, even red meat, are essential for healthy hormone cells. Jane needs to include some of these, along with monosaturated fats like olive oil and nuts to obtain a more correct balance in her body.

But, the best thing we like about fat is its satiety. It satisfies like no other food. Jane's constant cravings could be curbed by simply adding an appropriate amount of healthy fat and pulling back on the excess carbohydrates. Sugars stimulate the appetite while fats suppress it. Studies have shown that high-carb foods can cause people to eat 60-70 percent more calories at their next meal.

Jane's Turnaround

It's going to take some convincing for Jane to change. She'll feel guilty, almost sinful, by adding foods like real cheese, cream, butter, and even red meat to her diet. She'll worry it will end up giving her a heart attack, but in actual fact, her triglycerides will most likely come down while her HDL (healthy) cholesterol will rise.

Jane is not going to have to give up baking healthy treats with her older girls. She only has to be introduced to some new recipes that will be less stimulating to her hormone insulin. She'll love our *Trim Healthy Pancakes* (*Morning Meals*, Chapter 18) recipe. It will help satisfy her sweet cravings. At the same time it will help her slim down since it is much higher in protein and has a more healthy balance of carbs than the pancakes she is used to eating. She'll soon become familiar with new flours and her oven will be wafting all sorts of cinammony goodness. She'll find that she can still make delicious muffins and other healthy treats using flours from flax, coconut, or almonds. Switching to these forms of baked goods will help eradicate that thickness around her middle area. It will also have a more balancing effect on her blood sugar, suppressing the craving for dried fruit and sweets all day.

Her constant bloated stomach will be less of a plague her. Her skin will "plump up" while her body will "plump down" and she will easily slide into her size eights again. Come on, Jane, you know this is the time for change. Feeling satisfied, rather than bloated and stuffed, is going to feel fantastic.

Chapter Two

Drive Thru Sue

Let's meet Sue.

Sue is a mother of two in her late twenties. She's not that fond of cooking, but she's perfected mac n cheese from the box. Sue works part time. She is constantly on the go and her children's ball games and school activities keep her out many afternoons. Sue and children are regulars at their local McDonald's drive through where her children order their happy meals and she fuels her caffeine fix with a 32 oz. soda. This helps keep her energized until she gets home where she can grab a coke from the fridge.

Sue has never thought much about nutrition until recently, but doesn't know how to change on her own. The conflicting information she hears from TV and sees on the titles of magazine covers at the grocery store has her so confused she tunes most of it out and figures worrying about that sort of thing is not for her. She's just not the "health-nut" type. She figures that 10 pounds more on the scale will be the tipping point when she'll scramble the money together and join Weight Watchers or Jenny Craig.

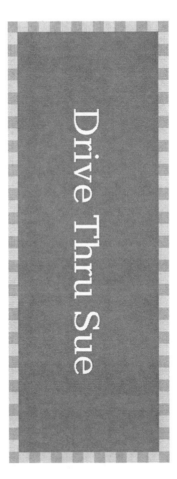

She eats what many call the SAD diet, short for Standard American Diet. It's sad because it leads to degeneration of the body, the common stereo type of a middle-aged person with too many pounds and too many prescription medicines. But, Sue's own mother worked full time and there was never much of an opportunity to learn about wholesome home cooking. The white bread, soda, packaged foods, and sugary cereals in her grocery cart have always been a regular part of her life. It doesn't dawn on her that they are such a problem. And, she wouldn't know how to replace them and wouldn't even know how to start. Should she buy rice cakes and smear them with margarine? Random thoughts like this cross her mind and leave her more confused than ever.

Eating Less No Longer Works

Sue developed a bit of a weight problem in her teens, but was able to keep it from getting out of hand by skipping meals. That may have worked in her teenage years, but it is making things worse now. Her weight has become more and more of a problem in the years since being married. Her metabolism has slowed down due to the habit of skipping meals. Now, it seems anything she eats goes to her hips, belly, and thighs.

She has always wondered why she is overweight when she actually eats less than many other people she knows. She's not a big breakfast person, aside from the occasional bowl of cereal, quick pop tart or a cup of coffee. She is still in the habit of skipping meals, mostly breakfast and sometimes lunch, but that causes her to eat most of her calories at night. This is when the munchies occur and she reaches for the Doritos or her children's goldfish crackers. Her appetite wakes up for pizza. They order in pizzas a couple of nights a week, or go out as a family to the pizza buffet in their area. It's not like Sue pigs out. She usually never eats more than two to three pieces of pizza, but she always washes them down with a refill of coke.

Missing Fruits and Veggies

Aside from the odd banana, or the lettuce that accompanies a fast food hamburger, fruits and vegetables are quite rare in her diet. Sue never developed a taste for them. This makes her bathroom visits for number two infrequent and painful. It's quite common for Sue to go two to three days without being able to have a bowel movement. It is annoying to feel constipated all the time, but she has lived with it for so long that not eliminating for days is quite normal for her. She often has to resort to laxatives to find relief.

Occasionally, Sue attempts to eat more healthily by opening a can of vegetable soup and throws in some fat-free oyster crackers. She even buys V8 juice now and then because she half believes the advertising that says it counts for a full serving of vegetables. She keeps orange juice in the fridge and tries to remember to have a glass or two for her fruit quota every other day or so. She'll eat a banana so they don't go bad when she buys them, but fruit is not her thing.

That Lovin' Feeling—It's Gone, Gone, Gone!

Sue may put on a happy face, but her diet is contributing to problems in her marriage. Although her husband eats similar food and much more of it, he doesn't struggle with his weight. Sue is frustrated with her own accumulating pounds and is more and more uncomfortable with intimacy in the bedroom. Her husband takes this as a lack of interest, and though it may be true, Sue's reluctance is more to do with her insecurity. She doesn't feel sexy and she purposefully sabotages intimate opportunities with her husband, blaming her indifference on fatigue and too much to do. She hasn't pulled out that lacy black teddy in a couple of years now. Sue's attitude to her sex life lately is "lights out, let's get this over with." She doesn't actually say that, but her body language speaks loudly.

Frequent headaches drag her down. A mild case of adult acne has set in, and this only adds to her insecurity. Heartburn is also a problem. She carries Tums in her purse and uses them frequently.

Her doctor has given her a prescription for depression, but she doesn't like taking it. While it numbs her despair, it also makes her feel numb in many other ways, and her husband notices the depression meds make her lagging libido even worse.

I Spy the Insulin Truck Again

Sue knows that sugary foods are "bad." Everyone has heard that, but she is probably not aware that white bread and crackers are the same as sugar in her body. Even her glasses of orange juice and V8 are basically sugar in a cup. The packaged foods with all their additives, dyes, preservatives, and excess sodium are not doing Sue any good, but her real problem is sugar in all its deceptive forms. She's not eating cakes all day, maybe a candy bar now and then, but the refined grains in her "get-n-go" diet are the major cause for her expanding waistline. She'd be surprised that the breading on her chicken nuggets, the pastry in her pop tart, the flakes in her Special K cereal are all sugar in her body. All these foods cause a higher level of glucose in her bloodstream than is optimum for lifelong weight control. The double whammy is that there is very little fiber in her diet to slow the rise of her blood sugar to anything other than a speed racer level.

Her Drinks Drag Her Down

A lot of Sue's excess insulin problems stem from her drinks. Carbohydrates in liquid form are the worst offenders. They rush straight into the blood stream causing the most rapid and dangerous spikes! Sue, like a large chunk of U.S. population, is getting fatter more from her beverages than even her food. Those drinks may even be labeled "fat free," but as we learned in Whole Grain Jane's case, it is all about sugar levels in the blood stream, not necessarily fat. In goes the soda or juice. Bam! Out surges the insulin to take care of the high glucose. Insulin knows where to put its load from constant, forced habit—right in her fat cells. Goodbye, youthful figure!

But there's hope. Sue can learn many delicious alternative drink choices to sugar laden soda that will contribute to a beautiful waistline and healthy skin. They will help purge her body from the onslaught of chemicals she has ingested over the years. They'll even taste good, we promise.

A Clean Slate

The good news is that Sue has not been indoctrinated with too many food theories that are going to be hard to shake. She has tried to eat less to lose weight, but that seldom works for long. If she ends up joining a weight loss program, counts her calories along with fat grams, and slims down for a little while, it's not likely to be a long term solution. Never feeling fully satisfied will bite her in the end. She will more than likely get sick of being constantly hungry and go back to Pizza Palace Buffet to get a fix. Nor will joining a weight loss club or ordering their expensive diet meals help to nourish the rest of her family. They'll still be eating boxed mac and cheese while she eats her own tinier boxed meal. Boxes everywhere, and who can get full on those puny meals?

The timing is perfect now for Sue to make lasting changes. She still has an open mind. She can easily learn new food lessons, tips, and tricks. The simplicity of these truths will make sense to her because they are not extreme. Once she understands how the foods she currently chooses on a daily basis destroy her figure and health, and learns how to wisely replace them, she will have direction. She'll have a foundation to build good health precepts, layer upon layer, for her and her family. Not only will she change her own health, but she'll break the cycle of the "junk food mothering" she grew up with. Her children will have a head start at finding lasting health and be able to pass this down to their own offspring.

Sue is not likely to change into a Granola Mom. In fact, she doesn't have to become the Granola Mom type. Don't worry, Sue, you don't have to transform yourself into the woman who takes recycled organic cloth grocery bags to the co-op and sings "Kumbaya" with your children in the big white van on the way home, all the while crunching on carrot sticks. But, you can learn simple, whole food cooking little by little and even find enjoyment in it.

Sue can take small steps toward getting her life back, rather than staying stagnant and floundering around in confusion. A few simple changes is all it's going to take. A few new habits to replace old harmful ones, and her family, along with her figure, can take on a new healthier path.

Baby-Steps

Sue can turn her racing blood sugar levels around with a little basic knowledge. She doesn't need to become a gourmet chef and spend hours in the kitchen. Instead, she will learn how to make quick prep meals that are centered around healthy protein forms, rather than relying on fast food chicken nuggets or frozen, breaded chicken nuggets. Sue will learn to use the crock-pot for easy and nourishing evening meals that will help draw the family together, settle her children, and bring their minds and bodies sustenance. Her husband and children will think she's become a fantastic cook, and she will experience great satisfaction watching them eat healthier foods with little effort on her part.

She needs to include more life-giving enzymes in her diet in the form of raw foods. She'll feel so much better when her diet no longer consists of dead foods. The addition of speedy, no fuss salads with a sprinkle or two of flax or chia seeds, and a handful of low glycemic fruits like berries will help cleanse her body and help her go poopy. Yay! These are easy additions, no rocket science required.

Creamy and quick protein-based smoothies in the morning will only take as much time as toasting a pop tart, but will help change her body from the inside out. They'll be just like a thick shake, filling and full of fiber, which will only benefit her more in the bathroom department, and will work with her "on the go" lifestyle. Or, if she prefers, she could eat our *Muffin in a Mug* for breakfast (*Morning Meals*, Chapter 18). Who doesn't love a big chocolate muffin for breakfast? Or, maybe she'll prefer a cinnamon muffin with a pat of butter. This muffin has ample protein, is full of fiber, and most importantly, is absolutely delicious. Sue will love the fact that she can easily make it from start to finish within three minutes. Even the most inept person in the kitchen can master this recipe.

Switching to whole grains in smaller quantities in place of the white burger buns, boxed cereals, and crackers, will lower her surging insulin problem and again add more fiber. She'll finally throw the laxatives away. She can add a natural magnesium supplement before bed each night which will help her nerve health and give added assurance for regularity in the morning.

Sue can take delicious and filling sandwiches with her when she goes out. She'll still be able to eat them with her favorite fillings such as deli meats, chicken, or egg salad. She'll just change her bread casings to smarter choices that are much easier on her blood sugar. No, she's not going to eat potato chips or pretzels with her sandwiches anymore, but she can get clued in to other great snacky sides that are just as delicious and give her that crunch fix she craves.

She's not the type to make her own bread. She has no desire to knead dough and grind her own wheat, but not to worry, there are some wise options at her local grocery store we'll steer her toward that won't cause the usual blood sugar spike in her body. She'll learn the brands that will help her stay slim. Our *Trim Healthy Pan Bread* recipe (*Muffins, Breads, and Pizza Crusts,*

Chapter 19), is so quick and easy. Sue might find herself becoming such a pro at making them that she will prefer them to buying store specialty items.

But, knowing our Sue, she won't want to make her lunch every day. Life gets crazily busy sometimes. Yep, she can still drive through while she's out and about. We'll teach her how to do it right in later chapters. She'll just have to make some little changes in how she orders her lunch in order to fill up without carbing up.

It All Comes Together

Next thing she knows, Sue will feel some vitality returning. Her husband will notice the happier girl emerging that he married eight years ago, the one who no longer feels so overwhelmed and down trodden. It won't happen overnight, but slowly and surely, her waistline will reappear. Sue's not going to weigh herself much, but she'll notice that her black pants are now too big and will start going to yard sales for smaller sizes. New blossoming confidence in her body, coupled with teaching on married sexuality, will help transform her bedroom into a spicier place. Yard sales have sexy lingerie, too!

Sue needs enough knowledge to give her a place to start and the assurance that "yes" she can do this. She doesn't have to feel that this change is beyond reach for her lifestyle and personality. A trim, healthy body is totally possible for her and all the other Sue's.

Do You See the Connection?

On the surface it looks as if Sue and Jane are opposites in their eating habits and approaches to life. However, there is a common thread in their diets—blood sugar spikes. They have both been taking different roads, but their unwanted destination is similar. A better way is in store for both of them.

Chapter Three

Raw Green Colleen

Now, we'll meet Colleen.

She wakes up in the morning, chugs back a glass full of Barley Green powder, and then dutifully assembles her juicer. She selects some carrots from the 50 pound bag in her fridge, adds an organic apple or two, and a handful of parsley. This is her morning detox juice. It is time consuming, but she is convinced it is worth the effort. To round out her breakfast, she'll slather some almond butter on a banana and call herself done.

As you might have guessed, Colleen is a health nut. But, she has good reason. Her mother and aunt battled breast cancer. Colleen doesn't want to be another statistic. Five years ago, she decided to get serious when her own health began to deteriorate. She had some benign breast lumps that scared her. Now, her diet is more than just a way of eating. It's her way of life.

Heavy Equipment Required

Much of Colleen's time is taken up with sprouting, juicing, dehydrating, and all the extra prep her meals require. Of course, she has to wash the juicer after each quart of juice, which only takes four times as long as it does to assemble it. Try that three times a day!

She eats neither meat nor dairy, consuming mainly live plant foods. Salads, nuts and seeds, superfood smoothies, fruits, dehydrated crackers, and occasional lentil soups, baked potatoes, and brown rice make up her diet. She shares some similarities to our first friend, Jane, in that she likes to snack on a lot of dried fruit. She's a whiz at making tasty balls from coconut butter, nuts, seeds, raw honey, and yes, more dried fruit.

She Doesn't Give Up

Her husband misses hearty hot meals at suppertime, but since he gets to eat whatever he wants at work for lunch, he tolerates the night time meal, which he affectionately calls "rabbit food." Concerned friends and relatives make comments that their children are too thin, but Colleen brushes them off thinking that with all the childhood obesity today, it is a good thing her children are not headed in that direction. She firmly believes the human body is not supposed to carry any extra fat. Her diet gurus assure her that one can get sufficient calcium from dark green leafy vegetables and carrot juice. They tell her that nuts, seeds, and sprouts provide sufficient protein for anybody.

The first couple of years eating this way, Colleen was over the moon with the changes she noticed on this diet. Her allergies left, she shed 20 pounds, gained abundant energy, and tried to convert anybody who would listen to her predominantly raw way of life. She became free of breast lumps since starting her extreme diet. The next two years were not quite as joyous. Strangely, her energy levels no longer bubbled over, but she put her tiredness down to the fact that this diet required so much work. She hung in there, determined this was best for her and her family.

In her fourth year of eating a predominantly raw diet, Colleen became pregnant. She struggled with low energy, but did not sway from her ideals. She gained less than 15 pounds which her midwife thought was not near enough, but she was rewarded with a healthy 7 ½ lb. baby boy. She felt relieved and justified. All those people who said she needed dairy and meat were wrong. Weren't they?

Tiny Seeds of Doubt

For the first time Colleen wonders if she is making the wisest nutritional choices for herself and her family. These seeds of doubt are worrisome since she has been fully persuaded for so long that nothing could be superior to her pure way of eating. It requires much self-denial, work, and determination. She is sure it is the pinnacle of all dietary lifestyles, and there could be nothing wiser or better. She cannot see herself going back to the Standard American Diet she used to live on.

However, now her baby is a year and a half, and Colleen feels a pit in her stomach when she looks inside his mouth and sees his narrow looking, brown stained teeth. Why are they like this when all her other children were blessed with strong pearly whites? Surely it couldn't be the pure, life-giving diet she lived on while she was pregnant?

Last week, she took her children to the dentist and was aghast to hear that her youngest already had cavities in his new teeth. "Have you given him juice bottles or allowed him to sleep with a bottle in his mouth?" she was asked. "Never!" she'd answered. "He was exclusively breastfed."

What left her feeling even more defeated was when she was told some of her other children would need fillings for cavities. Why, when they had started out with such healthy teeth? Cavities had never been a problem before this change to a more raw diet. It's not like she allowed them to eat candy or drink soda. Hey, they had baby carrots, fruit, and nuts for snacks. They also had regular brushing habits.

Colleen's idealistic world is beginning to crumble. Not only are her children showing signs of deficiencies, but now she has some concerns about herself. She's losing muscle tone, even though she walks a good hour every day. She's noticing more cellulite, even on her arms, which she can't understand. While she could still be considered thin, her figure has changed. Her scales don't reflect any weight gain, but her stomach seems to be protruding. She knows she's slouching more, and that doesn't help the look of her figure, but she can't work out why she looks three months pregnant when she's not.

Missing Food Group

Colleen doesn't realize, but she has a protein deficiency. Without adequate protein, our bodies start to age at a faster rate. Our muscles, organs, bones, cartilage, skin, and the antibodies that guard us from disease are all made of protein. Without sufficient protein, none of these can repair themselves, and they decline into cellular breakdown.

Chronic, low-grade, long-term protein starvation leads to a loss of face and body skin tone. Women notice their breasts beginning to sag faster. Their posture starts to stoop. But, she could change the way she looks and feels beginning with her next meal. With the addition of animal protein, she would begin to notice a visible lifting and toning of her skin on her face and body.

Colleen would argue that she gets plenty of protein. On a rare cooked meal, she combines rice and beans to try to make a complete protein. She makes lots of nut pates, and what about all the sprouted seeds in her diet? The problem with being mostly vegetarian or worse, even vegan, makes getting adequate protein a complicated affair. Animal protein is the only reliable source that contains all the essential amino acids. If our body does not have complete availability at all times to the full range of these amino acids needed for cellular repair, it deteriorates.

Carnitine, a potent antioxidant and cell rejuvenator, as well as taurine, are only found in animal sources. There are some amino acids that are critical for the brain and nervous system that are found most abundantly in eggs and meat. These are the sulfur containing amino acids, methionine and cysteine. Additionally, animal sources are our only dietary means for Vitamin A and D, and the newly discovered X factor (a protector against the ravages of toxins). Without these, hormones will become unbalanced and depleted.

Meat is not usually looked upon as a health food. That's a false perception, because meat contains all the necessary amino acids needed for life, all the essential fats, and 12 of the 13 essential vitamins in large quantities. Vitamin C is the one vitamin that is scarce in meat, but it abounds abundantly in leafy greens, the perfect companions to meat. Meat and greens complement one another completely.

In his book, *Slimmer, Younger, Stronger,* the author Sam Varner, who was former trainer of the U.S. Olympic team, talks from his experience about the importance of animal protein. He followed a strict vegan program for two years and did not notice any decline in health.

During his first year of coaching with the U.S. ski team, he had the opportunity to participate in a protein study with some of the Olympic athletes. The study measured nitrogen balance in the body. This determined if the athletes were consuming enough protein for their activity level. Mr. Varner was sure his results would prove his vegan diet to be superior. To his complete surprise, the tests showed he was in a negative nitrogen balance, meaning he was not consuming enough protein. A prolonged negative nitrogen balance is very harmful. It has been observed in almost every disease state. Sam Varner promptly changed his diet to include some animal products.

Animal Protein is Slimming

Colleen believes her mostly raw, high vegetable diet is the only effective way to remain slim. She dropped 20 pounds when she eliminated meat from her diet, and she does not want it back. She doesn't realize that adding protein in the form of animal products would be a better and easier way to manage her weight and keep her middle from protruding. Eating protein, especially animal protein, can boost the metabolism by as much as 25 percent. A recent 2011 study cited in the *Journal of Nutrition* reveals the body expends 25 times more energy digesting protein, such as chicken and low-fat dairy, than it does digesting carbs, or even fat. According to this study, women on a protein rich plan lose up to 21 percent more weight and 21 percent more belly fat than women on higher carb plans.

The animal foods in Colleen's previous diet were unlikely the reason for her excess weight. The real culprits were the processed grains and "Chips 'n' Dip" diet she used to eat. When people eliminate meat and dairy from their diet, they usually also eliminate foods like white buns and fries that accompany burgers, white toast that often accompany eggs, and sugar that most yogurts and ice-cream contain. They start eating more vegetables, fruits, and whole grains in place of these items and attribute their weight loss and improved health to the elimination of animal foods. They don't realize it's the diminished amount of refined, carby junk that is the real reason. Another recent study by Korean researchers found that dieting adults who ate more protein lost about two more pounds of pure belly fat than those who ate less protein and more carbs. It's hard to argue with such results.

Unknown to Colleen, despite all her tiresome effort in keeping up her diet, she has a lot in common with Whole Grain Jane and Drive Thru Sue. She has a glucose and fructose rich diet with all her dried and fresh fruit and large amounts of carrot juice. In addition, the only way she can get her protein is through protein sources that are in carbohydrate form.

Colleen's concentrated servings of grains and legumes are wreaking more havoc with her insulin levels. She could enjoy them in moderate amounts, but trying to make them a full protein source creates a monster. She would need to stuff herself with seven packed cups of brown rice to get the protein content of one puny chicken breast. She would have to eat two packed cups of beans to get the same amount of protein. And then she has to mix beans and rice together at every meal to ensure she is getting a complete protein serving. She needs at least this much protein at each meal for daily requirements. Can you imagine having to eat all that? Having to do this on a daily basis, Colleen would only be rewarded with a belly full of bloat, incomplete essential amino acids, and rising insulin levels.

Trying to get her protein through nuts and seeds also poses problems because these are highly concentrated foods, containing both fat and a small amount of carbs. Used as an additional source of protein in smaller portions, nuts and seeds are hugely beneficial. But, making a full meal of them can be fattening, especially when they are paired with other carbohydrates.

Lusterless Skin

Dr. Perricone, a renowned anti-aging dermatologist and author #1 best selling, *The Perricone Prescription* says, "Eating diets heavy in carbs to achieve your necessary protein affects the collagen fibers of the skin. Diets heavy in carbs create a highly visible, inflammatory effect of the face and the body. This is particularly apparent in my vegetarian patients who often appear years older than they actually are. Their skin sags more and their skin color tends to be dull, rather than rosy."

A Heart at Risk

Colleen believes that meat leads to heart disease. But, scientific research like a 1986 study cited in the *Canadian Medical Association Journal* indicates that inadequate protein, i.e. vegetarianism, leads to loss of myocardial muscle and may therefore contribute to heart disease.

Tooth Decay

Science also proves that Colleen's children's teeth issues are also caused by inadequate protein. Dr. Weston Price found that those whose diets consisted largely of grains and legumes had far more dental problems than those living primarily on meats and fish. A more recent study by Dr. Emmanuel Cheraskin backs this up. This doctor devoted 50 years of his life to natural health practice and research. His study, which surveyed 1040 dentists and their wives, revealed that those with the fewest problems and diseases had the most protein in their diets.

The myth that Colleen, and many of us have believed, that high protein diets will lead to calcium loss and consequently bone and teeth loss, is not backed up by science or anthropological surveys. The only studies that showed any evidence of that being a problem involved test tubes where proteins were isolated as amino acids, rather than in whole form. Meat and other dairy products in their whole food state are naturally enriched with high vitamin D and A levels. They do not leach nutrients from the body, but rather, add a layer of protection to bones and teeth.

Mops and Brooms or Bricks and Mortar?

Colleen's raw diet made her feel great for a while because she dropped the white processed food she'd been formerly eating and added a lot more vegetables. This helped to cleanse her body from the toxins she had consumed during her life. Yet, it wasn't long before her body became depleted of the protein it needed to build and sustain her against the daily wear and tear of life. Raw juices and foods sweep out debris, but they are not the building blocks that our bodies require for long term battle against the elements.

Colleen's distended stomach and constant bloat is due to living on an herbivore diet without the four stomachs needed to digest this constant barrage of roughage. She keeps brooming out her intestines when they actually need a break from all this spring cleaning. Meat eating mammals (humans included), all contain hydrochloric acid in their stomachs. Herbivore mammals do not have this acid. There is no need for it since its purpose is to digest animal foods. We need this acid, we are actually born with a small amount of it in our stomachs. It increases quickly as we grow and we are usually able to maintain healthy levels of it all our lives. However, it can be completely depleted after years of trying to live like an herbivore. The body stops making it if it no longer has to digest animal foods. This causes major digestive problems since it's a natural component of the human digestive process.

Splat!

Constant roughage and a decline of hydrochloric acid can be a setup for strange bowel habits. Colleen is under the impression from reading material by her raw gurus that she should be able to evacuate her bowels after each meal. This is happening to her, but there is now no form to her bowel movements. Instead, they splat several times a day. Colleen has been persuaded by her reading that this is great. It keeps her body clean she's told. Sometimes, at night, she even takes this a step further and gives herself coffee or salt water enemas. Purge, purify—then purge, purge, and purify some more. This is the raw food mantra. Vegetable matter is thought to keep the body clean; meat is thought to dirty it up. In reality, it is a more natural and healthy occurrence to have one or two well formed bowel movements per day than this constant dropping of waste products.

In a paper titled *The Myths and Truths about Beef*, the authors, Sally Fallon and Mary Enig write: "Meat does not putrefy in the gut. Humans are admirably equipped to digest meat. That is the main job of the human stomach, which unlike the stomach of the cow or rabbit, contains millions of cells that secrete hydrochloric acid. Our intestinal tract is much shorter than that of the vegetarian animals, but somewhat longer that of purely carnivorous animals. Man is an omnivore with teeth, stomach, intestines, and bowel all designed to handle both animal and plant foods."

Colleen's body is now becoming mineral deficient, as a largely vegetarian diet lacks the fat soluble catalyst need for mineral absorption. A teaspoon or two of butter or two would help her absorb more minerals from the vegetables she eats, but how to convince her of that?

Living Enzymes

Colleen sticks to eating as "high raw" as she can to get all the living enzymes that raw food offers. If she could only let go of her "no animal product" idealism, she could add even more enzymes to her diet in the form of cultured dairy. Fermented dairy products like yogurt and kefir have more enzymes than even a raw salad. A raw salad has enough enzymes to help digest one meal. Fermented dairy has an abundance of enzymes that not only facilitate digestion, but are utilized for other non-digestive metabolic purposes such as detoxification and proper functioning of the endocrine glands and other vital organs. Colleen is correct in her thinking that life-giving enzymes are the catalyst for robust health, but she needs to become aware of better options that are more powerful enzyme boosters.

Cooking Food Does Not Always Destroy Nutrients

Yes, raw vegetables are healthy, and most people need to eat more of them, but Colleen is missing out on some health promoting properties that are only released from cooked vegetables. According to a recent study in the *Journal of Agricultural and Food Chemistry*, steamed broccoli has higher concentrations of many carotenoids than raw. Amazingly, even after cooking, broccoli retains nearly 70 percent of its vitamin C, and virtually all of its kaempferol, which is a flavonoid that saves cells in the body. Steamed broccoli with butter would be very soothing for Colleen's digestive tract which is constantly dealing with harsh roughage.

Colleen would probably be surprised to learn that a recent German study published in the *British Journal of Nutrition*, found that 77 percent of 198 people following a strict raw food diet had plasma lycopene levels below what is considered optimum. Lycopene is a powerful antioxidant, proven to reduce the risk of several cancers. Tomatoes are an excellent source of lycopene, but Colleen is not receiving their full potential, because she believes cooking destroys them. In fact, cooked tomatoes have much higher concentrations of lycopene. Roasting tomatoes causes cell walls to burst, releasing more of this powerful flavonoid. Lycopene is fat soluble, therefore eating roasted tomatoes with coconut oil, olive oil, or even butter, should help bring Colleen's levels back to a health promoting level.

While this advice is not relevant to most people, Colleen actually needs to lower her raw vegetable and fruit intake and find balance with more protein-centered meals, including some healthy animal products and soothing cooked vegetables. Colleen does not need to keep punishing her body to attain long-term health. The meals she eats purge her body, but they do not nourish and soothe. A hot meal that includes fat releases oxytocin in the body. Colleen's body desperately needs more release of this chemical which fights stress and diseases in the body. We'll learn more about this important chemical in later chapters.

Hopefully, Colleen will learn that she does not need to be such a raw zealot to ensure optimum health. She should take a more gentle approach to food. Including some warming whole foods in her diet will not be the undoing of her health. In further chapters, Colleen will learn that God has quite a bit to say about what foods are supposed to be received by our bodies. Letting go of fears and trusting in His higher wisdom will bring peace and comfort to Colleen's entire family.

Chapter Four

Farm Fresh Tess

Meet Tess.

Tess feels blessed to live on 30 very usable acres. She and her husband always dreamed of being self-sufficient. That dream came true when they sold their house in the suburbs, bought their fixer upper farm, and got out of debt.

Tess receives great fulfillment gathering fresh eggs in the morning and overseeing her older children as they milk their goats. She makes homemade cheese, yogurt, and kefir from the milk. Most of their meat is farm-raised and Tess enjoys knowing that the aroma of her evening meal comes without mysterious antibiotics or hormones.

The family also tends a large garden. They reap enough to sell any extra produce at their local Farmers Market on the weekends. Tess believes in wholesome eating. She puts up food seasonally. Her children are robust and well nourished. As a whole, Tess and her family do not suffer from common colds and viruses as frequently as others do. Tess is strong and can work hard.

Whole Foods and Plenty of 'Em

They are a meat and potatoes sort of family. They eat a lot of pure protein like their home raised meat, eggs, and dairy, but always accompany the meal with hearty servings of starches. Items like potatoes, noodles, breads, and rice are staples at mealtimes.

Tess's husband loves to boast about his wife's wholesome cooking. She makes a mean lasagna (a potluck favorite), and you would die for her cinnamon rolls and fruit pies. Home fixed sweet tea with honey accompanies most meals.

Since Tess knows there are many nutrients in her diet and she is not missing out on anything, she doesn't mind treating herself. She doesn't relate to food Nazis. Life is to be enjoyed. She and her daughter both love to get in the kitchen and bake cookies for the whole family's pleasure. Homemade ice cream from grass fed cows . . . what could be better?

Strong and Sturdy

Tess has never been tiny. She stopped caring about her extra padding in her thirties, thinking it's better to be happy and healthy than forever trying to be skinny. Her husband has no complaints about her well padded body and loves her just the way she is. His slow accumulation of weight over the years has never bothered Tess either. She chooses not to dwell on her weight, which if she had to guess, is close to 40 pounds heavier than her wedding day, and she was no Skinny Minny then. There is so much else in her life to keep her busy, why focus on all that? She says every now and then that she wasn't born with "skinny genes."

A New Problem

Now that Tess and her husband are in their mid-forties, new concerns have recently arisen. Her husband has developed high blood pressure. It was first noticed at a recent doctor's check up. Rather than have him go on meds, they have tried many alternative therapies for blood pressure, but without too much success. Tess does not want her husband to have to go on medication for the rest of his life, but that will be the reality unless he follows doctor's orders and loses weight.

Along with the blood pressure issue, Tess's husband has also just been diagnosed with sleep apnea. Tess had noticed his loud snoring becoming progressively worse, but was still surprised at the doctor's prognosis after he ordered a sleep study. Their doctor suggested, as most doctors do, that her husband restrict salt intake and implement a lower fat diet. He prescribed her husband a CPAP machine to wear while he sleeps. It's uncomfortable, and both Tess and her husband are bothered by the fact that he must wear it every night. It's not very romantic and really interferes with spooning and cuddle time!

To support her husband, Tess is considering losing weight alongside him. She can't, in good conscience, feed him tofu and rice cakes while she chows down on the good stuff. The thought of counting calories or fixing fat free anything is abhorrent to her. Second helpings of good food are as much a part of their life as the sun rising. She also doesn't like the idea of having to give up the rich nourishing foods their farm provides when they have worked so hard to achieve them.

High Blood Pressure

Tess is unaware of her own health issue. Her fasting blood sugar is creeping up higher than it should be with every year. Both she and her husband, due to their heavy starch habits, are headed toward Type 2 diabetes within a decade.

High blood sugar and high blood pressure are very good friends. If one presents itself, the other will usually follow. Recent studies expose that excess insulin plays an important role in the development of high blood pressure. In fact, high blood pressure in itself can be a critical sign that the body is flooding itself with too much insulin. This is exactly what is happening to Tess's husband. His pressure readings are an obvious symptom of his excess insulin.

Excess insulin release can lead to blood pressure problems in a few different ways. It stimulates the nervous system, which makes the heart beat faster and causes the blood vessels to narrow. Another way it helps is to regulate salt in the blood. If you have too much insulin, more salt is retained, in turn, causing more water to stay in the blood stream. This greater amount of fluid causes higher pressure as it passes through the vessels and arteries. As we now know, insulin also stimulates the production of cholesterol and the buildup of plaque on the walls of blood vessels. This narrows the space for blood to flow, and there you go, you have a reading of 155 over 94. Not good!

Right now, Tess's blood pressure is okay. She is still ovulating every month and her estrogen is protecting her from hypertension. Once she reaches menopause in just a few years, things will most likely change quickly. Women are much less likely to suffer from hypertension in their child-bearing years, but when they lose their hormones during menopause, they join the men who suffer in equal numbers.

Don't Give up the Good Stuff

If only Tess understood they do not have to give up those wonderful eggs her free range chickens have been laying, or any of the nourishing foods her farm yields. Neither does she have to deny her husband healthy forms of salt and fat, the two things that make a meal tasty and satisfying and which release the wonderful "feel good" neurotransmitters.

Science is now finally proving that what is a natural human urge for salt is not wrong. Men are especially wowed by both the components of salt and fat in a meal. One recent study on the effect of a low salt diet made headlines, disclosing that a low salt diet increases mortality for patients with congestive heart failure. This study concluded there was not enough evidence to advise a low salt diet for the rest of us. Another 2010 *Harvard University* study linked low salt diets to an increase in insulin resistance.

Another Australian study that followed 638 Type 2 diabetes patients for an average of 10 years, found that lowered salt was associated with all increases of mortality. A similar study was carried out on those with type 1 diabetes and the same conclusion was reached. Yet another study published in the *American Journal of Hypertension* showed eating less salt will not prevent heart attacks, strokes, or early death. On the contrary, low sodium diets increase likelihood of premature death.

These new findings are all vastly different from the low salt advice that has been the norm for decades. Popular wisdom has told us that a low salt diet is crucial for people with high blood pressure. We have all heard the grave advice, "sodium should be limited to . . ." and at the end of the sentence is a number which immediately signifies bland food. Studies used to support this advice have only shown that reduced salt consumption can only lower blood pressure slightly, but now we know there are ramifications with constantly lowering salt intake. A large overview of 167 different studies were recently analyzed and published in the *American Journal of Hypertension.* The analysts made an overall conclusion that too little salt can be dangerous. They noted that salt restrictive diets may raise cholesterol and triglycerides (fat in the blood).

Dr. Dach, an MD who specializes in hormones, writes about this subject in an interesting article entitled, *Low Salt Diet Increases Cardiovascular Mortality*. In this article he discusses the studies on salt reduction. Referring to these studies he writes, "They show the low salt diet will in fact reduce pressure slightly. However, this effect is minimal, and is counteracted by compensatory mechanisms that release harmful substances into the bloodstream, hormones, and chemicals mediators that counteract the low salt diet. The released chemical mediators include insulin, epinephrine, norephinine, renin, aldosterone, etc. These are harmful and damaging to the vascular system."

In his book, *Salt Your Way To Health*, Dr. David Brownstein points out the difference between refined salt which is commonly used in all processed foods, and natural sea salt. Natural sea salt contains trace minerals that alkalize and benefit the body in many ways. Natural salt is necessary for the adrenal glands which regulate energy levels. It helps to combat elevated blood sugar, relieve muscle cramps, combat osteoporosis, and help manage cases of hypertension. Tess does not need to remove salt from her husband's foods, but make sure it is in natural sea salt form.

It is also important that salt contain iodine, an important nutrient for the thyroid and one that fights cancer in the body. Many iodized, natural sea salts can be found in food stores, so this will not be a hard switch for Tess's family. Her husband's blood pressure problems, along with his sleep apnea, can be greatly alleviated by weight loss in a healthy, hearty, and still tasty way. Rice cakes and salt-free bland tasting foods, who needs them?

Tess's own stout figure, which she has resigned herself to live with, can also naturally melt away to uncover a vibrant physique to match her personality. Tess is never going to become a primping Barbie Doll type. Why should she? But, there is a healthier and trimmer body underneath that extra padding that's waiting to be revealed. It will even surprise Tess herself. She may not have been born with skinny genes, but she was born with genes that are just right for her. Slowly and surely that "just right" will emerge without ever a rice cake entering the house.

Connecting the Dots

Now that we've met all four women, we see that despite their very different lives, they all share a common problem. What is the culprit? Too high blood sugar, resulting in surging insulin. The core of Tess's problems is the same as the other three women, even though her lifestyle looks vastly different.

To beat her challenges, Tess needs to rely more on non-starchy vegetables as sides to her free range meats, which are not the offenders. We're not saying she can't ever have a sweet potato in her life. However, rather than rice, potatoes, or bread (sometimes all three—aaahhh!) at every meal, how about roasted cauliflower with cheese, made from her goat's milk and herbs from her garden? She'd be just as satisfied with grilled zucchini, drizzled with olive oil, garlic, and sea salt than pasta salad on the side of her delicious grass-fed pot roast. Instead of buttering up starchy corn, she can toss some spaghetti squash in butter, sea salt, and parmesan cheese.

Her family will love these lower glycemic options. A few side dish swap outs is all that's needed for Tess to get her husband's and her own health back on track. If Tess only knew how close her diet is to being optimally slimming, as well as satisfying, she would no longer have to fret about the future of their farm derived foods. The core of her diet is spot on; she only needs to adjust the edges.

Tess can keep the ice cream made from her grass fed cows by changing to a sweetener that has zero impact on blood sugar and her ice cream treat becomes a slimming superfood. She will learn to eat it as a dessert after a vegetable/meat meal, rather than one with a higher carb count that includes big helpings of starch.

Tess can still bake bread. She'll love learning to catch the wild yeasts of the air and sour-doughing her bread, which will only increase her husband's and her health. But, she'll learn how to scale bread back to a more health promoting part of her diet.

Tess's family only has to learn the art of conscious carb eating. She won't have to give up her desserts or second helpings. They will take care of themselves. As her starchy carb intake goes down, so will her hunger. Sugar and starches create bigger appetites.

Tess can keep some of her winning dessert recipes for special occasions, but on a daily basis, she will learn to make delicious, healthful desserts that her husband will fall in love with, while his weight drops and his blood pressure finds more stability. He'll lose some of the fat that has accumulated around his neck and throat—goodbye CPAP machine. Welcome back queen bed cuddle time! Tess is soon going to notice that her husband's snoring is no longer a nightly occurrence and he'll start sleeping like a baby.

Tess doesn't have to change her whole lifestyle after all, only a few simple ingredients.

Chapter Five

Get Ready for the Plan

Did you figure out which woman you relate to most? We'll admit that we've had a lot in common with a few of them over the years. Yet, there's a new woman we want to introduce to you. It's you! Your metamorphosis as you come out of confusion. You are about to be **Satisfied** and **Energized.**

You are going to read these two words (**Satisfying** and **Energizing**) over and over again throughout the book. We'll shorten them to **S** and **E**. We have nicknamed our way of eating as **The S and E Plan**. Yes, a plan. But don't tune out. It's the way we have to teach it to you in the beginning. If you have some weight to lose, you'll need to learn to make each meal you eat burn one primary fuel source, rather than two.

The two primary fuel sources for the body are glucose and fats. It is crucial that protein be included with every meal, but it is not a primary fuel for the body. Once you focus your meals on one fuel source at a time, your body will be able to burn through that fuel, and then switch directly to the task of burning your own adipose tissue (body fat) for fuel. Results? Natural weight loss.

After a while, this won't feel like a plan. Eating **Satisfying** and **Energizing** meals will become as much a natural part of you as breathing in and out. First, you'll need to learn about these **S** and **E** meals and how they both deliciously help you find healthy weight and greater overall health.

Prep Time

Before we jump right into the specifics of the plan, it's important that you get prepared. This preparation is not a list of things you must do, or buy, before you start changing your eating habits. It is a preparing of your heart and mind. Even if you recognized yourself in one of the four women we described and realize there are changes to be made, don't charge into your kitchen and start throwing things out of your cupboards and refrigerator just yet. That may come later on. First, we want to chat to you for a little bit about the general ideas behind these dietary principles that work so well in our busy family lives.

Grab a cup of coffee, take a deep breath, relax, and open your mind to some new, and also surprisingly very old food ideas.

We hope the next couple of chapters will scrub away myths, lies, and confusion about nutrition that are imprinted in your mind. It will be easier to embark on this journey toward greater health and weight management if your mind is not ensnared by certain cages of thinking.

Any long term turnaround is not as likely to be sustained if you stay married to current beliefs about nutrition. Many widely held beliefs about certain food are simply myths. It's our hope that you will let go of unnecessary mind baggage that can easily hold you back. Weigh and measure our suggestions and ideas with an open mind and heart. We do not claim to know it all, and still have much to learn ourselves, but hopefully you'll soon discover that much of our culture's current, dietary beliefs are actually in direct contradiction to the Bible.

These current nutrition beliefs block progress to stable weight because they hold people captive to defeat. It's impossible to find an ease in life while trying to do as most modern food advisors tell us. If you think that having to constantly worry about counting calories, or stripping the fat and a large quota of animal foods like butter and red meat from most of your meals, is simply too hard to do—that's because it is. This sort of advice is bondage, and with God's help, you can shed the weight of it from your life.

Welcome to a new world, where the principles behind the words, **Satisfying** and **Energizing** can change your life. Get ready to fly!

Stabilize Your Blood Sugar

You will soon be eating in a way that is termed "Low Glycemic" and we're going to teach you exactly how to do it. You've probably heard this term thrown around. It simply means the foods you eat will have gentle impact on your blood sugar levels. It is imperative to stop the vicious cycle of too high, then too low blood sugar in your blood stream. You'll do this by learning how to be more carbohydrate conscious.

Our approach is not like other low-carbohydrate diets which are also low glycemic, but where people tend to get in the rut of constantly overdoing meats and fats. Often, they do not include adequate amounts of fruits and vegetables, and rely on chemical, artificial sweeteners. Very low-carb diets are successful in weight loss at first, but they can end up slowing down the metabolism as the body gets more efficient at metabolizing predominantly fats and proteins. We want to avoid this at all costs, and as this plan unfolds, you'll learn some tricks to kick start your metabolism into high gear.

Becoming carb conscious is the smartest way to live. It will enable you to take better dominion over the size and health of your body. You'll soon be a carb conscious mama and proud of it. You won't do this by counting every carb; that's more bondage. Instead, you'll learn to center your meals with protein, and learn the difference between starchy and non-starchy carbs. You'll choose more delicious non-starchy carbs to complete your meals, but will not eliminate the starchy ones, though they will no longer rule your plate. You'll find a healthier, wiser place for them in your diet.

A carb conscious approach to food, rather than a constant low-carb diet, is crucial to long term health because most of us cannot constantly live on a very low-carb diet and remain healthy. It is not long before glycogen (stored glucose in the liver and muscles) becomes depleted and stays that way. This can lead to a lack of energy. Also, long term, very low-carb diets can sometimes lead to other complications like a more sluggish thyroid and metabolism. This is why our plan works. We promote an inclusive diet, rather than an exclusive one. It includes all three essential macronutrients—fats proteins and carbs, even certain amounts of starchy carbs. We can enjoy all three and stay slim.

Focus on the Right Foods

The **S** and **E** plan focuses on non-starchy vegetables, both raw and cooked, often drizzled with creamy dressings or buttery sauces. We also want to encourage a lot of superfoods like salmon, berries, nuts, seeds, cultured dairy products, and super fats like coconut oil. These foods, alongside more natural sources of red meat, eggs, and chicken, with balanced amounts of whole grains, legumes, fruits, and sweet potatoes are the ultimate fuel for the human body and can bring much healing.

Do any of these foods sound like a deprivation diet? Nor do they come in tiny little boxes for only "mini me" people to eat. Staying satisfied is the name of the game now. These are foods on which the whole family can thrive.

This new approach to food will not send you into a constant state of ketosis (burning fat by using ketones for energy). Healthy weight loss easily occurs without this becoming a 24 hour state in your body. If your body naturally slips into ketosis now and then through eating **S** and **E** meals, it shouldn't pose too much of a problem as it won't remain in that state for long. Having said that, ketosis has occurred naturally in humans for centuries. People groups lived seasonally before export, import, and refrigeration were common. At times, they feasted on summer harvests. At other times, they had nothing more than dried meat and herbs which would have induced states of ketosis. Many of us get into a state of ketosis overnight and by morning we are naturally burning ketones for energy. It also occurs for brief periods after our body burns through the fuels in our meals, but ketosis is not a state we have to constantly seek to achieve weight loss.

Give Fat the Welcome Mat

Eating this **S**atisfying and **E**nergizing way will not be a low-fat lifestyle. In fact, many of the meals you'll soon be eating may include liberal amounts of healthy fats to help you feel satisfied. This makes life so much more enjoyable. Who doesn't like cream and butter? Yes, you can finally say, "I love butter" and not feel guilty about it. If you are like we were for so many years, buried under the dogma that butter is evil and fattening, you have some therapy ahead of you. You might need to say, "Butter is my friend," 10 times. Go ahead . . . we'll wait!

Feel any release yet? It may take a while.

We'll get to butter and its benefits again a little later on. For now, let's take baby-steps. If you're feeling shocked and shaky at the thought of giving butter more freedom, feel reassured that you won't be heaping it on every meal, but you will get to enjoy it often enough. People may see you smear it generously on your broccoli at a restaurant and wonder how you can do it and not be obese. They'll think you're one of the lucky ones who has never had to worry about weight a day in your life. Little will they know that you have simply acquired the knowledge of dietary, sensible science.

As we discovered by examining our first friend, Whole Grain Jane's diet, the low-fat approach wasn't helping her at all. Jane showed us how low-fat and high grain diets can often lead to cravings and constant hunger. Remember that good fats are not the enemy. Fat is essential for every function of our body, and too little of it for too long will cause depression, hormone loss, and accelerated aging. Fat is the only thing that really satisfies and curbs cravings. Try not to be too obvious about it, but look at anyone who has spent a good length of time limiting fat. You'll likely see that their skin looks aged beyond their years. Constantly trying to skimp on fat is not natural, and if you try it for too long, it will mess with ya.

The only way for fats to be stored in the body as actual body fat is when glucose rises in the blood and the hormone insulin has to rush out to take care of it. Remember the picture of insulin as the body's sugar delivery truck we talked about in Chapter One where you met Whole Grain Jane? Insulin puts the body in storing mode. It will store any excess glucose from the meal as fat, and not only that, when there is such an abundance of glucose for fuel, the body will be prevented from burning all the fat you just ate for fuel. It's double trouble!

Fat for Fuel

We must do the opposite when we eat fat. Here is something so simple yet extremely important to learn. You can eat generous amounts of fat in a meal if you don't stimulate your sugar delivery truck into loading off a bunch of glucose to your cells first. You avoid this by keeping starchy carbohydrates out of that particular meal. Two good things occur for fat loss when this happens. Firstly, your fat cells will not get fed any excess glucose (which makes them even fatter) since glucose will be scarce. Secondly, and even better, all the tasty and satisfying fat you ate in that meal will be able to be burned as fuel, rather than stored. It will become your primary fuel source.

Let's condense this into one sentence and make it so simple that you never forget.

EATING FAT DOES NOT MAKE YOU FAT IF CARBS ARE KEPT TO A MINIMUM.

If eating fat makes you fat, we'd be obese, because we eat a lot of it. Instead, we're thin, and that is not because of genetics. It's science. Look at a nice breakfast of fried or scrambled eggs in butter, turkey sausage, sliced tomato, and coffee with a spot of cream. It has fat, yes, but it does not contain the type of foods which create a high glucose state. As we have stated, your fat cells only get fed glucose when there is more glucose available than the cells in your muscles can take in for energy. A breakfast like this is not going to cause that issue. Results—a decadent meal, a satisfied mama ready to take on the day's tasks, and a flattening tummy.

If you keep starchy carbs to a minimum in some meals like this, your body must fuel itself instead from the fat in your food. That's great, as fat was designed by our Creator to be a wonderful fuel for the body. After your body has burned through the fat in your meal, it will turn directly to your own fatty tissue for fuel. You have to keep living, and in order to do this, you need constant fuel. Causing your body to turn to your adipose tissue like this is a good thing, because when your body fat finally gets a chance to be used for energy, it means it diminishes, and you become thinner!

Meals like the breakfast we described, allow the cells in your muscles that are designed to respond to insulin and accept the blood sugar it offers, to finally get the chance to empty out a little. Remember, these cells are often so full of sugar that they are becoming more insulin resistant. They need to use up the glucose with which they are already choc full before you start forcing more glucose down their throats.

Eating meals that have a good bit of fat in them, without a boat load of carbs, is the ticket to make this happen. You get to fill up and feel satisfied. There is no Twinkie craving at the end of this type of meal. Your body goes "Ahhhh" and is able to relax. This is the basic premise behind our **S** meals. The details you will learn further on.

Why the Opposite?

Dieticians on TV, articles in women's magazines, and most likely your general practitioner, will tell you to always trim the fat from your food to stay healthy and lose weight. You torture yourself and try to eat little to no fat for weeks as these low-fat advocates recommend, but you'll still likely create that delivery truck hurtling full tilt. Why? Because you're probably going to overdo carbs in place of eating fat. The body wants fuel. That's its natural survival instinct. People are carbing up too much because they're constantly told that fat is bad.

Foods that are commonly considered "weight loss friendly" like fruit flavored non-fat yogurt that is pre-sweetened or non-fat, lightly frosted cereal flakes with non-fat milk, or tinsy pre-packaged snacks of pretzels or cookies advertised as only 100 calories and "fat free" all contain loads of carbs and sugar which elevate glucose in the blood. High-carbs equals high glucose which equals high insulin. Brrmmm, brmmm goes that truck. It's going into super delivery mode now. Storing here (a little on the tum), storing there (a little on the butt), storing everywhere (a little more under the chin). Have a look around your local grocery store. Shelves are full of these low-fat low-calorie items, but the obesity epidemic is not slowing down.

Sure, some foods without any fat are lower in calories and certain people whose cells are not yet too insulin resistant, can lose some pounds by reducing their calorie intake this way for a while. But, the weight loss is usually temporary, because the body's metabolism lowers. And constantly lowering calories and stripping fat sure is no fun.

As humans, our bodies crave fat. Denying ourselves what we essentially need by using self control only lasts for a while. The resultant unbridled blood sugar that ensues from kicking fat out, while keeping carbs in, will still be a problem, even if pounds can be lost by some people in that manner. Insulin is still likely to overproduce, causing other problems in the body.

Created to Enjoy Food

In 2010, a self study by a professor at Kansas State University caught a lot of national media attention. He put himself on a convenience store diet of candy, nutty bars, sugary cereals, and Oreos, but reduced his caloric intake to 1800 calories a day. He lost 27 pounds in 10 weeks! The news headlines had a heyday with his results. The consensus boiled down to calories. Even junk food, if kept within calorie guidelines, can make you slim!

It's a good thing this diet was only a temporary experiment for the professor. The professor may have been able to use oodles of portion control for the experiment and eat only tiny candy meals so as not to exceed his calorie limit, but who could do that long term? We were created to eat! The eating experience is as much a part of living as breathing. The natural cycle is to eat, become satisfied, take a break—then eat to get satisfied again. There's no getting past it. We are wired to get satisfied from food, and a few gummy bears and half a Twinkie is not going to do that long term. We'll talk later about how calories fit into the picture and if we should pay them any heed at all. But we'll warn you now that the approach of pulling them back to a small number day after day is the gateway into yoyo dieting disaster. There is a smarter approach to the calorie debate and dilemma.

You can bet this professor would end up giving in to real hunger, sooner or later, and stop limiting himself to such stringent portions. Eating larger portions of those sugary foods would inevitably cause his blood sugar to spike. The consequent large surges of insulin his body would have to generate to clear that sugar would then become a long term problem.

In excess, insulin suppresses human growth hormone which is needed for youthful skin, muscles and bones. It also contributes to higher blood pressure as we learned from the example of Farm Fresh Tess's poor husband. It also has an inflammatory effect on all bodily systems. In the book, *The Schwarzbein Principle*, Dr. Diana Schwarzbein writes:

"When insulin levels are kept high too long, the result is a physiology that promotes excess body fat gain, a physiology prone to infections and all the chronic degenerative diseases of aging: osteoarthritis, different types of cancer, cholesterol abnormalities, coronary artery disease, less lean body mass with excess body fat, high blood pressure, osteoporosis, stroke, and Type 2 diabetes."

In the book, *Why We Get Fat*, author Gary Taubes makes his case very clearly about the hazards of high insulin. On page 124 he writes, "The bottom line is something that's been known (and mostly ignored) for over 40 years. The one thing we absolutely have to do if we want to get leaner—if we want to get fat out of our fat tissue and burn it—is to lower our insulin levels and to secrete less insulin to begin with."

Notice that both these authors mentioned the hazards of too high insulin. We need to stress again that when insulin is working for us, rather than against us, it shouldn't be blamed for fat gain.

One of the most concerning problems when insulin is stimulated to excessive levels by carby foods, is what it does to our feel-good neurotransmitter serotonin. When insulin is raised high very quickly, it causes a rush of serotonin to be released from the brain. This can make you feel good at first. You know the feeling of a sugar high? That's simply the result of serotonin flooding your body. But, over time, this causes increasingly more rapid drops in serotonin levels. That's never a good thing, because we need sufficient serotonin to avoid feelings of depression and apathy. Serotonin is also our natural pain reliever. Aches and pains in the body, like headaches and joint aches, become a major problem when we lack serotonin. We have to wonder if there is an obvious connection between our modern diet, its effect on serotonin, and the high amount of antidepressants (SSRI's) that are prescribed to help people with depression.

In the book, *Why We Get Fat*, author Gary Taubes argues the case against the commonly held theory that low-calorie diets work. The notion of calories in, calories out, doesn't hold water according to this author. He points to studies, history, and science to expose the shaky ground of this widely accepted theory (we disagree with the evolutionary part of his history and science, but there is much to be learned in his books despite that). Mr. Taubes discusses in-depth one particular large study that was part of the collection of studies called *The Women's Health Initiative* (WHI). This study involved 20,000 women in the early 1990's. These women were instructed to eat a low-fat diet, rich in fruits, vegetables, and fiber. They were also instructed to eat 360 calories less every day. That was 20 percent lower than what public health agencies advise women to eat. The woman cut their total fat consumption and saturated fats by a full quarter. They were even given regular counseling to help motivate them to stay on the diet.

Eight years later the study found these women did lose weight. A whopping two pounds! And, these study participants had a lot to lose. The majority were overweight, and about half were obese, which always makes losing weight quicker to shed. According to calorie reduction math, these women should have lost at least 22 pounds in the first year and continued a slower loss after that. Not only did that not happen, the kicker was that their average waist circumference (a measurement of abdominal fat) actually increased! This makes it more likely that the average of two pounds that they did lose was muscle, not fat. The disappointing results flabbergasted everyone. These women may have lost weight at first, but the eight year mark was the big truth teller regarding long term success.

History repeats itself. Zoom forward to the last decade. Television has spotlighted calorie counting in prime time on the show *The Biggest Loser*. We have both enjoyed watching the show now and then, even though we think the fast-forced weight loss is not a sustainable approach. The show's dietary approach is low-calorie/low-fat and semi low-carb. It works at first with sensational "TV worth watching" type results. But, have you ever done a little research follow up on the contestants?

A few of the contestants still look rather stellar some years later, but more often they gain some, if not all of the weight back. We watched an episode that looked at the lives of former contestants. One of them shared her struggle with not gaining the weight back by saying she had to exercise two hours a day to maintain her new weight, even sticking rigidly to her daily low-calorie limit. Who could sustain that long term?

A 2009 book called *Simple Swaps*, authored by the head nutritionist for *The Biggest Loser* showcased some earlier season contestant success stories. Most of these success stories had gained back at least 20 to 40 pounds. None of the failure stories were talked about, the ones who gain all or most of their weight back. Weighing portions and holding back fat grams in every meal is no way to live! No wonder this constant counting approach is not sustainable, even for famous TV contestants who feel like they're letting a whole country down if they put their weight back on.

Carbs Need Some Love Too

If we're going to stay nourished and stay sane, we need fat. Yay! We always need protein, that's a given. But, we also need some starchy carbs, too (Yippee Yay Again)! Let's not leave anything out.

Glucose for Fuel

Our bodies were designed to receive glucose for energy. If that were not the case, God would not have designed the process. Consequently, we shouldn't deny our cells from receiving adequate amounts of glucose fuel by constantly staying in a low-carb/low sugar state and trying to burn only fat for fuel. This is what constant low-carb diets attempt to do. Meals that include starches need to be eaten in a savvy way, similar to meals that include a nice amount of fats.

Healthy carbs that even include some starch, help to keep the metabolism revving, the brain working well, and energy levels up. Our **E** meals serve this purpose. They're the way to eat healthy starches and offer your cells glucose for fuel without fattening your body at the same time.

Hopefully, you now have it locked securely in your mind that your insulin hormone should not be triggered into a state of overdrive, always having to make more sugar deliveries than needed. But, we shouldn't try to suppress its natural function, either. It does a fine job when it's not acting like Martha in the Bible and constantly overworking. It needs some rest time, too!

However, it will keep overworking unless you order it to slow down. Tell it to chill a little. Insulin will only get the message to chill out by the food you send to it. You can tell it what to do by the content of your meal. It only drives around like crazy, making all these excess deliveries because it's been given the triggers to do so by carb heavy meals. You can stop giving the green light for all this excess activity by being more carb conscious in your very next meal.

It should be clear by now that attempting to completely prevent insulin from doing the job God designed it to do, should not be the goal. Enough carbs need to be eaten for insulin to work for our benefit, but for this to happen, we must first create a better cycle where our cells are able to empty out first and actually get hungry for blood sugar. They will then say to insulin, "Just what I needed . . . thank you very much!" rather than, "More gallons of glucose? No, no!"

A better way for your cells to receive energy from blood sugar is if they start from a cleared out state. Eating our **S** style meals causes this to happen. Then, you can naturally refuel your cells by eating what we call the **E** meal.

In this **E** meal, your sugar delivery truck will have a moderate amount of glucose from some healthy carbohydrates. The meal will also include lean protein and a little bit of healthy fat, just enough to aid digestion and assimilation of nutrients, but not enough for fat to be stored. This would be perfect! The delivery truck gets on the road since the whole grains have caused a medium rise in blood sugar. But, the protein, and the little bit of fat, actually help to slow down the force of this vehicle. There will be no need for a second glucose clearance and the consequent excess glucose delivery to fat cells. In a balanced meal like this, insulin will efficiently clear the sugar from your blood and make only one, well-needed and wanted, blood sugar delivery to hungry muscle cells for energy. Hungry cells will burn through this fuel more efficiently than when they are bloated and sluggish. This allows your body to get down to the task of burning your own fat stores for fuel. This is the premise behind our **E** meals. Details will come later.

Create a More Natural Cycle

Thus, we have two well-needed types of meals. **S** meals give your cells a chance to empty out since they involve less total carbs and allow you to use fat for your primary fuel. **E** meals help fill your cells up again, and because they have more carbs, they offer glucose for your primary fuel source. But, **E** meals do this in a manner that is much wiser and safer than force feeding large amounts of glucose to already overstuffed cells.

Now, you've got a bodily cycle occurring that works for health and weight management, rather than leading to weight problems and disease. Both meal types utilize one primary fuel source. After that is used up, your body can get right on to body fat burning.

The results of a recent 2011 study show support for the premise of this better and healthier eating cycle we advocate. The study was presented at *The San Antonio Breast Cancer Symposium*. British researchers studied 115 women at high risk for breast cancer due to obesity and problems with the hormone insulin. The study determined to find a diet that was not too hard to stick to for people in high risk health situations. The researchers found that women who eliminated carbohydrate rich foods like bread, pasta, potatoes, and rice just two days a week, lost an average of nine pounds over four months even while eating their regular diet the rest of the week. Meanwhile, women who ate a reduced calorie, Mediterranean style diet of 1500 calories per day for the same time period, lost only five pounds. It seems evident that people may be better off cutting back on carbs on certain days rather than constantly counting calories.

Why did eliminating starches like potatoes, bread, and rice only two days a week work? The answer is obvious. To us, at least. The women in that group were setting up a better cycle for their cells to be able to process blood sugar. After eating a few meals without high starches, their cells emptied out. In other words, they used up all the glucose with which they were previously bloated. This meant their bodies did not have to redirect glucose to fat cells after every meal due to being constantly engorged. Once these women returned to eating meals that contained starches, they could actually use that blood sugar rather than store it as fat since their muscle cells were empty and hungry.

We think that eating a regular SAD diet five days a week is still not the healthiest option, even though the women in that study did have some success. Nine pounds lost over four months is not too shabby, but the study mentioned that these women were obese, and weight is much swifter to shed when obesity is present. They could have lost more. We have a much healthier plan for you by using our **S** and **E** meals. Cycling two healthy style meals like **S** and **E**, rather than cycling lower carb meals with regular junky ones, is a much wiser idea. However, this recent study is a great example of how implementing a natural "carbs in–carbs out" cycle is important, and much easier to implement than constantly worrying about calories.

Avoid the Head-on Collision

Our **S** and **E** plan naturally avoids the dilemma that occurs when high amounts of carbs and fats are eaten together. Hopefully, by now, you agree with us that we don't want to kick fat out of the game. We need it. We can't live a great life without it. And we are sure you agree that we don't want to turn the cold shoulder on carbs either. The same thing goes, we need 'em, can't live well without 'em. We've already said you can't get fat by eating fat, but a problem occurs when you put together a meal consisting of both fats and carbs. If you throw both high-carbs and high fat into the mix, you are most probably going to get weight gain . . . uh oh! What's a girl to do?

The carbs and fat combo is fine for a very few people who have trouble maintaining weight, but for most of us, it's a sure fire way to go up in skirt sizes. Take a look at two common food examples, donuts and potato chips. They are both very high in carbs from their starch content and they get the insulin truck running hard. They are also both high in fat. It's the double trouble situation again— excess glucose, so some of it has to be redirected to fat cells. The fat cells are doubly fed because insulin, our delivery truck has the task of storing excess glucose, plus hefty amounts of fat. Fat cells accept both glucose and fat. They take whatever's offered them.

Smooshing both high-carbs and high fats together in one particular meal, or in one recipe, is not the best way for most of us to eat these macronutrients. That is, if we want to stay slim or become that way. The combination of high fats and carbs is not exclusive to junk food either. Everybody knows donuts and chips are fattening, but you'd be surprised that whole grains paired with fats can do the same thing. You can find yourself colliding into excess pounds simply from eating a plate of brown rice with beef and veggies.

Brown rice elevates blood sugar quite easily, even in normal serving amounts. Now you have fat from the beef on top of rising blood sugar from the rice—goodbye waistline! What about a salad with an olive oil dressing and a couple of thick pieces of homemade whole wheat bread and butter on the side? Sounds healthy, right? It is, except you've got enough carbs from the bread to stimulate a hefty surge of insulin to deal with rising blood sugar. Now, on top of that, is the fat from the butter, and the salad dressing. This combination is not kind to your hips or belly.

The science behind the fat and carb smoosh is pretty easy to understand. Meals that contain both these macronutrients in liberal amounts work to fatten us up because our bodies are designed to chiefly burn one fuel at a time, but glucose always gets priority. Let's say you eat a hamburger with fries. Your body burns the glucose first. Gotta get that sugar out of the blood so you can stay alive! It doesn't necessarily do this because it prefers glucose as a fuel source. It does it to protect you from the toxicity of too high blood sugar. Sugar must be cleared out of the way before dealing with fat. Out surges insulin and attempts to clean up the mess. It will take a while, and it will be a challenging task because the starchy fries and white burger buns caused a huge surplus of blood sugar.

Meanwhile, the fat in that meal (the oil from the fries and the fat from the beef and cheese) is shipped off directly to your fat cells for temporary storage. Your body intends to use that fat for fuel as soon as it has taken care of all the glucose. Fat is an awesome source of fuel, and your body will be only too happy to burn it once the glucose fuel tank says "empty" and your blood sugar gets down to more healthy, pre-meal levels. The intent is there, but will your body get around to accomplishing it? Sadly, no.

The Plot Thickens—So Does the Waistline

In this meal, the fat that was supposed to be stored temporarily and used up as fuel later, gets no such chance to do so. It ends up sitting there as forgotten old storage. Your body had such an abundance of glucose for fuel, it didn't have any reason to signal the fat to be released from its temporary storehouse to be used as a back-up fuel source. To make things worse, not only was the fat not used as fuel, it was pushed, more permanently, into storage because insulin tipped another big load of glucose down on top of it.

It's a sad ending to this story, don't you think? Despite its determination to play hero and fuel the body, the original fat from the meal never had a chance to do so from the beginning. It was smooshed in with high-carbs with every bite. The final nail on the coffin is that (if you are not *Trim Healthy Mama-ing*) your next meal would likely contain another big load of glucose, making it even less likely for that fat to get a chance to burn. Glucose will again take priority after that next carb laden meal.

Carb rich meals elevate insulin for up to four hours. If you have burger and fries for lunch, insulin will not finish the enormous task of getting your blood sugar down to safe levels until late afternoon. You're hungry again then, but you feel guilty for the take-out so you eat a pre-sweetened Activia yogurt for an afternoon snack. Up goes your blood sugar. Up goes insulin. Not a chance for the fat to be released and used up. It stays put.

That fat might as well make itself really comfortable in its new home with the rest of the unused fat cells in your body, steadily being added to every day. The moral to this story? Dietary fat is meant to only be a short term tenant in the body, but meals like that turn it into a permanent resident.

Our **S** and **E** meals help you avoid this head-on collision between carbs and fats. We'll get into the nitty gritty of how these two meals work soon. Basically, they allow you to eat fats, carbs, and protein without fattening your body in the process. They allow for glucose burning, but they also set the right conditions for fat burning. Both get to be fuel stars in the body.

It is not necessary to go to extremes and completely separate these macronutrients. We don't call our approach to eating "food combining." You can call it that if you want to get particularly technical, but we dislike that phrase. It conjures up images of a bunch of rules on a blackboard such as, "Don't eat fruit with protein, don't eat starch with protein, don't eat veggies with fruit." Forget all that. We can't be bothered with food theories of that nature. All those rules are too restricting and confusing for our busy lives. Surely God made our bodies able to handle more than one or two food groups at a time!

Our **S** and **E** plan is learning better ratios so each fuel source, either carbs or fat, can really shine. And we have a sneaking feeling you may find that focusing on one particular fuel for each meal allows greater enjoyment of that meal. A solo fuel shows off more when it doesn't have to fight against another contender for prominence. You'll come to value each one for all it's worth.

Once you understand this fuel science, your dietary life will never be quite the same. You won't have to be in the dark about what any particular meal may do to your body. You'll have the knowledge to naturally create wiser choices. No more eating hazardous meals out of ignorance.

Chapter Six

Truths from the Bible

Before we get into the specifics of how to implement this **S** and **E** plan, let's turn to the Bible and have a look at what it says on this dietary subject. We feel it's important to share with you some of the Scriptures that finally helped us let go of a lot of the false nutritional ideas we had formed over the years.

We don't want to be the next food gurus you should follow. If that is the case, any changes you make will likely be temporary. This plan will only be another fad and you'll eventually give up on us and return to the way you lived and ate before. Hopefully, God's Word will enlighten your mind and heart in ways that are impossible for us to do.

We freely admit we got caught up in some tangents over the years. We were always eager to find the healthiest ways to eat and raise our families and we followed others who said they had found the right or "only" way. Unfortunately, a lot of those ideas were folly. They didn't line up with God's Word.

We guess it shouldn't be surprising that the Bible has a lot to say about food. God is practical in nature. He is natural, but supernatural. It wasn't until we scoured the Scriptures for truth, with humbled hearts from all our mistakes that we were able to let go of the heavy burdens we were carrying. God's Word helped us lay them down. How good that felt!

Including much of the dietary principles we found in the Bible would be a whole other book, so let's just hit the highlights.

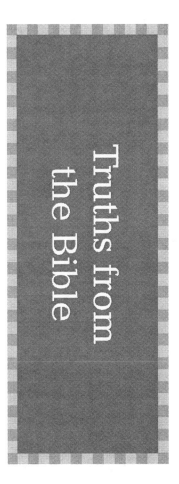

All Food Groups

We have established that we should not exclude any of the macronutrients that God created (carbs, protein, and fat) from our diet, but rather find a healthier balance for each one. It's also important to understand that neither should we eliminate complete food groups. Diets that eliminate food groups are dangerous and always result in negative consequences. We had to learn that lesson the hard way. We never want to be misled into repeating those mistakes again and we want you to avoid them too.

The Bible depicts the abundance of all food groups in Deuteronomy 32, where it describes God taking care of his people. In this beautiful passage of Scripture, He called the children of Israel the *"apple of his eye"* and described himself as an eagle fluttering over His young in the way He looked after them.

As a way to elaborate on how God took such good care of them, He mentions the foods he gave them. We can see that God, depicting himself as a caring, parent eagle was careful to leave nothing out of their diet. The passage, starting at verse 13 mentions how he gave the children of Israel *"the increase of the field"* (grains and greens), *"honey from the rock"* (glucose), *"oil from the flinty rock"*(fats/oils), *"the fat of the ram"* (meat and animal fat), *"butter of kine"* (butter from cattle), *"the milk of the sheep"* (dairy), and *"the pure blood of the grape"* (fruit).

If God did not approve of all these foods, He would not have mentioned them. Yes, there were times of fasting in the Bible when people abstained from meat. Those with vegetarian mindsets will remind us of the story of Daniel who lived mainly on vegetables and being healthier than everyone around him. We know those Scriptures well, and used to quote them to our meat-eating friends. Yet, fasting from certain foods or complete fasting are temporary states. Daniel turned down the king's meat because it was not killed according to God's laws and was also offered to idols. That is why Daniel stated that it *"defiled"* him, not because he thought vegetarianism was a better way of eating.

We are not living in the Garden of Eden anymore. You cannot go back to an Eden body state by simply avoiding animal foods. You cannot purify your body or heart through avoiding animal foods either. God sent Jesus Christ, and the shedding of His blood, to purify us. Nothing else can do it. And, going back to a solely plant-based diet will not enable you to live 800—1000 years as the early Bible heroes were able to do. God slew an animal to clothe Adam and Eve with its skin after they sinned. Since that time, animal foods have been an important part of human diet.

Gurus or God?

Vegetarian and low-fat diets were very popular in the eighties and early nineties. They fell out of the spotlight for a while, but have made resurgence with the raw movement, which is still gaining momentum. All these diets present scientific evidence to back up their ideas. For us, after years of following, and even promoting these sort of diets, it came down to the question of who were we going to believe. Would we trust in the Bible, which clearly says all the food groups are good and have been given to us for our health, or would we trust whichever health guru was the latest flavor of the month?

A very popular book in the last few years that continues pushing the "low-fat, no animal products" dogma is *The China Study*. It has been given much acclaim. It boldly says, "Eating foods that contain any cholesterol above 0 mg is unhealthy."

The China Study clearly infers by that statement that all animal foods cause health decline since that is the food group that contains cholesterol. Hmmm . . . strange that God thinks otherwise! Deuteronomy chapter 14 deals with the clean and unclean foods that God made *"to be received."*

Deuteronomy 14:4 says, *"These are the beasts which ye shall eat; the ox, the sheep and the goat."* It doesn't say, "Well, if you must eat meat, which is second best to plant food and might be unhealthy for you, then I guess you could go ahead and eat the sheep, ox, and goat since they're not quite as bad as other meats."

No, it uses the word *"shall."* It says you ***"shall"*** eat those particular animals. We will continue to offer information and scientific studies to counter refute the "plant foods are superior" viewpoints, but in the end, it comes down to where you place your trust. You could go around and around looking at the scientific evidence from both sides of the argument for days, months, and even years as we did. Take for instance the contrast between the book, *The China Study* that says all foods with cholesterol are harmful, and Dr. Schwarzbein's book, *The Schwarzbein Principle* where it says on page 71: "Eating cholesterol is one of the best things you can do for your body."

Opposite opinions, yet both books have received much clout in the medical and health communities. Who do you believe? Both sides can be rather convincing when they present evidence to back up their theories. For us, it finally comes down to what does or does not line up with God's Word. We don't have PhDs or MDs after our names, yet many of these authors, with a string of letters after their names, have written books full of so-called "facts" that don't line up with biblical common sense. You don't have to be a professor or a doctor to determine if something completely contradicts God's Word. We can either choose to believe an author of a book that causes fear about meat eating (doctor or not), or we can choose to believe God who has told us plainly that certain meats are to be received by the body. God designed every cell in our bodies and formed us in the secret of our mother's womb. That makes Him the foremost authority on the subject.

Whatever sides of the argument authors want to base their theories on is up to them, but if these theories differ from, or belittle the truth of God's Word, then we, as Christians, should quickly dismiss such advice.

Truth or Lie?

In light of Deuteronomy 14:4 and the verses following, which go into more detail about how to identify clean meats, we realized we had to make some grave assumptions about God if we were going to side with the anti-flesh food people and keep to our "meat fearing" mindset. Were we going to believe God to be a liar, that He deceives us into eating foods that are bad for the body, and doesn't know what He's talking about? Does God, the Creator of the universe, not understand that flesh foods are not good for humans? Don't know about you, but once we understood the magnitude of this line of thought, we made the decision to no longer hang our hats in that camp. We let go of it all and decided to trust God.

The New Testament even goes as far as calling abstaining from meat a doctrine of devils. 1 Timothy 4:1-3 says, "*Now the spirit speaketh expressly, that in the latter times some shall depart from the faith, giving heed to seducing spirits, and doctrines of devils: Speaking lies in hypocrisy; having their conscience seared with a hot iron; Forbidding to marry, and commanding to abstain from meats, which God hath* ***created to be received*** *with thanksgiving of them which believe and know the truth.*"

Harsh words? It's a good thing we didn't come up with them or you might think us rather mean. Notice the phrase, "*created to be received*"? Our bodies were designed to receive these animals for food. God created them with the thought of us eating them. Wow! The clean meats are not second best or inferior in any way to the other food groups that God has made to be received.

We want to offer you truth in love, but we don't want to judge and hammer you over the head if you're having trouble shedding some of these ideas about animal foods. We were right there with you for so many years and God gave us a lot of grace, love, and patience. It's important for us to keep in mind what Romans 14:1-3 says, "*Him that is weak in the faith receive ye, but not to doubtful disputations. For one believeth that he may eat all things: another, who is weak, eateth herbs. Let not him that eateth despise him that eateth not; and let not him which eateth not judge him that eateth: for God hath received him.*"

We certainly understand if you are still struggling and wrestling with what you believe concerning meat and dairy eating. However, we remember how great it felt when we were finally released into the freedom of knowing that all the food groups were created by God with His best intentions for our health. It felt fantastic to no longer harbor the fear of meat and to understand that it's not a second-class food.

God Knows what He's Doing

If we still had our vegetarian mindsets and were living back in Old Testament days, we would have been sore out of luck, or should we say, out of a miracle on the night of Passover. God told the Israelites to eat the whole lamb on that night. He didn't have a tofu alternative. Of course, there were spiritual reasons for eating of the lamb, but God is also practical. His people would be going on a long journey in the morning and they needed a lot of sustenance.

Lamb is high in vitamin B12 which supports red blood cell production and allows nerves to function properly. The Israelites were certainly going to enter some nerve-wracking situations—think of crossing the parted sea with the Egyptians chasing them. Lamb is also an excellent source of zinc, a mineral critical to immune function and wound healing. A healthy immune system was imperative to starting out on a long journey with challenging hygiene conditions. Red meat, like lamb, is a great source of carnosine, that potent antioxidant which renews cells and is good for the heart. Yes, we probably have to repeat that since it's news that is not widely spread in most media outlets—carnisone is only found in meat and is very good for the heart.

God was very specific to the Israelites the night before they embarked on their long journey out of Egypt. They had to eat the lamb with bitter herbs, which are dark greens. Lamb is a fatty, red meat. Many current nutritional gurus would be aghast that God told the Israelites to eat such fare! Shouldn't He have told them to load up on root vegetables and fruit? That would have given them lots of enzymes, fiber, and much less fat and cholesterol which could possibly clog up their arteries. No. God knew exactly what He was doing. And, thankfully, the Israelites didn't second guess Him. They didn't make turnip and leek stew instead of lamb, thinking they knew better than God and it would be a healthier option.

What about Jesus' own parable of the prodigal son? The Father in the parable told his servants to prepare the fatted calf ready for a feast when his son returned home. Of course, this parable was not told as a lesson on what to eat, but we need to pay attention to every red letter word in the Bible. We shouldn't gloss over any of Christ's words as trivial. There is joy and celebration in eating meat, and we are not any more righteous or holy, or even more healthy, if we deny ourselves red meat.

We say this only because we are very familiar with the mindset of abstaining from meat. There is a certain component to it that can deceivingly make one feel "cleaner" or more "pure" by not eating flesh foods. We used to think meat soiled the purity of the body because, after all, eating meat is ingesting dead animals, and meat stays in your system longer than plant foods. We didn't like the idea of dead animals festering inside us, making us less pure. However, that was merely a mindset, a misguided "feeling" since the flesh foods that God ordained for us to eat were designed *"to be received"* by our bodies. They do not dirty or defile our temples. It's all in how we choose to look at things.

The Lean and the Fatty

We are told by conventional wisdom to only eat lean meats, if we eat meat at all. There is a healthy place for lean cuts in our diet, but we should not exclude meats with healthy amounts of fat either. We need to eat both types and our **S** and **E** plan includes both. Our Creator has physically endorsed both kinds in both Leviticus and Deuteronomy, where He sanctioned more fatty meats like sheep and cattle along with lean flesh foods such as fish, certain birds, wild deer, and wild goat.

Our previously vegetarian indoctrinated minds were perplexed as to why Jesus himself prepared fish for the disciples when He cooked a meal for them on the shores of Galilee after His resurrection. Surely, some olives or fresh dates from the palm groves bordering the Lake Galilee would be superior to flesh food, even though it was of the lean kind!

Too bad we can't go back in time several years and awake to the truth! But, hind sight is rather useless. We have to guess that the soil of our minds was rocky ground for quite a while and we were not ready to receive these truths. Just think of it, the Savior of the world, Jesus Christ himself, making a meal. And He cooked fish! Shouldn't we take notice?

If Christ prepared fish over a fire and fed it to His disciples, and also fed 5,000 hungry people with it, then any theory we clung to that touted "you can get all the protein you need from plant sources," and "cooked food is unhealthier than raw food," cannot stand up to that. Once the soil of our minds became more fertile, we realized such notions were foolish, and to be tossed out of the window in light of the simple truth that Christ thought fish was good food to serve his hungry friends. Our **S** and **E** plan makes sure to include fish, especially superfood fish like salmon, as a frequent food.

Take the Blame off Dairy

Dairy has been given such a bad rap in the last quarter century. We urge you to reconsider it in its most healthful forms unless you have a real allergy to lactose. Kefir, especially from goats' milk, is sometimes tolerable to those with lactose allergies since the culturing process eats up the milk sugar. If God thought dairy products were less than optimum, why did He, in Proverbs 27, advocate goats' milk for the "*maintenance of thy maidens*"?

The word "maintenance" (Proverbs 27:27) in the *Strong's* Hebrew Concordance has the words, "fresh, life, living thing, alive" to describe its meaning. The word refers to the upkeep of our living bodies and keeping us fresh! This lines up with the science that shows animal protein maintains our bodies and repairs damage at the cellular level.

It's good to read Proverbs 27:26 and 27 together to get a clearer picture of how God talks about these animal foods.

"The lambs are for thy clothing, and the goats are the price of the field. And thou shalt have goats' milk enough for thy food, for the food of thy household and for the maintenance of thy maidens."

God clearly thinks dairy products are a good food for us.

Do you remember the story in the Bible when Abraham was visited by the Lord and two angelic beings to tell him the miraculous news that he was going to have a son? Abraham made a meal for his angelic visitors. The contents of the meal are interesting. Genesis 18:8 says, *"So*

Abraham took butter and milk and the calf which he had prepared and set it before them; and he stood under the tree while they ate."

Butter! Can you believe it? And milk! Two animal foods! And there's that dreaded red meat again! Make that three animal foods in one meal. It doesn't specify what kind of animal milk he used—it could have been cow, sheep, or goat for all we know.

Certainly, if the Lord did not think butter a wholesome food, He would not have eaten it. You maybe reeling that we esteem butter. Yes, we do. Abraham could have offered them olive oil. There was plenty of that around. Yet, a supposedly unhealthy, artery clogging saturated fat was the choice for His prestigious visitors. It's hard to argue with Scripture. Strong's concordance actually depicts the Hebrew word for "the angel of the Lord" used in that verse as "Jehovah." Yes, the Creator of our bodies, God Himself, sat down and ate butter! He also ate meat and dairy (most likely cultured).

A quick side step into the debate whether milk should be separated or left whole. Some people do not believe milk should ever be altered from its original full-fat state. The Bible gives us an easy one word answer for that subject too.

Butter.

The product of butter can only be obtained by separating the cream from the top of the milk. It would have been ridiculous to then throw away the skim milk. Historical research shows evidence that people in biblical eras curdled milk in skin bags. The history of kefir can be traced to inhabitants from the Caucasus Mountains, many of whom were scattered Hebrew tribes. The result of this curdled milk would have been very similar to our yogurt or kefir of modern day. This was a way of lengthening the life of milk since there was no refrigeration and it naturally reduced the sugar content of the milk.

Are any of us more knowledgeable than God? Are the latest health magazines, news headlines, books, or internet nutrition blogs better informed than God? That's the question that revolutionized the way we began to look at food. We cannot pretend to know better than God as to what is good for our bodies. His ways are infinitely higher than ours. The "beware of butter" mentality, with which many have been brainwashed, is the wisdom of man. It doesn't wash with God's Word.

Butter is Better

Feeling any freedom yet? We know that you hear that butter promotes weight gain and builds up cholesterol. Well, how about some science to back up our butter lovin'?

Butter consists of butterfat, trace amounts of milk proteins, and water. Butterfat is butyric acid, a short chain fatty acid which supports colon health. You may be surprised to learn this is basically the same substance that mothers produce to nourish their babies.

Butter is rich in antioxidants, and you thought they were only in plant foods! It boasts beta carotene, selenium, and other antioxidants which shield the body from free radical damage. It is an excellent source of conjugated linoleic acids or CLA's. These fight cancer, build muscle, and boost immunity.

Butter is also rich in iodine, which is essential to thyroid health and protective of breast and ovarian cancers. Butter is also rich with lecithin. This phospholipid protects cells from oxidation and may contribute to cholesterol metabolism. Many people actually take lecithin as a supplement to help lower their cholesterol. Lecithin is also a natural source of choline which promotes better brain function.

Butter contains the readily absorbable form of vitamin A which is required for endocrine health and for maintaining eye sight. It is also an excellent source of vitamin D. There is a widespread deficiency of this vitamin in Western People groups. Vitamin D helps your body absorb calcium to maintain strong bones and plays a big role in lowering the risk of heart disease, osteoporosis, and many forms of cancer.

Butter is also loaded with Vitamin E and Vitamin K. Vitamin E is anti-inflammatory, promotes skin health, speeds wound healing, enhances immunity, and may protect against diabetes, heart disease and Alzheimer's. Vitamin K ensures proper blood clotting and bone health.

There's more yet. Butter also enables us to better absorb vitamins from other foods. Consuming a pat of butter (36 calories worth), doubles the body's ability to absorb vitamins A, E, D, and K from cooked vegetables. So, butter and vegetables are the perfect natural combination.

Let's Party!

Maybe you felt a little stupid trying our "Butter is my friend" therapy. Well, how about you really let loose and say a few times, "Ooooh! I love me some buttah!"

Bet you can't say that and not smile or chuckle just a little bit. Let your hair down, mama! We offer you freedom and it comes right from God's Word. This feels good and we should celebrate a little because butter has been the evil villain for so long. No more!

Maybe we don't get to spend enough time in polite society out here in the Tennessee woods, but we just had the silliest time saying "buttah!" to each other while writing these last couple of paragraphs. Our children are looking at us like we are nuts! They should be used to it.

Caution!

But wait. We may have whipped you up into a butter-loving frenzy and you are just about to go slap a big pat on a piece of bread. Hold it. Remember, certain foods may be healthy, but you need to educate yourself on how to pair them up. We don't want a fat and carb head-on collision! Read on into the next few chapters and we'll show you how to use butter in your diet to aid weight loss, rather than causing the opposite effect.

Fat can be your friend or foe depending on how you use it.

The Other Extreme

We exercise equal caution toward paleolithic type diets as we do toward vegetarian diets. Paleolithic diets, more commonly known as "Paleo or Cave Man," and other similar diets like the primal diet, swing to the other extreme and suggest that primitive Stone Age man, affectionately known as "Grok" by followers of these diets, is the prototype for how we should eat.

Paleo diets teach that grains are a modern food and our bodies are not equipped to process them. Neither should we eat legumes, like beans or lentils, they say. Dairy products are a cultured food, often not in their original state so they are out, too. Goodbye, healthy Greek yogurt! Apparently, Stone Age man ate mostly fatty meats (i.e. a lot of pork fat), eggs, nuts, and fruit, and that's about all . . . well, maybe a few root vegetables now and then and we should do the same. You'd be surprised at how popular this diet is right now. There are millions following it and it is gaining momentum. Walk into your nearest Barnes and Noble and we betcha some paleo diet books are displayed in high traffic areas. "Grok" is rising from his paleo grave and teaching us modern folk how to eat like a cave man.

Some principles of the paleolithic diet do have some merit. Our culture overdoes grain and there are some people who have legitimate allergies to gluten and need to avoid many grains. But Jesus likens himself to the *"Bread of Life."* He fed over 5,000 hungry people with loaves and fishes. He broke bread with His disciples. Was He intentionally harming them? No. Did He not know better? Better than us, for sure. God included grains as *"the increase of the fields"* (Deuteronomy 32:13) as part of His food groups. Paleo diets teach that grains are toxic to our bodies. God obviously thinks differently. Who's right? That's a no brainer.

Now, if you have gluten intolerance, we have many bread recipes included in this book that don't use grains. They will be perfect for you. However, we do advise you to keep some wonderful gluten-free grains in your diet. Quinoa is one of the foundational foods we advise you to include in your diet, and it's naturally gluten-free.

The gluten-free industry is booming. Have you noticed the recent large additions of gluten-free products in your grocery store lately? More and more people are being diagnosed as gluten intolerant. Maybe it's because modern hybridized grains have become too abundant in the general western diet and people's bodies are starting to pay the price.

If you know that you truly cannot tolerate gluten, beware of filling up on many of these new gluten-free products that use rice and other grains in place of wheat. They are just as detrimental to stable blood sugar levels as regular products that contain gluten. They can just as easily make you fat!

Like we do, paleo diet advisors encourage people to use non-grain flours like coconut, flax, and almond flours instead of store-bought mass marketed grain replacements. However, our common beliefs stop there.

We want to emphasize a reliance on God's Word over the words of men. Real gluten intolerance is one thing, but looking down on grains because a fictitious Stone Age man, supposedly, did not eat them seems like a slap in God's face. Accepting this paleo theology is akin to accepting Darwinism and evolution. It does not make practical sense. Most Christians believe God created man from the dust. Most of us dismiss the theory that man evolved from an ape and became a paleo man at some point on that evolutionary time line. Therefore, shouldn't just the name of paleo diet be a red flag for believers?

When Abraham prepared a meal for his angelic visitors, we see that along with animal foods, he also served a *"morsel of bread"* to the Lord himself (Genesis 18:5). We should not fear grains, only the over doing of them. Nor should we despise dairy. It is a healthy source of protein for most people and is actually a healing superfood when cultured from a raw state into kefir or yogurt. It was definitely included in biblical fare. Beans and lentils, those other "no, no's" of paleo theology are fantastic foods and are mentioned frequently as biblical foods. God knows better than "Grok."

The Clean Meat Debate

We also differ from paleo diet followers who are advised to eat a lot of pork bacon. Paleo dieters are often encouraged to eat the fattiest of meats as the largest part of their diet and bacon fits that bill perfectly.

We don't want to make a big issue about pork in this book, but we should make mention that it is listed as one of the unclean meats in the Bible (read Leviticus chapter 11). Neither of us eat the meats God stated to be unclean as we think our Creator knows what He is talking about with regard to the health of our bodies. He must have good reasons for telling us to avoid them. When you think about the fact that pigs don't have sweat glands and most of the unclean meats are scavengers, this makes scientific sense. However, we don't ask you to sway to our beliefs in this matter. Some people believe The New Testament has more freeing guidelines toward unclean meats. Choosing to stick to clean or unclean meats is a decision for you and your husband, not for us to make on your behalf. But, it's good to think about these things.

If you are a shrimp lover or pork bacon fanatic, go with your own conviction. We don't want to vilify these foods for you if you have freedom of conviction in eating them. Our families eat turkey, chicken, or beef alternatives to pork in all forms, whether sausage, bacon, or even pepperoni, so there are choices for all of us in our various persuasions. We didn't eat shrimp growing up and never developed a taste for it, but there is no judgment from us if you don't want to give it up. You can still eat them and stay on our plan, even if we don't.

However, we firmly advise that you eat only the flying insects described in Leviticus 1:21-22 rather than the crawling ones without wings. God said only the flying ones are clean to eat and they are certainly more delicious—just kidding! Gotcha! Well, the Bible does deem these flying insects as part of the foods that are *"to be received."* Apparently, they are a good clean protein source.

Don't fret. We don't have any recipes with grasshoppers as the star ingredient. We think it's a good thing Leviticus 11: 22 says you *"may"* eat of the locust, rather than you *"shall"* as it does with the cloven hoofed animals like cattle and sheep and the finned and scaled fish of the sea. Just to be sure, we had to check the Hebrew word for each. Yes, they are different—sigh of relief. It's nice to have a choice to not have to partake of "Crispy Locusts on Toast," don't you agree?

No Snacks?

Many paleo followers try to adhere to the commonly promoted paleo principle to eat only two meals a day. Snacks are frowned upon because "Grok" would not have had access to lots of snacky foods. "Grok" would rise with the sun and sleep soon after it set, so he would have likely eaten only two meals a day some gurus say. We disagree with this limited snacking principle for many reasons, but if you are pregnant or nursing, it's even more important to not get pulled into this type of deception. Your baby needs frequent sustenance for which you are responsible. Ever notice that after feeding your baby you become ravenously hungry, even though it may not be long after a meal? That's a natural God-designed signal your body makes to keep up a full milk supply.

Even if you are not pregnant or nursing, you can end up with unstable blood sugar levels if snacks are continually restricted. A protein-filled snack is the perfect way to ward off the blahs, jitters, and moodiness that comes with going without food for too long. We believe snacks enable the metabolism to function better.

Raw Diets

There are two versions of raw diets—the vegan raw foodists who only consume plant foods and the omnivore raw foodists, more commonly known as primal raw folk.

Primal raw followers include animal foods, but make sure to eat them raw. For example, they pickle their fish in acidic lemon juice brine for several days to avoid the cooking process. We're not saying this is unhealthy. It may even be a yummy superfood, but Jesus cooked fish for his friends, and He partook of it Himself.

God told the Israelites to *"roast"* their meat on the night of Passover (Exodus 12:8-9).

In Exodus 16:23 God told the Israelites how to cook the manna He provided for them in the wilderness, *"And he said unto them, This is that which the Lord hath said, Tomorrow is the rest of the holy Sabbath unto the Lord:* ***bake*** *that which ye will bake today, and* ***seethe*** *that which ye shall seethe and that which remained over lay up for you to be kept until the morning."*

In Strong's Hebrew concordance, the word, "seethe" means "boil, or the act of cooking." Can we trust that God wasn't encouraging the Hebrews to completely spoil or devitalize their foods by cooking them? Sure we can.

Look what Numbers 11:8 says concerning the manna God sent the children of Israel to eat. *"And the people went about and gathered it and ground it in mill, or beat it in a mortar and* ***baked*** *it in pans and* ***made cakes*** *of it and the taste of it was as the taste of fresh oil."*

The Old Testament priests were actually commanded to cook and eat certain parts of the sacrificial animals. In certain instances, they were told to boil the meat of these offerings; other times they were instructed to roast the meat. Do you think God would allow the priests to experience degenerating health due to this cooking process?

The priests were to undergo many purification processes before they entered the temple, but abstaining from cooked food or animal flesh was not one of them. It's interesting to note that the priests were not to eat the fat of these animals that were set aside for sacrifice. The fat of sacrificial animals was always for God only and to be burnt upon the altar.

Genesis 8: 21 tells us that God smelled Noah's animal sacrifice offerings that were burnt on the altar as a "sweet savor." God was pleased with the smell of cooking meat. You can't really argue with that. Cooking is not only plainly stated in the Bible, but endorsed. Let's shed these burdens put upon us by man's rules. They are not God's rules and His opinion is the only one that counts in the end.

Recently, we were talking to a friend about many of these modern food theories. He'd seen a book on the internet by Dr. St. Louis A. Estes who is considered to be the "Father of the Raw Movement." The book, *Raw Food and Health* published back in 1927 is so highly valued it was selling for over $150. Interestingly, on this doctor's cause of death certificate was written "severe malnutrition" and "generalized arteriosclerosis." Yet, his ideas on diet are still praised.

We discussed the contrast of such food theories against the common sense of the Bible. How can the simple diet advice of the Bible be so easy for many of us to miss, or dare we say, dismiss? We can't judge. We missed it ourselves and chased down many of the new fan-dangled "best way to eat" theories for years in search of some sort of Holy Grail diet. After sharing some Scriptures about food with this friend, he commented, "It's so simple. It's so simple that it's profound."

Sometimes rediscovering the simplest things can have the most profound impact on our lives.

Too Much of a Good Thing

Now that we know more about what the Bible says about food, this whole diet thing should be a cinch, right? Let's eat a biblical style diet. Could it be that easy? Well, times are different. It is our modern lifestyle that has warped the simplicity of the way God designed us to eat.

In Bible times, they didn't have access to the amount of grains available to us today. Mass produced bread factories from harvests all around the world were not an option. Housewives could not go to Walmart to load up on packaged breads and cereals each time they ran out. Nor did they have the latest wheat grinders and bread machines. What grain they were able to obtain was usually sprouted, unleavened, or made with wild yeasts of the air (sourdough). These healthier grain sources could not be consumed in the same abundance as we do in our modern society and were much gentler on glucose levels. It is much easier to eat more of our puffed up, fluffy breads but they can cause dramatic blood sugar spikes.

Dr. William Davis, author of the book, *The Wheat Belly* writes regarding modern day wheat, "It is not the same grain our forebears ground into their daily bread. Wheat has changed dramatically in the last 50 years under the influence of agricultural scientists. Wheat strains have been hybridized, crossbred, and introgressed to make wheat plant resistant to environmental conditions, such as drought, or pathogens, such as fungi. But most of all, genetic changes have been induced to increase yield per acre."

Our modern culture is overwhelmed by the sheer abundance of these hybridized wheat products. Advice to eat more whole grains was issued by the *National Heart, Lung, and Blood Institute* in 1985. Coincidentally or not, we think not, that same year also marks the explosion of obesity and diabetes in the USA.

We're not living in Bible times where the macro nutrients in meals were naturally in healthier ratios, i.e. meals were much less sugar and starch laden. You can bet obesity back in Bible times was a rarity. This is obvious if we look again at the story about Abraham and the meal he prepared for his angelic visitors. In Genesis 18:5 Abraham says to his visitors, *"I will bring you a morsel of bread that you may refresh your hearts."*

It's interesting that the word "morsel" was used. According to the Strong's Hebrew Concordance, it simply means "a bite to eat."

Abraham told Sarah in Genesis 18:6, *"Make ready quickly three measures of fine meal, knead it and make cakes."*

There were three visitors, therefore three cakes. We can easily deduce that the angelic visitors were given one flat-bread each in a morsel-size helping. Abraham certainly did not carbo load his visitors, but gave them enough grain to *"refresh their hearts."* We love that phrase. The meal consisted of protein in the form of meat and milk (most likely the cultured milk of that time), fat in the form of butter, and a small amount of whole grain carbs. Sounds like a set-up for perfect blood sugar levels with a little heart refreshing to boot! It also sounds a lot like one of the meals on our plan that we call an **S Helper**—you'll find out about that later.

Get Proactive

Our modern age makes it necessary for us to be more proactive in our approach to food. This is the reason we have simplified our nutritional approach into a doable plan. In biblical times, they were not faced with the vast array of food choices we are constantly bombarded with today. Aside from not having to deal with the overabundance of refined grain items, fruit was not on the menu for every meal either. It was seasonal. You could not have imported oranges from Florida in the middle of winter. Fruit in our modern era has been hybridized to the point where it is much sweeter than it was originally. Fruit like wild blue berries and black berries are far from candy sweet. They have a different taste from their mass grown counterparts.

Meat was grass fed, not laden with hormones and antibiotics. Dairy was almost always cultured because there was no refrigeration, but this created more living enzymes and it broke down the sugar content.

Take Dominion

We need all the food groups, but as God told Adam to take "dominion" in the garden, we also need to take dominion over the foods we intake. We shouldn't stuff anything into our mouths at any time just because we have such an abundance of food. That leads to chaos in the body.

You may wonder why we are so earnest—that's being easy on ourselves. Let's be honest and use the word "insistent," maybe even "obsessive" about making sure we eat according to a plan that ensures both a trim and healthy body, and then bother to take close to five years to write it all into a book. You might argue that it is best to eat three sensible meals a day and not be too perturbed if that causes a little meat on the bones. Our response? We do not advocate that anyone should try to be skinny or too lean, but what are currently considered to be normal meals in our society are a far cry from the whole food diet of biblical times.

Normal is No Longer Natural

We cannot take a "normal" approach to food, because so-called "sensible meals" these days usually result in too much weight gain for most body types. The reason, of course, is that they are shockingly full of hidden carbs and sugars. Excess weight is never healthy, with the exception of fat roly poly babies who will naturally lose all their beautiful baby chub as they get to the toddler stage and start running around.

A "normal" breakfast in our culture (not donuts, pastries, or drive through sausage biscuits), might be a bowl of whole grain cereal featuring wheat with low-fat milk, a glass of orange juice, and maybe a boiled egg on the side.

A "normal" lunch (not burgers, fries, or pizza) might be a turkey sandwich on wheat bread, a bag of pretzels, and possibly a soda to wash it down. Only one, that's not excessive, is it?

The "normal" evening meal (not Kentucky Fried Chicken followed by an ice cream sundae) might be lasagna and a salad, a bread roll or piece of white, garlic bread on the side.

The carbs in these meals are well over the top of Bible time foods. Orange juice, cereal flakes, soda, pretzels, wheat bread (not whole rye or sour dough), white noodles, bread rolls—all these components of our common meals are in a whole new dangerous category compared to the simple foods of Bible times. Most of them are based on modern, genetically altered wheat which produces big, unnatural bellies. The "normal" diet we described is not even counting a packaged snack or two, and the sugar laden dessert after supper which most people have! We ourselves can't do normal. We are tall women with naturally healthy metabolisms, but these types of "normal" meals even make us fat!

The foods spoken about in the Bible, like a hunk of dark rye sourdough bread, raw goat's or sheep's cheese, kefir, or a bit of roasted meat or fish with herbs, were far gentler on blood sugar levels than our regular foods are. Sometimes, we read in the Scriptures about folk eating honey or a few dates, but those pure forms of glucose were much needed due to their more physically demanding lives. We ride in cars, they walked. We use a washing machine and turn on a tap for water. They beat clothes in a stream and had to haul water from a well. You get the picture? And cells that were not fed a lifetime of a too high glucose diet would have been much more insulin receptive, so a bit of honey now and then would have been quite acceptable and well needed.

Just Cut Back?

Others might argue why we don't encourage people to eat less of their regular food. Use temperance and cut back on portion sizes. There is a common diet tip thrown around that suggests people always leave a third of their plate uneaten—that'll work to keep you slim. Our response? Good luck with that! It is the nature of our modern, high sugar foods to make us want to eat more of them. You're going to have to have self-control the size of a big buff body builder if you're able to leave one third of your plate untouched every time you eat, long term. The low serotonin state that stems from excess insulin creates a cycle where a person craves that "fix" of sugar again. They feel lousy and want to feel better, so the body says, "Eat more carbs, I need the fix." It's hard to resist overeating when you're caught up in this vicious cycle.

It's okay to get filled up! We think it's unnatural to feel gnawing hunger at the end of a meal. We're not advising that we should stuff ourselves full at every meal time, but most often, that is the result of the type of foods consumed and the unnatural compulsions they cause in the body. Years of doing this leads to food addictions. Another name for those addictions is "carb addictions." Have you ever heard of anybody with an out-of-control protein addiction before? It's time to rediscover the foods that we can eat and then feel naturally satisfied without causing destruction to our bodies. Let's go after it!

Part II

Practice the Knowledge

It's time to eat the S and E way.

Here's how it works!

Chapter Seven

Go for the Plan

We are ready to get down to the nitty gritty of how our **Satisfying** and **Energizing** meals work as a lifelong way of eating. You have to learn to eat fats in a smart way, and you also have to eat some carbs in a smart way as both are necessary for optimum health. Pull either of these macronutrients out and you'll likely end up in an imbalanced state of health, craving so-called "forbidden" foods that God actually designed for you to eat. Fighting off cravings only lasts for so long. We want you to learn to indulge your cravings in wise yet yummy ways. Protein is the middle man in our plan; it needs to be solidly entrenched at the core of all meals.

We've talked about the dilemma that occurs when high fats and carbs are thrust together. That is why this plan is successful for a lifetime approach. You don't have to give up certain food groups, you just have to learn to pair them with the right foods.

Get Smart

While all the food groups we encourage you to eat are healthy, and many of them are superfood status, this does not mean they are also slimming (unless you are a rare, super high metabolism, ectomorphic body type), staying slim requires some street smarts. It doesn't work to only eat more healthy food and less junk food. Even healthy food can make you fat. Sounds strange, but it's too true. Remember Farm Fresh Tess, our friend who eats whole foods from the farm and garden? She was robust and had ample energy but her diet wasn't kind to her waistline. It's important to first understand, and then implement, a little of the science behind how food is metabolized by the body and the main hormonal players involved, and then make practical applications with that knowledge. This way we can make all these healthy foods slimming, as well as nourishing.

First Rule to Remember

Here's the bottom line. Both of us are united on this. There is only one rule to remember by heart. You might find us bantering back and forth later in this book on minor details, but here is one that is concrete.

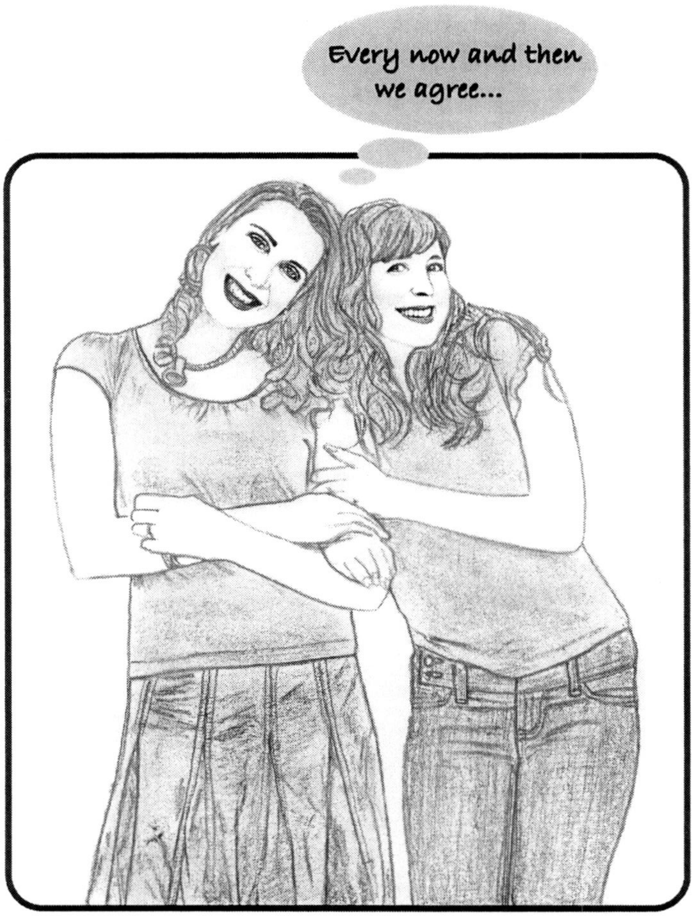
Every now and then
we agree...

otta get this. Don't bother with the rest of this book if you don't learn this rule. We'll wait ... e you get your fluorescent highlighter.

NEVER INCLUDE LARGE AMOUNTS OF BOTH FATS AND CARBS IN THE SAME MEAL UNLESS YOU ARE TRYING TO GAIN OR MAINTAIN WEIGHT. IN OTHER WORDS, DON'T TANDEM FUEL!

If you don't follow this rule, you will have no control over your body fat. If someone wants to borrow this book as a weight loss tool and you're not eager to lend it out, show them this page because it is what you need to know in a nutshell.

To make this rule work effortlessly with little thinking on your part, we have split this eating plan into two different types of meals. These two meal types ensure that glucose and fats, the two primary sources of fuel for your body, both get their time in the spotlight without having to play tandem to each other. Tandem fuel burning inhibits weight loss.

One meal type is called **S** (for **Satisfying**). The other is **E** (for **Energizing**). We've briefly mentioned a little about both so far. You will primarily focus on these two styles of delicious meals if you have weight to lose, while incorporating a couple of close relatives to **S** and **E** meals for variety and bolstered effect. This is how you'll get proactive and learn to eat skillfully in a culture that is bombarded with ridiculous food choices. This is how you'll easily put into practice those "street smarts" so you can successfully navigate a long term healthy path for yourself in this modern world.

If you are happy with your current weight, we'll show you a method of eating that maintains weight healthfully by combining these two **S** and **E** meal types. It enables tandem fuel burning so no weight loss occurs. You'll learn why most children need to burn tandem fuels at every meal and how this will help them grow strong and healthy without weight problems.

Chapter Eight

The Satisfying Meal
(S for Short)

Introducing the **S** meal! It is a higher fat meal so it chooses to use fat, rather than glucose as your primary fuel source. It is always lower in carbs. **S** meals basically consist of protein (usually animal protein), fats such as butter, oils, and cheeses, non-starchy vegetables, berries, nuts, and seeds. The good thing about this meal style is that it is very satisfying. Hence, the name. It deters cravings. It makes you slim! You're gonna love it!

We will give you so many examples of what an **S** meal could look like as you keep reading, but here is a quick visual picture of what an **S** evening meal might be:

Salad with creamy dressing and grated cheese
Baked chicken with crispy skin
Steamed or roasted veggies tossed with butter and seasonings

Sound good? Don't worry, you'll also get to eat plenty of desserts with **S** meals. There'll be no self-denial needed when it comes to chocolatey goodness. There are so many creamy and sweet **S** desserts to delight you included in this book. You won't feel sad or deprived as you bid sugar farewell.

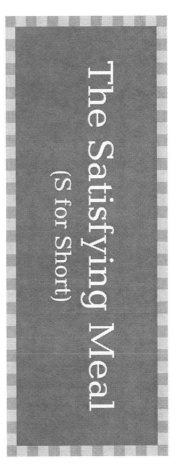

Since **S** meals are liberal with fats, they must have lower carbs if they are to assist in weight loss. It's important to remember to keep grains and most fruits (with the exception of most berries) away from **S** meals. That is the trick to make you trim. You can bring those back in small doses as accompaniments to your **S** meals later in your journey to goal weight.

All the wonderful, healthy fats in **S** meals cannot turn into pounds without high sugar in the body which is stimulated by such foods as potatoes, grains, and fruits. The fats in this meal will nourish you, feed your endocrine system, and leave you feeling greatly satisfied.

Think of a seesaw. **S** meal ratios look like this on a seesaw. Look at the difference in heights between carbs and fat. Notice that when fat is higher in a meal, carbs are lower. That's the visual you need to remember if weight loss is to occur. Protein always sits solidly at the core of the seesaw.

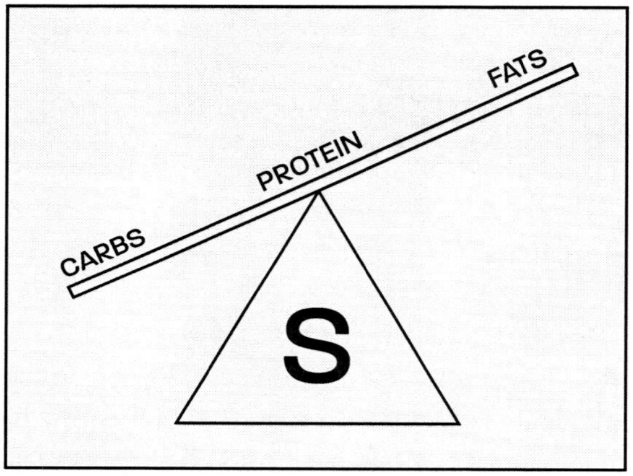

Non-Starchies! Where Have You Been All My Life?

They've likely been playing wall flower, overshadowed by sides like potatoes and mac n cheese. That's about to change. **S** meals should always be furnished with non-starchy vegetables. "What's a non-starchy vegetable," you ask? It's basically any vegetable that is not a root vegetable like a potato or a carrot, or a starch like corn. That still leaves you with literally hundreds of choices.

Non-starchy vegetables are very gentle on your blood sugar. They don't get that sugar delivery truck named "insulin" revving and rearing to go since they don't put much glucose into your blood stream. Anything that grows from the ground contains carbohydrates. However, although these veggies have a few carbs, their fiber levels are often almost as high as their total carbohydrate levels. This cancels out the impact their total carb levels have on your blood sugar.

Remember, we don't want you to get obsessed with counting the carb levels in all your food, including non-starchy vegetables. You should eat them freely. But, if you're interested, most non-starchy vegetables have between two to six net carbs per serving. They are all perfect for **S** meals.

Non-starchy veggies are low enough in carbs that they will not cause much of a blood sugar rise. This is important since we don't want blood sugar to be the chief fuel in an **S** meal. It is fat's turn to "burn, baby burn"! If you allow your blood sugar to trigger high enough from starches and sugars in a meal, there's no stopping it. The fat in that meal will stick to your belly and hips rather than fuel your body. Hence, these non-starchy veggies are the ticket to healthfully round out your **S** meals without causing fat storage. Instead, your own body fat will start to melt.

Lettuce and other leafy greens have less than one gram of net carbs per serving. That's ridiculously low. By making the most of them you can get more life-giving raw food in your diet. They are also super low in calories, so filling up on them makes perfect sense. Any form of tasty animal protein like chicken, beef, or salmon over a nice big plate of lettuce with succulent dressing, always makes a quick, complete, and slimming meal. You don't have to worry about portion sizes of lettuce when it makes up the bulk of your plate. Have as much as you want. The ample fat and oil from an olive oil or cream-based dressing will help satisfy you, along with savory meat topping the lettuce, and you can always add a sprinkle of cheese. Yes, all of those foods put together are weight reducing.

In a perfect world, it would be better if you made your own homemade dressings, but store-bought can work. Don't worry about how much fat the dressing contains for **S** dressings, but make sure your store-bought choice has no more than two grams of carbs per serving, one gram is a better choice. Check labels to make sure you're not buying dressings with hidden sugars—the lower the carb count, the less chance of sugars and other needless fillers. Ken's Ranch dressing has only one carb and although it is far from a superfood dressing, it works on plan. We do suggest one tip with store-bought dressings. Pour about one fourth of the dressing out (possibly into another container to avoid waste), add water to make up for the loss, and shake well. Store-bought creamy dressings tend to be overly thick anyway and we doubt you will dislike the slightly thinner consistency. Why overdo calories when they're not superfood ones your body needs?

The good thing about vegetables in an **S** meal is they don't have to be in the form of bunny food. Cooked vegetables like squash, broccoli, cauliflower, and eggplant are great **S** options even though they're a little higher in carbs than leafy greens. We expect you'll find yourself eating more vegetables than ever before because thanks to **S** meals, cooked vegetables can be yummified.

There is nothing worse than being told to eat more broccoli and trying to eat it dry and unsavory. Sort of goes against the human taste buds, we think. However, broccoli is delicious when it is made into a creamy casserole, or tossed in butter and sea salt. It is easy to slip in more servings of vegetables when they are drizzled with luscious, smooth sauces, or tossed with the delicate decadence of healthy fats. Our *Vegetable Sides*, Chapter 22 contains so many tasty veggie ideas for you. Remember, it's okay to say, "I love butter." Actually, for optimum mineral absorption, vegetables are best paired with fats like butter or coconut oil.

Yes, more saturated fat will be consumed in an **S** meal, from both animal sources like meat and butter and also from oils like coconut oil. However, as we learned through the Scripture examples, this is not the bad thing we have all been taught from "man knows best."

Pearl chats: Do you have trouble getting your children to like vegetables? I believe the reason so many children say they hate vegetables is because they are often prepared as unappetizing as possible. I'll admit, I actually dislike broccoli by itself. But, when I steam it until tender and toss it in butter, it becomes entirely different and I love to consume lots of it.

All my children love broccoli and cauliflower and ask for second helpings. This is only because I make it in an appealing way, not because there is any great love for the taste of the vegetable itself. I have always termed broccoli "little trees" and cauliflower "little trees covered in snow" when talking about vegetables in front of my children. They love imagining them in this way. Even the older ones still get a kick out of it.

There is an easy and quick way to make broccoli so yummy that even a fussy four year old will love it. Place the contents of frozen bags of broccoli and cauliflower florets in a steamer, or regular pot with a fold out steamer at the bottom. Steam the vegetables until tender. They don't have to be crisp like you hear some people say. Who wants to eat a half-raw piece of cauliflower? Just don't let them get so soft that they are mushy, or the broccoli turns from a deep green to an awful gray/green color. You could use fresh broccoli to steam if you'd prefer, but I don't like to chop and wash if I don't have to, so the frozen bags work best for lazy me. Add lots of butter, sea salt and pepper, and then sprinkle with a couple big handfuls of grated or shredded cheddar cheese. Stir all this into the florets and let the toppings melt. This simple combination should please the whole family.

Welcome Back Saturated Fat

Are you still persuaded that saturated fats can lead to an early grave? It's hard to shake deeply inground notions, isn't it? They have been given such a bad rap by the media and diet "dictocrats."

A lot of the anti-saturated fat notions some of us have a hard time shaking off were propagated by the hired lawyers of the wealthy soybean industry. A couple of decades ago, there was a forceful campaign to smear saturated fats as bad for our health. It worked. Saturated fats in the form of healthy tropical oils, like coconut and palm, were used widely in packaged baked goods until the soybean oil industry took over. Soybean oil, being unsaturated, did not have as high a shelf life. It became rancid easily and did not achieve the desired texture for foods. Therefore, scientists saturated the fatty acids (hydrogen atoms) and hydrogenated oil was born. Since then, American health has gone downhill and weight has gone up.

Only Cook with Saturated Oils

We stress the importance of using only saturated oils when cooking. On this plan you will cook only with saturated oils as these are the only ones that don't turn to trans fats when heated. Beware of modern marketing schemes which tout "No Trans Fats." The vegetable oils used prior to frying or baking chips were not trans, but once cooked, those so-called healthier variety of corn chips are a bag full of trans.

The only oils you should use for cooking are coconut oil, red palm oil, or butter. You can be quite liberal with them in your **S** meals. Olive oil may only be used at low heats, but is best raw. Butter is a short chain fatty acid that is very stable when heated. Please do not use canola oil to cook with, or oils labeled as vegetable. They turn into dangerous trans fats very quickly when heated.

Feel free to use red palm oil liberally. You can even fry with it! Its powerful tocotrienals fight cancer aggressively. Studies show it retains its powerful health benefits even after several sessions of cooking.

We realize it is an acquired taste, but its strong taste may be tempered while cooking by mixing it with other oils like coconut or butter. Don't bother trying it raw, yuck!

Okay, here is our first difference in ideas. You'd better get used to this.

Pearl chats: I sometimes sauté foods in extra virgin olive oil at low heats, making sure to never get the temperature to smoking point. There are many health benefits to olive oil, and while I agree that it is best to use it uncooked, the Mediterranean flavor is a great addition to certain recipes. Also, I like to include a healthy amount of olive oil in my diet as it was used liberally in biblical times and has great anti-inflammatory properties.

Serene chats: I agree with the health benefits of olive oil and love to drizzle it liberally on my salads. Oils like coconut, that are saturated, don't work well for salads (they tend to harden on cold contact). However, because I'm a bit of a perfectionist when it comes to eating, I don't like the idea of even a half-formed trans fat on my plate and I don't cook with it. So there, Pearl!

Nuts Are In

You are welcome to enjoy nuts with **S** meals or as **S** snacks. They are predominately made of protein and fat, with just a few carbs, usually between two to five net grams per serving. Like nonstarchy veggies, those amounts don't create issues with blood sugar. *Spicy Nuts* (*Snacks*, Chapter 24) and cheese are a wonderful snack when you need a little pick me up in the afternoon.

We don't give license to go crazy when eating nuts. Unlike non-starchy veggies, they are very high in calories so moderation is a good idea. They are also very filling and your body usually knows when to stop eating them. Note the word "usually." Some people don't have a stop button when it comes to nuts. Peanuts in the shell are a good idea for people with portion control issues. Shelling the peanuts takes time and you'll end up consuming fewer nuts than eating pre-shelled nuts.

We don't want to give hard and fast restrictions on how many nuts you can have when eating them in an **S** setting, but if you are one whose body does not signal well when you are satisfied, try not to consume more than a couple of handfuls. That amount should be fine for most body types in an **S** setting. If you find it hard to eat only two handfuls when there is a large container of nuts sitting around begging to be scarfed, put snack sized portions into baggies, and take a baggie out to naturally set your limit at snack time.

Nut and seed flours are going to come in very handy when you begin using them for making **S** style breads, muffins, and desserts. Do we have some goodies in store for you!

"Franken Foods" or Shortcuts?

If you take a more purist approach to eating, like Serene, you will be satisfied on **S** by simply eating all the delicious meals you can put together with whole foods like meat, cheese, butter, cream, vegetables, berries, nuts, and seeds and their ground flours. There are limitless ideas for meals and desserts that satisfy. You'll be content within these boundaries and will not feel you need to color outside these lines. But, we are aiming for a lifetime approach, and some may think the idea of not having pasta with a meat sauce is unbearable and "unsticktoable" (that might be a new word). Ordinarily, noodles with any kind of creamy, cheesy, or meaty sauce causes the dilemma of high-carbs and fats thrust together, and those two dreaded words—weight gain.

There is good news if you don't always want to stick to spaghetti squash or peeled zucchini as pasta, although we think they are yummy. Spaghetti squash creates delightful angel hair type noodles and it's delicious tossed with butter and parmesan cheese. However, we do want to educate you about some diabetic friendly pastas that don't raise blood sugar. They are perfectly approved for **S** meals, and they are delicious.

What about bread? Bread and butter? Bread and cheese? Buns and burgers? They fit in the "no, no" category of carbs and fats, right? Yes, if you're trying to lose weight. We have plenty of **S** bread recipes and alternatives in the recipe sections, which are nourishing and yummy and don't contain heaps of carbs. Feel welcome to smear butter on them. You can also purchase plan approved, low blood sugar impact pitas, tortillas, and breads, etc., that are fine to be paired with fats like cheese or mayo. You won't have to go without lasagna, BLT's, quesadillas, burritos, or even egg salad sandwiches.

Pearl chats: Serene is going to block her ears right now because I am going to talk about some items that I use to keep myself completely content following this eating lifestyle. Serene calls them "Franken foods." I think of them as shortcuts. Sure, I'll be the first to say these items may not be superfoods, but they are not destructive to the plan when used in moderation. Most of these specialty items are now available at your local supermarket, as the concept of elevated sugar levels is becoming more understood and accepted.

You'll still lose weight and won't feel like you are missing out while incorporating these standard foods that are too hard for some of us to give up.

Serene chats: For the purists who don't mind a little extra time (just a few minutes) and don't want to miss out either, we have included delicious recipes for muffins, crackers, breads, corn chips, etc. **S** meals can be fully enjoyed in a more superfoody way. These "franken foods" are not a necessary part of the plan, although I admit I'll use some of them for my husband now and then.

Pearl chats: Yes, I make and enjoy many of the recipes we have created too, Serene. But, there are many, like me, who want the ease of being able to buy these types of items pre-made for convenience. I try to keep my diet centered on whole foods, but throwing in a "shortcut" purchased item now and then can make life easier. There may be a preservative here or there, and a little soy flour included sometimes (a bit of a no, no), but these items are full of fiber and often high in protein. They will not act like regular flour based items and spike your blood sugar. We will include a full list of these acceptable specialty items, but I'd like to make special mention of Dreamfields pasta. It tastes great, and I don't know anybody who wants to miss out on genuine lasagna or spaghetti with meat sauce, or any other Italian style pasta recipe.

The creators of this product patented a way for the carbohydrates to leave the body the same way as fiber does. Basically, they ride on the back of the fiber on their way through the body. Under a microscope, this cooked pasta looks more like a protein than a grain, and it acts the same way in the body. Dreamfields is available at our local Walmart and Kroger supermarkets here in the South US, but it is also easily purchased via the internet.

I also make use of Joseph's brand pita and lavish breads for sandwiches quite often, and these are readily found at Walmart in the deli section. Gluten intolerant people should stick to our homemade recipes, as these bought items do have small amounts of wheat.

Serene chats: Can I unblock my ears, yet? Okay, I am very happy making noodles out of zucchini and spaghetti squash—super delicious. We have easy to follow recipes in the recipe sections. I don't eat Dreamfields myself since it's not quite pure enough for me, but go ahead and try it if you're an Italian food lover. You'll still be on plan, but don't eat it every day, please! Stick to real foods as often as you can.

There are some wonderfully healthy noodles made from the konjac root called shirataki or yam noodles and I would urge you to eat them as often as your budget can afford. They get my purism seal of approval and I do not call them "franken foods."

Now you know what an **S** meal looks like. Not only can you eat decadently from foods like ground beef burgers, chicken in all forms, broccoli and cheese, salad and creamy dressing, bacon and eggs, berries and cream, chocolate and peanut butter (in moderation), but you are also not going to be denied bread or pasta, if you use the right items. It sounds like you could simply stay eating **S** meals for life, right?

Wrong. That's a dead end.

What's missing? As we keep insisting, it is important to include other food groups for ultimate health. Chant the motto: include not exclude, include not exclude. Our **E** meals are going to provide you with more glucose which is an integral fuel for the body. We don't want you to completely leave out grains, beans, fruit, and some root vegetables. They are all important foods for your diet.

Here is a list of all appropriate foods for **S** (**Satisfying**) meals.

Vegetables

- cabbage
- cauliflower
- broccoli
- zucchini and summer squash
- pumpkin and winter squash
- eggplant
- mushrooms
- celery
- jicama
- winter greens; such as kale, collards, turnip greens, etc
- summer greens; such as lettuces, spinach, parsley, cilantro
- okra
- onions in moderation; including leeks and green onions in any amount
- tomatoes in moderation

- peppers of all kinds
- green beans
- green peas in moderation (not dried split peas which are a legume)
- asparagus
- sugar snap peas
- avocadoes (½ at a time)
- plenty of other non-starchy veggies

Avoid these veggies for **S** meals: corn, carrots, potatoes of all kinds, including sweet potatoes.

Fruits

- raspberries
- strawberries
- blueberries (stick to less than ½ cup)
- blackberries
- fresh cranberries (unsweetened only, and please do not drink cranberry juice)
- acai berry food supplements
- small amounts of dried goji berries and dried cranberries (unsweetened only)

These fruits may be added later on in the plan as **S Helpers**.

- ½ grapefruit
- ½ green apple
- 1 small cantaloupe wedge
- 1 small mandarin
- 1 plum
- 1 handful of cherries

Avoid these fruits for **S** meals: bananas, oranges, mangoes, pineapples, watermelon, pears, peaches, nectarines, all canned fruit even in own juice, all dried fruit except unsweetened cranberries or goji berries, and all fruit juice drinks even if label says 100%.

Dairy

- heavy cream, (raw is best, next best is pasteurized, ultra pasteurized is third, but still okay)
- half and half for coffee
- cottage cheese (full-fat and reduced fat are both okay)
- ricotta cheese (full-fat and skim ricotta are both okay)
- Greek yogurt, 0% (it has nine carbs per full cup, so one cup is fine if it is the main component of an **S** meal or snack, ½ cup is advised for an after meal **S** dessert)

- Greek yogurt, 2% or full-fat
- full-fat regular yogurt is okay in one cup servings if strained at home, but reduced fat regular yogurt does not work for **S**
- all cheeses, both full-fat and 2%, including goat, cow, sheep (raw is best, but harder to find)
- plain kefir (full-fat only)
- butter
- sour cream

Avoid all milk in **S** meals except a spot for those who prefer it instead of cream in tea or coffee. Even whole milk in a raw state is not acceptable. It is liquid carbs which fatten the belly. Unsweetened almond milk (although not a dairy product) is always welcome as it is a neutral fuel beverage.

Avoid pre-sweetened yogurt and all low-fat yogurts if they are not Greek style as they have a lot more carbs.

Meats

- all meats, both fatty or lean, that fit within your religious guidelines (hormone free and grass fed are best)

Eggs

- whole eggs (farm raised or omega-3 are best)
- egg whites (both carton and home separated whites from whole eggs are acceptable)

Grains and Beans

No grains at first (except for our non-grain **S** bread and muffin recipes, which are fine).

The following grain and bean servings may be added in later as **S Helpers**.

- ⅓-½ cup quinoa
- ¼ cup brown rice
- ⅓-½ cup oatmeal
- 1 medium *Trim Healthy Pancake or Pan Bread*
- 1 piece of bread (only sprouted breads like Trader Joe's or Ezekiel, whole grain rye, or sourdough breads).
- ½ sprouted tortilla or wrap
- ⅓-½ cup cooked beans like garbanzo, pinto, navy etc.
- ⅓-½ cup cooked pulses like lentils or split peas

Avoid corn bread, regular store-bought whole wheat bread, baked goods like muffins, bagels, pancakes, dinner rolls, tortillas, corn chips and pasta, unless specified in our specialty items or approved as an on plan recipe alternative.

Nuts and Seeds

- all kinds of raw and dry roasted nuts (in moderation)
- all kinds of raw and roasted seeds including flax and chia (in moderation)
- all natural peanut butter with no sugar added (in moderation)
- almond butter (in moderation)
- cashew butter (in moderation)
- sunflower butter (in moderation)
- tahini (sesame butter) (in moderation)
- coconut in all forms
- coconut flour
- all nut flours including defatted flours like Protein Plus Peanut Flour and Byrd Mill Peanut Flour Dark 12%

Condiments

- mustard
- mayonnaise (ingredients on label will usually include sugar, but this is a trace amount and doesn't count, carb count should be zero)
- all vinegars
- all oils that are cold pressed (remember to only cook with saturated oils)
- horseradish sauce (without sweeteners)
- salad dressings—full-fat is fine (if store purchased, try to buy healthy options keeping the carb count to two grams or less—French and honey mustard will not work, you'll have to make your own
- non-sweet pickles
- olives
- nutritional yeast
- chicken or beef broth or stock (free range is best)
- spices and seasonings (without sweeteners and fillers)
- unsweetened cocoa powder (both regular and extra dark)
- Bragg Liquid Aminos/Tamari/soy sauce
- ketchup (sugar-free homemade or store-bought reduced sugar with only one carb)
- hot sauce (stick to sugar-free preparations) Franks and Texas Pete are good

Sweeteners

- stevia—NuStevia Pure White Stevia Extract Powder, Truvia, or KAL and Swanson stevia drops
- xylitol and eyrithritol (natural sugar alcohols that have negative impact on blood sugar)

Do not use honey, sugar (white, brown, raw, sucanat, or rapadura), maple, agave, corn syrup, evaporated cane juice, fructose, dextrose, aspartame, or Splenda (unless you're not a purist and in a real bind).

Specialty Items appropriate for S meals

- plan approved whey protein powder, e.g., Jay Robb or Swanson Premium Brand Whey Protein
- unsweetened almond or flax milk
- glucomannan powder
- Joseph's pita bread or lavish bread
- low-carb tortillas such as Mission brand "whole wheat" style
- Dreamfields pasta
- konjac root or kelp noodles
- Lucienne's sugar-free chocolate (it is sweetened with our plan approved sweeteners)
- 85% regular dark chocolate squares in moderation (two squares)
- 100% cacao unsweetened baker's chocolate (for making homemade chocolate desserts)

Chapter Nine

The Energizing Meal
(E for Short)

Welcome the **E** meal to center stage . . . round of applause! **E** meals consist of a moderate amount of starch from foods like whole grains, beans, certain root vegetables, or natural sugar from fruit (fructose). They contain enough lean protein to help ward off any sugar spikes and to help increase the hormone glucagon which has a tempering effect on insulin's fat promotion. They also include just a little bit of fat. **E** meals will give you some pep since they offer your body glucose as your primary fuel source. They, like **S** meals, will also make you slim because of the way they're designed.

They are higher in carb counts than **S** meals, due to the inclusion of starch and fruit, but they are never a license to overdo carbs. They are designed to never spike your blood sugar too high, but they do offer a healthy amount of glucose to your cells for energy.

E meals allow for many carb choices, but none of those choices are refined or processed, and the carbs will give you energy without the later crash. Like **S** meals, they **must** be centered around a protein source, but this protein source will be leaner so that more carbs can be consumed without weight gain. Lean protein like chicken or turkey breasts; fish such as tuna, salmon, or any flaky white fish; or grass fed, leaner cuts of red meat like sirloin, or game animals such as buffalo or venison, are all perfect. Leaner dairy servings like 1 percent cottage cheese, skim ricotta or mozzarella cheese, light Laughing Cow or Weight Watchers cheese wedges, low or non-fat plain yogurt (specifically Greek, but regular is fine if that is all your budget can afford) and plain, low-fat kefir, are perfectly suited. Don't fret about the flavor of plain, yogurt, we offer you healthful ways to sweeten it up.

Here's a quick preview into what an **E** breakfast may look like:

> A stack of three generous sized *Trim Healthy Pancakes* (*Morning Meals,* Chapter 18), topped with blueberries, 0% Greek yogurt, and if you like, a swirl of light maple flavored syrup.

Sound good? You bet it is.

Let's have a look at what the seesaw ratio in an **E** meal look like. Notice how this **E** seesaw is the exact opposite of the **S** one? Now carbs are higher so down fat must go. Once again, protein anchors the picture.

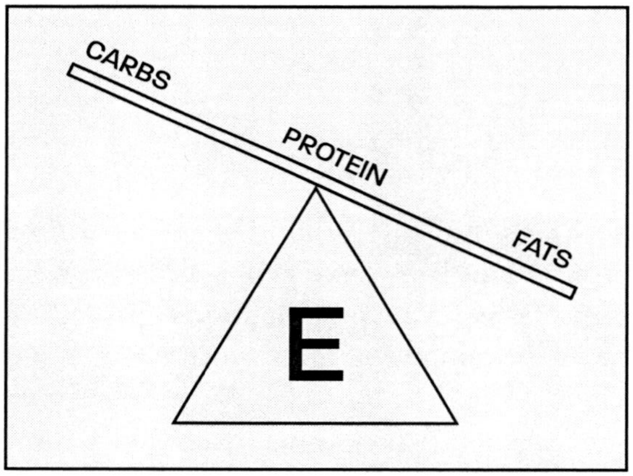

E Meal Carb Limit

It's so important to remember that **E** meals are not an excuse to gorge on carbs. Gorging on carbs will always result in weight gain around the belly, and lowers health whether the carbs are whole grain or not. Keep the starchy carb portion to a palm-size serving on your plate, unless you are eating beans and you can have more of those.

Keeping grains, fruit, and sweet potatoes to palm-size portions will naturally keep you around or under 45 g of carbs, which is the limit we advise. That amount gives your body glucose as fuel for energy, but it can be burned off without too much trouble. It then allows your body to give the signal to your fat to release some of its stores for fuel. In essence, an **E** meal allows you to first burn glucose and then burn some of your own body fat to keep you running. Making sure starches are kept to medium amounts is the only way this will occur.

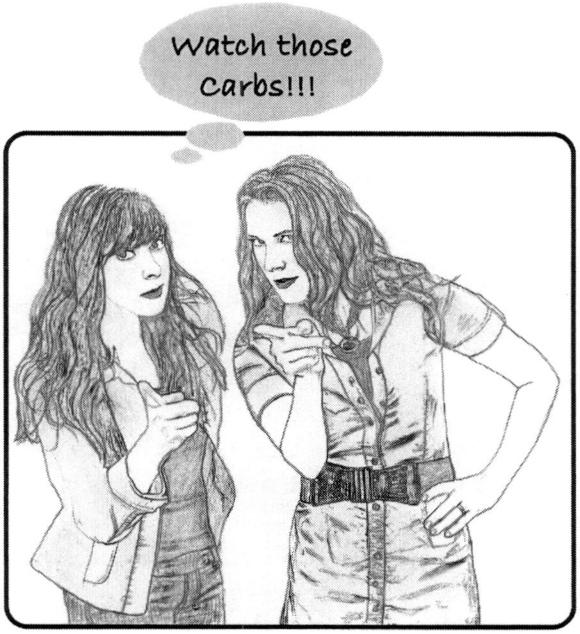

We don't want you doing a bunch of carb counting, which only leads to needless obsessions and detracts from happiness. The starch portions in our **E** list of approved foods are already allotted into safe helping sizes, so you won't need to think too much about it. Adhering to those portion sizes should naturally keep you from shooting past that safe 45 gram threshold. You won't have to do math in your head.

The threshold we advise for **E** meals can be more clearly understood by comparing low versus high-carb food. **E** meals stay in middle territory. Meat has the lowest carbs of all. It actually has zero carbs. This is why even fatty meat, when eaten in an **S** meal with other lower carb foods like non-starchy veggies, will not cause weight gain. A bowl of oatmeal, on the other hand, has between 20-30 net carbs. This is fine for an **E** meal. Your blood sugar should still be within healthy limits after eating it, and the oatmeal is a gentle burning grain that gives you a steady energy level throughout the morning. You can add some berries to the oatmeal and some low or non-fat yogurt to top it off, yet still come in just under 45 carbs. A perfect **E** breakfast.

Let's compare that oatmeal breakfast to a common evening meal that contains a baked potato around 60 carbs, a white dinner roll around 25 carbs, and a sugar laden dessert around 80 carbs. Put the three together like many people do, and you have well over 100 carbs in just one meal! That results in blood sugar racing out of control and extra releases of fat storing insulin to try to clean up the mess. We hate to implement rules, but we advise a 45 gram safety net to avoid health depleting situations such as this.

Fat Sits in the Back Seat

Since starchy carbs take more of a front seat position in these **E** meals, we need to scale the fat back to prevent the head-on collision that occurs with high-carbs and fats together. We don't want to be so cruel as to ban fat from attending the party, but with **E**'s we allow our blood sugar to rise more than what occurs in an **S** meal situation. Let's not double load our insulin delivery truck.

Even though fat is not the star player in **E** meals, it still has some importance. Naked carbs (those that have been stripped of all fat) cause faster sugar spikes. Protein slows this down, as does a little bit of fat.

One Teaspoon Only

That's the amount of fat we suggest you use with an **E** meal. Take an apple for instance. It is in the **E** category because it has more carbs than any of the foods suitable for **S** meals. One teaspoon of peanut butter (a little fat), combined with that apple helps to blunt any sugar spike, and it aids in assimilation of minerals. At only one teaspoon, it is not enough fat to become another whole fuel source for the body to burn. Too much fat will cause this unnecessary tandem fuel burning effect.

If you are used to putting a big glob of peanut butter on a plate and then dipping your apple pieces into it, you need to change your habit. Here's a tip. Take one teaspoon of peanut butter and smear each piece of the apple thinly with it. You won't miss the excessive peanut butter. It is still just as scrumptious and you are taking dominion over your food. Now, after the carbs in the apple are burned off, your body is naturally going to turn to your fat stores. Just what we want.

This one teaspoon of fat in the form of oil, butter, or nut butter is a good measure for an **E** meal, but it is not a strict rule. There may be certain times when you want to use one teaspoon of fat to sauté your protein source and you may want to use another on your salad. That would be the limit. Try to keep **E** meals under two teaspoons of added fat. Just this little bit of fat helps you absorb the vitamins and minerals from your food more efficiently. We are not for fat free meals. Forget that! There are small amounts of natural fats even in oatmeal, that's okay.

Salmon is lean enough for **E** meals, yet it has a little naturally occurring fat. We do not count the naturally occurring fat in lean protein. However, chicken with skin on and most red meat don't (with a capital D) work for **E** meals. That's offering fat fuel galore to your body. Save those protein choices for your scrumptious **S** meals.

You cannot be nearly as liberal with nuts in an **E** meal as you can with **S** since they are quite high in fat. But, we do use some nuts in our **E** recipes . . . just keep the portion size very low. When you're eating **E** style, always keep nuts to a very scant handful. Count that as your fat quota and you should be fine.

Your New Friendly Recipes

Our *Trim Healthy Pancakes* (*Morning Meals,* Chapter 18) and *Trim Healthy Pan bread* (*Muffins, Breads and Pizza Crusts,* Chapter 19) are your perfect **E** meal companions. These two recipes are quick and easy to make, delicious, and filling. You can eat the pancakes with fruit or berries and 0% Greek yogurt for breakfast. At lunch, you can make a sandwich or two out of the pan bread using a little light mayo, mustard, dijonaise or horseradish sauce, lean deli meats, or leftover grilled chicken breast and lettuce.

Foods, like pancakes, are usually incredibly high in carbs, have little protein, and quite simply, they make people fat. Our recipe may resemble IHOP pancakes, but they will help slim you down since they have just enough whole grains to aid in energy, heaps of protein to cause your body to burn more calories, and only a small amount of fat. They are perfect **E** style foods, and their carb count still leaves room for you to add a little fruit without going over the 45 gram carb threshold. Woohoo!

Pass The Beans

Beans are the cheapest carbohydrate to use in an **E** meal. If you have a tight budget, you'll love beans for their price alone. You can feed a houseful with a bag or two of beans or lentils for less than a couple of dollars. But beans have more than just bang for your buck going for them. They contain what is known as resistant starch, which has a much more gentle impact on your blood sugar than other starches. As a result, you can eat larger servings of beans than grains in your **E** meals, if you desire.

They are also very high in antioxidants, especially beans with vivid or dark colors like red kidney beans or black beans. While beans do have some protein, it is important to remember that they are predominately a carbohydrate. Adding a little bit of lean animal protein to your bean meal in the form of some diced chicken breast, a dollop of Greek yogurt, or a sprinkle of low-fat cheese will boost the protein content of your meal and keep you more satisfied.

Soak beans well as this resistant starch is known to cause a lot of gas for some of us. If you are not the "from scratch," type cook and prefer ease and speed, then canned beans are acceptable too, only avoid canned beans with sugars or starchy sauces. Also, endeavor to use cans without BPA—a chemical we'll talk about later in the book.

Be sure to check out the information we provide in our *Foundation Foods*, Chapter 17 on a legume/bean called chana dahl. It is a very low glycemic bean and is perfect for you if you are pre-diabetic or full diabetic and your response to most starches is poor. It is a great food for everybody else too.

Welcome Veggies, Except One

Can you guess which vegetable is not invited to the **E** table? Yes, it's the white potato. While **E** meals do allow some starchy carbs, the potato is going too far. It's like eating white sugar, especially when it is baked. It ignites your blood sugar! We want you to give it a miss if you have weight issues. You'll be able to bring it back in small amounts once you get closer to your goal weight. We don't think you'll really miss it with all the other foods you will be eating. It will be good for you to let it go so you can open your mind to all the other vegetable options available. Sweet potatoes can take its place in your **E** meals.

Sweet potatoes are loaded with goodness, vitamins and minerals, and are easier on your blood sugar. They are an awesome **E** food. An easy **E** lunch or dinner is a medium-sized baked sweet potato topped with one teaspoon of melting butter or coconut oil. If you like a sweeter version, sprinkle some cinnamon and Truvia on top. If you like it savory, drizzle Bragg Liquid Aminos, Creole seasoning, or sea salt and cayenne pepper over the sweet potato. Now, add a bunch of ripped up lettuce leaves to your plate, dump on a can of light packed tuna for protein, and drizzle on a light dressing. A superb meal with no fuss and little time required!

You'll notice on our approved **S** and **E** food lists that non-starchy vegetables are on both lists. Some foods like these are neutral and are included in both lists. In **S** meals, we encourage non-starchy veggies as fantastic replacements for more commonly eaten starchy sides, and for that purpose, these veggies can often be cooked. You may have cooked, non-starchy veggies with **E** meals too, if you desire, but you can't dress them as decadently with all those good fats. Most of us think dry broccoli is "yuck" and we don't want you to eat "yuck"!

We do have one recipe for cooked non-starchy veggies in a cream style sauce that will work for **E** purposes. Check out our *Creamless Creamy Veggies* recipe in *Vegetable Sides* (Chapter 22). It uses a neat trick that comes in real handy. Cooked non-starchy veggies also work well in stir fry sauces for **E** meals. We have a couple of good recipes for those that are tasty and do not contain lots of fat in our *Evening Meals*, Chapter 21.

On the whole, remember that an **E** meal will not work if you ladle on the butter or cheese, or fry or sauté your vegetables in any generous amount of oil. Think about it, you've already got a starch and a protein in an **E** meal. In most cases, (with the exception of stir fries), adding another cooked side is overkill and only more time consuming. The best suggestion is to save most of your cooked veggies for **S** meals and stick to raw veggies like side salads for the majority of **E** meals. If you get sick of salads easily, try out the recipes we mentioned.

Watch your Dressings

Salads work great with **E** meals because they contain a high amount of fiber which contributes to a slower insulin rise. Another thing that works to slow insulin rise is anything naturally sour, therefore a lemon or vinegar based dressing is perfect for an **E** salad. It helps to protect you from too high a sugar surge in your meal. In **S** meals you get to use creamy dressings or pour lots of olive oil on your salads. Don't do that when you're eating **E** style; it will kill your meal's slimming abilities.

Keep dressings lower in fat by using more vinegar to oil ratio if you are making your own, or try our *Hip Trim Honey Mustard* recipe (Chapter 25) or buy a reduced fat dressing that is not laden with sugar or chemicals. Italian styles often work best as do light vinaigrettes. Another option is to use less dressing and add more lubricating veggies like cucumber and tomatoes to avoid a dry salad. Wish-Bone Salad Spritzers come in handy and are readily available at most supermarkets (but they do have some ingredients to which Serene turns up her nose).

Fruit in Moderation

Fruit makes a great **E** snack. It can also be a refreshing **E** dessert. We still recommend that you eat it with a little protein, but that is not a hard and fast rule. If you want to chomp on an apple as a small **E** snack and don't feel like eating anything else, go ahead. However, we don't want you to eat fruit as a whole meal and call yourself done. That requires too much fruit to be consumed and floods your body with too much fructose (fruit sugar). Please, don't ever eat fruit only for breakfast. You need more protein to start your day.

Try to stick to one piece of fruit as part of any **E** meal or snack. If you're still hungry, fill up on some lean protein. Don't sit down to a whole mango, then a large piece of watermelon, and think you are doing yourself any favors. The body can only handle small amounts of fructose at a time. A large bowl of fruit salad might sound healthy, but don't be fooled. Skim forms of Cottage, ricotta cheese, or Greek yogurt are all perfect accompaniments to fruit, and they give your body some lean protein to help prevent too much insulin being secreted.

A word about bananas. God made them and they are a wonderful food. We buy them for our children, who are growing and still very insulin sensitive since they have young cells and run around all day. We very rarely eat bananas ourselves, as they are more like potatoes, and can easily fatten an adult. If you don't want to say a complete goodbye to them, stick to half a banana as a limit when eating **E** style. Fill up on something else and we have plenty of choices for you.

Time for a Sandwich

See how blessed you are now? You can eat sandwiches with both **S** and **E** meals! We're not depriving you of anything on this plan, except excess body fat. Your **S** style bread options always have less carbs, so you can have more fat in your sandwich and enjoy fillings like egg salad with real mayo. **E** bread fillings need to be leaner since your body will now be dealing with actual grains that are going to push your blood sugar a bit higher. If you have weight to lose, don't double load your insulin truck by piling fat like butter and cheddar cheese on your grain-based sandwich.

But, **E** sandwiches can still be delicious. You can fill them with lean meats, spicy mustard, horseradish spread or reduced fat mayo, lettuce, tomato, and a small amount of reduced-fat mozzarella. If you'd rather, you can make your own **E** suitable mayonnaise by mixing 0% Greek yogurt with a little lemon juice and a dash of salt and pepper. That goes great with lean deli meats.

We mentioned you can eat our *Trim Healthy Pan Bread* recipe as sandwich casings, but there are plenty of other options as well. One of the best grain-based breads for you to eat is Serene's sourdough recipe found in *Cultured Recipes*, Chapter 26. If you're not the bread baking type, you can purchase wonderful sprouted breads. If you're lucky enough to have a Trader Joe's store in your area, they have some great sprouted breads under their own brand name that are perfect for **E** meals. Make use of their Sprouted Seven Grain and Sprouted Rye versions. They are the best store-bought sprouted breads, in our opinion, as they have lots of fiber and fewer carbs than most grain breads. Ezekiel Bread is another good sprouted bread option and can be found in the Health Food sections of some regular grocery stores.

We prefer you to eat the breads we have mentioned because any bread that is sprouted or "sour-doughed" from whole grain is much easier on your blood sugar levels. Dark rye breads are another good option since rye does not have the same negative effect on blood sugar as wheat flour often does. Studies from Europe, where rye is a more common bread flour, have shown it keeps people feeling full for longer amounts of time than wheat. The grocery chain store, Aldi, has some wonderful dark rye breads from Germany that come in seasonally and are very inexpensive. The brand name is Deutsche Küche.

Stock up while they have them to last you all year.

Please, never eat more than two pieces of grain-based bread at an **E** meal. Any amount above that pushes grains above their safe limit. The exception to that is our *Trim Healthy Pan Bread* recipe which is high in protein and lower in starchy carbs than even most sprouted or sourdough whole grain breads. This means you can eat up to four bread-sized pieces of this recipe at an **E** meal. That's two whole sandwiches if you can handle that much food! Of course, you can save half a sandwich for a snack later if you get too full.

Cut each sandwich in half and you get to hold and eat four yummy sammies. It feels great, like you're a guilt-free little piggy with a lot of hand-to-mouth satisfaction. This is part of the reason we urge you to make fast and frequent friends with this recipe. It enables you to really fill up and that helps the psychological aspect of being able to stay on plan long term.

Waistline Killer or Healthy Snack?

It would be cruel to take popcorn from your diet. Popcorn fits into the **E** category as it is a starch and contains more carbs than **S** allows. Corn is used to fatten up animals and we don't promote it enthusiastically in this book. In too high amounts it won't do you any favors. But, we don't want to lose you by being popcorn Nazis. It is a natural, all American snack, full of fiber and gives a great crunch fix. There are two main glitches with it—overconsumption (easy to do) and fats and carbs collision. We'll tackle one problem at a time and offer solutions.

Popcorn is one of those foods we all love to sit and eat mindlessly. It doesn't fill the belly well so you can too easily eat oodles of it and generate high surges of insulin. Usually, most of us eat it without protein and with a lot of butter. Lack of protein makes for higher glucose surges without the mediating effect of glucagon and lots of butter equals fats plus carbs weight gain. But, let's be honest, popcorn is fantastic with lots of butter and that's okay for a real indulgent **Crossover** meal or snack now and then. "Now and then" means rarely—had to say it!

For your odd snack of popcorn, we're not going to harp on to you about protein. If you follow our plan correctly you will receive ample amounts of protein with virtually every **S** and **E** meal and snack you eat. We're going to bend our own rules just for popcorn's sake and say, "Okay, don't worry about eating protein with popcorn." There, that was hard for us, but we managed to type it in! If the amount of popcorn we suggest leaves you still feeling hungry, it might be a good idea to pair it with one of our whey protein smoothies. This will give you a greater fullness level and even more fiber to help combat any possible glucose spikes from the more starchy popcorn.

Sorry, but we must set up a few boundaries for popcorn if you want to eat it regularly with our blessing.

- Popcorn should not make a full meal, on plan it is always a snack.
- Keep a three hour distance between popcorn and an **S** meal. That will make sure a fats and carbs collision does not occur. (If you don't have weight to lose, you can bend that rule)
- Don't eat it as a snack every single day as you will miss out on more protein filled snacks.
- Limit portion size to four (or at the most five) cups of popped kernels, eating slowly. Over that amount and you'll jump right out of weight loss mode into opposite territory.

You can go the purist route and pop the seeds yourself in an air popper, or put two tablespoons of seeds in a brown paper bag, double fold and pop it for one and a half to two minutes in your microwave (Serene prefers you air pop). Popping in a saucepan with butter will not work for an **E** snack of popcorn because the butter required will need to be over our recommended one teaspoon allowance.

Pearl chats: If you care not a whit about food purism, you can buy microwavable, 100 calorie mini popcorn bags and eat one of those as an **E** snack. They're handy for portion control since they conveniently come in four to five cup servings. Be sure to stick to one bag. There is some concern that the lining of popcorn bags releases PFC's (perflourinated compounds) that are harmful to immune health but I'll admit we still use them in our house. Serene hates that I'm even mentioning these mini bags, but some of our Drive Thru Sue mamas might think the ease of these bags are worth the small risk. Some brands are now coming out with PFC free bags, so keep an eye out for those.

If you're popping your own seeds, they will taste dry and unappetizing without sprinklings and seasonings, so what do you do if you can't pour on heaps of butter? A good solution is to spray with a healthy cooking spray like olive oil. Non-purist types could use a butter flavored spray. This spray is only to allow your seasonings to stick. Don't spray 50 times, that will defeat the purpose. Once you have coated the kernels with a small amount of oil, season with sea salt, pepper, parmesan cheese, nutritional yeast, spices of your choice, or even a little hot sauce. You can also look at health food and online stores for a brand of popcorn called, Half Naked Popcorn. It is in bags already popped if you want to skip that step. It does not contain harmful ingredients and has appropriate fat amounts. Just be careful to remember our portion guidelines.

Popcorn is a great and very inexpensive snack for children if you home-pop the seeds. All of our children love to pop their own bowls and get very creative with flavorings. We don't worry about how much fat get poured on with the children in our homes that are still growing. They melt heaps of butter or coconut oil to pour over, but they are all lean and shooting up like weeds, so the fat and carbs collision doesn't hurt them a bit. If your children have weight issues, it may be a good idea to show them how to make **E** approved popcorn.

There is growing concern about GMO's, the genetically modified form of modern corn. We don't get too caught up with this fear as we try to feed such nutritious fare overall to our families and we cannot afford organic everything. But, if your budget allows more wiggle room and you have concerns about GMO's, purchase organic popcorn seeds and you will have nothing to worry about.

Here is a list for all appropriate foods for **E** (**Energizing**) meals:

Vegetables

- all vegetables, except potatoes (save potatoes for **Crossovers** or complete cheat meals)
- sweet potatoes, keep to one medium sweet potato per **E** meal
- carrots, both raw and cooked are acceptable

Fruits

- all fruits in small quantities e.g.,1 apple, 1 orange, 1 slice of cantaloupe (very high glycemic fruits like bananas and watermelon should be kept to minimum)
- all berries in liberal quantities
- all fruit jelly, we approve Polaner All-Fruit Jam with Fiber (for use with Greek yogurt and skim ricotta)

Dairy

Eat freely from the following forms of low-fat or non-fat dairy.

- low or non-fat plain regular yogurt
- low or non-fat plain Greek yogurt
- low or non-fat plain kefir
- low or non-fat cottage cheese
- part skim ricotta cheese
- skim mozzarella cheese (very small amounts only)
- reduced fat (2%) hard cheeses (very small amounts only)
- Light Laughing Cow or Weight Watchers cheese wedges
- low-fat sour cream (it is healthier to use low-fat yogurt, but is okay)

Meat

Eat freely from all lean meats, avoid all fatty meats

- chicken breast
- tuna packed in water
- salmon (both fillets and canned forms are fine)
- all other fish (not fried)
- leaner cuts of bison, venison and grass fed beef
- turkey breast
- lean ground turkey or chicken (96%-99% lean)
- lean deli meats (natural brands that don't use hormones or antibiotics are best)

Eggs

- egg whites only—no yolks (carton egg whites and Egg Beaters are also acceptable)

Grains

- brown rice—¾ cup cooked serving
- quinoa—¾ cup cooked serving
- oatmeal—up to 1¼ cooked cup serving
- *Trim Health Pancakes* and *Trim Healthy Pan Bread*—up to ⅓ full recipe batch serving
- whole grain bread, sprouted, sour dough, dark rye—2 piece servings
- Popcorn—4-5 cups of popped kernels

Legumes

- all beans and legumes including lentils and split peas—up to 1½ cooked cup cooked servings

Nuts

- nut butters (1 tsp. servings)
- nuts (very small handful servings, basically a sprinkle size)
- defatted peanut flour (we recommend Protein Plus Peanut Flour and Byrd Mill Peanut Flour Dark 12%—1 Tbs. serving for use in desserts, sauces, and to stuff celery)

Condiments

- reduced fat mayonnaise
- mustard
- horseradish sauce
- all vinegars
- hot sauce
- reduced fat dressings (keep fat grams to 4 or less and sugar low)
- soy sauce/Bragg Liquid Aminos/Tamari
- chicken or beef broth or stock (free range is best)
- spices and seasonings (without fillers and sugars)
- unsweetened cocoa powder
- cold pressed oils (one teaspoon servings—maximum 2 teaspoons)
- Fat Free Reddi Whip (for use with desserts)

Sweeteners

- stevia—NuStevia Pure White Stevia Extract Powder, Truvia, or KAL and Swanson stevia drops.
- xylitol and erythritol

Specialty Items

- plan approved whey protein powder, e.g., Jay Robb and Swanson Premium Brand Whey Protein
- unsweetened almond or flax milk
- glucomannan powder
- Joseph's pita bread or lavish bread
- Dreamfields pasta
- konjac noodles

Chapter 10

Mama, Meet the Relatives

You've now been introduced to both **S** and **E** meals. They are your primary caregivers. Picture them as mommy and daddy, providing you with all the care and nutrients you need. You need both a mommy and a daddy for the balance each brings. **S** is the more indulgent parent, treating you with creamy desserts and filling, sumptuous meals. **E** is the more practical parent, providing you with all your B vitamins and other energy promoting foods that enable your body to work efficiently for all of life's mundane tasks.

As different as they are, both are weight reducing meals, at least for the majority of people who do not have sluggish metabolisms. These **S** and **E** parent meals will always take care of you. They'll help you get to a healthy weight and remain your faithful supporters for the rest of your life.

However, no family is complete without relatives, even the odd crazy one, right? We've got three extended family members we want to introduce to you. They'll bring color, variety, and encouragement to your journey. Each of these three meal types has its own personality and talent and will lend you a hand whenever you need some extra help. After all, that's what family is for, isn't it?

First, we want you to meet the jovial cousin, **S Helper**. He's a rule bender at heart, but never goes too far. Next, you'll meet the generous doting grandmother, **Crossover.** She's a nurturer by nature, making sure you are never underfed. She loves to see you with a full dinner plate. However, we can't leave out the crazy uncle, **Fuel Pull**. He's a mad scientist to the core and has invented unique and effective ways to help lean out your body.

You may need to form a closer bond with one of these relatives. It's only natural to have tighter bonds with certain relatives more than others. You may have certain needs that require the help and guidance of one of these extended family members more than the other two. Some people with high metabolisms may need to spend more time with Granny **Crossover** so they don't lose too much weight eating **S** and **E** alone. Others, with sluggish metabolisms from years of yo-yo dieting, hormonal issues, or certain genetic body types, may need to visit with Uncle **Fuel Pull** more often than the rest of us. He's a miracle worker when it comes to stubborn weight problems. Cousin **S Helper** is a friendly guy to have around and he always brings a little sunshine when you need it most.

Cousin S Helper

This meal style is worth getting to know after you make some progress in your weight loss journey. It is an optional little blesser. We call it an **S Helper** as opposed to a hamburger helper. (Giggle). It makes life a little more fun and freeing along the journey. Basically, you add a little more carb to your **S** meals for pleasure's sake, but don't go near as far as a **Crossover**, which will be described shortly.

The amount of carb is not enough to cause fat storage for most people. Due to the addition of this small amount of starch or fruit, your body will go into glucose fuel burning mode first, before it burns the fat from your meal. But, this glucose rise is designed to be small. Your body should burn through the glucose rather swiftly then get right down to the task of burning all the nourishing fat in your meal. If you're metabolism is not in too drastic a state, you'll still likely burn a small amount of body fat after the fat from your meal is used up as energy. The meal won't be as weight loss promoting as a pure **S** meal, but it can happen.

The portions are quarter to half a cup of starchy foods or a small amount of fruit. We mean measuring cups, not huge coffee mugs or big gulp soda refill containers. Just making doubly sure, now!

We don't have **E** helpers. This is because an **E** portion of carbs naturally becomes a **Crossover** if you add any more fat than one to two teaspoons.

Here's a little glimpse into what an **S Helper** breakfast may look like.

Scrambled eggs with sausage and one piece of plan approved toast with butter.

Nice!

Here are your **S Helper** options that can be tagged on to an S meal:

- 1 piece of sprouted Trader Joe's, or Ezekiel bread, or 1 thin slice of homemade sourdough bread, or ½ piece of homemade regular whole wheat bread
- 1 medium *Trim Healthy Pancake* or *Pan Bread*
- ⅓-½ cup of cooked quinoa (it's more gentle on blood sugar than most other grains)
- ¼ cup (no more) of cooked brown rice or other starchy grain (it's harder on blood sugar)
- ⅓-½ cup of cooked oatmeal
- 1 extra small serving of fruit, such as ½ apple, ½ orange, or 1 mandarin
- ⅓-½ cup of cooked beans (you can use a more liberal and generous ½ cup serving of chana dahl)

Here is what **S Helpers** look like on our seesaw. Notice the seesaw is still tipped lower on the carb side, but not quite as low as pure **S** meals.

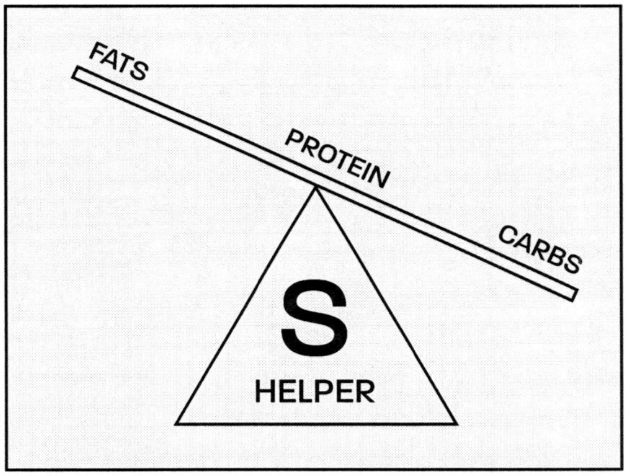

Make Progress First

S Helpers are only for people whose weight loss has already made a good start. You don't have to be at your goal, but should be noticing continuous results. This usually takes a couple of months to achieve. **Crossover** meals will allow you to maintain weight, but **S Helpers**, with their very small addition of healthy starches, still make room for weight loss.

WARNING! They will hinder weight loss if you become too liberal and start tossing starches on your plate, rather than eying or measuring first. Keep your quarter and half cup measuring cups handy, mama. You'll make frequent use of them if **S Helpers** appeal to you. Start out with a third cup of quinoa under your fried eggs at breakfast. If weight loss keeps going well for you, you may be able to increase to half a cup. Both of us easily enjoy half cup servings of quinoa as **S Helpers** with our fried eggs, but we have been at our goal weights for a long time. Easy does it when you first include these. Ramp starch portions up slowly.

Some people with more insulin resistance may notice a halt to progress if **S Helpers** are included too often. Women who have PCOS (Polycystic Ovarian Syndrome) may have to keep to pure **S** and **E** (using primarily quinoa and chana dahl as their **E** options) to see weight loss, with more heavy reliance on **S**. This is because PCOS can make the body less able to handle carbs in most forms. It induces a tough state of insulin resistance and only a couple of very slow burning starchy carb forms can be handled. Fortunately, chana dahl and quinoa are tolerated quite well, even by the most insulin resistant.

Why do we not suggest **S Helpers** at the beginning of this program? We want to make a clear distinction that it is high starches in combination with fats that are responsible for any body fat storage. You may be used to eating larger amounts of starches. Therefore, it will be more helpful for your progress to eliminate them from your **S** meals and focus on non-starchy veggies. This will train you to be more creative with these vegetables, without always having to include starchy carbs. Also, pure **S** meals help to clear cells that have been overstuffed with sugar for too many years. They will make them more able to handle and process blood sugar so greater weight loss is achieved.

Until all this happens, it may be much harder to enjoy quarter to half cup servings of a whole grain instead of the usual excess. Adding **S Helpers** later in the program will seem like an added treat, but not necessary for your satisfaction. We don't want you to look at **S Helpers** when you first start our plan as some sort of punishment like, "What do you mean, I can only have quarter of a cup?" Bringing them in too early could cause that response.

Once you have learned the satisfaction of filling up on non-starchy veggies (and it is a learned skill, but once mastered, very addicting) then adding a little starch should feel more like, "Wow, you mean I get to have a whole quarter to half a cup? Thanks, Serene and Pearl. I'm quite satisfied with the way I've been eating, but I may try adding it in!" (Wink!)

Having said all this, if you want to be stubborn and decide to include **S Helpers** from the outset, you may be okay. We say "stubborn," because we have a brother who insisted he would only follow our plan if he could keep in a certain amount of starch with all his **S meals**. He did not want to feel psychologically deprived in any way whatsoever. He wanted that piece of sprouted toast under his eggs in the morning, come what may! But, he needed to lose some weight in a healthy low glycemic manner as his fasting blood sugar revealed pre-diabetic numbers and his pants were too tight!

During the first six weeks of our plan and doing it in his own stubborn way he did not lose weight, although he told us he felt much better and his blood glucose numbers improved. We told him (in a sisterly "told you so" fashion) that he would have more success if he'd forego all the **S Helpers**. He ignored our advice and continued to enjoy his **S Helpers**. What do you know? Four months into the plan he'd dropped 15 pounds. Seven months later, he'd lost close to 30 pounds and had a much healthier fat distribution in his body. But, he's a guy. Men have less fat cells in their bodies and they usually drop weight faster and with more ease than women.

Ultimate S Helpers

If you are not familiar with the grain that is actually a seed called quinoa, or the legume called chana dahl, read about them in *Foundation Foods,* Chapter 17. They are the ultimate **S Helpers** as they are both very slow burning in the body, will not likely cause elevated blood sugar, and should be far less likely to halt weight loss.

Quinoa is yummy, fluffy, and very versatile. As an **S Helper** serving of a third to a half cup's worth, it can be used underneath your eggs for breakfast, tossed into your salad or soup, or layered as a bed under your salmon for lunch. It is also the perfect accompaniment to your curry or stir fry in place of rice. It cooks a lot faster, too.

Chana dahl is a legume that has a glycemic index so low that it's almost unbelievable. It is versatile, too. As an **S Helper** in half cup portions it can be used as a seasoned mash on the side of your plate with your evening meal, tossed into your salad or stir-fry at lunch, or used as part of soups and stews. We like the idea of quinoa and chana dahl as your first **S Helpers** as they are much gentler on your blood sugar than most other grains and beans. However, if they don't appeal to you and you are not pre-diabetic or have Type 2 diabetes, the other **S Helper** options that are listed should be fine.

No Extra Helpings

Once you start adding **S Helpers**, it's important to remember that they are not part of second helpings. It's okay to go back for a little more food if you are still hungry at the end of your meal. But, if you've already had your **S Helper** portion in your first round, put some more protein and non-starchy veggies on your plate, and skip that second piece of bread or other portion of grain. This, of course, does not apply to soup or chili where foods like quinoa, chana dahl, or lentils and beans may be already appropriately portioned into the recipe to fit **S Helper** standards.

The Winning Number

While we don't want you counting carbs meticulously, it is good to have a general idea of carbohydrate content. Our **S helper** portions are designed to stay under 15 net grams of carbs. But that's easy to manage if you remember to keep to one small piece of bread, or quarter to half a cup of a more starchy item. Don't become a counting freak! However, for interest sake, when counting net carbs, always subtract the fiber to come up with the correct number. For example, 16 grams total carb with four grams of fiber equals 12 grams net carb portion. That would work great for an **S Helper**.

Berries are not considered a carb portion on this program unless you have more than one cup's worth. Therefore, we include them in both **S** and **E** meals and do not consider their sugar levels high enough to be in this **S Helper** group. Blueberries are the exception. They should not exceed half cup portions when paired with **S** meals as they are a little higher in carbs than other berries—three quarters of a cup would be an **S Helper** portion of blueberries

The Choice is up to You

S Helpers are not a required add-on for most people. They are just a way to have more freedom on this plan. You get enough carbs with your **E** meals for overall health purposes; adding these helpers to your **S** meals is not mandatory. If you decide to add them, and they slow your weight loss down too much for your liking, or completely halt weight loss, forego them.

If **S Helpers** make you happy and content to continue this way of eating indefinitely, even if weight loss is slower, that's okay by us. Remember that this is a lifetime approach to healthy eating, not a race to shed 50 pounds within six months. It would be better to take a year or two to shed 50 pounds and enjoy your food and your life. That's a smarter approach than losing a bunch of weight quickly and then returning to your previous eating habits due to a stringent mindset.

We are all different. If you are one of those people with strong carb addictions, it's possible **S Helpers** might throw you off too much, especially bread. Some people have portion issues with bread. If you simply cannot eat only half to one piece of bread as an **S Helper**, due to strong carb addictions, you may need to tread carefully when you try to include this little 15 gram carb addition. You know your own weaknesses.

Once weight loss is well on its way after eating **S** and **E** alone for a while, give yourself a chance with some **S Helpers**. If adding half to one piece of bread with your **S** meal still makes you hanker to eat three more pieces, this will not be an **S Helper**, but an **S Killer**. It will swing that seesaw the wrong way! Go back to pure **S** and stay the course for a while longer. As this diet heals your sugar addiction, you may be able to try again later when you are stronger.

S Helpers for Hypoglycemia

There is one small group of people that may need to add these helpers to their **S** meals from the beginning of this plan and that is those who have a strong tendency to be hypoglycemic. Simply eating protein, fats, and non-starchy vegetables may not raise your blood sugar enough to get it into the optimal range. You become dizzy and faint due to blood sugars remaining too low. The inclusion of a small carb should help support more medium blood sugar levels. Adding **S Helpers** from the onset of this plan may slow down initial weight loss a little, but it will still happen, but at a slower pace. This will be a healthier approach for you.

However, before you say, "that's me" and label yourself hypoglycemic, do a self-check. You may be hypoglycemic only because you have spent years eating meals that are far too high in carbs. By now, you will understand that high-carbs elevate blood sugars to unhealthy highs, but after the spike, they fall too low. Give yourself a chance at **S** meals by themselves when you start the plan and see how you do. You may find the protein and healthy fats in **S** meals will balance your blood sugar nicely and you will no longer be hypoglycemic. Making sure your meal is protein-centered can, in itself, prevent hypoglycemia. But, there are always exceptions. Our bodies are all unique and we are prone to different ailments. People with chronic hypoglycemia, not due to initial blood sugar spikes, are the only ones that need to add in the **S Helpers** from the beginning.

In the early stages of changing to this healthier way of eating outlined in this book, your body may have a few withdrawal symptoms. Your body has been used to using high amounts of glucose to fuel energy levels. You may feel a little "draggy." It takes awhile to adjust to new energy pathways. Give yourself three weeks. If you still feel very fatigued, you can check your blood sugar two hours after a meal with a glucose monitor. If your blood sugar is much below 70, then you may need to add in **S Helpers** early. Remember though, hypoglycemia is not a ticket to constant **Crossover** meals if you have pounds to lose. Stick to **S Helpers** if hypoglycemia afflicts you. You can still shed the fat over the long haul.

Granny Crossover

This meal crosses over the lines that keep **S** and **E** foods separated from each other. It mixes carbs with fats so weight loss does not occur. But, once again, it is designed to ensure you never spike your blood sugar too high which is the pathway to degenerative health.

The concept behind the **Crossover** meal is to enjoy carbs in the quantities we suggest for **E** meals (not too high, but enough to gain energy) along with more liberal amounts of good fats in the **S** category. Just mix 'em together. Your body will first burn the glucose from the starch in the meal, then it will burn the fat contained in the meal. It won't get the chance to burn your own body fat because you are offering it back to back fuel sources. It will stay too fueled up and busy burning the two fuels it is offered to get around to burning your actual body fat.

This meal type is a far cry from the tandem fuel burger and fry combination we talked about earlier. That was a **Crossover**, but it was tipped too high in starches. Remember, the fat did not get a chance to burn as a fuel source, so it was stored in the body. **Crossovers** are well-balanced fat/starch combinations that allow both fats and carbs to fuel the body.

Here is a glimpse into a suggested **Crossover** meal:

salad with cheese and creamy dressing
beef and veggie stir fry over three quarters cup of rice or one cup of quinoa

Sound good? Of course it does! **Crossovers** are hearty fare.

Here is a picture of what **Crossovers** look like on a seesaw. Notice how carbs and fats are evenly balanced?

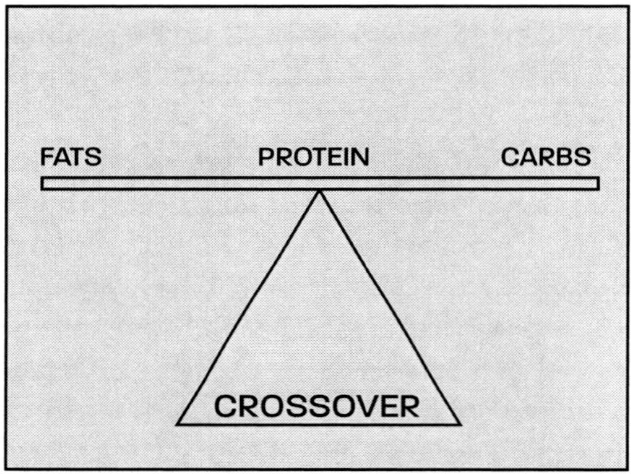

Key to Maintenance

Crossovers are the key to maintenance on the **S** and **E** plan. A lot of plans throw you to the wolves once weight loss is achieved. People don't know whether to keep eating according to plan and keep losing weight, or tentatively return to their old way of eating and gain back the weight. That is why we designed **Crossovers**. They enable you to incorporate the healthiest way of eating once goal weight is achieved.

Once you've reached your ideal weight, and don't want to lose anymore, we don't want to leave you in a situation where you have no place to go and where you resort back to your previous eating habits. Shock and horror! Please, don't do that! We're begging and pleading, DO NOT RETURN! DANGER! It will only lead you to the likelihood of common middle age issues like Type 2 diabetes. You don't want to go there.

Our **S** and **E** plan works so well that even when you reach your desired weight you may keep losing weight unless you incorporate some **Crossovers**. You'll never look gaunt or get that "skin and bone" look. Remember, your husband likes curves.

Female Fat Layers

A certain amount of fat keeps your skin looking younger and more supple. As females, we have 12 percent essential fat in our bodies to support our reproductive organs, brain, bone marrow, spinal cord, and complete nervous system. That percentage is high compared to men who only require three percent essential fat. We also need some non-essential fat. That is the fat that lies just below our skin layer and helps protect our bodies from injury and cold. It also provides us with a great source of energy and allows us to sit on something, rather than just a tail bone.

A healthy amount of body fat on a woman is not repugnant. Don't think you need to be "shredded" and try to eliminate all body fat. That is not healthy for your hormonal profile. Going too far below a healthy body fat ratio will disrupt your delicate endocrine balance, and if you are pre-menopausal, you may stop your period altogether. That is a dangerous set-up for bone loss, depression, skin aging, and cardiovascular disease. God did not design a grown female to appear like ripped muscle and skin as men are more apt to be. Desiring that appearance is a warped perception of how a female should look. Female fat layers in the right proportions are beautiful. The "too skinny" look is very aging for anyone over 30 years.

Most women should not dip too far below 20 percent total body fat if they want to remain healthy, with an absolute minimum of 17 percent. Our fat deposits communicate with our hormones. Too little fat and our hormones sense we are in a state of life and death stress. In this state, hormones decline and we will be less likely to conceive a baby. Survival mode kicks in and shoves reproduction smartly out of the way. Some experts believe a minimum of 22 percent body fat must be maintained for regular menstrual cycles to occur. That is up for some debate, but it is generally accepted that a young girl will normally come close to the 20 percent body fat mark before she will begin menstruating.

However, there is a growing concern today that young girls are growing adult bodies at much earlier ages than any other time in history. This is due, in great part, to carb-heavy lifestyles that promote earlier fat gain. Once a young female reaches a high enough amount of body fat, her body says to her ovaries, "Hey, I am now padded like a woman. Start your thing!"

How Often?

Once you reach your ideal weight, depending upon metabolism, **Crossovers** should be incorporated into your diet about 20 percent of the time so you can maintain a healthy body weight. You'll stay on **S** and **E** meals, throwing in some **S Helpers** now and then the rest of the time. If you find weight creeps up too much on this ratio, pull **Crossovers** back a little. Or, if weight continues to drop, increase their frequency. You will find your sweet spot.

If weight loss is going well, even if you have not yet reached your goal weight, you may incorporate **Crossovers** once a week or so. Just keep an eye on your progress, and you won't stall.

CAUTION! **Crossover** stage does not give you permission to eat "kid food," even whole grain nourishing "kid food." Children, unless they have a weight problem, are much more insulin sensitive than adults. If your growing boys are able to eat three bowls of whole wheat pasta, or four pieces of toast and burn it off within half an hour, and ask for more, do not follow suit. Even if your metabolism is high and you need to gain weight, that style of eating will put fat on your belly disproportionately. Growing children, especially boys heading into teenage years, often need upwards of 4,000 calories a day to keep up with their high metabolic needs. It's no wonder those of us with boys in the home have to constantly restock our cupboards, but there is no reason for us to mimic their eating habits.

Skinny Does Not Mean Healthy

You can be skinny, but not healthy at all. Maybe excess weight is not your problem. Take a self-check for a minute. Are you quite thin, yet find your belly protrudes? Start making your meals **Crossovers.** They will work to keep your blood sugar stabilized while maintaining your weight, and they will go a long way to create a healthier body fat distribution in your body. Remember, there is much more to health than a number on the scale. **Crossovers** help keep your youth as long as possible by avoiding insulin spikes from poorly proportioned meals. Spiking insulin causes that inflammatory response in the body that is the trigger point for disease.

If your energy is lagging, your skin and hair dull, and your emotions roller-coasting, who cares if you are a size four, you are still miserable as well as everyone around you. **Crossovers** are your way to better health and mood stability.

Balance the Seesaw

You will notice the majority of the recipes in this book are either **S** or **E**. It's easy to turn any of these meals into a **Crossover** by adding either more fat to the **E**, or more carbs to the **S**. This will even up the seesaw to avoid weight loss. For example, make one of our healthy and hearty evening meal **S** dishes such as *Creamy Cheesy Chicken* (*Evening Meals*, Chapter 21). Eat this **S** recipe with only non-starchy veggies if your weight needs to go down. If you don't have a weight issue, add some starch such as whole grain bread and butter, three quarters of a cup of brown rice, or a full cup of quinoa on the side.

For a lunch meal, make a delicious healthy salad topped with chicken, nuts, cheese, and lots of olive oil. Instead of stopping in **S** mode, chop up a big apple and throw it in with the rest of the salad. Easy. Now you have combined the two primary fuels of fats and glucose instead of opting for only one. If you eat the salad without the added carbs you will continue to lose weight. Prevent this by upping the carb count, but still have a nourishing meal that poses no danger to your pancreas.

Protein Priority

Again, with **Crossovers**, protein centers the meal. Never base a meal around a carb. Don't think because you are at **Crossover** stage, you can sit down to a lunch of four pieces of bread, butter, and sugar-free jelly. That's carb heavy. Your seesaw is off kilter, and where is the protein in such a meal? Continue to adhere to the good advice to not eat more than two pieces of bread at a time, no matter what stage of this plan you are on.

If you don't have a weight issue, please don't think you can snack on corn chips and salsa whenever you want. Again, where is your protein? You may be blessed with a high metabolism and don't have to worry about only eating our **S** and **E** weight loss style meals, but this snack will raise your blood sugar and cause an inflammatory state in your body which will age your inner organs, as well as your skin.

Always giving protein its priority is the key to a low-glycemic and anti-aging lifestyle. A better **Crossover** lunch than four pieces of bread and jelly would be two pieces of sprouted bread, butter, cheese, deli meat turkey or leftover chicken (for protein), and a handful of spicy nuts on the side. A better **Crossover** snack than the corn chips would be two tablespoons of peanut butter or some cheddar cheese with a large red apple. This way, you get a healthy amount of glucose (or fructose in the case of the apple), but round it out with protein, which is much healthier for your body.

What if you don't feel like an apple, but you've got the munchy crunchies? Go ahead and have some corn chips if you're at **Crossover** stage, only try to avoid trans fats by eating baked style whole grain corn chips. Sure, have some salsa with them, but increase the protein content by adding cheese, beans, and Greek yogurt (even full-fat Greek yogurt, if you like), or sure, plop on some sour cream. Now you've got some protein. You've got some fat. You've got some carb. You've got a **Crossover**. Enjoy!

Check Your Source

Like **E** meals, **Crossovers** are not an excuse to revert back to poor carbohydrate sources. Stick to sprouted or heavy rye sourdough breads. Choose lower glycemic grains like quinoa and oatmeal. Our *Trim Healthy Pancakes* and *Trim Healthy Pan Bread* are great for a **Crossover** if you want to have some nice pats of butter with them, or a dollop of whipped cream for extra succulence.

Choose brown rice over white, but don't overdo it. We want you to keep rice to no more than three quarters of a cup. Even though brown is much more nutritious than white rice, it is still rather high on the glycemic index. You should be fine using a whole cup of quinoa in a **Crossover**, or even a little more. We aren't worried about calories at all in **Crossovers**, so feel free to be **very** generous with more gentle burning grains like quinoa. Choose sweet potatoes over white. Not only do they contain more vitamins, minerals, and beta carotene, but they have less impact on your blood sugar, despite having a sweeter taste than regular potatoes. However, you could go ahead and enjoy a white potato now and then in a **Crossover**.

Be liberal including fat with all those carb options. You'll be able to have a banana with some peanut butter now and then, but don't throw two bananas, dates, and a big squirt of honey in a smoothie. Watch how that will swiftly give you a pooch, even if you have a naturally high metabolism and your arms and legs stay skinny. Why? Because, it's a carb binge! It's jumping right past healthy blood sugar margins.

Beans are an excellent **Crossover** carb choice as they contain some plant protein and resistant starch. You can be very liberal with beans in a **Crossover** meal.

Who Needs to Eat More Crossovers?

Growing children. We'll go into their needs in much more detail later on. But, there are some adults who need to focus more predominantly on **Crossovers** than on one fuel source at a time.

Ectomorphs

Some people can eat whatever they want and never put on weight. These people are true ectomorphic body types and actually have trouble keeping enough fat on their bones. If this is you, you're rare, and the rest of us don't like you very much! Pure ectomorphs are the uncommon types who have the opposite condition from most of us aging adults. Their muscle cells remain insulin sensitive and burn through glucose like wild fire, while their fat cells are more insulin resistant. Their fat is actually unwelcome to glucose deposits. How about that? Not fair at all! If this is you, skip **S** and **E** meals. You're going to have to live predominantly on **Crossovers.**

However, it doesn't give you license to fill up on sugary foods or munch on potato chips whenever you want just because you are skinny. Sometimes, we notice super skinny people eating all sorts of junk and pouring sugary sodas down their throats just because they think they can. It makes us shudder! Even though these foods may not fatten super skinny people, they devastate the body in other ways.

Crossovers are a much healthier and anti-aging eating approach for super high metabolism types. Center your meals around protein, carbs, and healthy fats. This will help blunt surging glucose and enable a gain of more muscle and healthier body mass than a thin layer of flabby fat. The healthy fats in **Crossovers** will nourish you and the medium servings of starch will enable your blood sugar to rise just enough so that whatever fat you eat is able to stick more easily to your bones. Throw out the food pyramid that we are all supposed to follow with the largest focus on carbs. Even if you are thin, do not let carbohydrates become the focus of your diet, whole grain or not. Think protein, protein, protein first.

Heavy Exercisers

Avid exercisers may also need to make **Crossovers** a bigger, rather than smaller, part of their diet. If you have no weight to lose and enjoy doing longer amounts of intense exercise, you may need to live mostly on **Crossovers** to maintain a healthy body weight. The exception would be times when you eat very large amounts of fat, i.e., a big marbled steak or homemade ice cream (made with real cream) since a high amount of saturated fat may produce its own glycogen. Only then would it not be quite as necessary to include some starch.

Some Nursing and Pregnant Mothers

Nursing and pregnant mothers may also need to include more **Crossovers.** Notice we use the word "may." Only include lots of **Crossovers** if you are losing too much weight while nursing, or cannot gain sufficient weight while pregnant. Be true to yourself. Some people need a lot of **Crossovers** while nursing and pregnant, others do not. Having said that, it is not a good idea for pregnant women to try and achieve weight loss.

Pregnant women who put on weight very easily may have to stick to **S** and **E** with very limited **Crossovers**. Some women have bodies that become very insulin resistant during pregnancy. This is due to the way their body reacts to the presence of high progesterone that pregnancy promotes. Pregnancy causes a mother to be more prone to insulin resistance, but some women have genetic components that make this worse. If you are in this category, your body will balloon up if you eat too many carbs during pregnancy. You'll have to be especially diligent to watch that you don't collide your fuels by eating lots of carbs with fat.

Women who are prone to gestational diabetes during pregnancy may even have to be careful about eating too many **E** meals. Your cells may not be able to handle the glucose our 45 carb threshold allows if it is in the form of bread or rice. You should be okay with chana dahl and quinoa, as both **E** and **Crossovers**. Aside from those two options, you may have to focus primarily on **S** meals with lots of **S Helpers** so that the fat in those meals can slow down your heightened insulin response during pregnancy.

Constant Crossovers are Rare

Now that we have mentioned the groups of adults that need lots of **Crossovers,** we can easily generalize and say they are more the exception than the rule. Most of us don't need to constantly eat **Crossovers** to maintain weight. Adding a few of these meals a week should do the trick to halt weight loss. Constantly crossing the lines between **S** and **E** makes ideal weight impossible for the average person. If you frequently fill your plate with potatoes and meat, bread and butter, grain-based crackers with cheese, or noodles with a cheesy meat-based sauce, you won't need to wonder why your baby weight is not shedding. Those combinations are **Crossovers** and designed to healthfully keep fat on you, not pull it off.

Serene chats: Both Pearl and I are genetically tall and reasonably thin people, but if we live on predominantly **Crossover** meals we notice our clothes get tighter. I like to keep **Crossover** meals to only a few times a week and make real good use of them around holiday times like Thanksgiving and Christmas. Turkey and stuffing, anybody?

Edit. Four years after writing this chapter, we both find ourselves in the position where we need a lot more **Crossovers** to maintain our weight. Several years of eating **S** and **E** meals with lots of **Fuel Pull** snacks have revved our metabolisms to the point where we now need to include more **Crossover** meals or we become way too skinny for even our own liking. That's how well this program works. And, our husbands like a little more than a little less to grab onto! We now make sure **Crossovers** make up at least one third of our diet. However, unless it's a rare "cheat meal," we never binge on carbs. Our **Crossover** meals are a healthy balance of medium-sized starch or fruit portions, protein, superfood fats, and greens.

Uncle Fuel Pull

Fuel Pull meals are the complete opposite of **Crossovers**. Instead of making sure you incorporate both primary fuels, these meals strip them both way back. We told you this Uncle comes across as a little "coo coo," but boy oh boy, his science works!

While **Crossovers** keep weight healthfully on you, **Fuel Pull** meals swiftly shed excess weight. They are faster fat shedders than your reliable **S** and **E** meals, but must not be abused and used too liberally for this talent. Included too often, they will harm your long term doable approach, rather than help. We'll teach you how to incorporate them into your life with judgment and respect.

An example of a **Fuel Pull** meal could be:

angel hair sliced cabbage sautéed in fat free chicken broth with diced chicken breast and our *Creamless Creamy* sauce

Don't think this is a small amount of food. It is a huge plateful and will leave you very satisfied.

On the following page you will see what a **Fuel Pull** looks like on a seesaw. Seesaws do not naturally bend down on both sides but **Fuel Pulls** utilize wacko science to defy the forces of nature!

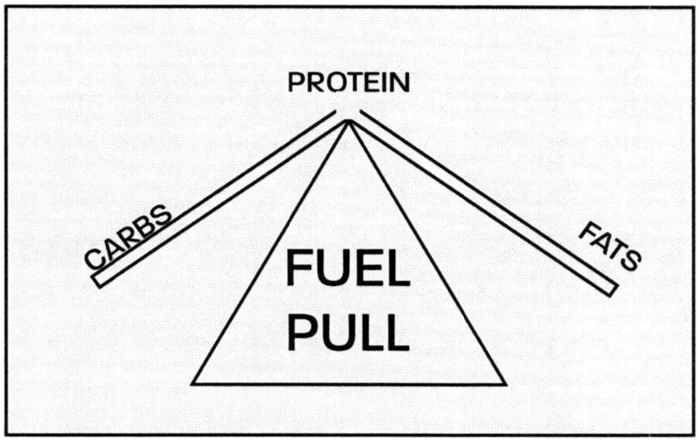

How They Work

As you know, your **S** and **E** parents make sure you have one healthy fuel of either fat or glucose to burn at each meal. The science behind the **Fuel Pull** is to strip both of these primary fuels almost fully away and force your body to immediately burn its own fat as fuel. This may sound like it goes against the premise of our whole book. In a way it does, and that's why the **Fuel Pull** does not have legal guardianship of your body. You visit with this mad scientist uncle on occasion, or a little more often if needed. You don't camp out at his house!

List Doublers

What on earth are you left with to eat if you pull the two primary fuels of fat and carbs away from your meal? That's easy—the foods that are on both **S** and **E** food lists. These are lean protein sources of both dairy and meat such as chicken breast, fish, lean ground turkey, egg whites, 0% Greek yogurt and 1% cottage cheese. Your non-starchy veggies are also on both lists (think greens, greens, greens), and you can fill up on them. Berries are also list doublers. We also encourage a bunch of whole food-based "trick foods" to make these **Fuel Pull** meals and snacks yummy and your tummy full. You'll probably be surprised just how delicious **Fuel Pulls** can be if put together smartly.

Speaking of trick foods, you'll notice konjac noodles are on both **S** and **E** lists. They can be an amazing tool to help make a **Fuel Pull** extra filling. Read more about their talents in *Foundation Foods*, Chapter 17 under the heading, Glucomannan. These noodles have no fats, calories, or carbs, yet they offer your body incredible health benefits. Take the example meal we mentioned of cabbage, chicken breast, and our special *Creamless Creamy* sauce. To this you can add a packet of glucomannan noodles. They'll blend in nicely and we'll be blown away if you do not feel overly stuffed if you finish all that food. Yet, the meal promotes weight loss galore.

Uniquely You

All of us drop excess weight differently. There is no cookie cutter ideal on how much you should lose in any certain period of time. However, in a *Life Long Approach*, Chapter 12 you will learn why fast weight loss is hazardous to your health and not something we encourage on this plan. As with the recommendation we made with **S Helpers**, too many **Fuel Pull** meals should not be included too often at the beginning of the plan, with the exception of using them as snacks and desserts. They can be used as easy breakfasts and a lunch or two, but not too often for evening meals.

Most mamas with excess weight will start to shed sensibly and surely eating predominantly **S** and **E** once they learn the ropes. It takes several weeks to become expertly familiar with the basic **S** and **E** core of this plan and the lifestyle changes it brings, so don't over stress yourself trying to include full **Fuel Pull** evening meals too early in the game. It won't do you any good to become an expert at creating **Fuel Pull** meals if you first do not have a good grasp on the core **S** and **E** plan. The core must take priority because it is your nourishing foundation and is more family friendly, even if, for whatever reason, it doesn't help you lose the weight you want. **Fuel Pulls** will defeat their own purpose if they try to stand alone or take too great a place in your overall diet. Once the core is learned, they can extend naturally to become a powerful addition to the plan.

If you get to the point where you have been doing the **S** and **E** core plan for three months or more without much fat loss to show for it, then it may be time to rely more on Uncle **Fuel Pull** with his big guns! Zero weight loss for much longer than three months can be discouraging, even if you are steering your home toward a healthier course. Negligible weight loss is not liable to happen on the **S** and **E** plan, but, it's possible. Some women have fat that doesn't want to budge. Usually this occurs when there are thyroid issues, sex hormone imbalances, or metabolisms that have slowed down from calorie restrictive diets. We will address hormonal issues in Chapters 33 and 34.

If your body refuses to burn its own adipose tissue after implementing **S** and **E** correctly, don't despair. **Fuel Pulls** will help you get to where you want to go, even in the face of tough challenges. Everybody needs to see some signs of progress; it's the hope that keeps us all going. And we don't want you giving up from disappointment!

For these very tough cases, we show how to do a structured fuel cycle in *One Week Fuel Cycle*, Chapter 28. This cycle forces your body to burn its adipose tissue, whether it wants to or not! It utilizes two full days of **Fuel Pull** meals back to back. Thankfully, they are safely sandwiched between full days of **S** and **E** so you won't be without primary fuels for too long. For these two **Fuel Pull** days, you'll eat only neutral foods like lean proteins, lots of non-starchy veggies, berries, and some other sanity saving helpers like whey shakes, glucomannan noodles, and puddings. Once you've finished a fuel cycle or two, you'll be very familiar with the way these meals work to help you through weight struggles and become an expert on how to naturally incorporate more of them into your individual **S** and **E** plan.

Fuel Pull in the Spotlight

These meals are still yummy and filling even though they sound like a science experiment.

A breakfast **E** meal of scrambled egg whites and veggies which would normally include a side of quinoa, toast, or a sprouted grain wrap can be stripped down to egg whites and veggies alone. Without the grain, it is now a **Fuel Pull**. You can still make it tasty with seasonings, spices, and a good sprinkle of Parmesan cheese (which doesn't have a lot of fat or carbs), or you can melt in a Laughing Cow cheese wedge for creaminess (another useful cheese without too much fat or carbs). Pair these scrambled egg whites with a whey shake made with a half scoop of whey, frozen strawberries, unsweetened almond milk, cocoa powder, plan approved sweetener, and ice. Now you have a tummy filling high protein breakfast without it containing a primary fuel. Although you are filled up from the good amount of food, your body does not have to burn glucose from the usual **E** grain before it gets down to burning your own body fat. You are purposefully removing one metabolic step to make your body burn up adipose tissue more swiftly.

Or, forego the egg whites and choose to indulge in our *Fat Stripping Frappa* or *Big Boy Smoothie* drinks for your **Fuel Pull** breakfast (*Morning Meals*, Chapter 18). These are sweet, creamy, and filling since they make a full quart or more and you get to drink all of that for breakfast. Wooah! We promised we'd never make you go hungry and these smoothies deliver.

Likewise, an **S** salad can also be stripped down to its core. Let's look at a typical **S** salad that might contain neutral grilled chicken breast as its protein source, but also include fats like cheese, nuts, or avocado, and a creamy or oily dressing. All good stuff for the core plan, but also easily converted to a **Fuel Pull**. Keep in the chicken breast for lean protein and all the non-starchy salad greens, but omit the full-fat cheese and nuts and utilize a much lighter dressing such as our *Hip Trim Honey Mustard* recipe. If desired, you could add some low-fat cottage cheese or a very small amount of skim mozzarella and a small handful of turkey bacon bits. Now, your body does not have to burn through a lot of **S** fat fuel before it burns your own body fat. Adipose tissue burning begins more promptly. Simple science for stubborn weight issues.

Short and Sweet

Is it now clear that removing these primary fuels causes much swifter reductions of weight? However, do you also see that you are pulling away much of the nourishment in the meal? **Fuel Pulls** are used as a good trick to ensure weight loss for stubborn cases, or even stubborn seasons in your journey. However, we stress again that they are **not** to be the constant part of your diet. We want you to achieve health at the cellular level rather than only on the bathroom scale.

Pulling the majority of fats and carbs from a meal will naturally lower the calorie content of that meal. This is only beneficial in spurts. Too low-calorie intake for too long and your body will start holding onto its body fat rather than shedding. Survival mode kicks in and your body won't want to burn through any calorie you eat. It believes it is in an emergency famine state and tries to preserve body fat to keep you alive. We want to avoid this at all costs, so **Fuel Pull** meals must be carefully infused into the nourishing **S** and **E** core of our plan if they are to be effective over the long term.

Here's the good news. Your metabolism will not slow down if **Fuel Pulls** are not overdone. Offer your body some nourishing fats and energizing glucose from **S** and **E** foods in the majority of your other meals and your body will have no reason to think it's being constantly undernourished. Our *One Week Fuel Cycle,* Chapter 28, goes into further detail about how often **Fuel Pulls** may be incorporated for very stubborn weight issues. We cannot tell you how often you will need to use them since your body and your weight loss journey will be unique. But, we do insist on putting a limit on their frequency to keep you safe and your metabolism from slowing down. Even for very tough weight loss cases, make sure that you keep at least half of all your meals per week made up of the basic **S** and **E** core of our plan.

Most people will never need **Fuel Pulls** to make up almost half of their weekly meals, but it is possible some could need close to that amount, particularly some postmenopausal women. This way, even mamas with seriously stubborn pounds can experience the progress and joy the rest of get to experience.

Snacks and Desserts

Fuel Pull snacks and desserts can be handy, even from the start of the plan. They're like Switzerland. They're neutral in fuel source, so even when eaten in close proximity to another meal, they do not care whether your upcoming or last meal was either **S** or **E**. In the next chapter, we'll show you how to naturally switch between **S** and **E** meals, but for now, we'll give you a little scenario on how **Fuel Pull** snacks can come to the rescue.

You arrive home late in the afternoon from the grocery store. You didn't get to eat your usual mid-afternoon snack that would naturally be about three hours away from your evening meal—the spacing we recommend when switching fuel styles. You are famished, but dinner is still a good hour away. You grab a piece of 85% dark chocolate and wolf it down while you put away the groceries, then gobble some nuts without even thinking. Then you remember, your lentil soup has been simmering in the crockpot all afternoon. You were planning to have an **E** supper, but now you've just **S'd** yourself. What to do?

Don't waste your lentil soup; it will be a **Crossover** night for you. Weight loss will not likely happen, but that's okay for one night. Remember, this is not a race to get skinny. You'll remember this lesson on what not to do for the future and probably won't repeat the mistake.

Fuel Pull snacks can help avoid the collision that just occurred. Grabbing a quick neutral snack, such as a half to full cup of 0% Greek yogurt topped with some berries or a teaspoon of Polaner All-Fruit Jam with Fiber, or munching on a stalk or two of celery smeared with a wedge of Laughing Cow cheese can keep you safely on track with whatever meal style you may have coming up. Our extra large *Fat Stripping Frappa* smoothie (*Morning Meals*, Chapter 18) is a wonderful, neutral fueled bridge between meals when hunger hits. Snacks that consist only of these neutral foods like lean proteins, non-starchy veggies, and berries are perfect non-committal foods.

Not only is 0% Greek yogurt a perfect **Fuel Pull** snack, our puddings made with glucomannan are another. If you came home from the grocery store knowing there was a glucomannan pudding in the fridge and all you had to do was spoon that deliciousness into your mouth, the nuts and chocolate gobbling would not likely have happened. Check out the glucomannan puddings and mousse recipes in *Desserts*, Chapter 23. Keep some made up in the fridge. Fast pudding hits can deter many an erroneous snack decision.

Low-fat cottage cheese is another great form of lean protein and can be yummied up with our plan approved sweetener and berries. Or, how about lean turkey deli slices wrapped around red pepper sticks? Or, a few *Joseph's Crackers* (*Snacks*, Chapter 24) with some tuna, and/or low-fat cottage cheese for an afternoon snack? Or scoop out the seeds from a cucumber and stuff it with low-fat cottage cheese or ricotta. A stevia-sweetened whey protein smoothie with water, ice, and quarter of a cup Greek yogurt or unsweetened almond milk is always good and fills the belly nicely. All these snack options are no brainers and won't interfere with the fuel burning of your next meal, whether **S** or **E**.

We don't recommend making all your snacks this neutral way. That could get very boring. It's a lot more fun to sometimes indulge yourself. What about an **S** snack of *Basic Cheesecake* (*Desserts*, Chapter 23) and coffee in the afternoon? Although, this works better when you have a little time to sit, savor, and enjoy.

Fuel Pull snacks are good when life gets very busy and you can't put a lot of thought into planning. They are also extremely weight-loss promoting, which can be either good or bad, depending upon your body type and ability to shed weight. Just because we are paring these neutral snacks with the words "extreme" and "weight loss," do not think they are always superior to our other **S** and **E** snacks. Remember, we eat to nourish our bodies, and although the foods in **Fuel Pulls** are healthy, they are not offering your body a primary fuel source, so they should not be your only constants at snack time.

Specialty Items

Pearl chats: Below is a list of specialty foods that help to make **Fuel Pulls** more doable. Most of them are healthy, but some are more short-cut inspired. Serene is leaving this list to me since her purism stamp of approval is not on all of them. Not all of them will be necessary, but we urge you to purchase glucomannan as soon as possible in order to include quick desserts on your menu. It is also the base to many of our sauces.

It's doubtful you'll feed your children full **Fuel Pull** meals, so some of these items may be purely for your own needs. You shouldn't feel like you have to purchase the fish and chicken items mentioned in the list since it may be more budget friendly to buy in bulk and cook up your own. But, if you're the Drive Thru Sue type and can spare the few dollars they cost, they might make quick prep **Fuel Pull** meals more realistic.

We have a couple of quick and easy **Fuel Pull** soups in *Lunches*, Chapter 20, but if five or 10 minute's prep is too much of a bother for you, consider any of the Light Progresso Soups you can buy from your local supermarket. They do not contain any artificial ingredients or MSG, and fit our **Fuel Pull** criteria since they are low enough in carbs, fat, and calories. Best of all, you can eat one whole can for a quick lunch and still easily be in **Fuel Pull** territory.

You'll notice some of the items are repeats since they appear on both our **S** and **E** lists. They really shine when involved in a **Fuel Pull** meal or snack so I think they need to be featured here again in their own setting.

A perfect example is konjac noodles, which are on both **S** and **E** lists since they don't contain a primary fuel. They are tasty with a sauce that contains fat for an **S** meal, e.g., a peanut based satay sauce. But, if you have stubborn weight, it is the smartest idea to save items like konjac noodles for **Fuel Pull** meals where they can do deep damage to defiant pounds. If you use them in a meal that strips back both fat and carbs, like our tasty *Sweet and Spicy Asian Stir Fry*, you will gain the most effectiveness. Add some diced chicken breast and Asian style veggies. Wow, a full bowl of this goodness is very filling, yet extremely low-calorie. This is called trick fasting! It's taking the idea of "dietary changes" to the fullest extreme to ensure a hotter metabolism! (I take my bow to all the imaginary applause)!

- unsweetened almond or flax milk (for puddings, smoothies, shakes, and coffee)
- glucomannan powder (for puddings, sauces and gravies, muffins, smoothies and shakes, available at www.netrition.com or www.konjacfoods.com)
- konjac noodles/yam noodles (available at www.netrition.com, www.konjacfoods.com, or international stores)
- fat free chicken broth (as the base to most **Fuel Pull** sauces and soups)
- 0% Greek yogurt

- 1% cottage cheese
- carton egg whites or Egg Beaters
- whey protein (Swanson Premium or Jay Robb)
- oat fiber (for making our **Fuel Pull** friendly muffin and other baked goods, available at www.netrition.com)
- defatted peanut flour (for adding in small amounts to **Fuel Pull** stir fry sauces, or to include in a our **Fuel Pull** friendly muffin, ice cream, and pudding recipes—we recommend Protein Plus Peanut Flour and Byrd Mill Peanut Flour Dark 12%, available at www.netrition.com)
- whole psyllium husk powder (for making egg white wraps, available online under Now brand or at health food stores like Trader Joe's)
- Laughing Cow or Weight Watchers light cheese wedges
- Wasa crackers (these work for snacks smeared with a Laughing Cow wedge and topped with tomato)
- GG crisp bread crackers (for snacks with lean toppings, available at www.netrition.com)
- Joseph's pitas
- Gorton's grilled Tilapia (handy low-calorie lean protein source that tastes great for an easy lunch idea, available at most grocery stores)
- Tyson grilled and ready chicken breast and lean steak strips (for use in salads or stir fries, half a package is one serving of 3 oz., the perfect amount for **Fuel Pulls**)
- Light Progresso soups
- Fat Free Reddi Whip (This goes great with some of our **Fuel Pull** desserts. While we don't approve of the Cool Whip product since it has a bunch of chemicals and high fructose corn syrup, Fat Free Reddi Whip is a healthier and overall more natural option, but still not up to Serene's purist standards. But, it tastes creamy, even though it has very little fat and is super low in calories. Used in moderation, it can make **Fuel Pull** desserts like our *Muffin in a Bowl* feel a lot more decadent. It also goes perfectly with **E** fruits).
- Zero or light calorie dressings. Green Valley Ranch is zero calorie, does not have sugar, fat, gluten, or artificial flavors and colors. It is available at www.netrition.com. Walden Farms calorie free dressings and Wishbone Salad Spritzers are more readily available at most supermarkets. They also work great for **Fuel Pull** salads, but have some less than pure ingredients.

Chapter 11

You Won't Miss Out

We hope you are making fast friends with **S** and **E** meals, and little by little, getting to know **S Helpers, Crossovers,** and **Fuel Pulls** as your own individual needs and journey takes shape. These five meal styles can ensure great body weight and improved overall health for everybody. Let's briefly sum up each meal for quick reference.

- **S** – Protein-centered meals that are always low-carb, but liberal with fats. They utilize fat as their chief fuel. (Weight loss.)
- **E** – Protein-centered meals that are medium-carb, but have less fat. They utilize glucose as their chief fuel. (Weight loss.)
- **S Helpers** – Protein-centered meals that are still lowish-carb and liberal with fats, but include a small amount of starch or fruit. They utilize fat as their chief fuel, but also briefly offer the body glucose first. (Slower weight loss.)
- **Crossovers** – Protein-centered meals that are medium-carb with liberal fats. They utilize tandem fueling, both fats and glucose. (No weight loss.)
- **Fuel Pulls** – Protein-centered meals that are low-carb and low-fat, which in turn cause overall lower calories. They utilize the body's own body fat for fuel since they do not contain a primary dietary fuel. (Fast weight loss.)

Goodbye Deprivation

Can you feel the freedom now? In the world of **S** and **E**, there is still a place for baking. We do not frown on homemade treats. This is a place where your female cravings won't be denied, but rather encouraged. Chocolate? Totally! Ice cream? Sure! In a few minutes these desserts can be whipped up with healthy changes that still offer wonderful flavor or texture.

It's a place for "man-food" like steak and buffalo wings. Bring them on! Your kitchen should be wafting delicious aromas that draw your family and guests. Here is a place where your husband will be satisfied with hearty meals without growing a big belly. Replace his baked potato with succulent, roasted summer squash—hopefully he'll love it! If not, there is usually one vegetable even picky eaters can learn to love if cooked up in a creative way.

This is all possible to enjoy while losing weight at a sensible pace. The key is to keep meals in their correct group, either **S** or **E**, and then depending upon your individual needs, **S Helpers**, **Crossovers**, and **Fuel Pulls** as you get further along in your journey.

Always keep in mind that if you want to lose weight, each meal or snack you eat must be one on our **S** and **E** plan, with **Crossovers** only making rare appearances. Don't decide to partially do this plan and only incorporate these meal styles every now and then. This plan needs to fully replace what you are doing now. It will take a little time to get the hang of it. We don't expect perfection from you in the initial days and weeks. You'll mess up sometimes, especially when you first start, but this way of eating is very forgiving. But, it's not so forgiving that it will be effective if you do it with a half-hearted approach.

Switching Meals

The fun thing in **S** and **E** land is that you can customize your own plan. If you are trying to lose weight, you do not have to switch these meal types in any synchronized order e.g., **S** then **E**, **E** then **S**—how boring!

What does your body feel like each day? Are you feeling tired? Prepare an **Energizing** meal. Are you craving comfort food? Heartiness? Go with **Satisfying**. We call this freestyling. As long as you are incorporating a good mix-up each week, you are fine. You will receive all that you need.

Please don't get obsessed with having to include 50 percent of each type of meal per day. You could change between the two meal types each day depending on how you feel, or do full days of either **S** or **E**. We caution against spending more than a few full days eating only one meal type—that's slipping into extremes.

If your personality type does not gel with freestyling and you'd rather follow a plan, we have dedicated *One Week Fuel Cycle*, Chapter 28 on how to do a structured and safe fuel cycle. We recommend it for short periods for a deep metabolism massage and very stubborn weight.

We don't want people to rigidly stick to the proposed confinements, as you have a family and a life, and we want you to learn how to steer this boat yourself. Freestyling your own changes can be as loose, or as rigid, as you would like it to be. Find your own rhythm.

Ideas for S and E Combinations

We don't know the patterns and "ins and outs" of your life, but here are some suggestions for implementing **S** and **E** into your life:

You may want to start out with two to three full **S** days to get to know this meal better, followed by an **E** day or day and a half. Then repeat. Grouping together a couple of days of the same meal type back to back assists in swifter weight reductions. It gets your body deep into one mode of fuel burning and then turns it upside down when you make the switch. Your metabolism loves that. After a couple of months of learning to implement **S** and **E**, you can also begin to throw some full days of **Fuel Pulls** in to the mix. That will be another huge step if you need help pushing off unmoving pounds.

This is not an absolute rule, but **S** is the best way to begin as it helps to get rid of extra sugar in your cells. They need to get emptied out, remember? This way you create a better cycle once you add in **E** meals and offer healthy amounts of glucose to more hungry cells.

But, grouping full days of one meal type is not the only way to lose weight with our plan. Simply freestyling **S** and **E** according to your wants, whims, or needs will still allow for solid weight loss. It might be a tad slower, but it will give you a lot more freedom.

Maybe you'll decide to do two or three full **E** days each week and let the rest be **S**. You could choose Tuesdays and Thursdays as your **E** days. Perfect! Or, you could choose to take three days each week and make them **E** style until the evening meal. On those three days, you would have **E** breakfasts, lunches, and afternoon snacks then switch to **S** on those evenings. That allows for more comforting, hearty food that most of us like to enjoy at supper time. It doesn't matter if you eat more **S** than **E**. Sometimes that's just more practical. We both prefer to have a few more **S** than **E** meals. We love being satiated by **S** meals and their creamier after-dinner desserts.

Perhaps you do not want your plan to be **S** dominant. You may be drawn toward eating lighter type **E** meals. Maybe you prefer lean meats, or, you may get addicted to our spectacular *Trim Healthy Pancake* recipe, which is **E,** and want to eat them almost every day. Go ahead. As **E** desserts, low-fat or 0% Greek yogurt sweetened up is always a yummy **E** option. Our puddings are perfect after **E** meals, so is our *Tummy Tucking Ice Cream* and our *Melt in Your Mouth Meringues.*

There is no right or wrong way to switch **S** and **E** as both meal types are healthy. Just don't get stuck in a rut eating only one type and miss out on all the nutrients God has available for you. Don't constantly eat **E** because it seems closer to what most conventional health gurus preach as acceptable. You'll miss out on the important fatty acids **S** meals give to nourish your brain, skin, nervous system, hormones and hair. Give some room for **S** in your life—your skin and brain will thank you for it.

It may suit your personality and family lifestyle better to have certain weekdays that are set aside for either **E** or **S**, then freestyle the weekend. Maybe you'll do Mondays and Tuesdays as **S**, Wednesday, Thursday will be **E** during the day, but then you'll switch to **S** for the evening meals on those days. Friday will be a full **S**. Then you can, more loosely, freestyle the weekend as you wish. If you want to wake up and have bacon and eggs for breakfast on Saturday just because you feel like it, grant yourself that wish—you are choosing **S**. Feel like a nice apple for a snack a few hours later? Go ahead, that will be **E**. You're naturally switching over.

All these ideas are examples. We leave it up to you. There are no strict rules as long as you receive the benefits from both meal types each week.

Winging it Versus Rigidity

Some people can take freestyling to the limit and completely "wing it." Maybe you love living on the edge and will decide to eat either **E** or **S** only when the time arrives to prepare your next meal. We all have different personalities. That option may horrify some; others may love the idea. There are those of us who like to be more spontaneous and not plan everything out. Pearl is more like this with her meal ideas. She plans out some of them and goes by the seat of her pants for others. Serene likes more structure and often allots certain days to one particular meal style.

If you do decide to be more of a "wing it" person, make sure you don't sabotage your weight progress by leaving meal prep to the last minute. Don't arrive in the kitchen at full hunger without a clue what to make. You're more likely to make poor decisions in that state and sabotage yourself. Get into your kitchen and start preparing your meal before hunger screams at you. Leaving things too late is a bad habit. If this is you, you may have to practice predetermining into which meal or day you will group **S** or **E**. Winging things too much could be your undoing. Jot down your choices and meal ideas for each day of the week. Magnet them on the fridge and they will remind you when you open it to retrieve food for your meal preps.

We have a friend who designed a weekly meal schedule with our plan in mind. She printed out charts with each meal and snack typed out for each day of the week, with either **S** or **E** written above it. Now, that's super organized. It was too rigid for us to implement, but some have the gift of organization, and this worked for her.

A Day in your Life

Starting out, a general day freestyling **S** and **E** could look a little like this:

For breakfast you could have a bowl of oatmeal, berries, and low-fat Greek yogurt – **E**.

For lunch, how about sautéed salmon in butter and a dash of red wine over a heavily dressed bed of greens, with balsamic vinegar, extra virgin olive oil, and crumbled goats' cheese. Follow with a decadent Vienna coffee, topped with pure whipped cream. – **S**

In the afternoon, don't forget your snack—perhaps a green apple with 1 tsp. peanut butter or almond butter – **E**. If you are still hungry (who isn't?), try a glass of low-fat kefir, or a glass of almond milk whipped into a shake with NuStevia Pure White Stevia Extract Powder or Truvia, vanilla, and raspberries. Throw in a scoop of undenatured, chocolate whey protein powder for a further protein and metabolic boost, or add some glucomannan powder to thicken it up into a pudding consistency—yum! You're still in **E** mode for this snack. Dangerous four o'clock munchies are cured and your body loves you.

Who doesn't like comfort food for supper? Meat loaf topped with a tomato glaze sounds good. Have a side of decadent creamed spinach or creamy mashed cauliflower with it. Don't forget your side salad with creamy dressing and a few toasted pecans – **S**.

There's no insulin delivery truck tonight, so we won't feel guilty about having dessert. *Chocolate Dipped Cream Pops* – **S**, or *Tummy Tucking Ice Cream* – **Fuel Pull**, whichever you desire. Check *Desserts*, Chapter 23.

Can you believe you can reach your ideal weight eating like this? It doesn't have to be as fancy as we described. We got rather carried away with the red wine and the goat's cheese. That's what happens when we sit next to each other and talk about food. It's an exciting subject for us and we tend to get overly enthusiastic. But, you get the picture. Decadent food need not be fattening.

You can make your meals as simple as you prefer as long as you stick to the principles. That salmon based **S** style lunch we were talking about could have been ready in less than ten minutes and simplified to the basics. Don't feel intimidated or overwhelmed if you are more of a practical person in your approach to food. It's as simple as one, two, three.

1. Sauté a thawed salmon fillet in butter and seasonings.
2. Rip up some organic lettuce, dump it on your plate, and pour on healthy, low glycemic dressing.
3. Eat and enjoy, then savor some healthfully sweetened coffee with a spot of cream.

Is that too hard?

We, and the many people we've helped, are living proof this way of eating works. People often ask how we stay so slim. What is our secret? The example day we just described is our very hard to follow diet! Honestly, we feel sorry for every person who doesn't eat like us! Now you know our delightful secret, you can spread the word to others. It's hard to suppress such good news.

Want to see another day of "diet doldrums and deprivation?" Here goes another day of freestyling:

In the morning, wake early and sip on your green tea or coffee while you quickly prepare two or three fried eggs in butter over caramelized onions and tomatoes seasoned with Spike and a little cayenne pepper – **S**.

Mid morning munchies are satisfied with a large cup of our amazing glucomannan pudding – **Fuel Pull**.

Lunch will only take a few minutes to whip up. You'll dine on leftover sliced chicken, sautéed in a non-stick pan with 1 tsp. coconut oil, a dash or two of Bragg Liquid Aminos or tamari, and black pepper. Throw into that pan ¾ cup of pre-cooked brown rice or a full cup of quinoa. Rip up some organic lettuce, add a few baby tomatoes, drizzle with a light vinaigrette, top with your seasoned chicken and rice or quinoa, and you have a great lunch – **E**.

For an afternoon pick me up, rev your metabolism with a delicious and refreshing cucumber boat. Scoop the seeds out of a cucumber and spoon low-fat cottage cheese into each half. Sprinkle with a small amount of finely chopped toasted pecans seasoned with Bragg Liquid Aminos and cayenne pepper. This is a **Fuel Pull**—a neutral snack as it's not going too far in either the fat or carbs direction. If you are still hungry, try our *Fat Stripping Frappa* (*Morning Meals*, Chapter 18) made with ½ scoop of whey protein. Trust us, you couldn't possibly be hungry after that.

The whole family will enjoy salmon burgers and cheesy broccoli tonight, starting with crisp celery stuffed with peanut butter. The children can have their burgers inside whole wheat pitas with mayo, but you'll have yours with an extra serving of that decadent broccoli – **S**.

You may want to end this meal with a creamy, sensibly sweetened decaf coffee or chai tea and a couple of pieces of plan-approved chocolate for dessert like our *Skinny Chocolate* (*Desserts*, Chapter 23) – **S**.

Pearl chats: A practical way to have quick and easy access to rice or quinoa for **E** meals or **S Helpers** is to freeze single servings in Ziploc bags. I steam up a big bag of rice or quinoa and separate it into ¾ **E** cup portions. To tell the truth, I have seldom used rice for myself in the last year as I think quinoa is nutritionally superior and have come to love the taste better. I also do **S Helper** portions of ½ cups for quinoa (you would use ¼ cups for rice). I put these in the freezer to pull out whenever I need them. The rice or quinoa will thaw quickly in the pan along with your other food, or let it defrost in a bowl of warm water while you prepare your other food. You don't have to think about measuring or staying under your **E** 45 gram limit or your **S Helper** 15 gram limit that way.

Serene chats: About that coffee we mentioned. The Swiss water process of decaffeinating coffee uses no chemicals and is the purest way to have a caffeine free cuppa. The only reason we suggested decaf is that we were describing an evening coffee used as a night cap, where the more stimulating effects of caffeinated coffee are not appreciated. You don't want to go to sleep wired up.

Three Hours Between S and E

It is important to remember to keep at least two and a half hours, three being more optimum, between switching from **S** to **E,** or **E** to **S**. This ensures that higher glycemic loads in **E** meals will not be digested along with higher fats in **S** meals, which cause the unwanted head-on collision. At first, switching may take some thought, but after a while, it becomes second nature. If you have trouble switching meal types, it might be better for you to start out trying full days of either **S** or **E**.

We don't want you to get too legalistic regarding which day you are on. Your husband may want to take you out to eat on a whim. It's your **E** day, but he's an awesome guy and wants to treat you to an evening out at the steak house—go with the flow. A steak means an **S** meal and you'll remember to have a non-starchy veggie side instead of the usual baked potato. Be **E**la**S**tic! That's what this plan is all about.

Match Your Desserts

If you are a dessert lover, this is the only time when there's not a natural pause of about three hours between snacks or meals like there naturally is between an afternoon snack and an evening meal. Dessert is usually eaten within an hour or two after a meal while whatever you had for that meal is still being metabolized. Don't eat an **E** evening meal and then reward yourself with an **S** dessert afterward. Clash!

All our **Fuel Pull** friendly desserts make this a non concern because they won't cause a fat and carb collision. But, you'll also want to try our delicious **S** desserts that we have included. Always remember to keep those for after an **S** meal. Please don't go eating heavy cream, *Basic Cheesecake,* or our *Skinny Chocolate* recipe after you've dined on **E** fare. You will only put yourself in **Crossover** territory and that inhibits weight loss.

After an **E**, if you feel the need to finish your meal with something sweet, enjoy one of our glucomannan puddings, our *Melt in your Mouth Meringues*, some sweetened skim ricotta with a few sliced strawberries, or some stevia-sweetened 0% Greek yogurt with a little fruit. Or, look in *Desserts*, Chapter 23 for more **E** and **Fuel Pull** dessert options, maybe starting with *Tummy Tucking Ice Cream* which is a cinch to make.

Our **S** only desserts are truly yummy and indulgent and we'd love you to get to try them out too. This is why we like to eat more **S** than **E** meals in the evening. Some of us just feel better about life when we can eat chocolate after dinner!

Make Sense with Snacks

As with most ideas about nutrition, there are two opposing mindsets when it comes to snacking. One side says to eat small meals no more than every three hours apart. Advocates of frequent snacking warn that going for too long without eating slows down metabolism.

The other side believes it's good for the body to skip snacks, and even meals. Some current popular diets like The Warrior Diet suggest a person forego food all day and then have one huge meal at night. A more moderate approach to this meal fasting concept is gaining popularity with the Eat Stop Eat diet. A dieter takes two 36 hour periods each week and fasts from all food, but is encouraged to eat sensibly the rest of the time. The Five Hour Diet has similar principles.

We don't believe skipping meals (unless for spiritual reasons) and then filling up with one or two big meals is the best thing for a mama. Diets that try to recapture the culinary life of historical hunting groups, who often fasted through the day and gorged on their catch at night, don't make too much sense in our lifestyles. Along with paleo diets, you may notice that primitive tribal diets are all the rage these days. But, they're another distraction from the simple dietary truths outlined in the Bible.

There is no need to esteem any diet, whether tribal or modern doctor derived, over the words of God. Thankfully, God has a lot to tell us about diet in the Bible, so we're not left wondering.

There is no relevance in these warrior or tribal type diets to the life demands of busy mothers. Some supporters of this snack and meal skipping approach point to the large cats of the animal kingdom who only kill and eat about once a day. Most of the day, lions, tigers, and leopards lay around conserving energy. They don't have to clean homes, run errands, homeschool, and cook meals for husbands and children, etcetera.

Again, there is balance. You don't have to have a snack if you are too full, but going too long without food can be the perfect set up for over-eating later. This causes a higher glycemic response from sheer portion size. We suggest you shouldn't go much longer than four hours without food during the day. Many an overweight person becomes that way by skipping breakfast, maybe even lunch, and consuming most of their calories at night.

But, we are all different. Some feel better snacking. It keeps blood sugar in healthier margins (especially protein rich snacks). Others feel better eating only three meals a day with the occasional snack thrown in. Once again, beware of extremes.

Eating every two hours or less will interfere with the fuel metabolism of the last meal. You don't have to cater to every little hunger pang you feel, unless you are nursing a baby very frequently and the pangs are true hunger. Hunger pangs that occur only a couple of hours after a meal for non-nursing women are not true hunger pangs. They're usually only the mind and a body that wants to please itself whenever it desires. True hunger is a healthy natural state for the body and enables you to really enjoy your next meal. It's healthy to have moderate hunger pangs before your next meal or snack. Allow your body to enter that hunger state before your main meals.

Warning! Don't wait until you are famished! Feeling extreme hunger is usually bought on by skipping meals. Overeating often follows as a result and that cycle does not do your body any favors.

Spacing meals or snacks every three to four hours is a well balanced approach if you are not out hunting with a spear in the jungle or striped like a tiger! Remember, if you are mothering children, or especially if you are pregnant or nursing, fasting is not a natural state for your body. Three medium-sized meals with a small snack or two is a perfect way to ensure a fired up metabolism all day long. If you are nursing a baby through the night, or exercising intensely, you may even want to incorporate another snack or two.

Our *Snacks*, Chapter 24, has plenty of great ideas to keep you happy in between meals. Many of them are labeled as **S** or **E**, but keep in mind all the **Fuel Pull** snack ideas which can easily bridge you from one meal to the other without having to match fuel styles.

Pearl chats: You don't have to eat a snack if you feel too full. But, be sure it wasn't because you over ate at the last meal. I don't usually eat a mid-morning snack unless I ate a very early breakfast. I don't usually eat breakfast as soon as I wake up. I know people say you should eat a big meal first thing in the morning, but I can't do it! I have a hot drink of either coffee, or green tea, and ease my way into the day and eat about an hour or hour and a half later. It's best to not go too much longer, after waking, without kick starting your metabolism with some good protein.

If I eat breakfast around 8.30 am, lunch at noon will be a perfect three and a half hours later. I can easily switch fuel styles by then if I desire. By 3.00 to 4.00 pm in the afternoon, I am very hungry again. I never, ever miss my afternoon snack. Again, I can enjoy whatever I like, either **S** or **E,** or keep it Swiss and have a **Fuel Pull.**

Serene chats: Because I have been either pregnant or nursing for the last many years, as soon as my eyelids open, I am ravenous. In fact, it is hard to concentrate on preparing the children's breakfast before I feed myself, but I make it somehow. I never miss a snack and always eat six meals about three hours apart. None of my meals are huge. I never arrive at a meal hour without having given it previous thought. I love food and love thinking about it and planning ahead.

This works out well as I make health conscious decisions for my next meal or snack while I am already satisfied. This safeguards against hasty decisions caused from meals too far apart that would normally make someone "grab a carb."Instead of reaching for quick fixes from desperate hunger, I have healthy pre-made snacks prepared like my protein *Fridge Fudge* (*Snacks*, Chapter 24) or have pre-prepped items for my next meal. I consistently ask myself these questions, "What is my protein for my next meal?" Or, "Have I had enough raw life-giving foods today?" Or, "Do I need to tweak my metabolism and refuel my glycogen with an **E** meal, or go lighter and have a **Fuel Pull** snack?"

This may sound like a lot of thinking about food, but they are quick checks I can tick off in a jiffy. They stop harmful food fantasies and destructive cravings.

Chapter 12

Life Long Approach

Although the **S** and **E** plan is designed to steadily shrink fat cells if they are too large, we want to caution you against seeking very fast weight loss. Fast weight loss should never be your goal and it is definitely not what we promote. You're reading the wrong book if you are hoping for large losses on the scale every week. Eating the **S** and **E** way is not a race to be skinny. It is a sensible way to restore food sanity back into your life and home and healthy weight will develop naturally.

Unless you are extremely overweight, which makes dropping large amounts of pounds naturally faster, we don't want you to lose much more than a pound a week. Rapid weight loss becomes catabolic, which means there is more breaking down of the body than building up. It goes against the anti-aging premise of this book. Run far away from magazine and book headlines that scream, "Six Weeks to a Bikini Ready Body!" Titles like that are the nemeses of this book. Don't think of this as a race, but a lifelong approach.

Mamas who only need to trim down a little (20 pounds or less to lose), will likely see even slower moves on the scale than a weekly pound. Do not freak out and become obsessed if things aren't happening fast enough for you! Please do not weigh daily; you'll feel like you're going insane. That practice is a joy robber.

Diets that tout ridiculously fast weight reduction tax the adrenal glands and mess with your hormones. The catabolic hormone cortisol, which comes from stress, will start to pump through your body if you shed weight too fast. After a while, this high cortisol state will cause your weight to plateau and your results will halt. You may have lost 40 pounds super fast, but the remaining 20 pounds may become stubborn and immovable, especially around your middle. This is because excessive cortisol, after it eats you up, will put on or keep weight in your mid-section.

Gently Does It

We openly admit that diets like Atkins, which even put restrictions on the amount of non-starchy vegetables you can eat, or the opposite extreme diets that are higher grain and restrict fat, may initially cause faster weight loss than this **S** and **E** plan. Eliminating whole food groups will initially shed pounds swiftly since they are shaking the body out of its usual metabolic processes.

The prolonged state of ketosis induced by Atkins is the reason weight will usually drop off very speedily in the beginning of that program. But, we don't want your body pushed into an extreme state. Remember, we are finally learning to not be snared by extreme diets. Hopefully, we are not coming across as Atkins bashers, because lots of people have made great body transformations by implementing its principles. There are certainly some things to respect about that diet, but we seek a more healthy balance of all the food groups that God created for our optimal health.

We want you to be nourished, to enjoy eating as much as we do, and to watch with satisfaction as your husband and children gather around the table to a delicious, healthy meal that will build rather than destroy health. Weight management will naturally occur as you learn to steer your home to a smarter nutritional destination where whole foods reign and sugars and starches lose their stronghold.

The Tortoise, not the Hare

We want to remind you of Isaiah 40:11, *"He gently leads those that are with young."*

You may be a mother with a lot of physical exhaustion and responsibility. It is important that you stay nourished and strong. Constantly spilling ketones into your urine from almost completely restricting carbs is not a nurturing state for your body. Neither is it wise to enter into other diet extremes and deny your neurotransmitters and endocrine system the healthy fats they need for optimum function.

We know people who have dropped a lot of weight doing the HCG diet. You may have heard of this diet which has become quite popular in recent years. The pregnancy hormone, HCG, is either ingested sublingually or injected into the dieter every day for cycles of about three to five weeks, while at the same time the dieter eats a 500 calorie a day diet during the cycle. The diet includes very little carbs and is also very low-fat. It is similar in idea to our **Fuel Pulls**, but more extreme. It strips away the body's two main fuel sources, but it does it for long periods of time. It is essentially a starvation diet!

The HCG hormone is supposed to help curb hunger and cravings, reset the metabolism, and eliminate some of the usual problems of extreme dieting like skin sagging and low energy. The jury is out whether all the negatives are actually avoided by using this hormone, or whether it is a placebo effect, but there is no denying the diet works, and works quickly. People are able to drop enormous amounts of weight in a short time since they're literally starving for fuel so the body essentially eats itself to keep living.

Despite claims to the contrary by promoters of this diet, the weight often piles back on after the extreme diet stops. The Medi-Weightloss diet is another one that utilizes a 500 calorie a day diet. However, it is doctor supervised. We know a few people who have kept their weight off after dropping fast weight on these extreme diets by adopting our plan, or other low glycemic plans. Instead of gaining back weight, they even lost more weight using the principles we encourage, but very slowly. On the whole, most people we have observed who did HCG or the Medi-Weightloss diet put the weight back on because they never learned how to eat for life and simply returned to their old ways. These diets do have maintenance guidelines, but they are not fun to continue, so back on goes the weight.

We want this to be a gentle road for you. Seek a slow and steady reduction of fat. The tortoise beats the hare every time. If you are a quick loser and consistently lose large numbers on the scale using **S** and **E** alone, we strongly suggest adding some **S Helpers** or **Crossovers** to steady your weight loss. You will save your skin from sagging. Too fast a weight loss does not allow your skin to shrink in harmony with your decreasing body shape.

Have Patience

If you're not drastically overweight, but you still have a bit to lose, we reiterate again, please don't expect miraculous, swift drops in dress sizes eating the **S** and **E** way. In the first month or so, you may notice your clothes are looser, but you don't see any changes on the scale. We have helped several people who did not see actual weight loss in pounds well into month two.

Other mamas start our plan after flip-flopping from other diets. Some of them had lost 30 pounds or so on eating programs that were both unhealthy and impossible to live on. Substantial drops of weight like these are almost always followed by a plateau. It's the body's way of surviving and holding on to its fat stores for dear life.

If you're starting **S** and **E** in a similar state, you may have to wait patiently for your body to realize you are not going to deprive it of nutrition. Gradually, it will let go of its vice grip on your adipose tissue. The scale will move eventually. If you find your clothes fit better, even without a loss on the scale, this indicates that all the healthy protein is strengthening muscles and making a healthier body, fat to muscle ratio. This is a great sign. Keep at it. Your body will let go of fat at its own pace.

Be aware that whenever you are losing weight, it never happens at a consistent pace. There is usually a very frustrating rhythm that goes more like—little drop, big drop, no drop, no drop, no drop, medium drop, little drop, big drop, no drop, and so forth. Your body will naturally pause after each loss of about 20 pounds Let it regroup. Try not to get mad or sad and want too much too soon. That mindset leads to defeatism where you may be tempted to go back to your old ways rather than being patient and staying the course.

Keep the overall, long term goal in mind. You are establishing healthy eating patterns now for your whole family. You are learning to include all food groups and understand the science behind how each of them impacts your body.

Time to Intensify

If you have not seen sensible weight shedding by the three month mark, that would be your green light to read Chapter 28 and get started on the *One Week Fuel Cycle*. Do the suggested cycles, then start incorporating more **Fuel Pulls** into your own freestyling approach to **S** and **E**. It will happen, Mama.

The Magic of Change

"Change ups" are what keep a metabolism fired up. Switching fuel sources between **S** and **E** and then sometimes leaving them almost completely out with **Fuel Pulls** keeps your metabolism hot and revved. Constantly consuming the same fuel over and over is a slim figure killer. In short, you should burn glucose at some meals (**E**), fat at other meals (**S**), purely your own body fat at certain snacks and meals (**Fuel Pull**), and don't forget tandem fuel meals (**Crossover)** as you get closer to goal in your journey. This way, no adaptation takes place. Even if you don't have a weight issue, a revved metabolism is important for more than weight issues. A highly thermogenic body is healthier and more youthful.

Never Adapt! The Answer to Calorie Confusion

We disagree with the folk who say weight loss is all about calories. Energy in, energy out—that's been debunked. Constant calorie monitoring makes for a miserable life. But, as always, there's the other side of the argument which says calories don't matter at all. This side believes weight problems are purely about hormones, namely, insulin and leptin. Diets like Atkins and paleo hold more to this theory.

We agree that hormones matter and make sure to incorporate metabolic hormonal principles into the core of our plan. We do this by preventing the over stimulation of insulin through carb heavy meals. But, this is not the full picture either. Calories do matter in the end. It's no good to bury our heads in the sand and pretend they don't exist. Nevertheless, people take the wrong approach when they set a low daily number and try to shoot for it. While you shouldn't have to meticulously count calories, it is very important to change them up so your body does not become too accustomed to a continual amount. Let this be your mantra: "Never Adapt!"

The beauty of our **S** and **E** plan is that not only do we have fuel change ups occurring between glucose and fats, but we naturally have calorie change ups going at the same time. **E** meals are usually lower in calories than **S** meals, due to their more lean protein content and medium amounts of starches. But, that doesn't mean they're better. If you constantly stay on a lowish calorie diet like many of our **E** meals offer, your metabolism will eventually adjust. That's no good, because that means you'll have to end up eating less and less food or you'll gain weight again.

And, it's certainly not better, worse actually, to stay on extreme weight loss meals like our **Fuel Pulls**. Too long a time eating extreme low-calorie meals like those and you'll have to eat like a bird for the rest of your life, or once again you'll gain weight.

Staying on **S** meals only, which are naturally higher in calories due to fats, is another metabolism dead end. Continual **S** meals for weeks, months, and years on end can be calorie abuse! There is only so much high calorie food the body can take before it says, "Yeah, this is good food, all this cream, peanut butter, red meat, and butter, but I don't care how low-carb it is, you're stuffing it down my throat every meal so I've decided not to burn it up in retaliation . . . so there!" The fact that fats are higher in calories is not a bad thing. Don't get us wrong, we love fats and creamy foods and want you to enjoy plenty of them. But, always remember with calories at any constant, high or low, your very smart body will catch on.

Constantly counting calories to keep them low, or the opposite approach of calorie abuse by eating constant fat-laden meals are polar extremes. There's no balance in either place. We wisely and happily meet in the middle by keeping to our mantra of "never adapt."

These two opposing calorie camps can be likened to many extreme arguments, but after some debate between ourselves, we agreed on using the example of two pregnant women. The first opts to have a c-section for no other reason than because she only trusts in conventional medical intervention rather than the natural flow and rhythm of her own body. The second believes only in unassisted home birth, even in the face of a situation where the baby is failing and she and her husband have no training on what to do. They're both extreme camps and neither are sound mindsets. In reality, there are times where medical interventions like c-sections are necessary and there are also situations where home births can be safe beautiful experiences. Both sides of these arguments have valid points; both have some nonsense. The same goes for extremes in calorie beliefs. We don't have to pitch our tents on either side of the divide. Yes, calories count, but if we're naturally changing up our fuels, we don't need to be bothered with constantly counting them.

Tossing Balls

Picture yourself throwing one ball up and down. It's quite easy, and once you've learned how to catch that one ball well, you don't have to burn much energy to do it. You can mindlessly throw up then catch. It becomes so easy that it's natural to become lazy with the simple process.

That's essentially what happens when you stay on a diet that utilizes only one fuel type or one setting of calories. Some diets like Atkins and the paleo approach throw a constant **S** ball at you. Others like the South Beach Diet or Mediterranean Diet use the **E** ball. These **E** type diets wisely warn you against spiking your blood sugar and encourage a focus on lean proteins and whole grains, but it's still the same ball over and over. Some extreme diets like HCG and Biggest Loser even want you to throw the **Fuel Pull** ball up and down, again and again, for long periods of time. Dangerous!

All these different diets that hit upon a certain metabolic principle have merits. They wouldn't become famous and offer results if they didn't work and we can learn a lot from most of them. But, they keep you doing a similar thing continually. One ball up and down. Your body can't help but get lazy with the process. However, with two or more balls (alternating **S** and **E** balls), your body has to get more active to keep catching. **Fuel Pulls** are the lowest of all calorie meals. Including some of these now and then throws a third ball at your body to juggle. Your body has to be constantly on its toes to manage the change ups. You'll be burning all sorts of energy trying to figure out what ball is coming at you next. The magic of alternating these meal types is how your metabolism becomes a furnace.

If you're in tune with your body, these changes can occur naturally. After a few high calorie meals, it feels natural for your body to crave lighter fare. After lots of fat, it's time for leaner foods. After several meals of glucose, it's time to give that metabolic pathway a break. After feasting, you can listen to your body when it whispers, "Give me refreshing light food for a meal or two."

It's the same natural inclination as when you crave savory or salty foods after too much sweet. After lots of work, you feel like resting; after lots of rest, you feel like working. In the exercise world, rest periods are as important as the days of light workouts and then heavier workouts. It's the cycle of life.

Do not make each day a constant diet.

While it's good to learn about this premise, and some people can naturally do it, our plan makes sure these changes will happen, even if you don't easily hear the inner whisper of your body.

The fantastic thing about not getting stuck using only one dietary principle is that your food options expand extraordinarily. You have a smorgasbord of healthy options open to you at every meal. You can choose to eat grains and lean proteins, or you can choose lots of fat and dine on red meat and greens. You can choose to pull your calories back and eat lightly with a **Fuel Pull**, comforted with the fact that you get to eat more heartily any time you choose. We find it's almost a delight to incorporate some very low-calorie meals because we are not being forced to do it. When your body is nourished so often with lots of fat in **S** meals and healthy grains in **E** meals, pulling them out sometimes feels like a natural pause—a healthy break. A **Fuel Pull** actually feels like a welcome change.

Downfall of Popular Diets

Not only do many popular diets have you throwing up the same ball over and over again, we don't like that they pull out complete macronutrients. Diets that center on an **E** meal premise alone, like South Beach Diet or Weight Watchers, cannot offer the same superfood approach as we propose. Nevertheless, we respect the work of Dr. Arthur Agatston, the founder of the South Beach Diet. His books have brought paramount dietary information to the general public.

But, healthy fats are one of the body's number one superfoods. Diets that do not contain certain fats that are essential for optimal health and longevity are not complete. Neither are they nurturing. If you lived on our **E** meals alone, your hair and skin would not reach the same luster, your hormones would decline earlier, and delaying the aging process would be harder to achieve.

The Mediterranean Diet is another similar approach. While these diets use some olive oil and small amounts of fish oils, they never bathe the body in the superpower of lubricating, rejuvenating fats. They are fearful of Bible-based fats like butter and some fatty meats. They dab a little oil here and there, but never really grease the wheel. They entirely exclude healthy saturated fats which are now realized to be fantastic foods for the body. Any diet that does not allow you to get your fill of healthy fats like butter will end up making you crave forbidden food. We were designed to want fat because we need it. That makes sense.

Fat Keeps You on Track

It is more difficult to stay on these lean diets indefinitely, because diets without enough fat are simply not as satisfying. Lean protein is not enough to fully curb hunger for very long. Fat is the key for satiation. "Lean only" diets do not feed and nourish the endocrine, neurological, and nervous systems of the body. Our hormones are made from cholesterol. Our nerves and brains are protected by fat and we should not deny the body of its basic needs. Dr. Mariano, a renowned anti-aging MD and psychiatrist, says that interfering with cholesterol production can impair brain function. On his website, he talks of how lack of cholesterol causes "memory problems, mood problems, and even frank confusion."

He goes on to say, "Cholesterol is the signal from astrocytes that tell neurons where to make new connections (synapses). Cholesterol is a hormone/neurotransmitter in the central nervous system. It is necessary to form memory. Cholesterol makes up half of the dry weight of the brain."

Also, it's harder to treat yourself without fat. You can try to convince yourself it tastes like the real deal, but it can't compare to the genuine article.

Celebrate Food

Each food group is a gift to us to enjoy for life. **S** and **E** meals provide all the nutrients needed for a long term sustainable way of eating. They also offer the pleasure of variety. This is crucial for success as it easy to get sick of the same foods over and over again. Including all macro-nutrients, all fuels, and a wide variety of caloric meals is the way to celebrate God's abundant gift of food to us. With this celebratory approach, we also keep in mind that we don't have to include everything in the same meal.

Chapter 13

The Real World

One of the main things that bugs us about many of the weight loss books we have read (that's a l-o-o-o-o-t of books), is that they are impractical if you are trying to raise a family. A lot of the recipes they include sound rather scrumptious. They're nice in idea, but in reality, they often use expensive ingredients and usually only make enough food for one or two people. And they often take time and expertise to achieve the end result. Who cares about gourmet when you have many mouths to feed? It's 4.30 pm in the afternoon, your boys are tossing the football in the house, the living room looks like a tornado hit, the baby wants to nurse, and your husband will be home and hungry in 45 minutes! Gourmet Shmourmet! Fast, filling, and yummy is the only goal that matters at this point.

We want to teach you how to eat **S** and **E** style while still being able to merge your needs with those of your whole family. You shouldn't have to make complete separate meals for yourself that involve leeks and parsnips while the rest of the family gets by on frozen pizzas. The exception is when you particularly want to eat your own thing.

Lunch is a good time for eating a meal that is different from your children's if your husband is not home at that time. You can have the option of preparing one of our super speedy soup, salad or salmon recipes especially for moms. The children (if they homeschool) can eat whole wheat mac n' cheese if that is what they are begging for. You can find a few minutes of sanity and sit down to eat something that makes you feel like you're an adult human.

The evening meal should always be for everyone. We'll teach you how to make that happen while on plan.

But, we have to preface with a caution. Even though you're going to be mostly eating the same core food as your children at many meal times, you must first have a mind adjustment and always remember that their requirements are different than yours.

"Kid Food Mom"

For the sake of convenience, it is easy to fall into the trap of thinking you can eat whatever your child eats, but it's devastating to a trim figure. While you can learn to merge your own and your children's needs skillfully, we want to show you an example of what not to do. You may have recognized yourself in one of the four women we introduced to you at the beginning of this book. You may know this next woman, too.

Scene opens . . . the action looks familiar. You've seen this picture before . . . maybe you were once the star of such a scene. It's a beautiful summer's day and the children are playing happily at a park. Mom sits under the shade watching them.

Time for lunch! Back run the children to mama. They're hungry. She takes out baggies of peanut butter and jelly sandwiches on wheat bread and gives one to each child, keeping one for herself. She had taken the time earlier that morning to wash grapes and put those in individual baggies, too. Each child gets a bag of red grapes and so does mom. Next come the cheese puffs, individual baggies of cheese puffs for the children and one for mom, too. Let's not forget the juice boxes. This sweet mama is prepared. She gives one juice box to each child and drinks one herself—it's a hot day after all. Little does she realize that this typical scenario will punish her waistline, and of mothers all over the world.

The packed lunch looks pretty harmless on the surface. Aside from the cheese puffs, the bulk of it is not considered junk food. Yet, it is all sugar in the bloodstream. Mom is more insulin-resistant than her children. The peanut butter and jelly on wheat causes high glucose in her blood stream, and the grapes add to it. The cheese puffs take it over the limit, and the juice is the final nail in the coffin. Carbs, carbs, all of it, with only a smattering of peanut butter to give any protein. An innocent looking child's meal caused mother's poor pancreas to surge more insulin, which will put fat on her belly and butt! Double drat! The children run back to play and burn up most of the carbs. Mom keeps on chatting to her MOPS group friends, burning nothing except her shoulders.

Your Different Needs

Human beings require different fuel sources at different times of their lives. You don't suck on a bottle of milk all day as babies do. Babies need those liquid carbs to grow fast and develop all that yummy baby fat that we love to squeeze. Neither should you go around eating exactly what your six year old eats. He's growing; you are not. He's naturally more active than you are.

Remember the picture we described of the baby birds with their mouths open and ready to accept food? Your children have cells like that, ready to accept insulin. You do not. If you are going to eat "kid food," you are very likely going to say goodbye to a slim figure.

While they're still growing, your children need more whole grain carbs than you do. They can handle white potatoes. But, since insulin resistance is now becoming an epidemic, even among children, creating a home environment where carbs do not rule the roost will help those children who have already developed weight problems. Growing children with weight issues should have **S Helper** servings of starches or even **Crossovers**, but never carb binges. Watch what happens when those excess starches are replaced with more proteins, non-starchy veggies and healthy fats—those children naturally lean out.

Take Two, Action!

Let's revisit the scene at the park starring our "Kid Food Mom." What could she have done differently? It's not complicated to turn this scene around. Mama could have still made a sandwich for herself using one of our **S** breads, such as *Bread in a Mug* (*Muffins, Breads, and Pizza Crusts*, Chapter 19). Or, if she had purchased a low-carb bread item out of convenience, like Joseph's pitas, she could easily have made an **S** sandwich from one of those, too. Any of those bread options could be enjoyed with any combinations of mayo, deli meats, or leftover chicken or beef, cheeses, and lettuce.

New scene continues**.** Mom hands out the peanut butter and jelly sandwiches to the children, but eats her own more low glycemic sandwich with a smile, knowing it is doing the right thing for her body. Now she has a little protein and has not triggered the insulin spike. Hooray!

To round off her picnic lunch, she could have brought along a little baggie of a handful or two of nuts and cheese for herself, instead of the packaged cheese puffs. If berries were in season, she could have brought some fresh strawberries to eat in place of grapes, which are one of the highest sugar-laden fruits. In fact, even her children would be better off eating nuts and cheese. A container of cheap, dry roasted peanuts or party peanuts would have fed them all and not have been any more expensive than the cheese puffs. Mom could have made some delicious stevia-sweetened lemonade for herself and the children. Or, if her budget allowed, bought some stevia-sweetened natural fruit flavored drink from the store and made up a big jug of that. Everyone's blood glucose would have been at healthier levels without drinking the fruit juice.

"Kid Food Mom" could have even opted to take an **E** lunch if that was the order of the day. She could have packed a sandwich using either our *Trim Healthy Pan bread,* some sprouted bread like Trader Joe's or Ezekiel, or homemade sourdough bread. She would have wisely used more lean fillings like lean turkey, lettuce and low-fat mayo with mustard or horseradish sauce. She could have rounded off her lunch with a little container of low-fat cottage cheese and an apple or cantaloupe slice. None of these options would have taken her any longer to prepare than her original sugar-loading lunch. And, if she had taken a walk around the park rather than just sitting, this mother, formerly known as "Kid Food Mom," would be making huge changes to her metabolic self! We would have to find a new name for her. How about "Smart Food Mom"?

Harmonious Meal Times

By harmonious, we don't mean your three year old won't spill his water cup twice and the baby won't choose to have her fussy, screaming hour coincide with your sit down meal. It means that both the metabolic needs of adults and children can be met without having to completely alienate one from the other.

Pre-packaged meal diets divide dieting parents from eating with their children and they don't promote the important family meal table. The adverts for these types of diets may look compelling on TV when the stars announce how much weight they've lost. But, it's one thing to be in Hollywood, having your personal assistant bring your pre-packaged meal to your movie trailer. It's another thing to gather the whole family around the meal table for nourishing food and bonding family time, while your only option is to pull back the plastic lining of your tiny micro-waved box and pretend it's satisfying and everything is okey dokey. Who wants to go to the effort of creating important family time around the meal table if good food is not at the center? It doesn't give your children much to look forward to when they are adults.

An enjoyable meal releases the hormone oxytocin, which is your natural stress buster, and which also fights all manner of diseases in the body. Later, you'll learn how lots of sex with your husband can increase your oxytocin levels dramatically. Eating good food releases this same hormone to a significant, but somewhat lesser extent. Mothers need lots of oxytocin to help fight the stress and chaos that sometimes threatens to overwhelm us in our daily family life. Opening a tiny diet boxed meal, devoid of fat and calories, is not going to get that hormone flowing! Good food, and enough of it to satisfy, along with the assurance that your children are also eating that good food, is a formula for a nice release of oxytocin.

An **S** and **E** lifestyle can easily work for the whole family and meet all the different needs. The evening meal is the perfect time to put this into practice. Let's say you've planned a roasted chicken (or two or three) for dinner (*Whole Baked Chickens, Evening Meals*, Chapter 21). Perhaps you're not a scratch cook, you're more the Drive Thru Sue type and you picked up a couple of rotisserie chickens from the store on your way home from running errands. Don't be down on yourself; that'll work too, (so long as the chicken is not breaded and fried). In fact, if budget allows, you could have driven through Kentucky Fried Chicken and purchased pieces of their grilled chicken which would have saved you stress and time. It only matters that you ended up with some carb free animal protein around which you plan the rest of your meal.

It's simple, really. This meal will be **S** because you plan on leaving the yummy skin on the chicken and eating both the dark and white meat. You'll have your chicken with a big salad, sprinkled with some cheese, bacon bits, and creamy ranch. Or, you could have lots of grilled, steamed, or baked veggies, tossed with butter, and maybe a smaller side salad if you like. Hopefully, you'll make sure your children have some salad and a serving of veggies, too. However, they'll need to fill up more with healthy, whole grain carbs, or creamy mashed potatoes in proportion to their metabolic needs. Most children without weight issues need to eat at least **Crossover** portions of healthy carbs. Rapidly growing teenage boys may eat carbs in far greater than **Crossover** portions. But, remember, if any of your children are struggling with weight, try to steer them to higher protein and vegetable intake rather than the carbs, but don't take the carbs away completely.

Pearl chats: At dinner time, all my family enjoys the same protein source, whether it be chicken, beef, quiche, or beans. My husband and I eat more of the non-starchy vegetables than the children. I make sure they get some, but I usually butter slices of healthy whole grain bread and place these on the table so they have enough whole grains for their metabolic needs. Or, I serve potatoes, brown rice, or whole wheat pasta. The bread and other carbs do not interest me as the rest of the meal is so good and I am completely satisfied with vegetables, fat, and protein in an **S** meal. Now and then, I use the grains as **S Helpers** to supplement my meals. I do find though, with the exception of quinoa, that my sensitive digestive system has an easier time if I leave the grains completely out of an **S** meal at night time.

All of my children that are still growing burn whole grain carbs efficiently and they are all wiry and strong. My oldest daughter's growth has stopped now that she is 17 years and she finds it more important to lay off high intake of grains, or she gains weight.

When it comes time to prepare dinner, I always ask myself a couple of questions to get started. First, what will be my protein source? Maybe I've got some ground beef handy. Good. I'll make a meatloaf. Now I'm in **S** territory so I ask myself what non-starchy vegetable I'm going to use as the main side. I look in the freezer and see two bags of frozen cauliflower. Good, I'll roast them in the oven with coconut oil and delicious seasonings while the meatloaf is cooking. Then I ask what carb can I have for the children? I spy a box or two of whole wheat noodles in the cupboard. Great, I'll cook them up and toss with butter and parmesan cheese. The children will be very happy to have a serving of those noodles on their plates. But, because the cauliflower will taste so good, it won't be too troubling to get them to eat that, too.

Lunches are when I often like to have a piece of salmon. I try to do salmon at least two to three times each week, although I slip up sometimes when things are crazy around here. For lunch, my children often like to eat whole grain noodles or grilled cheese on whole wheat. Hey, I get to eat grilled cheese sandwiches, too, if I feel like it, thanks to the plain version of *Muffin in a Mug* (*Muffins, Breads, and Pizza Crusts*, Chapter 19).

After reading our chapter on *Foundation Foods*, Chapter 17, you may be persuaded to also eat more salmon. It is very quick to make for lunch. Sautéing salmon, along with some finely cut vegetables for **S**, or broiling or poaching the salmon and including three quarters of a cup of brown rice or quinoa for **E**, is speedy and easy. You don't have to think of it as having to make a "another whole meal, poor me!" Right now, as we're writing this book, we have all our children together, plus an extra cousin or two around. That makes about 15 children. We're on a deadline, but lunchtime will be a snap.

The children will be happy if we heat up brown rice from the night before in coconut oil and seasonings, offer them each a boiled egg from the fridge, and pass out apples for dessert. At the same time, we will sauté our salmon and side it with an awesome salad with avocado and toasted nuts, thrown together in a jiffy. Not too hard.

We'll be back to you in no time, but right now we're going to enjoy this fabulous lunch. Serene and I love eating together and telling each other how we enjoy our good food. It's loud in here right now, though!

Serene chats: There is usually one part of the meal that overlaps for everyone. Our family enjoys a lot of yummy soups, like *Coconut Thai* or *Chicken Curry*, (*Evening Meals*, Chapter 21). I usually serve a big pot of steaming brown rice on the table. My husband and I either forgo the rice, or add 1-2 heaping tablespoons to our soup or stew as an **S H**elper. We round our meal with a heartier portion of the scrumptious salad.

At other times we may have a favorite family casserole or meatloaf that is glycemic friendly and which everyone can enjoy. Again, the big pot of steaming brown rice is on the table for the children, but my husband and I round off our meal with yummy veggies instead.

It's very simple at our house. There is almost always raw whole milk and brown rice on the table for the children and maybe a little "mummy and daddy" dish that is just for us. The main portion of the meal is enjoyed by all, but we compliment our meals with the different foods that support our metabolic differences.

Of course, there are times when the family requests something that is not on the "plan" or, I have made something in bulk which is easy to feed the crowd of them, like a big lasagna with whole wheat noodles, which would not suit a slimming protocol. Instead, I sauté a little salmon in five minutes, throw a delicate salad on the side, and

I am set to go as well. If what the children are eating does not work for you and you are not at **Crossover** stage what is a few minutes to protect your waistline?

Keep it foremost in your mind that "kid food" will make you fat. Like Pearl, lunch times are more often the time when I'll choose to eat something very different from my children. It is always a quick meal time for both the children and me. I may make tuna sandwiches for my children while I have a piece of salmon on a bed of lettuce. Salmon and salad is about the most slimming lunch you could ever hope to find.

Hate to Cook?

If you don't love it yet, it is time to learn the joy and art of cooking. Anyone who chooses health and vitality must make a conscious decision to prepare meals for home, or take on the go. Studies show that people who are willing to cook at home have the most success at long term weight loss.

It doesn't matter if this is something you have not done in the past. You may be more like Drive Thru Sue and want to take as many cooking shortcuts as you can. That's fine, but you'll have to get some basics happening for long term health management. God made us to be creative and adaptive people. Saying, "I don't cook," is a mindset you can change. Our recipes are easy enough for even clueless cooks.

Cooking doesn't have to take a long time. All the recipes in this book are designed for quick prep. We have busy lives with large families and don't want to be slaves to the kitchen. Crockpots can really make a difference. You can do a little ten minute prep in the morning, rush about all day, and know that your meal will be piping hot and ready to serve at supper time, with a quick salad on the side and some whole grain bread and butter as another quick side for your children's higher glucose needs. **S** meals are perfect for crockpots. Meat simmering in a creamy sauce all day, how can you beat that?

Learning to love, (or at least like), simple cooking at home also helps your budget and allows you to purchase more organic items. Try the easy recipes in our breakfast, lunch, evening meal, snacks and desserts sections. None of them are hard or laborious. You can get many more ideas from the forum section of www.lowcarbfriends.com. Click on the Recipe Help and Suggestion box for hundreds of ideas for low glycemic recipes and meals. You can ask questions and have a bunch of knowledgeable folk help you out.

Eating Out

We know there will be times when you won't be eating at home. Date nights, celebrations—sometimes plain laziness. This is life. Our plan is easy to stick to while dining out at restaurants. Even fast food can be managed correctly.

Hardees has a low-carb burger, great for an **S** meal. Their meat is not the usual nasty, low end stuff. They use pure Angus beef. Actually, you can ask for any of their burgers to be "low-carbed." They wrap the burger and the fillings in a casing of lettuce that you can hold in your hand and bite into—yum! You can always order a side salad too. Skip sweet dressings and go with Ranch or Caesar. In-N-Out Burger chains do a similar thing with their burger, along with a couple of other fast food chains.

Note: you won't be able to drive and eat the low-carb burger at the same time. You'll need two hands as it's a little messy.

If everyone is screaming for McDonalds while you are traveling on a family vacation, you can still achieve weight loss or maintenance, even though it may not be the healthiest meal you've ever eaten. Order a salad and a burger or two. Feed the ducks with the white buns, but never yourself! The meat burger with all the fixin's still tastes great without the bun. It's an easy **S** meal. You can utilize the dollar menu that way. Actually, this can also be a good save when you're out running errands and you have not a clue what to do about lunch to stay on plan. Buy a couple of dollar burgers. Take the buns off, but leave the yummy fixin's—you'll taste the flavors better without the buns. The meat will fill you up well, even if you feel a little strange doing the bun removal trick.

If you are on a family day out and know ahead of time that you will likely be stopping at a fast food burger joint, we suggest taking a couple of *Oopsie Rolls* (*Muffins, Breads, and Pizza Crusts,* Chapter 19), or pieces of flax bread and swap these out for the harmful white buns. The buns are the worst offenders, not the burgers themselves. Our **S** bun options will fill you up much more so you won't even need to consider the fries.

Traveling days can be saved by having a full **S** meal at Cracker Barrel with their menu cards that indicate all their low-carb food options. Even Kentucky Fried Chicken does not have to be your undoing. You can order the grilled chicken, rather than breaded or fried, and a double side of green beans. Avoid the coleslaw as it has too much sugar. At the time of this writing (things change quickly), they also have a double chicken breast sandwich without buns that could work fine.

A six inch whole wheat Subway sandwich can be used as an **E** meal. Yes, the bread is not sprouted or sourdough, but it's not like you will be eating it every day. Choose a lean meat, lots of veggies, part skim mozzarella, a light mayo, and lots of mustard and vinegar. A foot long sub is too many carbs, especially when the bread is suspect, so avoid ordering that. Subway also has fresh fruit packets that could be a good **E** side option. This should tide you over until you can get to your destination and eat a little more correctly.

Pearl chats: Or, if you are a purist like Serene, you pack your little cooler with all your crazy goodies. She's not likely to even walk into a fast food restaurant, but some of us will not be able to avoid it.

Serene chats: Too right!

Beware of Bars

We don't mean the type that serve beer. We mean the packaged kind. Don't be fooled into thinking that grabbing an energy bar while on the go (even from the health food store) is a slimming or healthy practice. Nearly all of these so-called natural bars are extremely high in carbs and rely heavily on dried fruits like date pastes, honey, and glucose syrups. "Raw" bars are notorious for this. The occasional one for a growing child would be fine, but your blood sugar will be less likely to handle it. They often have a high nut content, which may slow down the insulin response a little, but combined with dried fruit and the amount of honey used, balanced sugar levels will be highly unlikely. Any fat the bar contains will climb on the insulin truck and you have a double whammy packaged as an innocent health bar.

The other alternative is a protein bar. Most of these are soy based, and we know from earlier discussion that soy is high in phytates and phytoestrogens. Corn syrup (even worse than sugar) is often used to sweeten the bars. Sometimes these bars may be advertised as "no sugar" or "low-carb." In that case, sugar alcohols, like maltitol, are used. Maltitol is the least healthy sugar alcohol and has its list of side effects, especially digestive distress. If you are really in a pinch and not a purist psycho like Serene, these types of protein bars would be the best of the worst. Atkins' company makes such bars and they are readily available at most grocery stores. We urge you to keep them for emergencies. However, it would still be a much better decision when you are starving to eat a maltitol sweetened protein bar than a packet of potato chips, or a high glycemic energy bar.

In *Snacks*, Chapter 24, you will find many recipes for energy and protein bars that are super quick and easy to take with you. These are excellent on-the-go choices, or even for at-home snacks.

Sit Down Restaurants

We think sit down restaurants are best for **S** meals. It's harder to do an **E** meal because most restaurants do not have whole grains or sweet potatoes on the menu. Your starch would end up being white potato, white rice, or white noodles. Those won't work.

Here's how to order a healthy **S** meal while dining at a nice restaurant:

1. Try to avoid arriving too hungry. Eating a light snack at home a little while before leaving for the restaurant is a good idea—maybe an ounce of cheese and a few nuts, or quarter of a cup of glucomannan pudding (*Deserts*, Chapter 23). This way, you will be more in control of yourself when faced with so many options and won't be as tempted to eat any of those FATTENING white dinner rolls that suddenly appear on your table.
2. Here comes the first test. Say no to the bread or rolls they offer you. If you are vulnerable to those temptations, ask for them to be removed from the table so you can focus on ordering healthy items.
3. Choose your protein. Most restaurants have salmon (our favorite choice), other fish choices, chicken, or fine cuts of steak. Make sure your protein source does not come with sugar sweetened sauces or glazes. Butter, lemon, or cream based sauces are usually fine.
4. Check if your protein source automatically comes with a rice pilaf, potatoes, or a side of pasta. If so, ask for a double serving of grilled or sautéed veggies instead of the starchy carb. Sautéed mushrooms are a perfect choice. Your server will always be most happy to oblige you.
5. Your meal will usually come with a house salad. Remember to choose a dressing that is not sweet. Oil/vinegar, Ranch, or Caesar are usually the safest options. Don't eat the croutons.

Pearl chats: It may seem a little obsessive to worry about such little items as croutons, but they can turn a wonderful **S** weight loss meal into a fat-promoting meal due to their carb content from the white flour. If you are in a restaurant where the salad is a buffet, you can put a small sprinkle of sunflower seeds on your salad or ask the waiter for bacon bits to replace that crunch.

Serene chats: I never order a salad exactly as described on the menu. I ask if I can create my own side salad. Or, if I want it to be a feature part of my meal, I ask them to make it nice and large and skip one of my sides that comes with the meal. They are always delighted to help and have never charged me extra.

At Carrabba's Italian Grill, my favorite restaurant in Franklin, Tennessee, I ask for the field greens and a generous medallion of goat's cheese, plenty of kalamata olives, pine nuts, and sun-dried tomatoes, but to leave out the croutons. I ask for the virgin olive oil and balsamic vinegar on the side. This is my favorite salad in the world.

You can also order a very healthy meal at O'Charleys by ordering fresh wild caught salmon or steak with non-starchy sides of asparagus and broccoli.

Pearl chats: Restaurant waiters must want to run and hide when they see you coming, Serene!

The Dessert Menu

You'll be asked if you want to look at the Dessert Menu—that's how restaurants make their money. But, you just ate a perfectly slimming meal at a restaurant of all places—kudos to you! Why ruin it? Sugar laden desserts will undo all your good choices in a second. Even more than croutons on your salad, a sugary dessert swiftly turns an **S** slimming meal into a tandem fueled fattening one. If you opted for berries and whipped cream that would be different, but it's usually much too tempting to pass up the cheesecake or the chocolate volcano! We suggest rounding your meal out with a rich coffee. You could ask for whipped cream on top. That won't be a problem for your server. Bring a stevia packet or two in your purse, or some liquid drops to sweeten up your coffee into a dessert-like finale. Now you can relax, fully satisfied, and devote yourself to flirting with your husband over your coffee cup. Oh yeah!

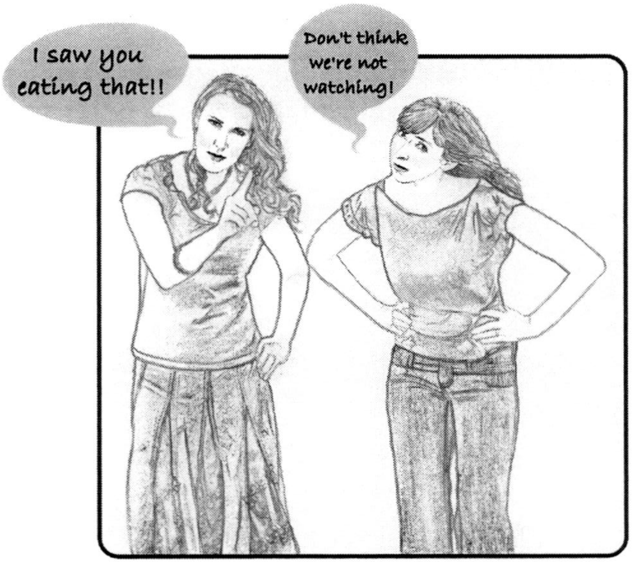

You can always think to yourself when faced with the dessert temptation, "I have yummy chocolates at home." Or, you could make a special chocolate cheesecake that is plan approved for the occasion, and you and your husband can share some when you're back home. The children will hopefully all be in bed, and you are not so full so you'll really get to enjoy it. Good foreplay.

Of course, if the occasion for eating out is a special anniversary, we are not going to judge you for splitting a dessert with your husband. Just don't make a habit of it.

What Would You Like To Drink?

Beverages at restaurants can be another trip up. Stick to good choices like Perrier sparkling mineral water with lemon. A glass of dry red or white wine would be fine, or a very low-carb beer if your husband likes that. Unsweetened tea (bring your own sweetener), hot tea, or coffee are all fine. Okay, if you haven't been able to completely kick the habit, a diet soda won't kill you. If you were able to baby step your way into choosing a suitable **S** meal from the menu, we won't be too mad that you just had to have a diet coke. Progress is what makes us happy. You get an "A minus" grade. Not too shabby.

Family Restaurants

You may not always be fine-dining alone with your husband, or out with adult friends on special occasions. Sometimes you're out to eat with your children. Or, other times, you're craving Chinese or Indian food. Let's look at four common restaurant favorites.

Mexican

Do not regularly go into a Mexican restaurant if you cannot say no to the corn chips they constantly refill at your table. Not only will they destroy your waistline, but they drip with trans fats that initiate degenerative diseases. You may be the type who will let your children have a treat and eat the corn chips, but please pass on them yourself (unless you are going to save your Mexican restaurant experience for a rare cheat meal then a few chips shouldn't hurt you too much). We find it is better to ask for a plate of cucumber slices and a side of guacamole to be brought straight away. Dunk and dip. It is yummy and fun. You won't feel left out this way while your children are having fun with chips and salsa. Cheese dip and cucumber slices are another option, but the cheese dip has moderate carbs since it is usually made with a little milk, so you'll be in **S Helper** territory.

The best item to order at a Mexican restaurant is Fajitas. Who needs refried beans, rice, and white flour tortillas, when you can have seasoned grilled meat with caramelized onions, peppers, and tomatoes? Tell the waiter you won't need the tortillas, rice, or beans. You can ladle on the sour cream, salsa, cheese, guacamole, and pico de gallo. Who would miss the bland starches? We certainly don't. Another option is Chile Relleno, which is a stuffed pepper with meat and cheese. Make sure it is not breaded. They are usually not made that way, but you might want to check first.

Avoid the margaritas. It is an alcoholic drink that is high in carbs from sugar. Mexican restaurants also serve a lot of Sangria, which is very sweet wine. Avoid this at all costs. If you like to have a glass of wine when dining out, ask them for their driest one.

For those who eat **Crossovers** occasionally, it would be fine to add a side of refried beans. But, adding the white rice would not be appropriate.

Chinese

We think Chinese restaurants are the hardest places to find a slimming meal, yet it can be done. Don't put the white rice, or the fried rice (that is white but looks brown from soy sauce) on your plate. Beware of the noodles, anything fried, breaded and crispy, and any sweet tasting sauce. What are you left with? Load up on lots of good vegetables like broccoli, cauliflower, green beans, and onions. Find which meat dishes are in non-sweet sauces. Beef and broccoli dishes are usually your safest bet. The sauces used for such dishes may have a little corn starch, but you'll survive; at least they won't be swimming in sugar. If you are ready to enjoy **Crossovers** or **S Helpers**, some Chinese restaurants offer brown rice.

Italian

You may be thinking, why even go, it's all pasta based. You have to get a little creative. Italian restaurants usually have nice grilled meats and vegetables. They also usually offer delicious steak on their menu. You can ask for a pizza to be made for you with a portabella mushroom as a base if they do not already have this idea on the menu. Stuffed eggplants or zucchini are often available. Don't forget the beautiful salads.

If you don't want to miss out on your pasta, we suggest this idea. Take a box of Dreamfields pasta and ask your waiter to tell the chef that you are on a low gylcemic diet for your health and should only eat this type (that's not a lie). There are so few digestible carbs in this delicious pasta, so you do not have to worry about **E** or **S** when choosing a sauce. Diabetics are known to do this quite often, so don't feel like a crazy person. The good thing about the USA is that restaurants desire to please the customer so you will keep returning.

Indian or Thai

Coconut or cream-based sauces from this cuisine are perfect for **S** options. Chicken Marsala or Butter Chicken are dishes that won't mess with your weight too much if they're eaten occasionally. If you eat them too often (more than a couple times a week), these cream-based Indian dishes can bring on calorie abuse because of their richness, but enjoy them now and then. With lots of veggies, you won't even miss the rice that **will** mess with your weight.

If you are brave enough and want to bring an **S Helper**, or make your meal a healthy **Crossover**, bring your own little Ziploc bag of correctly portioned brown rice or quinoa in your purse. Quinoa is probably better, because you can have more of it and still stay within **S Helper** guidelines. We are both known to do this very thing since we are crazy about Indian food. Again, beware of sweet sauces in Thai restaurants. Red and green curries are usually a safe bet.

Brown Bag Lunches

As homseschooling mothers, we are not out of the home much at lunchtime. The following brown bag ideas have stemmed from trying to find fitting foods to send with our husbands to work. These next ideas can really revolutionize your husband's life if he is struggling with weight issues or be handy ideas for yourself it you are out of the home during the day sometimes.

Pearl chats: Joseph's pitas are invaluable to me for making lunches for my husband. On the days he works outside the home, I often send him between half and a whole pita stuffed with either egg salad, tuna salad, natural deli meats, mayo, lettuce and cheese, or leftover chicken breasts as an **S** lunch.

If I send half a pita, I also usually add in five or six *Deli Meat Roll Ups* (*Lunches*, Chapter 20). He loves peanut butter and celery so I include a couple of stalks with natural sugar-free peanut butter. Some days, I change things around and fill the celery with ⅓ less fat cream cheese instead. I like to include *Cheese Crisps* (*Snacks*, Chapter 24) or a little baggy of spicy nuts and small pieces of cheese. He's a very happy guy when I send him with some glucomannan pudding in a jar ready to spoon out, some vanilla-flavored ricotta cheese, or even a piece of our *Special Agent Brownie Cake* (*Desserts*, Chapter 23).

For variety, I send him a couple of sandwiches made with *Trim Healthy Pan Bread* (*Muffins, Breads, and Pizza Crusts*, Chapter 19) with leaner fillings and light mayo for an **E** lunch. He really enjoys these. I make sure to include some sweetened skim ricotta cheese as a fitting **E** dessert to help him fill up some more on those days. Sometimes, I make him *Oopsie Rolls* (*Muffins, Breads, and Pizza Crusts*, Chapter 19). These gourmet looking croissant type rolls match perfectly with roast beef, cheese, and lettuce. They make a killer **S** style sandwich and he gets many comments from co-workers on how good they look.

Other days I send a huge **S** salad loaded with meats, cheese, grape tomatoes, onions, and a small container of water thinned Ken's Ranch Dressing on the side. This fills him up well. I'll let you in on a secret, though. More often than the **S** salad I just described, I try to send him off to work with **Fuel Pull** salads. He doesn't know this, so don't tell him! I do this because my husband eats lots of nuts almost every night as an after dinner snack. He loves to snack on high calorie **S** foods and doesn't naturally change to lighter foods on his own (but what man thinks about doing such a thing, right?)

Sending him a **Fuel Pull** salad once, or hopefully twice a week, really helps combat those night time high calories he eats and orchestrates a nice caloric change. The trick with a **Fuel Pull** salad is to make it extremely huge and then your guy does not feel like he is missing out on the tummy filling factor.

I chop up at least one big heart of romaine lettuce with green peppers, onions, and baby tomatoes. To that I add about 2-3 oz. of grilled chicken cut up into small cubes. I dress the salad with 20 sprays of Wishbone Ranch Salad Spritzer. That's a really light caloric dressing but it has a good flavor. It wets the salad greens well. I then sprinkle on sea salt, black pepper, and cayenne pepper which makes the salad taste even more flavorful. Or, I use Walden Farms calorie free Thousand Island dressing, which surprisingly, he actually likes! You could use *Green Valley Ranch* (another more healthful calorie free dressing) if you are leery of dressings with artificial flavors and chemical ingredients. I always add two to three good tablespoons of 1% cottage cheese to the top of the salad. Sometimes he cannot even finish the whole meal and has to save some for later. I give myself a pat on the back for job well done! On these **Fuel Pull** brown bag lunch days, I also send him some glucomannan *Choco Pudding* (*Desserts*, Chapter 23) in case he gets hungry in the afternoon, or his other favorite, glucomannan pudding made with banana extract and defatted peanut flour.

Charlie looks forward to his packed lunches and they keep him away from burgers and fries. His weight loss of nearly 40 pounds has been maintained for well over four years now, and these packed lunches have been the key—integral, crucial, and absolutely necessary!

I have to admit that I never feel like making Charlie's lunch in the morning. I am not a morning person. He has to leave early and I confess to being a bit grumpy when I have to get up with the alarm and make his breakfast and lunch, but I keep it to myself. Just the thought of the lunch choices he will make if he buys his own get me up and rising with that dratted alarm. It's a certainty that his choices will be pizza or a burger with large fries—scary thoughts for me.

After rising in the morning and trudging sleepily into the kitchen, I find myself thinking "I am going back to bed as soon as this is done, really, I am this time!" But, 25-30 minutes later he appears freshly showered at our breakfast bar as I have just finished making both his breakfast and lunch. By this time, my mood has improved, my kettle is whistling for my green tea, or my coffee is ready to pour, and I am ready for the day. The idea of going back to bed is no longer tempting. He sits in the kitchen to eat his breakfast and we get a nice couple of minutes to chat before he says goodbye.

Serene chats: Not only does it help our budget by sending my husband food from home, it also settles my worries about protecting his health. My husband enjoys stuffed Joseph's pitas, but he dislikes my pre-filling all the stuff inside. He likes moist goodies like pickles and says it becomes soggy and gross by the time he eats it. To solve this problem, I purchased two Tupperware containers that are divided into three spaces. I fill each space with different fillings like natural turkey slices, cheese, fresh tomato, Vidalia onion, lots of organic romaine lettuce, healthy pickles, jalapeno pickles, yogurt based dressing, and mustard. This sounds like a lot but it takes only a minute or two for him to put it together. I send him with a couple of low-carb pitas or Joseph's low-carb lavish bread and he fills them himself when he wants one.

I also send him a green apple and a Ziploc baggy with a handful of raw walnuts for a snack later in the afternoon. Sometimes I send him *Oopsie Roll* sandwiches. Lately, his favorite sandwiches are made with *Trim Healthy Pan Bread*, (*Breads, Muffins, and Pizza Crusts*, Chapter 19). He calls them "Manwiches" because he thinks they appeal to his male tastes more than other types of breads. He really loves it when I make them with Southwestern style Egg Beaters.

The most important part of Sam's lunch in the warmer seasons is a gallon of either homemade Nunaturals stevia-sweetened mint tea or lemonade. He drinks the entire gallon every day when working hard manual labor. He cares about his drinks even more than his food. This was a real problem in our early marriage as I hadn't yet formed the habit of sending his lunch with him. He would drink regular sweetened tea or sodas all day long. When I found out about this habit, it motivated me to take the extra few minutes to make alternatives for him.

In the winter, when he needs to be warmed up, I send nice hot soups in a Coleman's thermos. This is warming and soothing as he often works outside in the cold.

When I take the extra effort to prepare lunch for him, I notice his belly goes flatter and he looks more radiant in his complexion. When I go through less motivated seasons, such as when I have morning sickness and I don't fix his lunch, he gains weight and looks more tired.

My husband leaves very early in the morning, and especially when I am pregnant, I do not like getting up when it is still dark. To remedy this, I try to make his lunch the night before (after dinner when my children are doing chores) and have it ready for him to pull out of the fridge.

Cheating

The temptation to cheat is part of everyday living everyday in the real world. We just spent several minutes disagreeing with each other about this subject and what we should suggest in this book. We both think our points are more valid of course, so we'll give you both of them and try to get to the truth of the matter.

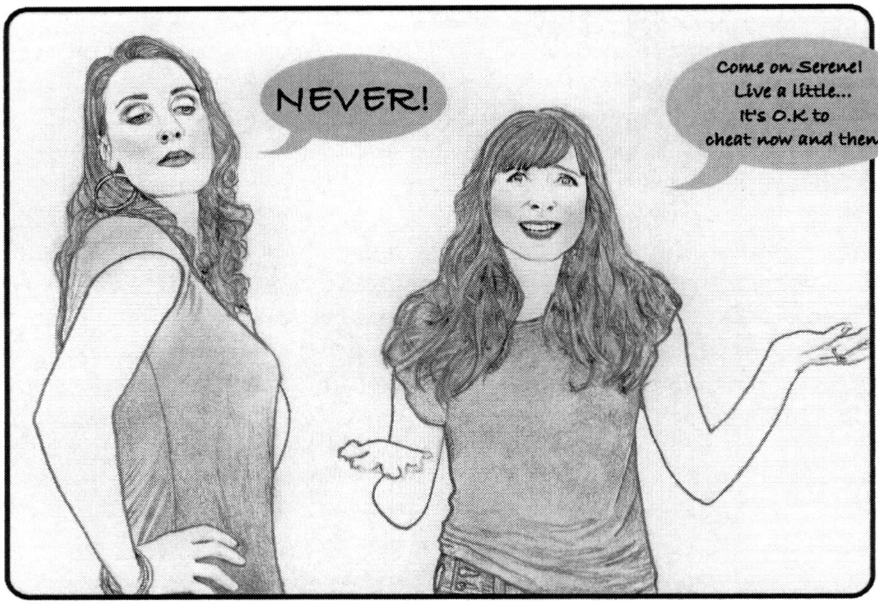

Pearl chats: Serene, cheating is bound to happen. You can't pretend life is perfect and that nobody will fall off the horse occasionally. I don't think we should say, "never cheat" to our mamas."

Serene chats: So you're calling me a nobody? I'm not going to fall off the "horse." And why are you calling healthy eating a "horse"? Some people like me cannot enjoy a cheat. How does something feel like a treat if you know you are poisoning your body, adding to the aging process, and having to work out harder tomorrow?

Pearl chats: They're unique thought processes to you. I don't have those thoughts when cheating. I'll have a bag of popcorn when my husband and I do movie dates about once a month or so, (even with that fake butter stuff they pour all over it). I'll eat a small bag of potato chips when I'm on vacation, or a real sugar brownie or two every now and then, and I am not going to spend the two days of Christmas and Thanksgiving denying myself anything, and I mean anything! Most people feel this way, and it is so easy to start back on plan the next day. I have had no problems doing this. Life should not be all about rules and restrictions.

Serene chats: Pearl, why does a treat always have to be junk? Why do you have to say you are denying yourself to not partake of junk foods? I splurge at Christmas as well, but with more expensive and gourmet foods that I normally would not purchase. These treats are not going to damage me. Christmas and Thanksgiving can be full days of **Crossovers** which make me more than satisfied.

Pearl chats: Well, we agree to disagree. Serene, you've always had super human self-control when it comes to what you eat. Most of us are not born with such ability. Feeling weighed down with shame for cheating can create a worse situation for some people. I know a few people who feel so awful about themselves for messing up now and then that they start to self sabotage. Healthy progress is hindered from self punishing choices. They figure, "I can't get this right, I already messed up so I might as well drive through and order a large Fry and a Frosty to dig a deeper grave."

For those who want to eat some forbidden foods once in a while, I say it is fine if you can handle it. Make sure this doesn't become a way for you to slip back into your old habits though. Serene has a point. Some cheats I wouldn't do because they are so unhealthy for the body. If at all possible, I urge you to stay away from fast food fries or onion rings, large amounts of potato chips, or other trans fatty foods. But, if you do find yourself eating birthday cake and loading up on all that other crazy stuff I just mentioned, do not say, "Well, I might as well throw this whole program away now. I just can't stick to it."

No, way! Our plan is forgiving and you must offer yourself that same forgiveness. Shake yourself off and make sure your very next meal is right on plan. You don't even have to wait until the next day. Getting back on target is a meal away. Please, don't beat yourself up too much. If I find myself cheating, I make sure to have eggs alone the next morning. I fry up two or three eggs in butter and this somehow tells my body to get back in line, thank you very much. This is a sure way to help reduce the excess sugars in my cells and get me back on track.

Serene chats: If our readers aren't going to beat themselves up, I will do it for them. Why? Because sometimes love has to be tough. They may say they only cheat on birthdays, but family birthdays can come several times a month. If they are part of a large family, or even extended family, they could end up cutting loose all the time.

How can you enjoy the holiday season if you know you are getting heavier and out of shapier! Okay, I just created a new word, but I am getting heated up on this subject.

Pearl chats: On that you are right, Serene. I agree we shouldn't take whole seasons to cheat. Choose the one or two seasonal parties or occasions and use a sense of commitment to plan the rest of the time. Many people get colds and flus around the holiday seasons because they binge on sugars, and this lowers immune defenses.

Some may know how to cheat well and have no problems getting back on plan. For others, cheating may be a ticket to disaster. Figure out who you are and know your limitations. Be honest with yourself. It seems I can cheat and jump back on plan easily. My husband can do this, too. He takes at least three full days over Christmas and eats to his heart's content all the things he normally wouldn't eat. I think he goes overboard and I'm always relieved when that time is up. I constantly have to zip my lips and not nag, although somehow my lips open and nagging just pops out—oops!

There will always be temptations. You cannot live in a sheltered balloon. On a daily basis there will be candy at the gas station . . . yeah, it even calls to me sometimes. Instead, I tell myself it is not real food and say to myself, "I don't eat that." Self talk works for me.

There will always be cupcakes at a friend's birthday. There will be all kinds of ridiculous options at the church pot luck. We can't cocoon ourselves away from it all. But, it's not like you can't make commitments and keep them! And the great thing is that we have wonderful options of healthy "cheat like" food on our plan. That's why you can stick to it; you can have all the indulgences at home.

On the whole, this is a good mindset to keep: be faithful to the plan, but if you cheat, forgive yourself and don't dwell on the "Oh No's" and a mindset of failure that prevents you from jumping back on the horse—just wrote that for Serene's sake.

Chapter 14

The Way to Do It, Mama!

We don't want you to be even slightly puzzled, doubtful, or left wondering about all the details once you begin implementing the **S** and **E** plan. Therefore, it's time to get really practical and give you a detailed look at what **S** and **E** meals actually look like. We'll contrast them with a meal that does not work, for example, an **S** or **E** meal gone wrong. We'll also take a look at examples of what well balanced **Crossover** meals look like for people who need to maintain or slow down weight loss. We're going to really get nitpicky here and enjoy every bit of it!

It will be a waste of time to focus on **S Helpers** and **Fuel** Pulls here. All you need to know for **S Helpers** is that they will be exactly like **S** meals with the addition of the allowed starch of fruit. **Fuel Pulls** are featured in greater detail in *One Week Fuel Cycle,* Chapter 28.

E Breakfast Example (the right way)

Bowl of stevia-sweetened steel cut oats or Old Fashioned Oats with 0% Greek yogurt and berries, or 1 tsp. coconut oil mixed with ¼ cup boiling water, cinnamon, and a little sprinkle of golden flax meal.

Pearl chats: Perfect! In place of the Greek yogurt or coconut oil thinned down with hot water, you could use either regular low/fat free yogurt or unsweetened almond milk.

Serene chats: Optimally, I love to make my own yogurt from raw milk after I have skimmed off the cream which naturally makes it low fat and perfect for **E** needs. I save the cream for wonderful **S** treats. But, I also buy *Greek* yogurt since I can't always make my own. It is so much better than most foods in a grocery store. Also, check out how to make the oatmeal with the one teaspoon of coconut oil in *Morning Meals*, Chapter 18. I think you'll love it for a change.

E breakfast Example (the wrong way)

A bowl of instant cinnamon and brown sugar oatmeal, with raisins, sliced banana, and non-fat milk. A glass of orange juice on the side.

Pearl chats: The carbs are simply too high in this meal. Please do not purchase the pre-flavored oatmeal in the little brown packets and think they are a healthy option for you. They're not. They are full of sugar and excess carbs. The person who eats this breakfast will be hungry in less than a couple of hours and seeking more sugar fuel. There is not enough protein to sustain brain concentration and it promotes belly fat.

Serene chats: Instant or quick oats are absorbed much faster into your bloodstream, so their carb content is more damaging. Even if you sweeten this breakfast with honey instead of brown sugar, your insulin surge would skyrocket, not to mention the sugary fruit choices you added. It is a very fattening breakfast. The worst part is that this type of breakfast is applauded by the American food guidelines and promoted by most diet dictocrats due to its high fiber and three fruit servings. What a load of bunkum!

S breakfast Example (the right way)

An omelet, made with omega-3 eggs and your choice of cheeses and veggies like onions, peppers, mushrooms, and tomatoes. Optional side of berries. Organic coffee with a dash of heavy cream.

Pearl chats: This is a good one. Omelets are my husband's favorite breakfast. I use cream cheese and finely diced onion to make them extra succulent. He lost his weight while eating these several times a week along with other healthy meals.

Serene chats: The egg-based breakfast is perfect. Research has shown that people who eat hearty proteins like eggs for breakfast are less hungry and battle less cravings throughout the day. Eggs, fried, poached, or boiled are the perfect start to the day.

S Breakfast Example (the wrong way)

An omelet, two pieces of buttered wheat toast spread with grape jelly on the side. Coffee with milk, honey, or sugar.

Pearl chats: All the goodness of the egg is ruined by the wheat toast. Some studies have cited more health concerns in people who eat eggs numerous times each week. It is not the eggs. Our culture usually puts eggs with junk carbs like white toast, bagels, or orange juice, etc, which all give rise to diabetes. Coffee, sweetened with honey or sugar causes fat gain.

Serene chats: You are creating fat gain by combining a hearty portion of protein and fat with an equally hearty portion of carbs. This is made worse by using carbs like wheat toast, which is really not much better than white toast. The label must read 100% to be whole grain and not list 50 unpronounceable ingredients after that. Even adding two slices of healthy sprouted toast to this meal is too many carbs for weight loss. It would be a **Crossover** instead of a slimming **S**.

Crossover Breakfast Example

Two fried eggs in coconut oil on one or two buttered pieces of super healthy toast, such as sprouted Ezekiel or Trader Joe's, homemade sourdough, or dark rye. One orange on the side, or an apple with a big scoop of peanut butter.

Pearl chats: You'll be nourished on this breakfast. The carbs are not high enough to spike your blood sugar, yet they will not allow a fat melt. The fats keep blood sugar nicely balanced.

Serene chats: To keep to a good weight, I enjoy a breakfast like this a couple of times a week.

E Lunch Example (the right way)

A sandwich made from two slices of sprouted or sourdough grain bread and smeared with light mayo, mustard, lean deli meat turkey slices, a thin slice of part skim mozzarella, tomato, lettuce, and onion; half a cup of low-fat cottage cheese; and a wedge of cantaloupe on the side.

Pearl chats: If you feel a little low in energy, this meal has just the right amount of carbs to help get you going again. It incorporates whole grains and they are well balanced by the protein in the lean turkey and cottage cheese. It is yummy, too!

Serene chats: You can see by this example meal that no more than two slices of bread at a time is ever recommended, even for **E** meals. If bread is included, keep the fruit portion smaller. Cantaloupe is a good choice here because it is a medium glycemic fruit. If your meal already includes two pieces of bread, it's a wrong decision to have larger portions of fruit, or even small portions of very sweet fruit like watermelon or pineapple.

E Lunch Example (the wrong way)

Turkey, ham, or baloney sandwich made from regular wheat or white bread, slathered with regular mayo, head lettuce, and one slice of American cheese. Side of pretzels or potato chips.

Pearl chats: This meal is so common and is a chief cause of expanding waistlines all over America. Don't fall into its trap or even believe that the pretzels are much healthier than the potato chips. They both spike insulin and guarantee that the fat from the mayo, baloney, and cheese is carried to your belly. This is simple tandem fuel burning science. It might not be more food than the first meal but the double fuels cause fat gain for most people.

Serene chats: I agree with Pearl that tandem fuel burning is a problem here, but there are other contributing issues. Even if you chose lower fat healthy turkey slices, and used a lighter mayonnaise to take out fat, two slices of regular bread alone, or with cheese, is already insulin producing and therefore fat promoting. Pretzels just make it worse.

S lunch Example (the right way)

Sautéed salmon in butter and coconut oil with a large decadent salad, dressed liberally with olive or hemp oil and lemon vinaigrette, and your choice of goodies such as avocado, toasted nuts, bacon bits, cheese, or boiled egg. You can have any, or all of the above. Finish with organic coffee with cream.

Pearl chats: This is a very quick meal, ten minutes at most. Deliciousness doesn't have to take long to prepare. This salmon could easily be made into **E** by pulling back the oil and opting for a nonstick pan, throwing in ¾ cup of brown rice or quinoa, and dressing your salad more lightly.

Serene chats: I love this meal. I confess I don't need much variety in my diet and eat this lunch many times a week. It is my favorite, and its super slimming! I love not having to hold back on the fats and the salad is so scrumptious. Salmon, being a superfood, is my preferred lunch choice.

S lunch Example (the wrong way)

Breaded fish fried in butter on rice pilaf, a side salad with full-fat ranch, and some sweet tea.

Pearl chats: Breading anything with normal breading ingredients like flour or bread crumbs is a major problem. The carbs mix with the fat for frying which creates an invitation for weight troubles. Instead of breading flours you can substitute parmesan cheese, store-bought coconut flour, or *Joseph's* pita bread crumbs.

Serene chats: Even choosing whole grain brown rice, unless eating only ¼ cup or less can cause weight gain alongside any rich, fatty dressing. Even if you chose whole grain bread crumbs for your breading and sweeten your tea with natural honey, it's just too many carbs. Plus, the added evil of combining it with a rich, fat sauce will do you in. But, I am not being fooled into believing this meal may be fish sticks with parboiled white rice and regular sweetened tea!

Crossover Lunch Example

Sautéed salmon in coconut oil with a medium-sized sweet potato and salad on the side. The sweet potato may be heavily buttered and sweetened with stevia and cinnamon if desired. The salad dressing must be full-fat.

Pearl chats: Indulgent and delicious. I have to eat this meal now and then (poor me, right?) to keep my weight up. If this were to be made an **E** meal, you would simply use way less fat.

Serene chats: I love **Crossover** meals with sweet potatoes. I heavily drench them with about two heaping tablespoons of raw virgin coconut oil and then liberally sprinkle on Celtic salt, cayenne pepper, and curry powder. It tastes divine, like a rich gourmet Indian curry. Having so much healthy fat helps stop any spike from the sweet potato, which is rather low glycemic anyway, but there will be a sufficient amount of carbs to give this meal a maintenance effect instead of weight loss. Anything over one medium sweet potato would go past the medium gylcemic point and be detrimental. This is especially true on an **E** meal where there is not a lot of fat to blunt the sugar climb.

E Evening Meal Example (the right way)

Mini Meat Loaves, made with extra lean ground turkey, (*Evening Meals,* Chapter 21) and a side of *Waldorf Cottage Cheese Salad* (*Lunches*, Chapter 20).

Pearl chats: These two recipes are high in protein and leave you feeling full. Since this is your **E** meal and the salad is your only carb portion, remember to make sure you put enough energy foods in the salad. One apple per serving makes it sweet and delicious and fills the salad out to ensure very big servings. Or, you could use half an apple per serving and toss in a handful of goji berries or currants. Two spoons of pineapple would be okay, too.

Serene chats: I love meatloaves and these minis look so cute on your plate. Sometimes, I make meatloaf with grass fed ground sirloin. It is also a very lean meat and a little more superfoody. You could substitute lean grass-fed beef, buffalo, or venison, but never regular ground beef in an **E** meal, please.

E Evening Meal Example (the wrong way)

Grilled chicken breast, corn on the cob, buttered dinner rolls, and salad with a sweet French dressing.

Pearl chats: There is so much wrong with this meal. This person may be under the impression that the nice lean chicken breast is going to help control weight. The corn will stop that. Corn works well to fatten up animals before slaughter and it can have the same effect on humans. The buttered dinner rolls are usually processed and devoid of fiber. French dressing will spike sugar unless it is homemade with a no-carb sweetener.

Serene chats: This meal is a typical dinner in our western culture. Not many people enjoy a meal without buttered bread, especially at a restaurant. However, margarine would be even worse. Even whole wheat yeast rolls are not a good choice on a low glycemic lifestyle as they are made with flour which is quickly absorbed into the blood as glucose. The only time we use any form of wheat flour in our recipes is with sourdough bread, which is fermented. This lowers the sugars while the sour lactic acid slows down an insulin response. The rolls were bad enough; but add the corn, which is genetically modified unless organic, plus a sugar laden dressing, and you're in for trouble. Sometimes people tell us, "I don't know what's wrong, I don't eat very much." You don't have to eat very much. It is deceivingly harmful meals like this that do the damage.

S Evening Meal Example (the right way)

New Mexican strip steak topped with melted cheese and green chilies with steamed broccoli tossed in butter on the side.

Pearl chats: This meal is a goodie. My husband and I cannot afford steak very often, but eating it at home occasionally feels like a special date. Like ours, most families cannot afford to feed everybody steak, especially organic or grass fed. Once in a while we'll let everybody in the family have a steak, but we usually throw on burgers for the children, and cook up one extra steak for them all to share so they get a taste of the real thing. Don't think that you have to eat exactly what you feed your children. They have different metabolic needs and get to eat some "special" items that you don't, so it evens out.

Serene chats: Those of us with large families know we can't afford steak for the whole family. I buy it at Costco for my husband, and an occasional treat for myself. It is fairly well priced when you don't feed it to the whole gang.

I'd like to add to what Pearl mentioned about specialty foods for the adults. When daddy eats his nice big steak now and then after a hard day at work, the children know he did not get to enjoy the heaping portion of the creamy mashed potatoes they ate. Children learn that they have their own treats. In our house I buy honey, raisins, bananas, white potatoes, whole wheat noodles, and other healthy glucose rich foods for the children only. They need these to grow. We buy grass fed milk that only the children drink. They get to enjoy organic jellies for their bread. Keeping steak for dad, and occasionally for you, should not affect your conscience.

S Evening Meal Example (the wrong way)

Grilled steak with large baked potato on the side, topped with sour cream and butter. Tossed head lettuce salad, with ranch dressing.

Pearl chats: This is a common one. The loser here is the baked potato, yet it is the main side offered with steak in most homes and restaurants. We urge you not to do this combination. It makes a wonderful steak meal fattening when it doesn't need to be.

I cut up yellow squash, season it well, and bake it in the oven with butter. My husband likes this with steak as well as any old potato. Broccoli is always good with steak, too. White potatoes are like white bread; they are straight sugar in the body. We don't recommend white potatoes for adults, even on our **E** meals. A small one now and then won't kill you in a **Crossover**, as long as you are already at, or near, your desired weight.

Serene chats: It's not only that a white potato has carbs enough to send your insulin revving to the moon, but people always dress them up with large amounts of fatty toppings because they are so dry without them. This is a double whammy. Eating the baked potato dry, just to be diet conscious, is still a bad idea, as you have learned that a naked carb is a blood sugar swinger. Plus, dry potato—yuck!

Crossover Evening Meal Example

Coconut Chicken Curry (*Evening Meals*, Chapter 21) over brown rice or quinoa. A side salad with olive/balsamic dressing.

Pearl chats: You can do a full cup or more of quinoa here if you like; much less than half a cup of grain will not likely help to maintain weight. In this meal, the fat and the carbs merge in a sensible synergy.

Serene chats: I love coconut anything! If you are trying to lose some extra weight, it may be a while before you will be incorporating **Crossover** meals. You can easily make this into an **S** meal by leaving out the rice and having this dish over *Cauli Rice* (*Vegetable Sides*, Chapter 21) or even some hemp seeds if you have any handy. An **S Helper** of quinoa is always another option.

Chapter 15

Thirsty Mama

Learning the art of keeping beverages glycemic friendly is crucial to the success of this plan. Anything you put into your body in liquid form is more easily absorbed into the bloodstream. If your drink contains sugar, your blood glucose levels will immediately sky rocket. This rapid sugar high is worse for your body than a regular sugar high from food, which is already bad enough. It is basically fat in a drink. With every gulp, you pour on the pounds.

Juice, the Great Deceiver

Many people think they are doing themselves a favor by opting for juice instead of sodas. Even 100% juice drinks are 100% fattening. Juice is liquid carbohydrate, the worst kind for weight management. The fiber has been removed. It has usually been pasteurized, or worse, made from a concentrate.

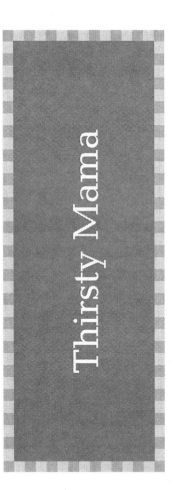

Even if you took the time to make all raw fruit juice at home with a juice extractor, it is still fat in a glass. How can we say that? There is never a good reason for the fiber to be removed from fruit. God put it there to slow down the insulin response. You may wish to detox now and then with fresh juices, or include them if you are fighting a grave disease. If so, always stick to green juices with a base of mild cucumber or celery. These are more cleansing and healing than sweet juices. Watch out for the myth of carrot juice. It has a similar effect as fruit juice on blood glucose. High sugar imbalances the body by promoting yeast and parasites which create the perfect environment for cancer growth and all disease. These pathogens and harmful microbes are like weeds which overtake the body's ecology or inner garden.

Better than juicing is to make *Serene's Earth* Milk (Chapter 27) which has the same healing and cleansing properties as juices, but tastes better.

The Naughty List

We know that sodas are fattening. Now you can place fruit juices in the same category. Here are some other drinks which are equally dangerous to your waistline. Excuse our Sergeant Major attitude for a minute. Hang in there—excellent options are coming.

- Sweet tea—fattening.
- Naturally sweetened healthy type green teas—fattening (the word "naturally" on a food label always means using sugar).
- Sports drinks like Gatorade—fattening.
- Energy drinks like Red Bull—fattening.
- Natural cane juice sweetened colas—fattening.
- Any store-bought or naturally sweetened lemonade—fattening.
- Vitamin water—fattening (except those sweetened with stevia).
- 100% juice spritzers—fattening.
- Any pre-packaged or deli made smoothie (usually contains apple juice, and or banana)—fattening.
- Most Starbucks concoctions—double fattening, due to fat and sugar combined (you'll be fine with their regular coffee with half and half or a little heavy cream).
- Hot tea with honey—fattening (good for rare medicinal occasion).
- Coffee with sugar—fattening.
- Overdoing diet sodas—fattening (long term use may mess with metabolism and endocrine system).
- Milk as a beverage—fattening (we'll explain why later).
- Beer—triple fattening (the highest on glycemic index). Ever heard of a beer belly?
- Sweet wines—fattening.
- Mixed alcoholic drinks—fattening

We feel like big ol' meanies after completing this list. Are you feeling a little chastised and deprived? It is depressing to write this, but we care enough about your success to get tough. Don't freak out! There is a superb replacement for each one of these no-nos.

Sip Ups or Slip Ups

We had to be thorough with all the "naughties" because the thought of someone starting our plan with gusto, then wrecking it with one needless slip up (or should we say sip up), ruins our day. We can't shake the following picture of a newly inspired *Trim Healthy Mama* throwing out all the high glycemic foods from her cupboards. She drives to a natural food market and excitedly fills her cart with omega-3 eggs, grass fed red meat, and lots of non-starchy vegetables. She's on a roll. On the way out of the store, feeling a little thirsty, she stops by the juice bar for a healthy pick me up drink. No more soda for her! She chooses one called Mango Madness and opts for a shot of wheat grass for good measure since she's now on a health kick.

Little does she realize her glucose levels surge through the roof on her drive home due to the so-called "healthy" drink, and her pancreas has to send out extra insulin to get rid of all that blood sugar. Her first day on our program becomes a disaster. There was nothing wrong with the wheat grass, but it doesn't have any sugar disabling properties to compensate for the contents of the rest of the smoothie. It was a waste of good money.

Don't let this be you. Get smart about your drink choices. There is no reason for you to feel deprived even if you have strong addictions to sweet drinks. Our recommended stevia products solve this problem. They'll be discussed in detail in *Foundation Foods*, Chapter 17. Please don't turn your nose up at the idea of stevia if you've tried it in the past and hated the bitter after-taste. We'll soon tell you about new products that taste just like sugar without that after burn.

Ideas for Juice Lovers

If you are a juice lover, we suggest purchasing berry teas such as Celestial Seasonings raspberry, orange, or blueberry flavored, and making them into iced tea sweetened with our recommended stevia sweeteners. This also works well with regular or mint teas and they are perfect over ice for hot days.

If you can't be bothered doing all that and have a little wiggle room in your budget, there are a couple of great new options to consider. In the future, there will surely be even more options since more companies are learning about the health benefits of sweetening drinks with stevia instead of sugar, corn syrup or other artificial sweeteners. However, we already know of a couple. Sobe brand has a beverage called Life Water. You can pick it up almost everywhere. We can even find it at our local hick gas station, out here in the Tennessee woods for about a dollar and a half a bottle.

The awesome thing is that since this Life Water is only sweetened with stevia and erythritol, it fits perfectly on plan and has zero impact on blood sugar. It is refreshing, fruity deliciousness and has no artificial ingredients. It offers many wonderful flavors like Fuji, Apple, Pear. Here in the South, Kroger grocery store chains also carry a drink that tastes like juice with no artificial ingredients. It is Kroger brand and is called, Zero Calorie, Vitamin Enhanced Water

Beverage. It comes in 12 bottle packs for a reasonable price and the Orange Starfruit flavor tastes like orange juice. Check to see if your local grocery store has something similar. The main thing to check with flavor enhanced waters is that the sweetener used is stevia, erythritol, or a combination of both. Be diligent when selecting, because while some beverage brands are starting to use stevia, most "sugar-free" brands of vitamin water are still using artificial sweeteners and other unhealthy ingredients.

Another good juice replacement can be found at Walmart, Kroger, and other popular grocers. Walk down the tea, coffee, and beverage isle where they sell Kool-Aid type packet mixes. Keep an eye out for a small box of dry packet mix called Hansen's Naturals Fruit Stix. It's a powder you mix with water to make a fruity tasting beverage. It is sweetened with stevia and includes only natural flavors. We heartily endorse it if you can afford it. It gives wonderful flavor and color to water, or sparkling water. It comes in a variety of refreshing fruit flavors.

Lemonade lovers can be happily satisfied using natural lemon concentrate or the juice from real lemons, which are both very low in carbs. Or, if you have some more budget wiggle room, most supermarkets now sell Pure Lemon packets. They consist of lemon flavored powder which is easily dissolved in water. They taste wonderful and don't have artificial additives. Adding these options to a pitcher of pure water and sweetening with our on plan sweeteners makes divine tasting and incredibly healthy lemonade. The same can be done with small amounts of unsweetened cranberry juice concentrate. Those who like juice spritzers could do a similar thing using sparkling mineral water instead of regular water.

Pop, Soda, Coke

Whatever you name them, we call them the death of a trim waistline. Thankfully, more and more companies are coming out with stevia-sweetened sodas. Kroger supermarkets carry three such brands in their health food section. One brand, called Zevia even has a cola flavor that contains caffeine. We know some of you may drink coke or diet coke for the caffeine hit. We're not going to bury our heads in the sand and pretend you don't exist. If you're a soda addict, switching to a brand like Zevia can be one way to drink your soda without growing an insulin belly from all the sugar in coke, or consuming the harmful artificial sweeteners in diet sodas. This might not be a purist approach but it offers a practical solution.

There has been quite a buzz lately about Pepsi bringing out a stevia-sweetened version of coke. So far, it's not on the market, but will probably happen before too long.

Pearl chats: My children love to drink Virgil's Zero Root Beer. They like it so much that they save their own money to buy it since it's not on my grocery list. It is stevia-sweetened, zero calorie, zero harmful ingredients, yet absolutely delicious. We find it at our local Kroger store.

No More Coffee?

Coffee and tea. They've been around for centuries. Our official stance is, go ahead! Shouts and cheers! Fist pumps and high fives all around. We join you in a resounding, Yay!

We know there is much controversy over whether or not coffee and tea are healthy. We have kept a close eye on the studies. Latest research has exonerated coffee and tea from their bad reputation. Studies show that coffee does not leach minerals from the body. It is not a great idea to take your vitamins with a cup of coffee, but it will not deplete your entire system.

You cannot count coffee as part of your water intake for the day, but it is a myth that coffee will cause dehydration. Tea may be counted as water intake. Both tea and coffee have wonderful benefits, but we still caution moderation since overdoing caffeine can raise cortisol levels and tax the adrenal glands. In moderate amounts, coffee and tea are beneficial because of their extraordinarily high antioxidant levels and mood lifting abilities. In fact, tea, and green tea, can be consumed more liberally than coffee since they have less caffeine and both offer benefits to the brain and body. Green and black tea can aid in weight loss, calm nerves due to their theanine content and are anti-aging tools. The caffeine in green tea is neutralized because of theanine, a natural de-stresser.

Coffee elevates dopamine levels, which contributes to a feeling of happiness and lessens the chance of getting Parkinson's. Numerous studies indicate that coffee consumption is associated with a sharply reduced risk of developing Type 2 diabetes, including an 18 year follow up study on Swedish women released in *J Intern Med* in 2004. A 2009 study published in the *Archives of Internal Medicine* reported that each cup of coffee consumed daily dropped the risk of this disease by seven percent. Another very recent study carried out in China at the *Huazhong University of Science and Technology* suggests the likely reason why coffee has this preventive effect against Type 2 diabetes. The researchers discovered that coffee is able to inhibit toxic amyloid proteins that are normally found in the pancreas of people with Type 2 diabetes.

One has to weigh up these findings with the rise of Type 2 diabetes. Most Americans drink coffee, yet Type 2 diabetes is on the rise. However, consider what they put in their coffee. Sugar, or some other sweet *Starbucks* concoction? We doubt even high amounts (4-6 cups) of plain black coffee daily can completely combat a diet that is too high in carbs and sugars. Yet, these beneficial compounds in coffee cannot be discounted. Logically, it seems best to eat low glycemic foods and also include some wonderful daily cups of Joe.

Coffee is now also considered by researchers to be an anti-cancer beverage. Laboratory studies show that it has an anti-tumor effect against ovarian, colon, liver, and other cancers. A recent 2011 study released in a May edition of *Breast Cancer Research* showed that post menopausal women who drink moderate to large doses of coffee are also at significantly less risk for an aggressive type of breast cancer known as "estrogen receptor (ER) negative."

Pearl chats: I look forward to my one cup of coffee each day, two on Saturdays. I jokingly call coffee my "paci," nicknamed for pacifier. It soothes, comforts, and lifts my spirits. I am thankful for this "paci" when my boys are extra loud and crazy and I finally shoo them out the door to play backyard football. What better way to de-stress than with a comforting mug of coffee? My coffee with cream helps me get through the rest of the day. Sure, it's a vice, but God knows we need that little extra help sometimes or He wouldn't have made the coffee bean! Having only one cup a day is not a rule, but I find I can become overly stimulated with more and push my body to do too much. I'm not particularly interested in becoming a super woman.

I find it helps to have a nice hot drink in the afternoon with a snack. Eating on the run, or while multi-tasking, often causes you to be unaware of what and how much you are eating. Devoting a little time to unwind with a cup of coffee or tea, and some yummy plan approved cheesecake, makes you stop and realize life is pretty great. You receive more pleasure through food by relaxing and are more able to stop eating when satisfied. Somehow, sipping on a hot beverage makes that more likely to happen.

Serene chats: When I first started researching on the benefits of coffee and how it is one of our highest dietary sources of antioxidants, I really wanted to be a believer, but I had been indoctrinated by dietary gurus who looked down their noses at coffee. It was difficult, with my purist approach to eating, to even put coffee in my shopping cart at first. I felt like I was starting to smoke cigarettes or something equally unhealthy (crazy me, huh?). Since finally allowing myself this wonderfully healthy indulgence, I have taken a step closer to comfort and the ability to nurture myself.

I have always enjoyed the deep aroma of coffee and tried to savor its flavor by using coffee substitutes made by roasted chicory and grains. They didn't have the depth and fullness I knew came from real coffee and I was always left unsatisfied. Living with a low glycemic approach, I didn't like the extra carbs in the grains (even though they weren't over the top) as I prefer to save my carbs for food.

At first, I didn't do regular caffeinated coffee as I was still trying to heal my adrenals after some lifestyle stressors. Regular decaf is unhealthy because of the chemical processes used. Here's the good news. There is a healthy way to decaffeinate. It is called the "Swiss water method." This removes the caffeine, but keeps the bold flavor and antioxidants. You can find this at any natural food store. I still love my Swiss water decaf coffee, but also enjoy the "real thing" now without any ill effects.

Now, along with my eggs in the morning, you can picture me enjoying real organic coffee with cream. Care to join me? What a yummy way to stay young, slim, sane, and healthy.

I like to research the best and healthiest approach to everything. Coffee and its different preparations has been my latest hot subject. Pearl laughs at my obsessive personality in this area. You could serve her Joe "any old how," as long as it's real coffee. She could probably even drink it lukewarm! Horror! When it comes to coffee she simply enjoys it without all the fuss. Me? I like to fuss. I am a complete coffee snob . . . well, perhaps a "wannabe snob." All my coffee gadgets come from the Goodwill thrift store. If I can't have a nice, potent, organic, freshly roasted "cuppa," then I'd rather go without.

I don't mind a cup of French press or filtered organic coffee, but I prefer to dive in deep and drink my coffee closer to the core essence of this antioxidant loaded bean. Behold, the espresso—the most potent way of receiving the antioxidant properties and bold flavor from the coffee bean. Surprisingly, it is also the best way of avoiding too much caffeine.

Espresso is made by forcing a small amount of hot water through the coffee very quickly. It is this rapid and pressurized contact with the water that extracts concentrated amounts of coffee's benefits without over extracting caffeine and breaking down the oils. In all coffee preparations, the best part of the coffee is extracted in the first cup of water that flushes through the grounds. This is like the first pressing of a good quality olive oil or wine and contains most of the incredible benefits we hear about coffee. When you brew a pot of coffee, you run multiple cups of water over these same grounds. More bitterness and acidic content of the coffee bean is extracted and you get a boatload more caffeine and diluted benefits.

The longer the contact time with water, the more caffeine is extracted. It is a misunderstanding that espresso is the stuff that gets you totally wired. Yes, it has a stronger and deeper flavor, but a 2 oz. double espresso has only 50 mg of caffeine, whereas an 8 oz. cup of brewed coffee has 2.5 times that much caffeine, sitting around 135 mg.

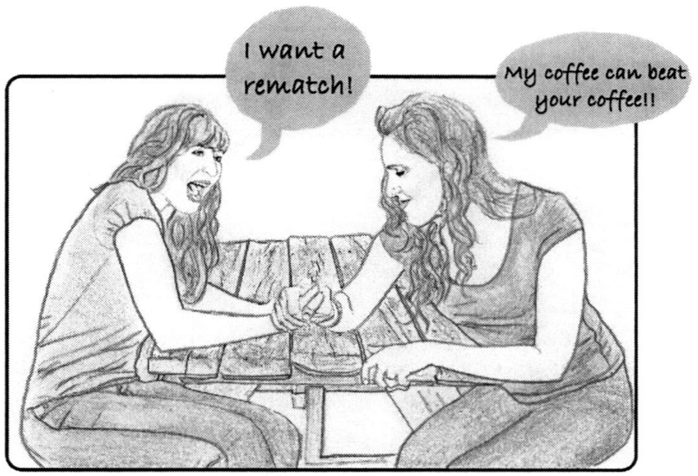

I don't want to come across as fearful of a moderate amount of caffeine. In fact, most of the studies show the benefits of coffee are associated with the real thing, not decaf. But, keep in mind we are not encouraging you to be a "caffeine junkie." Over-stimulating yourself is not beneficial.

I don't like to take my espresso in a quick shot as I love to savor a full mug of Joe. Therefore, I dilute my morning double espresso with the same amount of hot water and a dash of organic cream, if budget allows. Superb! This is called an Americano. It rocks with a quiet moment— the baby napping or nursing and my Bible or another meditational book in hand.

I found my espresso maker at Goodwill for five bucks. It does the job, but would probably make an espresso connoisseur completely dissatisfied. I am hinting to my husband about a Vev Vigano for Christmas. It runs around $40-50 for a small one. It is purported to make the best espresso unless you want to spend up to $1000. It carries an old world charm of being a stove top original Italian design. What makes it better than most stove top espresso makers is that it is made from stainless steel and not aluminum like other Italian models.

Pearl chats: Thanks for the loooooong coffee 101 class Serene. I still "like me some Dunkin' Donuts" brewed coffee. And yes, I can drink it any temperature.

You can drink your coffee with full cream or half and half for **S**, and either black, or with a dash of milk or almond milk for **E.** Please stay away from non dairy creamers. They are filled with trans fats and do not work for our plan or your health. If you are completely lactose intolerant, health food stores have coconut coffee creamers which work for our plan. Do not use pre-sweetened ones. They will counteract the wonderful health benefits coffee gives.

Also, please stop using flavored coffee liquid creamers like vanilla, caramel, or Irish Cream. They are full of sugar and cause your middle to expand. You can buy flavor infused coffee beans or ground coffee instead. Starbucks has a line of naturally flavored coffees. Watch out though, because most other brands of vanilla, caramel, or other flavored coffee beans are artificially flavored and add needless toxins to the body. If you love flavored coffee, purchase naturally flavored beans or grounds then add your own cream and on plan sweetener. You'll have the same end product, but a much healthier and trimming version.

Coffee Buzz or Sugar Buzz?

Some people pride themselves on the fact that they don't do caffeine. We often notice these people get buzzed through other means—namely sugar, often in the form of fructose. Many of these people are juice drinkers or like to eat way too much fruit. Sugar, even too much natural sugar, will give a feeling of energy at first, but is always followed by a slump a couple of hours later. These people then fuel up on sugar again. It may be in the form of a candy bar or the more deceitful trap of another banana or glass of orange juice. It is a vicious cycle and a lot worse for your health and waistline than a little caffeine in the antioxidant rich environment of coffee.

Coffee or Chai tea can be most useful after a meal when you are almost satisfied, but looking for that extra something. Following an **S** meal, you can add some cream, even whipped cream. Sweeten it up with a plan approved sweetener. It feels like a decadent dessert. You will no longer be hungry. Knowing you have this to look forward to after the meal helps to stop that compulsion for second or third helpings.

Just holding such a drink can be a great psychological aid when doing something that usually gives you the munchies, like watching a movie. Sipping contentedly, you won't feel deprived when others are reaching for the carby snacks. Treat yourself to stevia-sweetened icy Frappuccinos, hot coffee delights, and exotic chai delicacies.

The Milk Drinker

Now, let's tackle milk. There's a lot of confusion as to whether it's healthy or not. The reason we see it as a problem is because it is carbs and fat combined together in liquid form. Remember, liquid carbs are the most potent fat promoting form. Even if you drink skim milk, there will be an insulin response because the fat has been removed, leaving a pure liquid carb. The exception to this is when dairy is fermented as in kefir. The carbs are significantly reduced, and this is healthful rather than harmful. Fermented milk in both skim and full-fat forms was likely the way most milk was consumed in biblical times since they did not have refrigeration.

Raw whole milk is a healthy superfood with its high enzyme content and whole food nutrition profile. However, here's the problem. It is excellent for growing children, pregnant women who have trouble gaining weight, or high metabolism husbands. For the rest of us, it only fattens us up. The aforementioned people are the only cases for whom we recommend drinking milk.

Pearl chats: The only time I can endorse low-fat cow's milk is for having a splash in tea or coffee, pouring a little over oatmeal in an **E** breakfast, or having some with Uncle Sam's or other plan approved cereal every now and then. Half cup portions of low-fat milk shouldn't cause a problem used with these grains as the fiber and protein will help slow sugar responses. You may not always want to use yogurt, almond milk, or a teaspoon of coconut oil or cream with water on your oatmeal. Therefore, a small amount of low-fat milk is an okay option with an **E** breakfast if you can't tolerate our better options.

Serene chats: Raw, grass fed cow's milk and raw, farm fresh goat's milk which my family acquires from nearby farms are superfoods in my children's diets. They all do so well on this raw milk and are robust and healthy. My toddler drinks it all day long and I am not exaggerating. He has a nice, fat, gushy belly of which I'm proud. I know he will grow out of it when he does not consume such large amounts.

My husband loves milk, and when we were able to acquire this wonderful raw food, he started drinking it by the quarts and gained the same gushy belly. Once he stopped, his belly flattened again. Now, he enjoys unsweetened almond milk for his smoothies, or we scoop the cream off our lovely raw milk and mix that with water for a yummy extra creamy **S** smoothie.

I don't use low-fat regular milk on my **E** breakfasts, but Pearl's more practical balanced approach may work for some of you. I am a food zealot—you know that already!

Unsweetened Almond Milk

We'd love you to consider unsweetened almond milk. It is our favorite milk replacement and you'll notice we use it in a lot of our recipes. It is available at most grocery stores in cartons right next to regular milk. Unsweetened almond milk typically has zero net carbs, only a little fat, and more incredibly, only about 30 calories per cup. Lay the red carpet out for unsweetened almond milk in both your **S**, **E** and **Fuel Pull** meals. You can use it for your smoothies and on your morning oatmeal or quinoa. We like to use Silk brand. It tastes smooth and delicious.

Please do not buy sweetened almond milk. It's higher in sugar and carbs and therefore contributes to weight problems. Buy only unsweetened almond milk and add our plan approved sweetener.

New Kid on the Block—Flax Seed Milk

It's not as readily available as almond milk yet but keep your eye open for unsweetened flax seed milk under the brand of Good Karma. We predict it will become extremely popular in the next couple of years. The unsweetened version can be used for either **S**, **E** or **Fuel Pull.** Like unsweetened almond milk, it is both low in fat and carbs. It tastes great and is only 25 calories per cup! If you prefer the taste over almond milk you can replace it in any recipes that call for almond milk.

Coconut Milk

You'll notice in future chapters that we use canned coconut milk in some of our recipes. It makes great creamy curries, sauces for meats and vegetables, and is great for smoothies when frozen in ice trays or diluted with water. But, canned coconut milk does not make a great drink alone. The consistency just isn't right and its flavor and texture is too powerful.

Similar to almond milk, coconut milk is now packaged in a carton for drinking and is becoming a common item in everyday grocery stores. The problem is that this sweetened coconut milk is too high in carbs. You can purchase unsweetened coconut milk, but because it has more fat, keep it in an **S** setting.

If you would like to save money and enjoy the health benefits and taste of drinkable coconut milk, go to www.healthylivinghowto.com where it describes how to make easy and delicious coconut milk from unsweetened shredded coconut. Just remember, this homemade coconut milk recipe is approved for **S** purposes, not **E,** if you're seeking weight loss. The originator of this web site, Vanessa Romero, also gives an easy step by step guide on how to make this milk into delicious ice cream. We love her site because she has wonderful information on the benefits of a low glycemic approach to food and she breaks everything down into quick, easy, and doable steps. The pictures are incredible and you want to reach through the computer and gobble the coconut ice cream up.

Adult Beverages

Like coffee, wine can also be a healthful addition to an anti-aging diet. In excess, it is destructive to the body and dangerous to the liver. European countries that use it as a balanced accompaniment to their meals enjoy great health benefits. Several new studies back this up. A glass a day extends life. One reason may be its effect on inhibiting plaque in the brain, thus preventing age related neuronal disorders. It also helps the breakdown of collagen in the skin, consequently moderate wine drinkers are at less risk for an aging and wrinkled face. How about that?

One glass per day for women, and up to two for men, lowers harmful LDL cholesterol. Be careful though, mama, a recent, major 2011 study published in the *Journal of the American Medical Association* showed that women process alcohol differently to men. Drinking more than one alcoholic drink per day for females can go against health, rather than promote it. Women who drink more than one glass a day showed a modest 15% higher risk for breast cancer compared to women who drank less. Therefore, sip slowly and stick to no more than one 5 oz. glass.

Of course, you do not need to become a wine drinker on this plan. And please, don't even begin if you know you have the genetic potential to abuse it. If there has been alcohol abuse in your past, or in your family, you are probably best to stay well away from wine altogether.

There is exciting information coming out about a substance called resveratrol, which is found in the skins of the grapes in red wine. It turns on the life extension gene in our bodies, previously only known to kick in with reduced calorie diets. Resveratrol aids in weight control, especially in the mid section, and energy function. This supplement may be a great idea if you want to stay away from wine.

Never drink sweet wines! Always opt for dry, as these have very few carbs. Red wines, like Pinot and Cabernet Sauvignon are excellent. Dry, white wines can also be used, but they do not have the incredible resveratrol factor. If you'd prefer less alcohol content, a half glass of dry white wine mixed with sparkling water is a good alternative. Please do not send us letters about the evils of wine. Jesus performed miracles with it and wine was definitely a biblical beverage. This was not grape juice as some like to argue. Fermentation played an integral role in enabling populations to have enough to eat and drink in that day as there was no refrigeration.

Some wives may have husbands who like to have beer sometimes. It is very detrimental to a macho body. Beer tends to end up making men look pregnant once they are over 30 years and their cells are more resistant to insulin. You could suggest the idea of dry wine to your husband in place of beer. If sipping wine doesn't appeal to his manliness, and he would still like to swig a beer on the odd occasion, we only approve ultra light beers because the carb content has been greatly reduced to less than three carbs. Of course, your husband may not care a whit what we approve or do not approve, that's fine too. But, you could gently share the science with him. You don't need to say, "Serene and Pearl say . . ." He might get sick of hearing sentences that start out like that (if he's anything like our husbands). We're sure you could find creative ways to share the information with him that will not turn him off upon hearing our names, or this plan.

Chapter 16

Mama Saves Money

In Chapter 17, you will learn more about the foods that make up the core of the **S** and **E** plan and the reasons we encourage them. Some of these food items will be new to you and some very familiar. Most of them are affordable, while others cost a little more. Don't be overwhelmed. You don't have to include all the foods we write about. The way you steer this **S** and **E** plan includes as little or as many of these foundation foods as you can afford. Start slowly and introduce yourself to them one at a time as your budget allows.

A small food budget should not deter you from starting our plan. You may not be able to afford all the superfoods or specialty items we write about, but do what you can. Start very simply. We both have big families, tight budgets, and have learned to do this on a shoe string. You can too.

Cart Watching

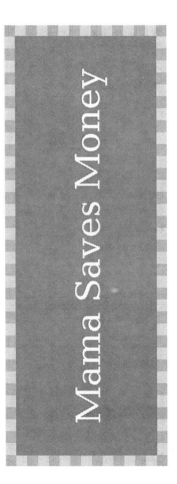

Yes, it's true that proteins cost more than starches do. We have to admit that white pasta, cheap, fluffy white sandwich breads, Ramen noodles, packets of pretzels, and generic brand chips are relatively cheap. People sometimes fill their carts with this sort of junk in the hopes of getting a lot of food items without spending a ton of money. This practice might save you a dollar or two, but you haven't bought any food. They are essentially non-foods. They might be cheap on your bank account, but will be expensive to your long term health.

When we "cart watch" (a term we coined to describe the past time of observing the contents of people's carts while waiting in the checkout line), we notice that it is not only cheap carbs that fill carts. There are almost always expensive ones too. Items like frozen lasagna, frozen pizzas, boxed cereals (ouch, those will cost you), or those silly little frozen packaged diet meals that don't fill anybody up and leave you wanting to eat potato chips afterwards.

We notice patterns when we cart watch. We often see women buying diet type foods like those little low-calorie boxed meals. But, they have potato chips in their cart too! Doesn't make a lot of sense, but it's extremely common. You will hopefully reduce or completely eliminate these more expensive carb-laden, frozen items. They should be completely deleted from your grocery list. Items like these are not cheap at all, so get rid of all such crazy carbs, whether they're labeled diet food or not. Replace them with healthy proteins, more veggies, beans, and whole grains and the switch should make very little impact on your budget. It should even itself out and you might even save a dollar or two on the total.

If you are on a severely restricted budget, look at what you can buy rather than what you can't. Foods like Old Fashioned Oats, eggs, cans of tuna, lettuce, cabbage, brown rice, beans, and butter are affordable for anyone.

We don't mean boiling your cabbage unless you actually like it that way. Cabbage is such a versatile, cheap vegetable that can be made in so many delicious ways. Think about sautéing or roasting it with delicious seasonings in butter or coconut oil. Nothing could be better. Cabbage is full of cancer fighting abilities and is the non-starchy vegetable that goes the longest way for the smallest amount of money. Frozen cauliflower florets are very inexpensive also, and when creatively prepared, can replace rice and potatoes very deliciously.

Treat yourself to a container of cooking coconut oil (Louanna brand from Walmart is cheaper than extra virgin brands) and buy some unsweetened cocoa powder. Adding plan approved sweetener, and you've always got chocolate to eat.

You could almost do our whole plan on these few inexpensive food items we're suggesting if you threw in a few berries, a piece of salmon now and then, and some green apples, as long as you don't mind not having a lot of variety.

Serene's Budget Tip

Serene chats: It costs just under a buck at any grocery store for a bag of dried beans and this is good news for a large growing family. When my children have growth spurts, they eat all day and I run out of ideas for snacks. Sometimes they have already had enough fruit, bread, eggs, popcorn, smoothies and the like to fill a battle ship. I need another healthy staple to fuel their tanks. Out of desperation, I came up with this very affordable idea and it is now one of their favorites.

I soak a couple of bags of their favorite dried beans overnight and cook them up the next day. After they become lovely and tender, I drain out the water and add a little sea salt. Once they are cool, I put them in a tub in the refrigerator and they are available for the creativity of budding chefs. When my children say they are hungry, I tell them they can fry up their beans with their favorite spice. They love creating their own specialties.

The older ones go at it on their own, and the little ones sometimes pair up with an older one and help stir or suggest seasonings. Some of my children fry them up with exotic curries and red palm oil while others prefer butter, parmesan cheese, and black pepper.

Personally, I have come to love garbanzo beans sautéed with virgin coconut oil with nutritional yeast and sea salt—great for a **Crossover** salad. Garbanzo beans are also great first finger foods for older babies (without the hot spices), a healthy whole food that grows strong children instead of sickly ones.

Check out our *Secret Agent Brownie Cake* which is made from beans (*Desserts*, Chapter 23).

Pearl chats: I have adopted this bean idea from Serene and my children love it, too! They often ask if we can have "bean fry ups" like the Allisons. That's often what they eat when they spend time at their home.

Bean days really help our budget. We often do these fry ups at lunch time since it works well for hungry homeschooling children. I fry up the pre-cooked beans for my younger ones in a little coconut oil, all purpose seasoning, and parmesan cheese, but the older ones take great pride in doing it themselves. They all have their own "best flavor" ideas. My oldest son, Bowen is a spice lover. Nobody else would be able to eat his version of beans because they are so heavily seasoned with cayenne pepper and Cajun seasoning. I don't know how he handles the heat, and I am a spicy hot lover! Because they are pre-cooked, it only takes a couple of minutes for the beans to heat up and so I make them all wait to use the same fry pan. Paper plates and one fry pan—clean up is not too bad.

I also make use of these beans. It's a great way to merge both the children's needs and my own at lunchtimes. I'm not always eating **Crossovers**, so instead of frying up my pre-cooked beans in generous amounts of coconut oil like the children, which would be a **Crossover**, I often take out a cupful of beans and make a tuna and bean salad as an **E** meal for myself. It's really quick prep and still cheap—add a can of tuna to the beans, some diced onion, and a delicious light dressing.

Lentils help our budget, too. My husband is not a big soup lover, so I often make lentil soups for lunch while he is at work or on nights when he has to work at his second job. Lentil soup is cheap and easy. Charlie also understands that when I'm at the end of my grocery week and there's nothing left, then it's lentil soup to the rescue. While not his favorite, he always eats two bowls full. My children love it with lots of cheese and whole wheat crackers. I adore lentil soup and eat it **E** style usually, without the crackers and with a little mozzarella sprinkled on top.

Don't forget to check out our information on a legume called chana dahl in *Foundation Foods*, Chapter 17.

Inexpensive Meat

We'd like you to have meat in your diet. If you cannot afford it from the store, inquire into a hunter's association in your area. Many hunters kill extra deer and they are only too happy to give it to families who need it. Venison is very healthy and great-tasting after cooking long hours in the crockpot.

Chicken thighs and legs are the least expensive parts of chicken and big frozen bags can go a long way. Buying frozen rather than fresh is usually quite a bit cheaper. You just need to keep thinking ahead of your next meal for thawing purposes.

If your budget is not too tight, we always recommend organic meat over regular, the best kind being grass fed. The benefits are widely known. Regular grain fattened beef is much higher in omega 6 fats, which are inferior to the omega-3 fats in grass fed meats and are much lacking in today's western diet. Grass fed beef is naturally very lean and can be purchased more economically when some families decide to buy a cow together and share in the meat.

Even if your budget is very tight, attempt to seek out better meat sources. Is there a farm near you which sells grass fed meat? Go thirds with other families to purchase a side of beef. Pastured beef, chicken, and eggs raised without antibiotics or hormones are always the best for your whole family's health. Google for Weston Price co-ops near you.

Are there Amish farms within driving distance of your area? They are willing to sell almost anything they grow or raise. Take a drive and knock on doors. There are many alternatives to paying high prices for grass fed organic beef at health food stores. Even Walmart carries some healthier brands of meat. Tyson, Perdue, Harvest Land and Laura's are all considered cleaner sources.

But every penny counts these days, and if the cheapest brand of meat is all you can afford, don't beat yourself up. As long as you stick to our plan, you're still supporting good health. The hormones are contained in the fat of the meat so if you cannot afford organic or grass fed beef, always drain the fat after browning.

If you become too much of a "meat snob" without the budget to back you up, you may jeopardize your health. Trying to feed a big family on only organic meat may give you only about one tablespoon or two on your plate. That causes you to fill up on more carbs which only fattens you up. Aside from weight, over-carbing causes inflammation throughout your entire body and earlier aging.

People often feel better about themselves when buying boxes, cans, and packets of food that are labeled organic. Unfortunately, they do their bodies no favors if they are high-carb items. It costs them twice as much, and they are still spiking their blood sugar, which promotes today's disease epidemics. You can eat organic macaroni and cheese until you are orange in the face, but it will rev up that insulin delivery truck and you're no better off.

It's quite sad to go to stores like Whole Foods and Trader Joe's and watch people spend oodles of money on foods that are still doing them harm despite their earth colored packaging and labeling. Even though the labels tout healthier ingredients, the end result on blood sugar in the body is the same. It's actually smarter to eat something like regular non-organic ground beef from Walmart with some non-starchy vegetables than a bunch of high priced organic carbs.

Exceptions

There are a few items we recommend paying a little more for if you can.

Lettuce

We strongly advise you to stay organic with your salad greens if at all possible. Walmart sells three Earthbound Farms organic romaine hearts for just a few dimes more than regular romaine. Another good brand is Living Lettuce. It is a nice, buttery Boston lettuce in hydroponic form. However, it is more expensive and doesn't go as far with a big family.

Walmart even has organic iceberg head lettuce. While this isn't the most nutritious type of lettuce and has less chlorophyll and vitamins than other leafy greens, it is still a great filler. Remember, all lettuce is low-carb and low-calorie, and if iceberg is the only one you like, use it freely to help you fill up. Pour on heaps of olive oil in your **S** meals and you'll still be doing your body a great favor. We don't want to be "lettuce snobs" either.

Eggs

Try hard to avoid eating the regular battery hatched type. You will consume too much omega 6, which is a prevalent imbalance in our modern way of eating. Walmart carries Nature's Harmony omega-3 eggs and other equally healthy brands that are not very expensive. Search locally for farm-raised eggs. But hey, if you have a large family and you go through a lot of eggs, buy any eggs you can afford and don't agonize over what you can't control. They are a cheap protein source with many benefits. You can trim down eating regular ol' eggs just as easily as with healthier ones.

Canned Goods

A study by *Harvard University* that was released late in 2011 shed a horrid light on the amount of BPA contained in common canned goods. BPA (Bisphenol A) is a synthetic estrogen used to harden polycarbonate plastics and epoxy resins. Sadly, it has been used in canned goods for decades, but more and more information is now being released on the hazards it causes in the human body.

It is a known endocrine disrupter, so it hampers the body's natural hormones responsible for metabolism, reproduction, and development. It has been documented to trigger a wide range of disorders like impaired brain function, cancer, diabetes, early puberty, and cardiovascular damage. Pregnant women should be especially careful about ingesting BPA from canned goods and other products like plastic water bottles, as BPA can pass from the mother to baby and cause a greater risk for abnormalities.

The *Harvard University* study gave a 12 oz. serving of canned soup to a group of subjects for five days in a row. At the end of the five days, they were tested for BPA. Compared to a control group of people who were given a 12 oz. serving of fresh soup every day, the canned soup group showed an average level of BPA in their blood stream that was 1,221 times higher than the control group! Scary stuff!

Thankfully, there is good news. More and more companies are now using BPA free cans for their food products. In May of 2011, Kroger supermarkets announced they will no longer be using cans made with BPA for all of their house brand items. That's excellent news, as they have great coconut milk and inexpensive tomato and canned fish products. You can get basically any canned goods that you need under their house brand. We applaud Kroger for this move. Hopefully Walmart will follow suit. As of now (2012), Walmart Great Value brand still uses BPA in their cans. They do carry Hunts which uses BPA free cans for their plain tomato products only. Let's hope they will follow through with the rest of their products. Walmart also carries Del-Fuerte which have tomato paste in BPA free cans.

If you have a Whole Foods close by, you can be assured that their 365 house brand does not use BPA in their cans. Again, this is great news because we love their coconut milk and many of their other canned products. Trader Joe's confirms that their house brand is also free of BPAs.

Other brands known to be BPA free in at least a lot of their products are Eden Foods, Native Forest, Vital Choice, Muir Glen, Wild Planet, Ecofish and Oregon's Choice. As we learn of more, we will post on our website the companies who are kicking out BPA.

Deli Meats

It is easy to purchase brands without harmful additives or preservatives, even at regular supermarkets. Hormel and Oscar Meyer natural versions are great. However, do what you can with the money you have. If stretching to more natural versions is too hard on your budget, at least search for more affordable deli meats with only one carb. This means they have less fillers and you will be better off.

We are less concerned about nitrates in cured meat as some people warn about. This is because brands that advertise, "no nitrates," still use celery extract as a natural nitrate. It is the same thing in our bodies as regular nitrates. Most vegetables naturally contain abundant nitrates, but also contain antioxidants like vitamin C which cancel out the harmful effects of nitrates in the body. If you are concerned about the nitrates in cured meats, take some vitamin C when eating them and this should go a long way to protect you. Having said that, brands which advertise "no nitrates," often use healthier raised meats and put less fillers in their products. You might be better off buying them if your budget allows.

Salmon

Salmon is only a superfood in "wild caught" form. Most farm-raised fish are fed soy and corn based feed which destroys the omega-3 benefits. They are also high in PCBs. Wild caught salmon can be inexpensive. It is easily found in the frozen foods sections of most supermarkets. We buy ours from Aldi, a budget chain supermarket that carries four nicely-sized, individually packaged wild salmon fillets for less than $4. Serene also buys a large style fillet of wild Alaskan salmon with skin on from Walmart. Both versions are affordable. Another cheap source is canned wild salmon. It's just as healthy and great for coconut Thai soups and salmon burgers. Purchase in cans that are BPA free.

Yogurt

Always buy unsweetened yogurt and add your own stevia. Greek strained yogurt is preferred because the whey water has been strained off, leaving fewer carbs. It is much creamier and has twice as much protein. But, if it stretches your budget too much, buy plain yogurt and strain off the water.

Other Essentials

There are a few essentials you will need to purchase from either the health food store, the natural food section of your supermarket, an international supermarket, or online. We'll talk in more detail about them soon, but here's a quick list.

- NuStevia Pure White Stevia Extract Powder.
- Bragg Liquid Aminos.
- Nutritional yeast.
- Glucomannan and xanthan gum.
- Dreamfields noodles. They are good for all noodle purposes including Italian and Asian style. Carried in most Kroger and Walmart supermarkets. If you cannot find them at your local supermarket, order online.
- Konjac noodles. Good for noodles in Asian style dishes and fantastic for **Fuel Pull** dishes. Available at www.konjacfoods.com or www.netrition.com. You can find cheaper versions at international stores. They are often called yam noodles. The ingredients will list "yam root" as the main ingredient. This is not the yam like a sweet potato, but is actually the konjac root itself, sometimes mixed with seaweed.
- Kelp noodles. Good for noodles in Asian style dishes. Available at international stores and online.
- Chana dahl. Great for a lower glycemic bean option. Cheapest at international stores but available at some Walmarts.

Chapter 17

Foundation Foods

Our plan is a superfood lifestyle of which certain foods make the core. Soon you'll be making our recipes and using these foods on a daily basis. First, we want you to first understand their health, anti-aging benefits, and experience the sense of well being they bring.

Salmon, King of Sea Food

Dr. Weston Price's worldwide research on traditional people groups revealed that those whose diets were high in seafood had the most robust health. Fish eaters' bones were more dense and thick. He observed their entire skeletal structure to be stronger and better set.

Coronary heart disease is reduced with just one serving of fish per week. Wild caught ocean fish, like salmon, are our best food sources of macro trace minerals, such as iodine and zinc. Eating wild seafood has become more important with the depletion of many minerals from our soil. Fatty fish, like salmon, also provides an abundance of our fat soluble vitamins A and D.

All wild caught fish are wonderful, but salmon is the king of all. It is our highest food source of DMAE (dimethylethanolamine), the richest source being found in Red Sockeye salmon. DMAE firms and lifts our skin and brings tone to our appearance. It is essential for brain health and has been shown to be very effective in combating disorders like ADD and lack of concentration.

The Mercury Question

Many people are worried about mercury from fish. This is only valid when eating fish caught very near the shores of industrial areas or polluted fresh waters. Avoid fresh water fish if you don't know their source. Catfish, carp, and other scavengers are not healthy choices.

The problem with farm-raised fish is that they are fed a diet of pesticide laden soy pellets. Their fatty acids are no longer healthy omega-3, which are crucial for brain, mood, and nerve health, but the over consumed omega 6. Farm-raised salmon is often fed a dye to make its flesh the lovely pink color that is truly only obtained in the wild. However, farm raised fish is probably better than no fish at all. It is still a good protein source, but we can't call it a superfood.

Breathe easy about deep sea fish like salmon. Flounder and Sole from clean shore line areas are also good choices. Mercury from these types of fish is not really an issue. Sally Fallon, author of *Nourishing Traditions* says, "Small amounts of mercury occur naturally in these fish. They contain substances that bind with mercury to rid it out of the body."

You won't find any mercury from industrial pollution in deep sea Alaskan salmon. It is truly a pure superfood to be safely consumed by modern man. Try to eat salmon at least three times a week. Serene eats it almost every day.

Pearl chats: I try to eat salmon a few days a week, and believe me, our budget is tight. I take my fillet out of the freezer by mid-morning and have it defrosting in its packet in a bowl of warm water while I continue to homeschool. By lunch time it is completely defrosted and only takes a couple of minutes to sauté with some veggies or enjoy on a salad.

On special nights, I give the children a whole salmon fillet each, but mostly, I use wild caught canned salmon and make *Crabby Patties* (*Evening Meals*, Chapter 21), as this is cheaper to feed a whole family. They love these patties.

Serene chats: The words "canned salmon" don't sound very healthy. But, this is far from the truth. Wild caught, canned salmon from Alaska contains both skin and bones. Servings of salmon in this form give even higher amounts of calcium and other minerals.

Canned salmon is the perfect food for growing children and nursing mothers. My family lives on curries and Thai soups with canned salmon as my preferred choice for these recipes. We also love to eat *Crabby Patties*. Dining on salmon regularly does not mean you have to be rich. Even large families can have their fill, and seconds too.

For lunch, I sometimes mimic what Pearl described, but more often, I whiz up gourmet garden soups using salmon. These take about five minutes from start to finish. Check out my quick soup recipes in *Lunches*, Chapter 20. Homemade fast food can be superfood!

Berries

Bite for bite, berries offer more antioxidants than most other foods. In a recent study published in the *American Journal of Clinical Nutrition*, blackberries ranked as number one for antioxidant content. Strawberries, raspberries, and blueberries all showed up in the top ten. But, this is only the beginning of their benefits.

Chock Full of Flavanoids

Women should consume lots of berries as they contain a flavonoid called quercetin, which helps regulate cell growth and protects against estrogen related cancers such as breast and endometrial cancer. Quercetin also helps prevent plaque from sticking to arteries and clots from forming.

Life Extending Abilities

Berries are an excellent source of phytochemicals that help fight cancer. Ellagic acid, one such phytochemical, is now being touted by world renowned anti-aging doctors as one of the most important substances we can consume for health and life extension. Blackberries, raspberries, and strawberries all have high amounts of ellagic acid. Studies show it inhibits lung, skin, and liver cancer in animals. Ellagic acid also wages war on arteriosclerotic lesions (plaque buildup). One study showed a 1000 percent decrease. That's better than any statin could do.

Do you notice the bright colors of berries? Fruits and vegetables that have vibrant hues are the ones that go on record for remarkable health benefits. Anthocyanins are responsible for the deep hues of berries. Foods high in these are particularly effective at counteracting the effects of aging, especially in neurological disorders such as Alzheimer's disease and macular degeneration, a leading cause of blindness in the elderly. Anthocyanins directly protect blood vessels, reduce blood pressure, and lower harmful type cholesterol. They also help fight diabetes, arthritis, and allergies by reducing inflammation.

The Brainy Berry

Studies have shown that berries help maintain a healthy brain. Only one handful of blueberries a day significantly decreases inflammation in the brain. They prevent a decline in memory and motor learning. Blueberries can also improve balance and coordination.

If you are a homeschooling mom, you may like to assign your older children and help your younger ones to search out the benefits of each berry. Each berry has something different to offer.

The Practical Berry

Berries are hits in our homes because they are sweet, exotic, and won't cause a sugar spike. You can buy them fresh, but it is usually cheaper to buy them frozen. This way, you can have them all year round.

Remember, berries are neutral ground. You can eat them with both **E** and **S** meals as their carb content is not too much higher than most non-starchy veggies, although blueberries are a little higher.

Pearl chats: My youngest daughter, Autumn, loves to eat berries as frozen treats by the bowlful. I prefer them thawed. I usually buy two frozen packets of berries every week from Aldi. I put the first packet I am going to use in the refrigerator to thaw. This way, the berries are delicious, juicy, and always accessible. I love to pour a nice amount of berries, along with some of the runny juice, into my Greek yogurt. It streaks it red and the strong colors let me know I am eating God's goodness. I enjoy them in my muffins, too. Check out our muffin recipes in Chapter 19.

Serene chats: I've found a berry trick that works for a snack on the run. I put some frozen berries in an empty peanut butter jar that has a lid. I fill it with my yummy homemade kefir and whatever flavorings I desire, screw on the lid, pop it in my bag, and away I go. The frozen berries keep the kefir chilled and the liquid thaws out the berries to succulent morsels—a perfect marriage.

Our family love berries so much that if we run out it feels like the kitchen is bare. I throw them in nearly everything. I eat them for a yummy **S** energy snack straight from the freezer, mixed with dry roasted almond butter. Delicious!

One of my family's favorite yearly highlights, looked forward to almost as much as birthdays, is blueberry picking season in our area. The whole family picks and eats, and picks and eats as this farmer doesn't mind eating while picking. My youngest is usually almost blue by the time picking is done. Look for farms within an hour's driving distance from your home. They are usually cheap and delicious, and it is a fun outing. Check out my *Whip of Wonders* (*Snacks*, Chapter 24). It is the ultimate superfood snack or dessert.

If you want to eat purely organic, you will be pleased to know that blueberries are raised without spray, even if they are not labeled organic. I found this out from a local berry grower who sprays everything except his blueberries.

Omega-3 Eggs

These perfect little ovals of gold and white are rich in nearly every nutrient and are the perfect brain food. Here are just a few of the amazing health-promoting nutrients of eggs:

- Fat soluble vitamins A and D.
- Sulfur, containing proteins crucial for cell membrane integrity.
- EPA and DHA, responsible for nervous system and mental health.
- Choline, found in the yolk. It is a B vitamin necessary for keeping cholesterol moving in the blood stream.
- Lutein, an antioxidant important for many reasons, including muscle repair.
- Leucine, one of the three very special branch chain amino acids. It stands above them all for muscle building. The highest source is found in eggs.
- Vitamins E and B12.

The Cholesterol Myth

Do not be too concerned about the cholesterol scare. Sugar and trans fats are the worst offenders, not eggs. God provided choline, found in the egg, as the perfect built-in cholesterol aid. It helps to raise HDL cholesterol, or what is known as the good cholesterol. This is needed for proper hormone production. It is actually dangerous for total cholesterol levels to be too low. This increases the risk of heart attack since adequate cholesterol ensures adequate hormones, and without adequate hormones the immune system breaks down.

Pearl chats: I eat eggs on a daily basis and absolutely love them fried with butter. I often eat two or three per day. I recently had my cholesterol levels checked and was pleased to find that my HDL levels (healthy cholesterol particles) were an outstanding 87! My triglycerides were nice and low, around 50. My total cholesterol ratio came back as one of the lowest risks for a dangerous cardiovascular event on the scale. Obviously, eggs are not doing me any harm. I know a man who eats at least 40 eggs a week (his cheap protein of choice), and his cholesterol is excellent. He is fit, trim, and proud to call his cholesterol "eggtastic."

Serene chats: I'll admit I'm more extreme than Pearl, an "all or nothing" sort of girl. I sometimes eat up to four to five eggs a day, but I know I am doing my body good as they are gathered from my free range chickens running around our property. The yolks are bright orange. Remember, it is the brightest and most colorful foods that hold the best goodness. I also have a great lipid profile.

I throw my golden egg yolks into smoothies, but the whites never go to waste. I use them in scrambles with veggies and cheese. Also, some of our **S** bread and muffin recipes call for whites alone as this allows fluffier textures and saves on needless calories.

Eggs, glorious eggs. They are a good cheap protein source for the entire family when you can't afford meat. Have a look at my idea for a soft-boiled egg based dinner which I describe in *Morning Meals*, Chapter 18. Let's say you use a dozen eggs to feed a medium to large family as the sole protein for a meal. That is around \$2–\$2.50 for omega-3 eggs. Not bad at all.

Stevia, Nature's Sweetener

You can keep your sweet tooth. Why try to deny it? Life would be too dull without dessert, and what woman can go without chocolate?

Some people say sweet tasting foods should be avoided because giving in to decadent food pleasures may train your taste buds in unnatural ways. We think that's a load of nonsense. That's like ignoring a beautiful spring day and thinking that if we enjoy it too much we'll despise every other day. Wrong. We can be awed with spring yet still enjoy the colors of fall, the coziness of winter, and the barefoot fun of summer. Similarly, we should be able to enjoy sweet foods as well as spicy and savory.

Who makes all these rules? What about the other rule that is frequently tossed around, "Eat to live, don't live to eat!" Blah! Eating is joy! When you do it smartly, you can wake up in the morning and actually feel excited about your breakfast. Why not a muffin or some cheesecake for breakfast if that's what you love? Last time we checked the Ten Commandments, avoiding sweets was not included.

We'd like to introduce you to stevia. This is our plan approved sweetener of choice. It has zero calories and zero carbs so perfect for any fuel style meal. Now, before you say, "I've tasted that and it has a bitter after taste, no thanks," give us a minute and we'll change your mind.

The two brands of stevia we recommend are Nunaturals and Truvia. These brands use a safe process to remove the bitterness of the stevia. We felt the same way as you when it came to that awful aftertaste for which stevia was known. We kept trying different brands, but still no luck. Once we finally came across Nunaturals, it was a whole different story. Their product tastes very much like white sugar with none of the bitterness. Since it is heat stable, you can bake with it. It is perfect for all our dessert recipes. Then Truvia hit the stores and that was equally as palatable.

Thankfully, Truvia is a recent staple in almost every grocery store so that makes it easy to put on your regular grocery list. It comes in packets or more recently, in a little jar to make spooning it out a cinch! However, please do not purchase the new baking blend product Truvia has recently released. It contains sugar and will do your waistline no favors. Stick to the original Truvia which is suitable for all your baking needs.

We actually like to use a combination of these sweeteners, depending on the need. Some recipes like our *Secret Agent Brownie Cake* (*Desserts*, Chapter 23) require a real sweet flavor, but using too much Truvia can be hard on the budget. Instead, add a dash (⅛-¼ tsp.) of NuStevia Pure White Stevia Extract Powder and you'll achieve the desired sweetness you want without breaking the bank buying truckloads of Truvia.

There is a wonderful website we recommend you visit if you want to save money and make up your own Truvia type sweetener. The site is www.healthyindulgences.net. The site owner, Lauren Benning, believes her homemade Truvia is better tasting than store-bought. It can be made for fraction of the store-bought cost by combining the correct amounts of NuStevia Pure White Stevia Extract Powder with bulk erythritol. She also has a lot of fantastic **S** recipes on her site and uses a whole foods natural approach to low-glycemic eating.

NuStevia Pure White Stevia Extract Powder is potent and a little goes a long way. Some people think it is best used along with Truvia for baking or mixed with another healthy sweetener called erythritol, which we will discuss shortly. Other people use it on its own and love the results. This extract powder is the only Nunaturals dry product we use, although the brand does have some other stevia products with added fillers. When you read "Nunaturals" in our recipes, you will know that we are referring only to this pure white extract powder.

If you have an extremely tight budget, you could try using NuStevia Pure White Stevia Extract Powder alone without ever bothering to combine it with Truvia or erythritol. This will save you some money since so little is needed to provide sweetness to recipes. Because it is quite difficult to spoon a tiny bit from the jar, Nunaturals has now made it available in a spice jar so you sprinkle a shake or two into your recipe. This makes it much easier. If ordering online, make sure to purchase one of these spice jars. You can buy it in bulk to save money, just keep filling the jar once it has emptied. You'll notice most of our recipes use both sweeteners as Truvia helps to add some bulk to baked goods and is easier to figure out exact measurements. You'll have to use some trial and error if you want to use Nunaturals alone.

We also recommend Swanson brand stevia drops, available from www.swansonvitamins.com. These drops are inexpensive and have no bitterness. If you don't want to purchase online, KAL liquid stevia drops work well too. This brand is found at health stores and even some supermarkets. In our opinion, KAL does not have that bad aftertaste many other stevia products seem to have. Liquid stevia is handy for puddings, smoothies, sweetening up plain Greek yogurt, and very handy to take in your handbag if you want to sweeten tea or coffee when you are out.

Serene chats: Final edit here. To help tighten our budget I have recently switched to using only NuStevia Pure White Stevia Extract Powder for all my sweetening needs. My husband drinks gallons of sweetened tea per week and trying to sweeten it with Truvia proved too expensive. Where Truvia is listed in our recipes, I use a few shakes of the Nunaturals extract. Always start with a little, taste, and add more if needed. Too much does not help the flavor. This sprinkling method works great for me even if I sometimes have to taste-test my uncooked batter before baking.

If stevia is new to you, you may want to start with Truvia and as you develop more expertise, opt for NuStevia Pure White Stevia Extract Powder.

Aids Health

Stevia doesn't only sweeten up your life. You should feel good about yourself every time you use it as it is impossible to get fat while "stevia-izing."

The sweet taste that God put in the stevia leaf does not come from carbohydrate molecules but through glycosides. These have a beneficial effect on the pancreas and help stabilize blood sugar. Stevia actually helps diabetic and hypoglycemic folk rather than causing more problems for them as most sweeteners do.

It is a great digestive aid. It lessens bouts of gas and soothes upset stomach. A hot cup of chamomile tea, sweetened with stevia, is perfect for anyone in your household with a stomach ache.

It is estimated that more than 500 scientific studies have been performed on stevia, and still there are no negative documented side effects. The news keeps getting better. A recent study at the *Institute of Chemical Biology* showed that stevia has high antioxidant levels that help protect against DNA changes which can lead to cancer.

There is a persistent rumor that keeps popping up when we talk to people about stevia. Sometimes women tell us they have heard on the grapevine that stevia can have a negative effect on fertility. We haven't met anyone yet who says stevia was directly to blame for their inability to get pregnant, and there are no scientific studies that give any credibility to this rumor, even though it continues to spread. We think it must be an urban legend that keeps repeating itself somehow. Serene has become pregnant three times while enjoying liberal amounts of stevia in her diet. We personally know many other women who use stevia and have had no trouble getting pregnant. Infertility can be caused by so many things, but we have yet to see any credible evidence that stevia should wear the blame. It has been used for thousands of years by women of childbearing age, and it was never used in history as a means for birth control, or to lessen fertility.

If we learn anything that changes our stance on the safety of stevia, we'll let you know about it through our website, www.trimhealthymama.com. If you have concerns and do not want to take our word for it, go to www.Stevia.net/safety.htm and look at all the studies provided. They address a study performed 32 years ago that suggested rats given extremely high doses of stevia liquid in place of water had less offspring than other rats. This study may be what instigated some of the fears certain people have about stevia and fertility. The site does a good job on shedding some sensible light on the study.

In fact, the recent studies on stevia keep showing positive benefits. It strengthens and protects teeth. According to research conducted at the *Hiroshima University School of Dentistry* and the *Purdue University Dental Research Group*, stevia reduces plaque formation by inhibiting reproduction of bacteria that cause gum disease and tooth decay. This makes it perfect for child appealing treats without damaging young teeth. Some people even like to use it mixed with water as a healthful mouth wash.

Those with elevated blood pressure should consider stevia for its ability to lower hypertension. Stevia will not lower blood pressure that is normal.

It is useful for healing a number of skin problems. Mixing the extract with water to make a face mask is helpful against blemishes like pimples and eczema due to its antibacterial properties.

If all this wasn't enough, it naturally increases energy levels. This makes it easier for people changing from sugar to stevia who are used to the artificial "sugar high" created by soaring insulin levels. However, stevia avoids the slump that always occurs a couple of hours after a sugar high.

Pearl chats: I buy my Truvia from Walmart where it can be purchased more inexpensively than a specialty health store. Strangely, I come across people who have been told that Truvia is an artificial sweetening product. This is not the truth. Truvia is non-bitter stevia mixed with erythritol, which is a naturally occurring sugar alcohol that has no impact on human blood sugar.

People can also get confused since Truvia says three grams of carbs per ¾ tsp. on the label. They worry that using Truvia in baking will produce high carb baked goods. Those carbs have to be numbered on the packaging, but they only reflect the erythritol which is inactive in the bloodstream. Essentially, you don't count those three carbs since your body doesn't register them. Ignore that number and enjoy your desserts as sweet as you would like them. Truvia should be considered zero impact carb—perfect for our desserts.

My little container of NuStevia Pure White Stevia Extract Powder lasts me months because it only takes a sprinkle or a pinch to get things really sweet. I have found both NuStevia Pure White Stevia Extract Powder and Truvia to be a godsend for my husband, Charlie and myself. Charlie's sustained weight loss eating **S** and **E** wou… never have been accomplished, or even more importantly, never maintained if he could not enjoy dessert every day.

I have always been astonished at the strength of Charlie's sweet tooth. In the past, the sugary foods he craved, and ate, on a daily basis took their toll on his moods and body. Now, he doesn't have those problems. The desserts I make with Truvia and Nunaturals are his absolute favorite, especially *Chunky Cream Pops* (*Desserts*, Chapter 23). Whenever I make a new batch he gives me the biggest hugs and tells me I am the best wife in the whole world, I don't mind that, of course! Sweet foods are definitely his love language. He also loves our *Tummy Tucking Ice Cream* (*Desserts*, Chapter 23). I'm sure glad about that because it is a **Fuel Pull** and a powerful tool to help keep his weight in check.

I tried so many different forms of stevia in my recipes before finding these forms of non-bitter stevia. Charlie would say, "It's still a little bitter," or "That was okay, but I really miss the sugar taste." He never complains anymore, just offers me his cute grin over dessert. I seldom have to go shopping for these items anymore. He often stops to purchase more at the store to make sure we keep a good supply in the home. For him, life without dessert is no life at all.

Serene chats: My husband's downfall is liquid carbs—sweetened iced tea. He can easily drink over a gallon a day. I had tried every healthy sweetener and version of stevia that was around, but they only made him grimace. I made him a batch of tea with Nunaturals and he thanked me for not putting any weird stuff in it. He could not tell the difference between this and sweetened tea with white sugar.

Some people look at stevia powder and think it is too processed. I have looked into the processing of stevia powder and cannot figure out why some other purists poohoo it. The extraction of sweetness from stevia leaves is a gentle and simple process.

Xylitol and Erythritol

These are two other acceptable sweeteners on our eating plan. They are both in the sugar alcohol family. They are not intensely sweet on their own and that is why they are often mixed with stevia. If you don't need a really sweet taste in your desserts, these two sweeteners might be perfect for you. They have zero impact on blood sugar, so you can utilize them to make all our creamy desserts without worrying about weight gain. Erythritol is the only sugar alcohol which has a zero glycemic index reading, whereas xylitol is very low on the scale and is therefore still plan approved.

While some sugar alcohols like maltitol and sorbitol can cause major gastric issues like gas and diarrhea, xylitol and erythritol are better tolerated by most people. However, the odd person with extreme stomach sensitivities may be affected and may need to stick to Nustevia Pure White Stevia Extract alone.

Agave

This sweetener is the latest craze since it's considered "natural" and a good alternative to artificial sweeteners. It is hitting super market shelves like wild fire. Many people now use agave thinking they are doing their body a favor since it is often advertised as raw. This promotes the notion that it is very healthy. Sadly, this is not true. While it is promoted as a low glycemic sweetener and safer than sugar for diabetics, we don't recommend it. Here's why.

It is somewhat lower than sugar and honey on the glycemic index, but it still contains around 16 carbs per tablespoon, these carbs count. In our opinion, that's a lot of carbs for one tablespoon! We want you to be able to enjoy creamy desserts, but the success of this plan lies in keeping carbs low when using liberal fats. Agave doesn't cut it. Our delicious, healthy recipes would turn from fat-melting to fat-gaining if you use agave.

There are other problems with agave. Due to processing, even at lower temperatures, it has an unnaturally high concentration of 90 percent fructose to10 percent glucose. Nowhere in nature does this ratio occur naturally. One food that contains a similar concentration of fructose to glucose is high fructose corn syrup, which you know is very unhealthy.

Research suggests that fructose in unnatural ratios like this may actually promote more disease than glucose itself. Table sugar is about 50 percent each of glucose and fructose. While we don't recommend white sugar, your body knows how to process that ratio better than sweeteners like high fructose corn syrup and agave. Glucose is metabolized by every cell in the body, but fructose must be metabolized by the liver. This can raise triglycerides (blood fat) significantly.

Unnatural ratios of fructose interfere with copper metabolism. This causes problems with collagen and elastin in skin which leads to sagging. Pure isolated fructose contains no enzymes, vitamins, or minerals and may rob the body of these nutrients in order to be used. There is concern over whether it may help contribute to diabetes as it reduces the sensitivity of insulin receptors. Don't be fooled by the advertising hype. Save your dollars, because agave is not cheap. Switch to stevia and/or the two safe sugar alcohols, erythritol and xylitol.

Honey

Did you know that honey can make you very fat? Sure, it contains vitamins and minerals and was a natural sweetener used in the Bible. But, as we've mentioned before, our world and lifestyles are now vastly different from biblical times. Honey has a high glycemic index and produces a similar effect in the body as regular table sugar. The honey that you buy at your supermarket has been pasteurized and will do your pancreas no favors.

Raw honey is the exception. It is very healthy, but we only recommend it for medicinal purposes. It has some undeniable healing properties. A little goes a long way. You could use half a teaspoon as a holistic allergy medication. It is anti bacterial, heals wounds, and is an excellent moisturizer whipped with shea butter. But, please **do not** use it as your sweetener unless you are trying to fatten yourself up. Your waistline will expand.

Honey can be a great sweetener for your children that are growing. They do not have the insulin resistance that age and a lifetime of high-carb eating accumulates. Let them have it on their whole grain bread and old fashioned oatmeal. Teeming with enzymes, raw honey will help pre-digest these grains and make them easier to assimilate. If you can't afford raw honey, regular supermarket honey is fine for children who have no weight issues. It is nutritionally superior to white sugar. Though nowhere near the health tonic that raw honey is, it still boasts minerals and vitamins. If any of your children have weight issues, limit usage to a little raw honey now and then for robust health promotion, and steer them toward our stevia options.

Sugar in the Raw

We also urge you not to be fooled by sugars packaged as "organic," "raw," or "cane juice crystals." These are often dressed up in more natural looking earthy colored boxes and are given more expensive prices. Don't be fooled. They will deplete your pocket book and still elevate glucose as much as regular white sugar.

Artificial Sweeteners

Next on the list of sweeteners to avoid is the billion dollar fake sweeteners industry. Aspartame, also known as Equal or NutraSweet, has constantly shown dangerous side effects in independent research. It is a known neurotoxin that causes over excitement in brain cells that lead to their death. Aspartame is banned in many countries.

Splenda has been thrust forward as the healthier alternative, having a similar profile to table sugar or salt, although researchers say that it has more in common with pesticides like DDT. There are grave concerns that it disrupts the endocrine system. Scientists call Splenda a 'mild mutagen," depending on how much is absorbed. In light of this, daily use is not a smart thing to practice.

Pearl chats: I don't like to be a legalist. Sometimes, little treats sweetened with popular artificial sweeteners can help out if you're in a bind. I believe it is regular usage of these substances that potentially cause health problems. I like a Splenda sweetened low-carb Breyer's ice cream bar every now and then, but I do not make this part of my everyday life. Sure, it's sweetened with Splenda, but it doesn't mess with my weight or raise my blood sugar to the extremes that sugar does.

Now and then, my husband will have a diet soft drink (he probably has more than I know about). Or, if I've been too busy to keep a surplus of healthfully sweetened desserts at home, he'll buy some sugar-free chocolates at Walmart, sweetened with Splenda and maltitol. I don't nag at him about this too much. At least these treats don't cause him to gain a bunch of weight and they go a long way to make him psychologically feel he can have variety in his diet. However, maltitol can cause a lot of digestive upset in certain people. If my husband eats too much chocolate made with maltitol, he always regrets it. I find it gives me very gassy stomach aches.

I know some people would rather choose to use pure sugar than chemical sweeteners. I see people opt for regular soda over diet as they do not want to introduce more chemicals into their body. I understand how they may arrive at their viewpoint. The way I look at it is that sugar and artificial sweeteners are both poisons, but one causes fat and the other does not.

Don't feel like you are making wise choices having the "real thing" over diet options. Once upon a time sugar was natural when it was growing under the sun as sugar cane. Fattening, but natural like a banana. If you want my opinionated opinion, the sugar in most sodas or packaged items today is every bit refined as opium is to the innocent poppy flower. Sugar, in my mind, is as much a poison as artificial sweeteners as it reduces white blood cell phagocytes that fight diseases. That's only one of its problems. Therefore, why feel high-minded about using it over chemical sweeteners? Neither is optimal, but being overweight causes diabetes, stroke, and causes cardiovascular disease. I choose to avoid those even if I have to have a little Splenda now and then. Oh my, here comes Serene! Always the purist vigilante, I'm sure she'll disagree with my viewpoint.

Serene chats: Pearl chooses to avoid all that, but would she mind the twitch in her left eye or growing another limb from using artificial substances? But, Pearl, you know I love you, girl!

Of course, I don't agree with her viewpoint at all. Life is not a dull bore when you can quickly and easily whip up healthy and delicious alternatives for you and your family. On this plan, you are already being treated on a regular basis. I personally would advise using a little self control and waiting until you can have a treat that doesn't cause any damage. When dealing with chemicals, I say, don't let it pass your lips. Chemicals, even in tiny amounts, can build up in your system. They are too much of a gamble when we already have to deal with the onslaught of environmental chemicals and toxins.

But, each to their own. If a little Splenda keeps you from slipping off the track, I won't be too upset.

As far as ice cream is concerned, check out our quick *Tummy Tucking Ice Cream* treat in *Desserts*, Chapter 23. You could never feel deprived eating this treat. And, for a rare treat, Whole Foods carries erythritol sweetened Coconut Ice Cream under the Brand "So Delicious." It is sweetened with erythritol and is fine for an **S** treat—yummy too. I like the chocolate mint version. And if you have a few spare dollars, you can buy Lucille's chocolate from www.netrition.com. It is sweetened with stevia and erythritol. Why eat artificially sweetened chocolate when you can eat healthier yummy chocolate like that?

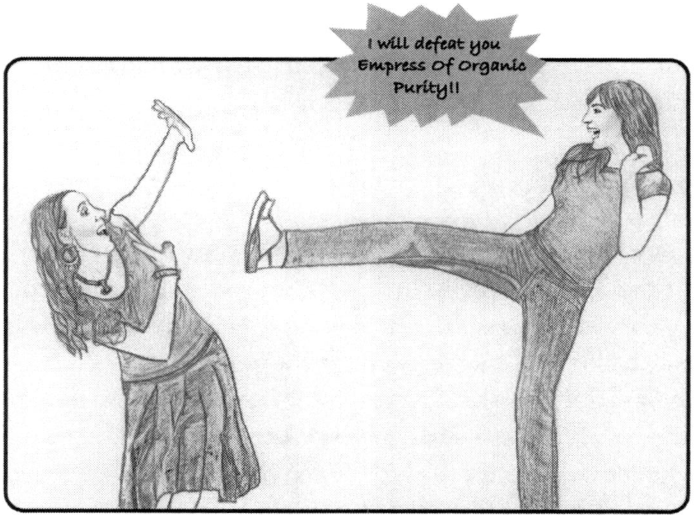
I will defeat you Empress Of Organic Purity!!

Note: If, for some reason, you try our recommended stevia sweeteners and do not like the taste, please do not let this throw you off embracing the entire **S** and **E** plan. We have a friend who was simply determined to stick to her Splenda because she was accustomed to the taste. She hated the taste of stevia in her coffee and was not convinced or concerned that Splenda could pose any grave risks to her health. After a while, we stopped nagging her, because while Splenda does not get our seal of approval, we would rather see you use some of it and eat everything else on plan, rather than feel you don't belong with others who are *Trim Healthy Mama-ing*. Stay with us and feel welcome.

If you do use Splenda, it is best to purchase a liquid Splenda since this removes all the other unnecessary fillers and reduces carbs. You can buy a brand called EZ sweet online where one drop equals one packet of Splenda. It is also suitable for baking.

Fermented Dairy and Vegetables

By enjoying our meal plans, you will lower and balance your sugar levels, but with the addition of fermented foods, you can actually heal the havoc of overgrown yeast that years of sugar consumption has caused. Other illnesses, like allergies caused by the absence of a healthy bacterial inner ecology, will start to clear up. More than that, they are yum, yum, yum.

By eating freely of these fermented foods such as yogurt, kefir, and sauerkraut, you will not only preserve, but replenish your enzyme count. Here's a quiz. Which meal has the most enzymes?

Meal one consists of a grass fed grilled steak, steamed asparagus with rosemary and feta, and a few tablespoons of pickled veggies on the side, or, if you prefer, a small glass of kefir for dessert.

Meal two is a large raw salad topped with raw nuts and a bowl of raw fruit for dessert.

You may be surprised to learn that the first cooked meal provided more enzymes and was much more enjoyable. The lacto fermented additions were so potent with enzymes that there were enough to digest the cooked food, leaving some leftover to replenish your body supply. The fully raw meal with no lacto fermentation had only enough enzymes to digest the food you ate. Nothing lost, but nothing gained.

Raw Foods on Steroids

Lacto fermented dairy such as kefir, yogurt, or vegetable preparations such as sauerkraut or pickled beets are living foods teeming with live nutrition. They are raw foods on steroids.

Not only does this fermentation enhance the digestibility, it also greatly increases the vitamin content of foods. These foods contain beneficial bacteria and provide a natural antibiotic and anti-carcinogenic effect to the body. Be aware of regular sauerkraut and pickles that are on the shelves of your supermarket. These are usually prepared with a canning process laden with white vinegar and table salt. They do not have living enzymes. It's not harmful to buy pickles this way, but don't think they are the superfoods we have been talking about. A good brand to keep an eye out for is Bubbies. It is fermented in the more traditional process and is found only in the refrigerated section of a supermarket or health food store.

If you are interested in making your own fermented vegetables, go to *Cultured Recipes*, Chapter 26 where Serene gives you simple steps to make these and other basic cultured recipes.

Kefir and Yogurt

Those who are lactose intolerant may be able to tolerate well prepared kefir which can be described as a drinkable yogurt. Kefir contains a different bacteria profile than yogurt and can be more powerful in healing the inner ecology of the body. The lactose is nearly all consumed by the fermentation, and the naturally occurring enzyme lactase will digest what remains.

Plain yogurt, especially Greek style (which is strained), is wonderfully healthy. Homemade yogurt from raw goat's milk or raw cow's milk is the optimum superfood. It takes a raw source of this milk to heal persistent allergies, but don't despair if you can't picture yourself going to the lengths it takes to prepare. Even yogurt, prepared from regular pasteurized milk, is brought back to life by the process of fermentation and is still hugely beneficial to many bodily processes. Think of it as "born again."

There are many healthful brands of kefir and yogurt that can be obtained from supermarkets these days if you do not want to make your own. Always remember to buy plain versions and sweeten them at home with stevia. Pre-sweetened yogurt and kefir go against the science of our **S** and **E** plan.

Greek yogurt has twice the protein content of regular yogurt and far less carbs. This is why we recommend it over regular yogurt, not to mention it has a more creamier texture. But yes, it is a little more expensive. Regular yogurt can be mixed with cottage cheese to further up the protein content, if your budget is extremely tight.

Pearl chats: I cannot always afford Greek yogurt, but I try to make it part of my grocery list as often as possible as it tastes so creamy and is full of protein. We go through a lot of yogurt in our home. The children are constantly into it, and I love it on my *Trim Healthy Pancakes* with berries and sugar-free syrup. If sometimes I can't afford Greek, I purchase cheapo non-fat regular yogurt from Aldi for my **E** pancakes.

I don't bother buying organic yogurt due to price. I just pretend that my yogurt does not have any pesticides or unknown hormones that were fed to the cows. You just gotta do the best you can, mama. Either way, you're getting healthful flora for your intestines and more protein in your breakfast by including regular Greek yogurt with your oatmeal. I am fully persuaded that the health benefits of non-organic Greek yogurt outweigh the negative that it may not bear the label "organic."

If you want full-fat yogurt for **S**, but can't afford Greek, remove the whey water. This reduces excess carbs since the milk sugar is in the whey water. Strain the yogurt through some cheese cloth in the fridge for a couple of hours. The creamy curd that is left is Greek style yogurt and you have saved yourself some money. I'm a little lazy to remember to do this, so when I buy full-fat regular yogurt (which is rarely since 0% is more versatile for my needs), I tip the whey water out each time I use it and hope for the best.

Serene chats: My husband had a painting contract business in the past and came up with a good idea. I used to use cheesecloth like Pearl mentioned which can be messy and annoying to use. In the paint stores, for mere pennies, they sell paint filtering bags made out of pure nylon. Some even have elastic on the top which fit perfectly over a bowl. They are my best cheese and yogurt making secret weapons and very easy to clean. You can easily strain whey water out of plain yogurt using them.

Nuts and Seeds

Nuts and seeds are powerful beauty foods. They provide needed nutrients for the skin and body. Did you know that it only takes a few Brazil nuts to give an entire daily serving's worth of selenium? Selenium, among its many attributes, is an affective cancer preventative. It halts the harmful effects of heavy metals like mercury in the body. If you have any thyroid or adrenal issues, make sure to consume Brazil nuts frequently, as selenium is an important nutrient that helps the body's energy levels and metabolism.

Almonds and sesame seeds are loaded with calcium. Hummus, with its main ingredient being ground sesame, also known as "tahini" is a high calcium snack. Almonds and walnuts are both helpful at lowering LDL or lousy cholesterol. Walnuts are a happy nut and raise serotonin levels, which is another of our "feel good" hormones. They are a reliable source of omega-3s which bring beauty to the skin and hair. Did you ever notice the walnut's shape? It looks like a brain and it helps to increase brain function. Sometimes God gives us little clues about what foods are good to eat for particular bodily functions.

Raw nuts are healthiest and soaking them creates the perfect snack food.

Serene chats: I suggest soaking nuts and seeds overnight in a small bowl of water with a generous toss of sea salt and throwing them in the dehydrator, or in a low oven, until crisp and dry. The soaking removes the phytates (which leach minerals from the bones) and enzyme inhibitors. Not only will they be more delicious this way, (you can add cinnamon and stevia, or savory herbs and hot pepper), but soaking aids in digestibility and puts less strain on the thyroid. Check out my *Dehydrated Nuts* (*Snacks, Chapter 24*).

Pearl chats: I find soaking interferes in my life. I say, relax and live a little, but if you want to soak, more power to you. Along with making my own easy *Spicy Nuts* (*Snacks*, Chapter 24), I sometimes buy dry-roasted spicy nuts from the store. They are a hit in my family. Our favorite is Blue Diamond Jalapeno flavor. I agree with Serene that soaked nuts are much easier on the digestive system. I have a sensitive stomach and if I eat too many un-soaked nuts I will be sure to get a stomach ache. I have to use a little more discipline and stick to only a handful or so, then I'm fine.

Serene chats: Since we are at your place today Pearl, and you are boasting about your Spicy Nuts, I think it would be most sisterly of you to make us a batch right now! We've been writing for hours. Our eyes are computer-glazed and our bottoms fused to the chairs beneath us. I say it's time for 15 pushups and a protein rich snack break.

Flax Seeds

These little guys are a wonderful and helpful addition to this **S** and **E** plan, not only because of their huge health benefits, but also because of their versatility.

Flax seeds carry one of the biggest nutrient payloads on this planet. Flax is not a grain, but it has a more similar vitamin and mineral profile to a grain than a seed. Like grains, flax is high in most of the B vitamins. That's just what we mamas need, because they aid mood health and help increase energy. Flax also boasts high amounts of magnesium. This mineral calms the body and is essential for nerve health and balanced hormones.

Full of Fiber and Lignans

Flax is full of fiber. In fact, its fiber level equals its carbohydrate level, so it is essentially a carb free food regarding the effect it has on blood sugar. The fiber in flax is responsible for its ability to help lower LDL cholesterol (that's L for lousy, flax only lowers the bad kind). This fiber acts like a broom in the intestines and sweeps out toxins from your digestive system. Flax can be thrown liberally into just about any **S** recipe to increase fiber levels. It's especially great in smoothies. One teaspoon of flax is also fine for **E** meals.

Flax contains lignans which help balance female hormones. There is evidence that these lignans may promote fertility, reduce pre-menopausal symptoms, and possibly help and prevent breast and colon cancer. Flax seeds are also rich in omega-3 fatty acids which are a keen force against inflammation in our bodies.

Amazing Flax Flour

The primary thing we love about flax is what happens when you grind it up. That's another way it's like a grain. It's the perfect baking flour with zero net carbs and therefore no sugar spike. And all you need is a coffee grinder. Grinding is the only way to extract all the nutrition out of flax. Whole flax seeds are good sweepers in the intestines, but they pass through the body without yielding any of their other wonderful health benefits. Consequently, ground flax seeds yield two great punches. In this form, you receive all the nutrition; and you also get to make yummy treats like muffins, crackers, breads, and even pizza crusts, and stay trim while eating like piggies!

If your budget is tight, and you cannot introduce all the foods we talk about here, consider flax as one of your first additions. It won't break your budget. Even if you are "cooking impaired," we have a great muffin recipe made with flax that will only take two minutes to prepare and one minute to cook! How about a chocolate, cinnamon, or blueberry muffin for a breakfast or afternoon snack that is delicious, healthy and takes less time out of your day to prepare than slipping on your shoes! All the kudos for this muffin goes to the amazing flax seed and a couple of other healthy ingredients. It will rock your world and make you think you can continue with this eating lifestyle forever. You'll find *Muffin in a Mug* recipe in *Breads, Muffins, and Pizza Crusts*, Chapter 19. The oven baked *Easy Peazy Cinnamon Muffins* are excellent also and will feed many more mouths than just your own.

Do not worry about soaking flax as it is naturally low in phytates.

Pearl chats: The great thing about flax is that it is cheap. I urge you to use golden flax over brown flax for your baking. It has a lovely flavor, texture, and color when used in baked goods.

Serene, that hard workin' sister of mine, always grinds her seeds in a coffee grinder, as it's cheaper to buy whole golden flax seeds and do your own grinding. I do that now and then when I am very financially challenged, but mostly, I am too lazy for that extra step.

I buy ground golden flax seed from Walmart. It is Wild Roots brand, which I find in the cereal aisle. It only costs around $3.50 for 16 oz. which is do-able for me. It is a non-GMO product and guaranteed cold milled processing. Walmart also has ground golden flax in their gluten-free section under Bob's Red Mill brand, but it is a dollar or so more for the same amount. I know Serene's flax seeds from the bulk bin are even cheaper, and you may want to home grind to save money, but it's good to know there are readily available alternatives for short-cut people.

While there is a good seal on the bag of flax seed I purchase, it is important to take further measures to prevent rancidity. Keep your bag of ground flax in the freezer since ground flax is rather delicate and prone to quickly go rancid if you don't.

Peanuts

These guys are loaded with serotonin (a "feel good" brain chemical) and even more antioxidants than green tea! We heartily endorse them, not only for their health benefits, but because if you buy them in their shells, it helps with portion control. Remember, nuts are high in calories and should be eaten with respect and moderation.

Peanut butter is a substance that can be the undoing of some of us. We want you to be able to enjoy it with **S** meals, but it can be easily consumed in too high amounts if you're not careful. One tablespoon, which can be gulped down pretty quickly, is a whopping 100 calories. Some women have metabolisms that can easily handle that calorie density quite frequently, but others need a good replacement for constant peanut butter in the diet. It's super yummy stuff and we don't want to deprive you.

Hello, defatted peanut flour! Thank you for saving us from calorie abuse! The two brands we recommend are Protein Plus Peanut Flour and Byrd Mill Peanut Flour Dark 12%, available from www.netrition.com.

Used in our recipes, both desserts and main dishes, this protein flour extracted from the peanut, can sanely offer peanut butter flavor without piling on needless calories. Check our *Tummy Tucking Ice Cream* (*Desserts,* Chapter 23). Amazingly, it's a **Fuel Pull** ice cream and therefore can be eaten any time for a snack, or for a dessert after any meal style. One tablespoon of defatted peanut butter makes the most delicious flavor in this ice cream—it's one of our favorite flavors. Defatted peanut flour works great as a glucomannan pudding flavor also.

This flour also helps produce a deep and slightly nutty flavor in our **Fuel Pull** *Sweet and Spicy Asian Stir Fry* (*Evening Meals,* Chapter 21). It can also be combined with a little water and sea salt and made into a paste. While not quite as good as regular peanut butter in your celery, it does a fair job for **Fuel Pull** or **E** needs.

Quinoa

To clear up the confusion, quinoa is called a grain, but it is actually a seed and the reason we have included it in this section. It is related to the spinach family.

If you're not yet acquainted with this superfood, hopefully both you and your entire family will do so soon. It packs powerful health promoting punches. It's a complete protein, containing all nine amino acids, and it has twice the protein of rice and most other grains.

It has a light fluffy texture and a slightly nutty flavor. It can be used in both sweet and savory creations. It makes the perfect breakfast porridge, sweetened with stevia and moistened with almond milk, but is also great to eat in the evening, because it promotes a relaxing night's sleep and is gentle on the digestive tract. If your stomach is sensitive, you know evening time is often when tummy troubles are at their worst. Quinoa can be substituted for couscous in tabouleh or whenever rice or barley would ordinarily be used.

Headaches to Asthma

Let's hit some of quinoa's health highlights. It's full of fiber. It increases brain function due to high folate levels. It is gluten-free and easily digestible, actually aiding the ecology of the digestive tract by feeding the microflora (good bacteria) in your intestines. Like flax, it contains powerful lignans which are known to reduce the causes of hazardous cancers. It is full of photonutrients and antioxidants which give it its superfood status.

It is impressively high in magnesium. People who suffer from migraines are urged to include quinoa in their diets by many holistic physicians. Magnesium, along with riboflavins of which quinoa also boasts, helps to relax the blood vessels at the base of the brain which decreases constriction and relieves tension. Magnesium also helps improve the elasticity of blood vessels and relaxes them. This is why quinoa is thought to be an excellent food for those with high blood pressure. It's these same high magnesium levels that are the reason it is recommended for asthmatics, especially childhood asthmatics as it decreases bronchial spasms and relaxes the whole bronchial area.

Gentle on Blood Sugar

Another reason quinoa is usually called a grain is because it has carbs in similar quantities to other whole grains. It's not a low-carb food on paper, but don't fret, as there is one redeeming difference. Quinoa is much lower on the glycemic index list than other grains. Its high protein and magnesium content have a positive influence on the glucose and insulin secretion in the body during digestion. Quinoa burns off much slower than other grains in the body and many diabetics find they can eat it without a bump on their glucose monitor after meals. In fact, it is a recommended food for type 2 diabetics. Although it's not terribly low in calories, it is considered to be a weight reducing food due to the way it slowly metabolizes. This slow burning effect makes it fit perfectly with our **S** and **E** plan. It may be added, as often as desired, in third to half cup servings as **S Helpers**, and in full cup servings for **E** meals.

Pregnant women should make frequent use of quinoa since pregnancy is a time where a woman's iron levels are easily depleted and quinoa is an excellent source of iron. Remember, it is related to spinach which is also high in iron. During pregnancy a woman is naturally more insulin resistant, so quinoa is one of the wisest carb choices to aid in energy levels during those nine months. It should be a preferred choice over rice, bread, and wheat. We're not saying you can't eat those other options, but try to reach for the quinoa first when you desire a carb side on your plate.

Quinoa is also known to be stimulating to mother's milk, so it is the perfect food while you are nursing.

Rinse Well

If your quinoa does not say "pre-washed," make sure you rinse your quinoa in a colander before cooking because it has a coating of saponins in its natural state. Saponins have a bitter taste, so rinse the quinoa well, using your fingers to swirl the grain around under the water, then pour off the water. Quinoa cooks up quickly in 12-15 minutes with two cups of liquid (water, stock, or broth), to one cup of grain. For ultimate digestion and assimilation of nutrients it should be soaked for seven to eight hours. Check out Serene's instructions for the way she soaks and cooks her quinoa in *Morning Meals,* Chapter 18. It's also a great idea to always keep baggies of pre-cooked, individual **E** and **S Helper** sized servings of quinoa in the freezer. This way, you can pull them out and add them to your meal whenever needed.

Hemp, the Happy Seed

Hemp seeds are one of our personal favorites. We are addicted to them (in a good way). You can use the seeds for a base in sweet nut-ball protein treats, or use them as a nutty rice substitute to pour various curries over the top. They not only pack a healthy power punch, but are delicious when thrown into smoothies or eaten straight from the bag.

Our favorite brand of hemp is Manitoba Harvest Hemp. In our opinion, their best product of all is Pro 70 Hemp Protein Powder. It tastes so earthy, yet completely heavenly. It gives that rounded taste in the mouth. It is such a smooth tasting treat when mixed in Greek yogurt, berries, vanilla, and stevia. We have not found another hemp product that can compare. Many of them taste too gritty.

We also enjoy Manitoba Harvest Hemp oil in salad vinaigrette. It gives a beautiful bright green hue to liven up a homemade dressing.

Hemp seed has a remarkable amino acid profile for a plant food. As an addition to healthy animal foods, it adds impact to your dietary protein. It contains high amounts of phenylalanine, an amino acid which converts to PEA in the body and makes you feel happy. This is the very same brain chemical which is released when you fall in love. It induces feelings of bliss, contentment, companionship, and even passion. You feel a natural and healthy buzz with daily consumption. If you're feeling down, add some hemp!

Hemp is high in healthy dietary fiber, rich in a synergistic balance of omega-3, and six essential fatty acids. It is a good source of hard to find gamma linolenic acid (GLA) and stearidonic acid (SDA). Hemp has a touch of class with its gourmet nutty flavor.

Serene chats: Would you like to know the funny story of how we began to enjoy the Pro Hemp 70 protein powder? Pearl and I were the guests at an *Above Rubies* retreat in Manitoba, Canada. The husband of one of the ladies attending the retreat was founder of Manitoba Hemp Company and she was kind enough to bless us each with a jar of Pro Hemp 70.

We were sitting in our room late at night and got the snackies. We opened up the jar and tried it out with a little Greek yogurt. I don't know if it was the jet lag from traveling in planes and cars since 3:30 am that morning and we were silly beyond tired, but that hemp and yogurt snack sure gave us the giggles and a surge of extra happiness. Apparently, hemp naturally raises dopamine levels, one of the "feel good" hormones. It has been tested to be completely free of any of the chemicals or other negatives related to its outlawed cousin. These natural hemp products are made from the little seed, not the leaf, and the plant used is from a different variety in the hemp family than the outlawed drug. We had a real fun time, regardless!

Note: Hemp products, such as these, do not make a person "high." They simply elevate your moods by gently raising dopamine levels in your body. We are apparently so pure that we were easily affected!

Chia

Chia seeds are a nutritious powerhouse. The food value per volume is very impressive. They are an excellent supply of calcium and boron. This is a double blessing, as calcium is absorbed best when boron is also present. Chia seeds have the ability to increase your brain power and body strength.

These powerful little seeds love water and can soak up ten times their weight. When chia is allowed to sponge up water before ingesting, like in our *Tapioca Pudding* or *Cookie Bowl Oatmeal* (*Morning Meals,* Chapter 18), its abilities start shining. The chia actually causes your body to stay hydrated longer and retain more electrolytes in your body fluids.

It was known as the "Indian Running Food." This legendary seed is described as having the ability to enhance endurance and stamina. The ancient Aztec warriors used chia seeds during their conquests and no wonder, because the nutrients inside chia travel to the cells very quickly. Aside from keeping these warriors hydrated, they provide quick and stable nutrition. Chia builds and regenerates healthy body tissue.

Chia is easily digested. The outer shell is easily broken down, even when swallowed whole. This is a one up over flax, which is usually passed through your system whole if not chewed very well or ground. They are also an aid to weight management by their bulking action which signals a full satiated signal. But, like flax, they have incredible cleansing fiber action which helps rid your intestines of rotting matter.

You may think chia seems expensive, but since it expands with so much water, a little bit goes a long way. In the long run, it works out to be quite reasonable. However, you might want to keep your chia *Tapioca Pudding* as a treat for yourself while your children have a milk and honey smoothie.

Chia and Hemp are great foods, but if your budget is tight, save purchasing them for a time when you have a little more room in your budget. They are fantastic superfoods that we'd love you to get acquainted with at some point, but are not necessary first additions.

Coconut—King of Superfoods

Coconut is king among superfoods. Bring it on, baby! It nourishes, protects, and heals. It is also a potent medicine. It wages war against aging and degenerative diseases, yet it is gentle enough for babies.

As a kitchen staple, coconut can morph into a myriad of wonderful creations—foods such as gourmet chocolate, baked goods, pudding, custards, pies, ice cream, creamy Caribbean coolers, hot winter nogs, palette waking curries, and ethnic delights. And these are only the beginning. It is hard to imagine the brown hairy bowling ball that a coconut resembles, or the dried flakes that come from it, are responsible for such a flavorful fare, but you better believe it! Coconut flour, coconut cream, coconut milk, coconut butter or oil, coconut concentrate, and young coconuts with their custard like flesh, are all our favorites. In our recipe sections, we will show you how to enjoy incredibly healthy food from the very versatile coconut.

Along with its powerful yeast fighting effect, it touts exceptional fiber content. One measuring cup of shredded coconut provides nine grams of fiber, which is three to four times as much as most fruits and vegetables. It may seem a daunting task to eat one cup of dried coconut, but when you make our *Blueberry Coconut Muffins* (*Morning Meals*, Chapter 18), this amazing digestive aid goes down as easily as a fluffy white Twinkie, not that we advise eating Twinkies—ever!

Coconut meat is also a source of vitamin B1, B2, B3, B6, C, E, folic acid. It also contains the following minerals: calcium, iron, magnesium, phosphorus, potassium, and zinc.

Coconut Oil is a Must

One of the main reasons for coconut's acclaim is the almost magical oil that it contains. It is the most saturated of fats, making it highly stable and resistant to oxidation through heat and light. Even at high heats you are assured of no trans fats or free radical formation when cooking with coconut oils. We don't want to spend a lot of time on this subject, but if you are still worried about saturated fats, recommended reads are *The Coconut Oil Miracle* by Dr. Bruce Fife and *Eat Fat, Lose Fat: The Healthy Alternative to Trans Fats* and *Nourishing Traditions* by Mary Enig and Sally Fallon. These are great sources to get you started.

We recommend using cooking coconut oil rather than extra virgin for frying and baking. It has a neutral taste and no coconut smell about it so the flavor of your food is not altered. It also saves money as it is a lot less expensive than the raw virgin alternative. You can order it in bulk from an online supplier such as tropicaltraditions.com, or go to Walmart and purchase the Louanna brand inexpensively. It is non-hydrogenated and due to coconut oil's stable qualities, using a more refined source like this does not affect the integrity of its fatty acids. Of course, raw virgin oil is more medicinal, so save it for recipes that are not heated like our *Skinny Chocolate* (*Desserts*, Chapter 23).

Coconut oil is unique and differs from other saturated fats. It contains medium chain fatty acids that are anti-bacterial, anti-viral, anti-fungal, anti-protozoal, anti-parasitical, and anti-microbial. It also raises the thermogenic temperature of the body, which boosts the metabolism as an effective tool for weight loss. It supports a sluggish thyroid and is an excellent energy source, fueling the brain and supporting intense exercise. It prevents premature aging of the skin and helps heal many skin conditions such as eczema and psoriasis. Coconut oil builds the immune system, improves digestion, and has multiple weapons against digestion problems.

Serene chats: I add coconut oil to most of the smoothies I make. If I get an earache, in the ear it goes. If I have a stuffed nose, I lay on my back and in it goes. If my children or I get a bite or a rash, on it goes. If I get a toothache, I swish the virgin oil around my mouth. After a bath or shower, all over my body it goes. After bathing, it is important to replace the natural oils from the skin with coconut oil as human skin sebum has the same protective middle chain fatty acids as coconut oil. If I am feeling run down, I increase my daily dosage since it is a natural energy source and immune booster.

Don't be without it during intimate times with your husband. It's the best lubricant available and you don't have to worry about foreign chemicals entering the vagina. Also, it kills yeast and that's a fun way to medicate this area of your body. Plus, it has an exotic smell, like sunscreen on a sultry summer's day on a deserted island. That should help get you in the mood.

When I am pregnant and nursing, I try to eat as many coconut and coconut oil products as possible as breast milk is meant to be a rich source of middle chain fatty acids. These protect the vulnerable baby from bacteria, viruses, and super germs. Sadly, with common deficient diets, mother's milk has been tested to be much lower in these important fatty acids. Dining on decadent coconut oil is a yummy way of reversing this problem and shielding your baby from the sicknesses lurking around. The most decadent way of ingesting large amounts of this oil is eating our *Skinny Chocolate* (*Desserts*, Chapter 23).

Pearl chats: Sometimes, I like to put a teaspoon of virgin coconut oil in my coffee, along with a dash of cream. I enjoy my coffee more, knowing I am getting more super-food mileage as I sip.

I learned a trick from reading the book, *Eat Fat, Lose Fat: The Healthy Alternative to Trans Fats* by Mary Enig and *Sally Fallon* where the authors suggest taking two tablespoons of virgin coconut oil before meals to speed up metabolism. The authors mention weight loss cases where people had trouble losing weight no matter what they did, but with the addition of coconut oil before meals, the pounds began to melt away. When I remember, I take one or two tablespoons before an **S** meal. I really don't mind the taste, and it tends to make me less inclined to over eat due to the satiation of the fat. You wouldn't do this before an **E** meal, of course.

If you are feeling cold in the winter and cannot warm up, try a teaspoon or two of coconut oil. It raises the thermogenic temperature of the body and may help warm you up.

When you start adding raw coconut oil to your diet, begin slowly. It can really loosen the bowels in some people. That can also be a good thing if your body tends to stay bound up. Eating some coconut oil off a spoon in the morning, or including it in your coffee may help sluggish bowel function.

Red Palm Oil

While we are on the topic of tropical oils, we should make mention of coconut oil's cousin, red palm oil. This deeply pigmented oil was prized by the Pharaohs of ancient Egypt as a sacred food. In Southeast Asia and Africa it is as widely used as olive oil is in the Mediterranean.

Reverse Heart Disease and Cancer

The orange/red hue is due to being nature's richest source of tocotrienals, tocopheryls, and carotenoids. This makes it a super antioxidant, proven to reverse heart disease and fight cancer. We could write another entire book to tell you about the merits of red palm oil. We recommend a great read called *The Palm Oil Miracle*, by Dr. Bruce Fife.

Dr. Fife describes how palm oil can be regarded as a brain food because it helps maintain proper blood flow. It causes the brain to receive the nutrients it needs by increasing blood circulation in the arteries that feed the brain. It supports neurological health and prevents stroke. It fights schizophrenia, depression, Parkinson, and Huntington diseases. It is one of nature's highest sources of Coenzyme Q10 (CoQ10), which feeds the mitochondria of the cell responsible for energy in the body.

Not only does daily use of palm oil help prevent cancer, but it is powerful in treating active cancer as well. It reduces chronic inflammation and is a high source of squalene, which strengthens and protects the skin. In Dr. Fife's book, he mentions that one of the most important therapeutic effects of palm oil is its photo protective properties against UV radiation. The protection you receive from applying palm oil to your skin is comparable to commercial SPR sunscreen. Pre-cancerous skin lesions have been reported to disappear with the daily use of this oil.

Pearl chats: This is off the topic of palm oil for a brief minute, but concerning skin cancer, look into a formulation made from extracts of egg plant called Curaderm BEC5. It has been studied for over two decades as a cost effective alternative to surgery for non-melanoma skin cancers, and now the results are clear. It is highly effective at treating basal cells carcinoma and unsightly keratosis. It selectively destroys skin cancer cells without harming normal skin cells.

This cream is not available in any stores. It is not a snake oil lotion that "just might" do the job. It is a powerful weapon against skin cancer that results in full restoration of healthy skin. Phase I, II and more recently, phase III trials have been carried out on this product. Results of the phase III trials determined that Curaderm BEC5 successfully cured non-melanoma skin cancers in 78 percent of patients when applied twice daily under occlusive dressing for eight weeks. When treatment was extended to 12 weeks, cure rates were 100 percent. Patients were then followed for five years post treatment and not a single recurrence of a treated lesion occurred.

You can ask your doctor to prescribe it. If he or she is unfamiliar with this cream and is not willing to do so, it can be purchased online. The cream may be ordered from the dispensary at The Tahoma Clinic in Washington, www.tahomaclinic.com.

Serene chats: Great news on that skin cancer cure, Pearl. Red palm oil is a great prevention for that disease. I like to put it on one slice of sourdough bread with a sprinkle of sea salt as an **S Helper**. I think you may find the flavor a little too earthy to eat like that. However, the flavor unites perfectly, even heavenly, with curries, stir fries, and ethnic soups. It is great for roasting meats in a deep dish pan, and for frying eggs.

It is a pricey item in a health food store, about $15.00 for a pint. The secret is to find an African food store in your area. You'd be surprised at how you can find them in most cities. Red palm oil is as common to them as potatoes are to the Irish. You can purchase a gallon of the pure stuff for under $20. While you are there, pick up some cans of the palm fruit called Palm Butter.

Like coconut oil, the integrity of the fatty acids is not changed during high heats with palm oil. In fact, the anti-cancer properties of palm contained in the orange color have still been found to be potent after seven uses of frying with the same oil, not that we suggest ever re-using an oil.

Canned palm fruit product is still very medicinal. Palm butter soup is the most delectable food if you like exotic flavors. Look for my palm butter recipes in *Lunches*, Chapter 20 and *Evening Meals*, Chapter 21. One is for the whole family which we enjoy in our home at least twice a week; the other is a five minute superfood soup for a mother on the go.

Pearl chats: I would use palm oil a lot more often, but my husband dislikes the very earthy smell and taste. If he is not going to be around for a meal, I will use it since I enjoy its flavor. Sometimes, I fry up a big batch of potatoes for the children in palm oil. I feel good that they can have fried potatoes without any trans fats and they love it.

Serene made a skin cream that she named *Sunshine Mousse* and gave it to me for my birthday. Palm oil is one of its key ingredients and it gives a nice sun-kissed glow.

Chana Dahl

Anybody with blood sugar issues such as diabetes, pre-diabetes, or hypoglycemia should use this legume as often as possible as a major carbohydrate source for their **E** meals. The reason? The healthy carbohydrates this dahl contains burn extremely slowly in the body. Amazingly, it has three times the fiber of most other beans and legumes, and it's common knowledge that beans and legumes already contain a lot of fiber. But, despite its high fiber levels, it has a very creamy mouth feel. In our opinion, it cooks up smoother and much creamier than other legumes.

It's almost unbelievable, but chana dahl has a rating of only eight on the glycemic index! That's insanely low. While this dahl contains carbohydrates in more similar amounts to other beans, it does not raise blood glucose in the same way. Most other beans and legumes have glycemic indexes in the thirties to fifties which are more medium glycemic levels.

You can feel very confident about incorporating the carbs contained in chana dahl for your energy levels without the risk of any sugar spike in the process. Make soups with it, mash it up for a side, or toss it with vegetables and chicken. It is a perfect **E**, **S Helper**, or **Crossover** carb option.

We'd love you to make very frequent use of this bean. It's actually more like a split pea, but rather than green, it is a lovely golden color. It is not yet widely known in this country, but has been a staple of East Asian cooking for centuries. It is sometimes known by its other name of "Bengal Gram Dhal." Begin to enjoy it in curries, burgers, and even pancakes and you will be one of the rare Westerners who makes smart use of this wonderful food. Along with quinoa, it is another excellent choice for pregnant women, to help avoid gestational diabetes.

Guess what? Our local Walmart now sells chana dahl in their international section. Who woulda thought it? Hopefully your Walmart will carry it, too. You can ask them to order it in if they do not already have it in stock. It can also be purchased online less expensively. Visit www.mendosa.com to find more information and lots of great recipes.

Whey Protein

- Whey protein's list of benefits is too long to go into great detail. We will briefly touch on some of them.
- Its protein has the highest biological value of any known naturally occurring protein. It helps sustain high energy levels—physical, mental, and emotional.
- It stimulates the release of hormones that enhance fat burning. Studies show that people trying to lose weight will always lose more when whey is incorporated. It helps train the body to burn fat for fuel.
- It helps to eliminate sugar cravings and hunger by promoting a stable blood sugar.
- Whey protein, above other dietary sources, raises glutathione, a detoxifying compound in the body which helps excrete toxins and heavy metals.
- It boosts serotonin levels and mood. Feeling down? Make a shake with whey.
- It fights breast cancer.
- It contains the entire essential and branch chain amino acids, plus all other naturally occurring amino acids.
- It is a powerful immune booster, containing lactoferrin, and other important immunoglobulins, which support and stimulate the immune system.
- It is a needed supplement during time of physical or mental stress, as well as post surgery, or after working out.

To receive any of these benefits, whey protein must be undenatured and cold-processed. You will not do yourself favors buying cheap whey protein that is sweetened with inappropriate sweeteners and has been heated to high temperatures. Make sure the whey you purchase has only one carb or less. Any more than that indicates incorrect sweeteners, or the use of other needless fillers.

We have found an inexpensive source for undenatured good quality whey protein. It is called Swanson Premium Brand Whey Protein. It has no sweetener so you'll have to add your own to your smoothies, but it is infused with a natural vanilla flavor. It is less than half the price of any other quality whey protein and is available from www.swansonvitamins.com. Swanson also has a more expensive whey called Bioactive Whey Protein. If you are fighting a serious disease, or are in need of an immune boost, it would be worth purchasing as it is a super healer for the body. It is the highest source of glutathione (a potent free radical destroyer and immune enhancer) found in nature. It is purely medicinal, to be consumed without food, and not to be blended. Other similar bioactive versions often cost double the price of this one so it is a good deal.

However, we want you to purchase the regular undenatured whey protein which is highly beneficial and works with our recipes. Other suitable brands are Jay Robb and Energy Pro. Jay Robb is easily found at most health food stores and even many grocery stores. Kroger carries it in their health food section. Both of these brands use only stevia to sweeten, they are undenatured, and have different flavors. Energy Pro is only available online, but it is slightly superior in that it is made from the milk from grass fed cows. Our recipe chapters include shakes, treats, and bars made from whey.

Whey Every Day

Well, let's be realistic. Not all of us are going to be able to afford whey every day, especially if you're trying to feed it to the entire family! But, we liked the way that slogan sounded. More seriously, some of these foods we mention like whey, hemp, goji berries, and salmon fillets cannot be fed to an entire family if you are on a tight budget. We have different needs as we grow older. Sometimes health issues arise. With increasing years, we must start preventing them. As women, we may be in our child bearing years, pregnant, or nursing around the clock. More is demanded from our bodies at these times. It's important to feed children whole foods and a highly nutritious diet. However, unless there is a health concern, we usually reserve these more expensive items, like whey, for ourselves.

We do not believe this is selfish. Our children need vibrant moms and dads who are filled with energy and not too exhausted to input into their lives. They will also learn from our example that when they enter these seasons there may be need for greater supplementation.

Pearl chats: Our finances go up and down. Sometimes, I cannot afford whey, so I make sure to have it on my birthday and Christmas wish lists. This way I get a stockpile. I really love Jay Robb's chocolate brand. After my workouts, I throw a scoop into the blender, with some ice, water, and one tablespoon of coconut oil. Or, I pre-make little frozen cubes of coconut milk and throw these in with some water and whey. Sometimes, I add frozen berries and/or glucomannan to thicken—best smoothies ever! They're like thick shakes.

A new problem I have now is that my boys like to work out and beg me for my protein powder. They want huge muscles, of course, and they're somehow convinced that whey will help them achieve that dream. It's hard to say no to their cute faces after they have completed 40 pull ups; not all in a row—sets of five and 10. But, they're tough and work hard. They also like to have it after football practice. My oldest daughter, Meadow also wants some after her workouts. Whey goes fast around here since it's so hard to say no to my sweet children. Consequently, there are times when we have whey, and times when we run out and go without for a while.

Serene chats: Whey is a constant with me, but not because I always have the money to buy it. I order it by the bulk case online about three times a year—when our budget allows for a splurge, Christmas time, or my birthday. Some women ask for jewelry on these occasions, I ask for whey. I don't keep up with all the things I would like to take as supplements as we would never afford it. However, whey is a biggie for me because I do resistance exercise with kettlebells and I want to guard against muscle wasting as I age.

Another good tip is to keep a serving or two in a Ziploc bag in your purse. If I am out and need sustenance, and there is nothing else around, I add it to a bottle of water, shake, and drink. It tides me over until I get home.

Nutritional Yeast

We love nutritional yeast because of its wonderful cheesy, nutty flavor. It is awesome sprinkled on eggs, or as you will notice in our recipe chapters, almost everything. Our children would think popcorn without nutritional yeast would be as wrong as bread without butter.

There is more to this incredible condiment than merely taste. It is also prized as a superfood. It contains 18 amino acids and is a complete protein. However, you'd have to eat too much of it to get enough protein to equal what animal food provides, so this is not an "out" for vegetarians. It is also a very good source of vitamins and minerals. It is a plentiful source of vitamin B complex which helps in managing stress levels.

Mineral Rich

Nutritional yeast is also rich in manganese, copper, vanadium, molybdenum, and lithium. Lithium is a very important trace mineral for brain function. Studies reveal that there is more crime and violence in areas where lithium is low in food and water. Lithium is a powerful brain nootropic (brain protector/enhancer) and has a positive effect on memory. Medical journals call lithium a "robust neuroprotective agent." Studies show that lab animals given lithium, and then toxins, always have less neuronal damage than animals that don't get the lithium. It helps protect our brain from the daily onslaught of environmental toxins. Lithium is one mineral that combats damage from glutamate toxicity. That alone is a good reason to make nutritional yeast a regular part of your diet since most prepared foods you purchase will have MSG (monosodium glutamate) as an ingredient.

What makes nutritional yeast fit so well with this eating plan is another trace mineral it supplies called chromium. This mineral's other name is GTF (glucose tolerance factor). This substance is highly effective for those with high blood sugar levels like diabetics, those with insulin resistance, and pre-diabetic conditions such as hypo and hyperglycemia. Chromium is also used to help lower cravings for carbs and sugary foods.

The Good Yeast

We know there are good fats and bad fats, good bacteria and bad bacteria. There are also good yeasts and bad yeasts. Nutritional yeast is one of the good yeasts and has no connection with harmful fungi like candida albicans. It will not promote the growth of bad yeast in your body. Nutritional yeast is the deactivated form of a yeast called Saccharomyces Cerevisiae which has no correlation with candida albicans. It is also a gluten-free food.

Just as sourdough bread captures good wild yeasts from the air and the process of kefir fermentation also uses yeast, we clearly see that not all yeasts are to be thought of as monsters. Nutritional yeast actually helps maintain ideal intestinal ecology in the body.

More Positives

This yeast also improves blood production, helps maintain optimum cholesterol, and improves liver health and function. It supports a healthy metabolic rate, beautiful skin, and is also touted as a preventative measure for cancer of the pancreas.

In light of all these benefits, even if nutritional yeast tasted like dirt, we might be tempted to include it by holding our nose and swallowing. The good news is that this is a delicious condiment which can completely replace tasty stock or broth in many dishes. It provides a deep savory taste to the mouth. We stock up from the bulk bin at our local *Whole Foods* store a few times a year. It is not found in regular grocery stores in our area.

Glucomannan

Glucomannan is probably a new word to you, but it will bring both pleasure and health to your life. We use it as a thickener for everything from gravies to puddings. It works fabulously and fits perfectly with the low glycemic premise of this plan. You will no longer need white flour for your gravies or starchy thickeners for your desserts. It's even an ingredient in our

Tummy Tucking Ice Cream (*Deserts*, Chapter 23) so if you want to be eating lots of trimming treats, it'll be a good idea to try to fit it into your budget.

What is this stuff?

It is a white powder that looks a lot like corn starch. It is derived from an amazing food called the konjac root. Ground up into powder, this root becomes a **s**oluble fiber which helps lower blood cholesterol and systolic blood pressure, slow glucose absorption, lower the glycemic index of meals, and promotes regular bowel action. Most of all, we love this powder because it makes a wonderful chocolate pudding in a jiffy.

Glucomannan has zero carbs, zero calories, zero flavor, and blends into recipes really well. Usually thickeners, like corn starch and flour, are laden with carbs, so gravies and puddings are in the fattening foods category. Glucomannan turns all that upside down. Puddings and gravies can now be super slimming and healthy for you. We are officially putting glucomannan in the public spotlight for the regular mama. This ancient traditional Japanese food can be your modern "can't do without" tool. Check out our *Fat Stripping Frappa* recipe (*Morning Meals*, Chapter 18). We discovered that when glucomannan mixes with whey protein and ice a magical reaction takes place. It fluffs up to become the most creamy consistency that would fool any diehard Dairy Queen addict.

Glucomannan powder does not need to be heated to thicken liquids although it acts as an even more potent thickener with heat. It also has about 10 times the thickening power of cornstarch, so a little goes a long way.

Super Powers of Glucomannan

This ground up root has an extraordinary water holding capacity and is the most vicious of all known dietary fibers. In the body, this creates a feeling of satiety or fullness through its water binding effects, and therefore curbs needless hunger. By creating a thick gel, it delays gastric emptying and slows the release of sugar into the bloodstream which helps to lower levels of insulin and blood glucose. This slower digestion time enables more nutrients to be absorbed from other foods in the meal. Studies using glucomannan reveal that it enhances the weight loss effects of diets. Amazingly, even in the absence of a calorie restricted diet, glucomannan stands by itself as a weight loss tool.

When obese adults consumed one gram of glucomannan fiber one hour before each meal for eight weeks, with no other changes to their eating or exercise patterns, they lost an average of 5.5 pounds of body weight. Experimental studies also indicate that it may protect against certain types of cancer. When elderly people are given glucomannan powder and fiber, the bacteria in their gut changes and encourages the growth of good bacteria such as bifidobacterium.

Increases in good bacteria are associated with a reduction in pro-cancerous nitrosamines, proteins thought to be responsible for the development of liver cancer and other cancers.

Glucomannan is a very alkaline food. Consider the alkaline levels of some foods compared to konjac. An apple equals 3.4, cucumber equals 2.2, carrot equals 6.6, and cabbage equals 4.9. Konjac comes in with a whopping 56.2! This is only surpassed by one food, which is a seaweed called wakame. For its alkalizing effects alone, konjac is a smart addition to our diet, but it offers so much more.

Studies on diabetic rats indicate that long term supplementation with konjac glucomannan may help prevent heart attacks and strokes in people who have diabetes.

We contacted Konjac Foods to make sure glucomannan was a safe food during pregnancy. The representative told us to not be concerned. He said the root has been used as a food for hundreds of years in Asia, and is eaten frequently by pregnant women in most Asian countries without problems. Konjac noodles have been a big part of the mass diet in these countries, especially for the poorer people. He assured us that konjac root is a natural food, not a herb. He did say that people who take medication may not want to take it at the same time as they eat something made from glucomannan since konjac slows down digestion and the medicine may not be absorbed into the blood stream as quickly as usual.

A warning. Keep glucomannan powder on a high shelf away from children. If swallowed without water it can form into a gum in the throat and cause choking. This doesn't happen when it's used in recipes, or when mixed with liquids, only when swallowed dry.

Where to Get it?

As far as we know, konjac powder (glucomannan) is not currently available at supermarkets, or even health food stores. It has to be purchased online. It costs about $20 dollars for one pound, but a little goes a long way. It should last you many months unless you go on pudding binges, which we've been known to do.

A good site for this powder is www.konjacfoods.com. You can also purchase it from www.netrition.com. Both sites also sell noodles and "rice" made from konjac root which also have zero carbs and calories.

Wonderful Konjac Noodles

These noodles and "rice" made from glucomannan can be heavy hitters in the fight against excess pounds. They are perfect for all fuel styles but do their best work in **Fuel Pull** meals since they have no fat, carbs or calories. Be prepared for a slight fishy smell when you open your bag of konjac noodles. This is due to the type of water they are packed in. You need to rinse the noodles well in a colander before cooking. The smell completely goes away once they have been

...d and cooked. They are best used in Asian style dishes but are also great with curries and peanut and coconut based sauces. They do fine with cream based sauces too. If you don't mind the different texture, they'll even work with tomato based Italian style sauces, but you have to have a little mind adjustment on the change of texture.

After rinsing, place konjac noodles in a dry hot skillet and dry-fry for several minutes (or microwave for one minute before commencing your recipe). This helps to eliminate excess liquid and any rubbery texture.

Konjac noodles are sometimes known as "yam noodles" in international food stores where they can be purchased less expensively. Check the ingredient list for the word "konjac root." Thankfully, we found a store about an hour away and their konjac noodles cost only half what they sell for online. We stock up and purchase 20 to 30 bags at a time.

Don't be confused by shiritaki noodles. These look quite similar to konjac noodles and are newly available in health food stores like Whole Foods. They are not zero calorie, or zero carb, but are very low-calorie and low-carb. They are made from tofu, not yam root. They will still fit into any of our fuel style meals. Give them a try if you desire, but they are not our first choice for you.

Xanthan Gum

Xanthan gum is another natural fiber-based thickener. It has zero net carbs and can be used in combination with konjac powder, or alone. It thickens sauces and gravies quite well, but is not very useful to make a quick pudding. When used alone, some people do not like the slightly slippery feel in their mouth. It is more readily available though and found in the gluten-free section of Walmart. You can purchase little packets inexpensively, so you could try it out before spending $10.00 on a pound bag. We use it in some of our recipes. It helps egg whites stay very stiff once they're beaten which can be handy for baking.

Pearl chats: I used xanthan gum as a thickener for my gravies for a couple of years before I became aware of glucomannan. My family is accustomed to xanthan and we do not notice the sliminess. If you can't afford glucomannan, xanthan is a good place to start. It won't make puddings the same way, so that's a bummer. Now, I use glucomannan more often, as I think the konjac powder is a more talented thickener and much better to make quick puddings and yummy thick smoothies, but xanthan is still handy to have around.

Serene chats: I am one of those who can detect sliminess in a gravy made with xanthan gum. I prefer glucomannan, but I do use xanthan in some of my baking as it helps to create a better texture in some **S** baked goods.

Part III

Join Us in the Kitchen

Novice or Foodie,

you can have success with these recipes!

All our recipes have been categorized into three groups. They are **S**, **E** and **Fuel Pull**. Some of the recipes match only one category, either **S** or **E**. Keep these with their correct food partners. Some recipes match all three. Mostly, the multi-matching recipes involve primarily lean proteins and non-starchy veggies, but occasionally they involve a very small (pulled back) amount of grain or beans. They can stay as **Fuel Pull** only meals for a stronger weight loss effect, or be paired with either **S** or **E** foods.

Chapter 18

Morning Meals

It would be dishonoring to start this recipe section without giving first place to eggs. For **S** breakfasts, the rich protein of whole eggs set the perfect start to a day of balanced blood sugar. A study performed by the *Rochester Center for Obesity* proved that eating eggs for breakfast helped women lose weight. In this study, two groups of women consumed the same amount of calories and protein every morning. One group ate bagels, and the other group ate two eggs for breakfast. The egg group reported feeling less hungry at lunchtime, despite the same amount of calories, and over the next 36 hours consumed a minimum of 400 calories less than the bagel group.

A *Louisiana State University* study found similar results, again comparing breakfasts of bagels versus eggs. The study group that ate eggs for breakfast five mornings a week lost 65 percent more weight after eight weeks and almost twice the amount of inches from their waistlines than the bagel group. They also reported greater energy levels.

Quick Egg Refresher

Aside from the weight loss benefits of eggs, there are more amazing benefits. These sunny sides up are going to give you the following:

- a boosted immune system
- lowered risk of cancer
- lowered risk of heart disease
- reduced osteoporosis
- maintained eye health

However, for those of you who have egg allergies, or for some strange reason don't like eggs, there are plenty of other healthy high protein breakfast options included. We'll get to you. Hang tight.

More Therapy Ahead

You may have the notion beaten into you (we did) that a fruit and whole grain breakfast is far nutritionally superior to eggs, coffee, and cream. That's a hard one to shake since this doctrine is constantly pushed by so-called "diet authorities." The myth of always having to have a grainy, fruity breakfast weighed heavily on both of us psychologically, and physically as pounds. We are now very glad to no longer wear that bondage.

We give you permission to finally release yourself from this deception. We think our "Love me some buttah!" therapy was pretty good. If you have been deeply indoctrinated with the "fruit and grain is best breakfast fare" notion, we think you ought to memorize this little poem to keep you on a track.

Fruit and grain every morning
Makes body fat start a-storing
I can't do something so deploring
As fruit and grain every morning

While this poem may not put us into the halls of poetry fame, its premise holds truth. Of course, you can still include some fruit and whole grains into your breakfast options. You are welcome to enjoy the yummy approved **E** style grain-based breakfasts we include in this book since most of them are paired with good sources of protein. It's the touted notion that naked fruits and grains are superior breakfasts that we want to shake from your psyche. The commonly esteemed bowl of whole grain cereal, splashed with skim milk and a side of fruit as the ultimate breakfast is a wolf in sheep's clothing. Learn to focus predominately on proteins as your first choice to start to your day. Grains and fruit need to fall into line rather than be Top Dog.

Hopefully for you, the "fruit and grain" myth won't end up being as hard a notion to shed as it was for us. Somehow, it felt wrong when we tried to switch from our fruity based breakfasts such as banana based smoothies to more protein based breakfasts that included some animal products. These new breakfast foods felt sinfully satisfying. It was hard to shake the guilt. Thankfully, we eventually got over it and embraced the freedom.

Even bacon and eggs can be a healthy breakfast. This does not mean you have to eat pork if you follow the clean meat laws outlined in the Bible, as we do. Turkey and beef versions of bacon and sausage are available, but be sure to find healthy versions of sausage that don't have more than two carbs. Unfortunately, some sausages are made with sweeteners and fillers that increase the carb content too much to fit well with **S**. If you have a healthy pork source, maybe a pig fattening in your back yard, then aside from religious reasons, chow down, but always keep bacon in an **S** setting.

While we encourage you to frequently eat whole eggs for breakfast, remember the **S** and **E** plan is about never getting into a rut. Enjoy some **E** breakfasts too, only be sure to include some lean protein in them as well. Our *Trim Healthy Pancake* recipe is chock full of protein. It's a fantastic breakfast (or lunch), but since it is **E**, the protein source in this recipe is egg whites instead of whole eggs, and low-fat cottage cheese. This leaner protein allows the oats in the recipe to give you some energy without sticking to your belly as fat. Changing your macro nutrients this way keeps your metabolism guessing. While eating three of these pancakes may make you nice and full, you may notice some other **E** breakfasts, such as a simpler bowl of oatmeal, may not keep you as full as an **S** breakfast. You might not make it to lunch without getting hungry. That's okay. Have a protein-centered snack mid-morning. It's part of the science that higher carbs with less fat trigger more hunger.

Avoid Fruit Only Breakfasts

Fruit, such as berries for **S,** or some frozen mango or peach in your light coconut milk smoothie for **E**, may still be enjoyed as part of your breakfasts. However, never have fruit only, or overdo fruits in the morning, or for that matter, at any time. Most fruits, except very high glycemic ones like bananas, are good for **E** in the mornings in small sized portions**.** The idea of fruit alone until lunch time is old school now. You must include protein if you're going to finally get control of your weight and long term health.

Fruit alone as a meal is detrimental to weight loss because it prevents stable blood sugar. Too much fruit is a slippery slope for weight control since fructose (fruit sugar) makes the body's glycogen storage signal "full" a lot sooner than glucose from whole grains, beans, or starchy vegetables. Due to this bodily process, any excess fructose turns immediately into fat to be stored as adipose tissue. It's a good thing to remember that fruit sugar storehouses are small in the body, so we should have small servings of fruit. We want to include all of God's foods in moderation. Yes, fruit is good for you, but don't overdo it.

Now, having those little breakfast reminders and cautions, here come the long awaited recipes:

Egg Recipes

Simple Fried Eggs – S

Basic Ingredients: eggs ✦ sea salt and other seasonings ✦ butter or oil

1. Heat a good pat of butter, coconut oil, or red palm oil in a pan on medium-high heat.
2. Crack eggs into hot fat and season with sea salt and black or red pepper. Optional: sprinkle with nutritional yeast (this makes the eggs taste much yummier).
3. For soft yolks (which preserves most of the omega-3's), turn over for only a few seconds at the end of cooking.
4. For firmer yolk, turn over half way.

Optional sides are caramelized onions (sautéed until golden brown), sautéed diced zucchini, or a mix of other veggies such as red peppers or mushrooms, or breakfast meats like sausage or bacon. Alternatively, you can toast one of our appropriate **S** bread slices to go under the eggs.

Once you get to **S Helper** stage, you can have the eggs over either a third to quarter of a cup of quinoa, one medium *Trim Healthy Pancake,* or one slice of approved sprouted or sourdough bread. But hey, if you want to keep things simple and eat two or three fried eggs by themselves for breakfast, go ahead. We often do that.

Pearl chats: I know we're talking breakfasts, but I have to tip my hat to fried eggs as a lunch idea too. If I did not eat eggs for breakfast, and instead had an **E** breakfast like *Trim Healthy Pancakes*, I will often switch over to **S** for lunch and fry up some eggs in the way we've described above. For lunch, I usually have them over lettuce with a sprinkle of cheese. It's a good option if you arrive in the kitchen a little late and your brain is fuzzy about what to eat. Eggs are always good to fall back on when you are not in an organized mode, a state I find myself in quite often.

Some people might think that hot fried eggs with yolks a little runny and piled on top of lettuce is a weird sort of lunch, but I love it. You can use a Caesar dressing (thinned with water) if you like since that's usually a very low-carb store-bought **S** dressing and its flavor works well. I prefer indulging with generous amounts of extra virgin olive oil which, by the way, has excellent pain relieving qualities (similar to ibuprofen), and countless other health benefits.

I pour the olive oil over my plate of ripped or chopped up organic lettuce and drench the lettuce well. I swirl on some balsamic vinegar and a dash of Bragg Liquid Aminos, or a pinch of salt. Sometimes, a tiny sprinkle of Truvia gives a hint of sweetness to the dressing I'm seeking. This is the lazy person's way to make a dressing as you don't even have to use a separate bowl! Less dishes and less time works for me.

I toss the lettuce well to help mix the dressing together, then ladle on my hot eggs glistening with butter. Super yum! Who could feel deprived eating this way? I get a big fat fix eating this combination of foods and I'm left very satiated. This is a very slimming lunch, give it a try. But if you think it sounds nuts, ignore me and my fried egg fetish, and focus on all the other lunch options we offer you.

Serene's Steamed Omega Sensations – S

Basic Ingredients: eggs ✦ coconut oil ✦ nutritional yeast ✦ sea salt and other seasonings ✦ optional sardines

1. Melt 2 tsp. virgin coconut oil in pan on medium/low heat.
2. Crack in 3 omega-3 eggs, season with nutritional yeast, sea salt, and black pepper.
3. As soon as the whites turn opaque, cover pan with lid and immediately turn to low. Steam for 5-10 minutes, according to how soft you like the yolks.
4. Once ready, do not divide the eggs but lift whole onto plate.

Optional: to raise the omega-3 value, two minutes before steaming is complete, arrange half a tin of drained wild caught sardines in extra virgin olive oil on top of the steaming eggs to slightly heat for the last couple of minutes. When the eggs are plated, sprinkle on walnuts which are the highest nuts in omega-3. Finish with a dash of hot sauce and a dollop of extra virgin coconut oil.

Serene chats: This is one of my favorite weekend breakfasts, followed by coffee with cream. The omega-3 fats in the eggs are not destroyed by the high heat of frying with coconut oil. I feel like royalty when I'm eating it, and the omega-3s from both the eggs and the sardines are through the roof.

Pearl chats: More power to your zaniness, Serene. I could never eat sardines for breakfast! They have too strong of a smell for me at that time of day.

Zuchinni Fritter – S

Basic Ingredients: zucchini ✦ eggs ✦ sea salt and other seasonings ✦ butter or oil

1. Grate 1 firm small zucchini or ½ a large one into a bowl (using your hands to squeeze out excess water).
2. Crack 2 eggs into bowl containing squeezed out zucchini.
3. Season with sea salt and black pepper to taste.
4. Whisk thoroughly.
5. Pour mixture into greased nonstick skillet and cook on medium/low heat until firm enough to flip.
6. Cook fritter on other side until golden brown.
7. Carefully lift the whole round fritter onto your plate with an egg flip and drizzle with extra virgin olive or coconut oil and nutritional yeast.

The above recipe can also be a quick lunch, along with half a sliced avocado and a favorite side salad. Or, you can make a bigger batch of the recipe and bake it in greased muffin tins at 350 for 20 minutes.

Egg White Omelet/Scramble – E or Fuel Pull

Basic Ingredients: egg whites ✦ veggies ✦ sea salt and other seasonings ✦ optional light Laughing Cow or Weight Watchers cheese wedge, parmesan cheese or skim mozzarella

1. Crack egg whites in bowl or pour in some 100% Liquid Egg Whites from a carton.
2. Add diced veggies of your choice such as green peppers, tomatoes, mushrooms, and onions.
3. Season with sea salt and black pepper and optional onion powder, then whisk together.
4. Pour into nonstick pan with just a smear of coconut oil or butter (far less than 1 tsp.).
5. Add either 1 wedge of light Laughing Cow cheese, 1 Tbs. of parmesan, or a very small amount of skim mozzarella. Let cheese melt into egg whites.
6. If making an omelet, fold in half once mixture is sturdy enough. For a scramble, simply toss around in pan until ready.

As you begin to see consistent weight loss, you may graduate to using one full egg for every three egg whites.

This recipe is **E** only when it is eaten with one of the grain sides we recommend. Egg whites are a perfect protein to pair with a whole grain, but by themselves they are a neutral food and can be eaten with either **S** or **E** fuels. If using this recipe as a scramble for **E** purposes, you can either place it over quinoa, wrap in a sprouted tortilla, or place over two pieces of plan approved grain-based toast like Trader Joe's or Ezekiel. If you would rather use fruit as your **E** side instead of a grain, consider a nice piece of cantaloupe, a whole sliced orange, or pear.

For really stubborn weight issues, consider having this egg white recipe alone sometimes, without the **E** fuel side. Add more whites and veggies to fill up and add a **Fuel Pull** friendly whey smoothie for extra sustenance.

Note: If you are using egg yolks in your smoothies or other recipes, keep a jar in your fridge to save egg whites. You can then use them for this **E** style scramble. Otherwise, you can use 100% Liquid Egg Whites from the store-bought carton. Yolks contain the most nutrition, so hopefully you'll still be eating plenty of whole eggs in your **S** meals. Yolks are very nutritious when eaten raw. It is the white that must be cooked through. You can enjoy your sunny side ups with runny yolks if that's the way you like it.

Whites are a good protein source and it might be more practical for you to buy the carton whites to save time and effort. Raw egg whites contain a substance called avidin that ties up biotin and prevents its absorption. Biotin is important for many reasons, one of which is to help convert our food into energy. Cooking egg whites deactivates the avidin. Liquid egg whites from the store have been pasteurized to 135 degrees which is lower than when scrambling eggs for breakfast. Purists don't need to be put off by the fact that the carton whites are pasteurized because you need to cook them anyway. If you identify more with Drive Thru Sue than any of the other women, feeling free to use the carton variety may also help you stay on plan for convenience sake.

Egg Beaters products add some seasonings and natural coloring to their egg whites product. They have a Southwestern flavored product that is quite tasty.

Light Baked Custard – S, E or Fuel Pull

This is another neutral recipe that does not contain a primary fuel of either fats or glucose. You can enjoy it drizzled with cream for **S** or nix the cream and include a fruit side for **E**. It is also perfect by itself without a side fuel as a breakfast, snack, or dessert to help with more stubborn weight issues.

It's good to remember that removing primary fuels every so often enables your body to dig into a deeper level of fat burning. This custard is a good recipe to keep in mind if you have the sort of weight that does not want to budge, even doing **S** and **E** correctly. It is also a perfect recipe for the two **Fuel Pull** days specified in *One Week Fuel Cycle*, Chapter 28. It is chock full of protein and you can have a full quarter to third of the entire recipe as a serving. Did we mention it tastes fabulous? In our opinion, of course.

Basic Ingredients: egg whites ◆ unsweetened almond milk ◆ sweetener ◆ vanilla ◆ optional pumpkin pie spice or cinnamon

1. Place 1 cup egg whites in a blender (carton kind is fine, or use 7 egg whites).
2. Add 2 cups unsweetened almond milk.
3. Add 7 tsp. Truvia and 2 tsp. vanilla.
4. Blend all ingredients well.
5. Pour into a lightly greased small baking dish or 4 ramekins and bake for 1 hour at 350.

If vanilla flavor is not desired, try adding spices like cinnamon or pumpkin pie spice.

Cheesy Omelet – S

Basic Ingredients: eggs ◆ cream cheese ◆ onion or other veggies ◆ sea salt and other seasonings ◆ butter or oil

1. Crack 2-3 eggs into bowl and whisk.
2. Add 1 oz. cream cheese and some grated or small chopped cheddar cheese.
3. Add a little finely chopped white or green onion. Optional: bacon bits, leftover cubed meat, diced green pepper, mushrooms, or whatever you love.
4. Add sea salt, black pepper, and a little cayenne if you like it hot, and combine all ingredients well.
5. Pour into a pre-heated medium-sized pan, greased well with butter or coconut oil.
6. Once bottom of omelet is slightly browning, fold in half, flip over, and cook for another couple of minutes.

Golden Soft Boiled Eggs – S

Basic Ingredients: eggs ◆ water ◆ sea salt and other seasonings

1. Boil omega-3 eggs for 7-8 minutes so yolks are still slightly soft.
2. Peel and place eggs in bowl.
3. While eggs are still steaming hot, break them in half and melt butter or virgin coconut oil over top, adding a dash of cayenne pepper and sea salt on each egg.

If you have already graduated to using **S Helpers**, this recipe is delicious with third to half a cup of quinoa added to your bowl. This gives a lovely chewy texture to the warm spicy eggs.

Serene chats: This recipe rises to an entirely different planet compared to boring hard boiled eggs. I often use this soft boiled egg idea as a basis for a cheap, easy, high protein evening meal—with no complaints from anybody. I boil a whole pot of eggs and cook a big pot of brown rice ready for the children. I place a variety of different condiments on the table so they can season their own eggs. I add a big salad, a pitcher of raw milk for the children—and everybody is well fed and happy.

Any leftover hard boiled eggs can be used the next day in a fried rice scramble or egg salad with bread for the children; or in cucumber boats or *Joseph's* pita for yourself.

I keep my little baggies of quinoa **S** helpers in the freezer in half cup portions. On boiled egg nights, I take out my quinoa and thaw it out while I am preparing the children's rice. Before we sit down to eat I quickly toss my quinoa into a skillet with a little coconut oil to throw in with my eggs.

Crepes – S

Crepes are great for big families because they make eggs go a long, long way. If just for yourself, you can make a batch for a few days use to pull out of the fridge for a quick breakfast, lunch, dinner, dessert or snack. They are even a good replacement for tortillas. While your children eat whole wheat tortillas, you can use these crepes, fill them with all sorts of goodies and not have to miss out.

Basic Ingredients: eggs ✦ cream ✦ water ✦ glucomannan or xanthan gum ✦ sea salt or sweetener

1. Depending on how many people you are serving, whisk thoroughly between 3-10 eggs in a bowl with just a pinch of glucomannan or xanthan gum.
2. Add dash of cream and some water (not too much, but until mixture is quite a bit looser).
3. Smear a nonstick skillet or griddle with coconut oil or butter and turn to medium heat.
4. Ladle some crepe mix into pan, pick up skillet with an oven glove and move it around until mix thinly covers a large area of the bottom of pan or griddle. Otherwise, spread the mix out thinly using your egg flip.
5. Turn crepe over once when slightly browned on one side and then lightly brown the other side.
6. When cooked, stack crepes in oven to keep warm if making multiple servings.

These crepes can be used for either sweet or savory creations. Add stevia, vanilla, cinnamon and an optional scoop of protein powder for a sweet version. Use salt and pepper, etc. for a savory flavor.

After typing this recipe, we felt hungry for an afternoon snack. We decided to whip up some crepes to eat with whipped cream and berries. However, they smelled so good and we were so hungry, we just sprinkled cinnamon, Truvia, and butter over them and wolfed them down—absolutely yummy. Now we are full and can concentrate again.

Some sweet filling ideas are whipped cream, berries, diced pecans or walnuts, melted butter, Truvia and a little squeeze of lemon. Hot chocolate sauce, our melted *Skinny Chocolate* recipe (*Desserts*, Chapter 23) with cream is another delicious treat. Roll up and devour.

For a savory breakfast, try these crepes filled with ⅓ less fat cream cheese, sliced sausage or deli meats, jalapenos, and melted mozzarella. They can also be filled with other foods that are more lunch or dinner appropriate such as leftover diced chicken breast or ground beef. Add sour cream, hot sauce, sliced avocado, tomato, sautéed veggies, etc. Leftover stews and curries work great folded up in these crepes.

Pearl chats: Visiting my sister-in-law, Monique one day for lunch, she served me one of the most delicious **S** meals I have ever eaten. She made these crepes and filled them with leftover warmed-up coconut chicken curry she had made the night before. She makes the most superb coconut curries. I could not stop raving about it.

My husband likes these crepes best as Mexican style burritos, stuffed with ground seasoned beef (or ground turkey), sour cream, and sautéed onion and tomato. We skip the lettuce, as it doesn't work quite as well with the delicate crepe texture. These crepe style burritos melt in your mouth.

Savory Protein Muffins – S, E or Fuel Pull

Basic Ingredients: eggs ✦ veggies ✦ meats ✦ cheese ✦ sea salt and other seasonings

1. Grease muffin tray and fill muffin holes with veggies such as green peppers, onions, mushrooms, and meats such as bacon bits, diced sausage or turkey, or leftover ground beef.
2. Whisk 8-10 eggs and season well with sea salt and black pepper.
3. Add 1 cup of grated cheese to eggs.
4. Pour egg mix into each muffin hole ¾ way to top.
5. Bake at 350 for 20-25 minutes.

These are great for a busy morning. If you have some already pre-made in the fridge, grab a couple and go. They're good either cold or quickly reheated, and perfect for husbands in a morning hurry. These can also be made with salmon or tuna and work great for brown bag lunches or an afternoon snack.

Savory Protein Muffins can easily be made **E** or **Fuel Pull** by using only egg whites, very lean meats like turkey or Canadian bacon, and much smaller amounts of reduced fat cheese such as mozzarella. They then make the perfect accompaniment to a small bowl of fresh fruit as an **E** breakfast. Or, to help with very stubborn weight, they can be eaten without a fuel side and instead accompanied by a **Fuel Pull** friendly whey smoothie such as *Big Boy Smoothie* or *Fat Stripping Frappa* (*Morning Meals*, Chapter 18).

Corned Beef Hash & Eggs – S

Pearl chats: You will be able to tell this is not a Serene inspired recipe because it uses corned beef out of a can, but my husband and I enjoy it sometimes on a Saturday morning with fried eggs (serves two). I'll record this one and she can go feed her baby.

Basic Ingredients: corned beef ✦ eggs ✦ veggies

1. Finely dice an onion and throw it into a well oiled or buttered fry pan.
2. Add one finely diced zucchini to pan and continue sautéing.
3. Add ⅓ can corn beef and brown along with vegetables.
4. Serve with eggs of any style.

Sunrise Grains

If you feel like a muffin for breakfast, go to the next chapter where you will find our recipes for *Muffins, Breads, and Pizza Crusts*. We have fabulous **S** style muffins that are made with flours that are not grain-based. They are perfect for breakfast, but this chapter would be too long if we included them here. You are welcome to enjoy them for your first meal of the day whenever you desire.

You'll notice we don't have a wide assortment of grains in the following recipes. This is because our **S** and **E** plan is not grain centered. Your new style of eating will now focus on more protein-centered meals with grains rounding some of them out. Certain grains are slower burning in the body and they induce a lower blood glucose response. Oats and quinoa are good examples. These types of grains are the ones on which we want you to focus.

If you are not an oatmeal fan and feel rather stubborn about your stance, go to the end of this chapter to a recipe called *Cookie Bowl Oatmeal.* It's doubtful you could still be an oatmeal despiser after trying this one.

Trim Healthy Pancakes – E

We're thrilled to share this recipe with you. It's a staple in our homes since it makes eating on plan such a delight. Who wouldn't want to eat white fluffy looking pancakes whenever desired? These taste and look like the fattening kind of pancakes we know we shouldn't eat and yet still want to. In contrast, these trimming healthy pancakes will be one of your new secrets to a slim waistline.

If you are gluten intolerant, you can easily buy oats from the gluten-free section of your grocery store that have been processed in a gluten-free environment. That way you can enjoy these pancakes too!

Trim Healthy Pancakes are a cinch to make with only three main ingredients—one cup each of oats, egg whites, and low-fat cottage cheese. What could be simpler? There are no bowls to wash because everything goes into the blender. Afterwards, put water into the blender, turn it on again and that should wash it well for you.

Who cares if it is not breakfast time? You'll probably want to make some right away, just to see if we're telling the truth.

Basic Ingredients: Old Fashioned Oats ✦ low-fat cottage cheese ✦ egg whites ✦ baking powder ✦ sweetener ✦ vanilla

1. Put 1 cup Old Fashioned Oats into blender and blend until oats turn into powder.
2. Turn off blender and add 1 cup of 100% Liquid Egg Whites from the carton and 1 cup low-fat cottage cheese (1% is best, but 2% is okay), or non-fat cottage cheese.
3. Add 2 tsp. aluminum free baking powder, 2-3 tsp. Truvia, and dash of vanilla. Blend well.
4. Heat a nonstick griddle or nonstick fry pan to medium temperature. Spray the pan or skillet with a tiny bit of oil spray, or moisten it with the slightest amount of butter.
5. Ladle mix onto skillet or pan in desired pancake sized shapes. You may use an egg flip to help spread the pancakes out a little since the mix is quite thick.
6. Once bottom of pancakes are golden browned and tops have bubbles, carefully use your egg flip to free circumference of pancakes from sticking then turn pancakes to brown on opposite sides.

7 Transfer pancakes to a paper towel for a minute before placing on serving platter.

It's less fuss to use 100% Liquid Egg Whites for this recipe since it only uses the whites for fluffiness and protein. There is no use in wasting whole eggs. However, if you don't have a 100% Liquid Egg Whites handy, one cup equals about seven egg whites.

You can have a full third of this batch for your **E** meal. That means you can eat one extra large pancake (rather huge), or three medium ones (medium ones are easier to turn on the griddle). If you make up the full batch at one time you should have nine medium-sized pancakes. If so, you'll know they're about the right size. You can put the other six in the fridge between paper towels for subsequent meals.

Top your pancakes with a handful of blueberries, raspberries, or small amounts of any fruit you desire (even small amounts of canned peaches or apricots in sugar-free syrup would be okay). Add a couple of generous tablespoons of plain 0% low-fat Greek or regular yogurt and swirl on a little sugar-free syrup. Delish!

Remember, with a full **E** serving of these pancakes, don't use butter. You won't miss it with the delicious toppings we suggest.

Check out the sister recipe to this one called *Trim Healthy Pan Bread* (*Breads, Muffins, and Pizza Crusts,* Chapter 19). It is the unsweetened bread version and makes great sandwiches. You can also use one of the pan breads as an **S Helper** to a more fat-filled breakfast. Fried eggs taste great with one of them.

Serene chats: I am not thrilled about the idea of store-bought sugar-free syrup! But, Pearl thinks we may lose some of our mamas if we don't give the go ahead for it. We certainly don't want you using regular maple syrup as that would undo the lower glycemic make up of this recipe. Go ahead, and pour some sugar-free syrup on if you feel inclined, only don't choose one that uses aspartame. Many sugar-free syrups use sorbitol or maltitol which are better options since they are natural sugar alcohols. They can cause some gastric distress for some people when used in large amounts, but a swirl of sugar-free syrup shouldn't be too much of a problem in that area.

I would never use regular sugar-free syrup on these pancakes. There are some other great options, depending on what your budget allows. If you're not penny pinching, there is a fantastic stevia-sweetened line of syrups available online. They are called Ali's All Natural Syrups with flavors like maple, blueberry, banana, boysenberry, and strawberry. They can be purchased at www.alisallnatural.com or at www.netrition.com. There is yet another line of plan approved syrups called Nature's Flavors. This brand uses xylitol as their chief sweetener and that's completely fine in our books. They also have a variety of flavors and can be purchased at www.naturesflavors.com.

Since I'm in the penny pinching boat, I prefer to make my own. *Go to Slim Belly Jelly* in Chapter 25. This recipe is quick and easy. I also love these pancakes dolloped with Greek yogurt, sweetened with stevia and a little natural maple flavoring. Natural maple extract can be found at some regular grocery stores, but if not, it should be available at your local health food store, or online. Sometimes, I squeeze lemon juice into the yogurt for variety. Both options make wonderful pancake toppings.

Pearl chats: Most seasons, frozen blueberries and raspberries are cheaper than fresh, so I keep either of these berries thawed and handy for topping the pancakes. In the summer, fresh are superior.

We can't take the acclaim for originating this recipe, but hopefully we'll make it famous as we have been given permission to share it with you!

I have an inspiring friend who suffered from carb eating addictions. She'd tried every form of diet available but always reverted back to her old ways. Finally, she diligently researched a diet for ultimate health, not only to lose weight quickly. She realized that protein was important while white refined foods and sugars were out. She realized that whole foods like meats, non-starchy vegetables, fruits, and small amounts of whole grains were the way to turn her health around. But, she wanted things to be sweet and yummy, too.

She was given a protein pancake recipe to try by a friend, but thought it tasted like cardboard. She knew if she could eat delicious pancakes on a daily basis, it would go a long way to help her make permanent changes toward a healthier lifestyle, as she craved foods like sweet pancakes. She continuously tweaked the ingredients until she came up with this recipe—and it didn't taste like cardboard.

Before these pancakes, she had seldom cooked a meal in her life, eating almost all of her meals from restaurants. She realized this recipe was something she could continue to do and actually prepare in her own kitchen. They turned out well each time and she ate them every day. Her body naturally dropped excess weight—20 pounds, then 30 pounds, and finally 40 pounds dropped off as she changed her food habits. She transformed her body through adding exercise and continues to treat herself by filling up on these yummy pancakes as one of her meals each day.

I did not get overly excited about the recipe at first as I had tried many versions of similar "protein pancakes." None of them tasted any good or had the right texture. I had been very unimpressed with all my attempts. The word "cardboard" fitted well, until I finally tried her recipe. I couldn't believe it when it resulted in IHOP looking pancakes. She told me how she eats them with Greek yogurt, berries, and a little sugar-free syrup. Now, I love to eat them exactly the same way. It makes you feel like you are eating decadent dessert for a full meal.

I make these pancakes frequently so I try to get the ingredients inexpensively. My children love them too and sneak my pancakes from the fridge! I buy 1% cottage cheese at Aldi (cheapest I can find). They carry carton egg white/egg beaters inexpensively also. For my own use, I cook up full batches, or more than one batch at a time, and keep the pancakes in the fridge, separated by paper towels (that's important as they sweat). A large, nonstick pancake skillet or griddle comes in handy. My sister, Mercy bought my mother one for Christmas that does not require any oil spray or butter at all—I'm jealous!

I reheat my next **E** quota of pancakes in the microwave for just a few seconds when I'm ready for them. If you'd rather, you could make your pancakes fresh each time. Remember, each batch gives you three full individual **E** meal's worth. Sometimes that's even a bit much for breakfast if you don't have a huge appetite in the morning. You can save one of the three for an afternoon snack if you get too full. I have a heartier appetite at lunch so I finish the full quota at lunch time.

You can store leftover mix in the fridge if you only want to make one third of a batch at a time. The batter thickens up quite a bit, but you can always add a little water to it and blend once more before cooking. Actually, if you care about phytates and such, keeping the mix in the refrigerator is a way of soaking the oatmeal grain to break down the phytates. Serene makes sure to make up her pancake batter and leave it in the fridge overnight to ensure added health benefits. She tells me it becomes more of a cultured food that way. Her husband, Sam is crazy about these pancakes and calls them "mancakes."

Morning Quinoa (basic recipe) – E

Quinoa cooks up quickly with one part grain to two parts of water or broth. Make sure quinoa is rinsed well before use if it is from a bulk bin or if your packaged quinoa is not labeled pre-rinsed. The following instructions can be used for breakfast, lunch, and dinner uses. If you want to make the grain taste more savory, use stock or broth in place of, or along with the water, and add salt to the water before cooking.

Basic Ingredients: quinoa ✦ water

1. Place any amount of quinoa in saucepan and add double the amount of water to pot (e.g. 1 cup quinoa to 2 cups water).
2. Bring to a boil. Cover with lid and simmer for 15 minutes.
3. Fluff with a fork.

Quinoa is made even more nutritious by soaking beforehand. Serene remembers to do this, so here's her recipe.

Serene chats: I soak my quinoa in a saucepan overnight, an inch below water level. In other words, the water should be an inch higher than the grain. I splash 1 Tbs. of apple cider vinegar into the water (if you are only soaking a little bit, reduce the vinegar accordingly) to help the soaking process break down phytates in the grain. In the morning, I pour off any excess water until the water covers the grain by a scant one centimeter. You don't need to throw out all the water because the phytates have been broken down.

I put the saucepan on high heat and bring it to a boil. I put the lid on, turn the temperature to low, and steam for ten minutes. Next, I then take the pot off the element, but keep the lid on for another five to ten minutes so the quinoa becomes extra fluffy.

Sweet Cinammon Quinoa – E (single serve)

This recipe works either cold or warmed up.

Basic Ingredients: cooked quinoa ✦ unsweetened almond milk ✦ sweetener ✦ cinnamon

1. Put 1 cup of cooked quinoa in cereal bowl.
2. Add Truvia or Nunaturals, cinnamon, and unsweetened almond milk.
3. Stir and eat.

Warming Quinoa Porridge – E (single serve)

Basic Ingredients: cooked quinoa ✦ water ✦ xanthan gum or glucomannan ✦ sweetener ✦ cinnamon ✦ Greek yogurt

1. Put 1 cup of cooked quinoa in small saucepan.
2. Add ½ cup water and turn heat to medium/high.
3. Add Truvia or Nunaturals to taste and generous sprinkle of cinnamon.
4. While porridge is heating, sprinkle in a little xanthan gum or glucomannan and whisk like mad so no lumping occurs. The amount of thickener used will be very slight, quite a bit less than ¼ tsp. This step is only to help all ingredients bind loosely together into a porridge consistency.
5. Once porridge is nice and hot, pour it into a bowl and put a nice dollop of 0% Greek yogurt on top. Eat each bite of porridge with a smear of Greek yogurt.

Creamy Quinoa – S Helper (single serve)

Basic Ingredients: cooked quinoa ✦ heavy cream or full-fat coconut milk ✦ unsweetened almond milk ✦ golden flax meal ✦ unsweetened shredded coconut ✦ sweetener ✦ frozen or fresh berries

1. Put ½ cup of cooked quinoa into a cereal bowl or small saucepan, depending if you want to use the microwave or stove to heat the quinoa.
2. Add 1 Tbs. golden flax meal, 1 Tbs. unsweetened shredded coconut, and Truvia or Nunaturals to taste.
3. Add 1-2 Tbs. heavy cream, butter, or full-fat coconut milk, 2 Tbs. unsweetened almond milk and stir all ingredients.
4. Heat on stove top or in microwave.
5. Once hot, add fresh or frozen berries to the bowl. The heated contents of the bowl should thaw out the berries in a minute or two.

Old Fashioned Oatmeal or Steel Cut Oats – E (basic recipe)

Don't buy Quick Oats as they break down faster in the body, causing a higher insulin response.

For ultimate mineral absorption, soak desired amount of oats overnight, keeping the water level an inch above the top of the grain. Add either 2 Tbs. of apple cider vinegar or kefir. These act as an acidic agent to help break down phytates that naturally occur in grains which bind with minerals and leach them from the body. By soaking your grains overnight, sprouting, or using a sourdough starter when making bread, you safely remove phytates and also make your grains a lot more nutritious and easy to digest.

Serene chats: Soaking sounds annoying, but all it takes is a little pre-thought and a few extra seconds. I automatically do this nearly every night before going to bed as my children usually eat soaked oatmeal every morning.

In the morning, if the oats have absorbed most of the liquid, I add more water right before cooking so the mixture is not too thick. It should be soupy. Don't drain the soaked liquid as you will cook your oats in the soaking water.

Basic Ingredients: oats ✦ water ✦ sweetener ✦ golden flax meal ✦ coconut oil

1. Turn saucepan on high heat using a lid until oatmeal starts to boil.
2. Turn temperature to low and add sea salt, vanilla, and cinnamon to oatmeal. Stir and return lid to the pot. Continue steaming the oats until fully cooked, approximately 10 minutes later.
3. Spoon out your desired portion and add Truvia or Nunaturals to taste, 1 tsp. ground flax meal, 1 tsp. coconut oil or heavy cream, and a little boiling hot water (about ¼ cup) to your bowl.
4. Stir thoroughly until smooth and delicious.

Adding a little whey powder to your oatmeal offers additional protein. However, oatmeal is one of the unique grains that already has five grams of protein per serving. You could also add thawed berries to this yummy breakfast. Frozen berries, like raspberries and blueberries, are fine to put in your bowl of hot oatmeal. They will thaw quickly. Don't cook them with the oatmeal as they will lose their living enzymes. Frozen strawberries will not work because they're too big.

For your children's portions add butter, honey, raisins, and optional coconut flakes to the oatmeal in the pot and serve with milk (preferably raw or kefir, but regular milk will do). If your children have any signs of insulin resistance like weight issues, nix the honey and use a stevia-based sweetener.

Pearl chats: The above is Serene's preferable version. I usually forget to soak my oats, so when I'm hankering for a bowl of oatmeal for breakfast, I quickly cook up the oats and hope for the best with the phytates. Or, I eat my delicious bowl of *Cookie Bowl Oatmeal* which is naturally soaked overnight. If you miss milk with your oatmeal, you may think the idea of one teaspoon of coconut oil mixed with boiling water sounds strange. But, it is delicious as it gels with the ground flax and becomes almost a tapioca pudding consistency.

I alternate between using the coconut oil and boiling water as liquid on my oatmeal and topping it with low-fat yogurt (Greek is best) and berries. This gives added protein to the meal. If you really miss milk with your oatmeal, you could probably get away with a little low-fat milk since you are not drinking a full cup. I also enjoy unsweetened almond milk.

Anabolic Oatmeal – E (single serve)

This is a high protein breakfast and fuels a great workout.

Basic Ingredients: cooked oatmeal ✦ egg whites ✦ golden flax meal ✦ sea salt ✦ vanilla ✦ sweetener

1. Take 1 cup cooked leftover oatmeal and place into small saucepan.
2. Whisk in 2 egg whites from cracked eggs or ¼ cup from 100% egg white carton.
3. Add 1 tsp. flax meal, dash of sea salt, splash of vanilla, sprinkle of cinnamon, and Truvia or Nunaturals to taste.
4. Add 1 tsp. coconut oil and enough water to whisk well into desired thickness.
5. Turn stove to medium and begin heating, stir often.
6. Turn off heat once egg whites are cooked through. This should only take a couple of minutes.
7. Optional: when you pour this anabolic oatmeal into your bowl, add a ½ scoop of whey protein powder.

Serene chats: There is another way to eat this breakfast which acts as an **S Helper,** instead of an **E** meal. It is an excellent way to use up a small portion of leftover oatmeal. Use only quarter to third cup instead of a full cup. Whisk in two whole omega-3 eggs instead of egg whites and add the same additional ingredients as in the above recipe.

Using this recipe as an **S Helper** does not restrict its fat, so now you can use more coconut oil. Personally, I like to have it with raw cream and a generous sprinkle of omega-3 walnuts. This really satiates me. Adding a little ground coconut is also delightful. Since I don't use any more than a third cup of oatmeal, I will not store the fat on my body. Remember, **S Helper** meals are not for beginners on our plan, but are utilized once weight loss has been established.

The above recipe can also be used with cooked leftover quinoa.

Cottage Blueberry Porridge – E (single serve)

Basic Ingredients: blueberries ✦ low-fat cottage cheese ✦ cooked oatmeal or quinoa ✦ sea salt ✦ cinnamon ✦ sweetener

1. Place ½ cup frozen blueberries and ½ cup reduced-fat cottage cheese into food processor and process until smooth.

2. Place 1 cup hot cooked oatmeal or quinoa into a breakfast bowl. Add cinnamon, sweetener, and sea salt if it wasn't already added during cooking.
3. Garnish some of blueberry cottage cheese mix to the sides of the bowl that contains the oatmeal or quinoa. Don't mix it in with porridge, but scoop some up with each bite.

If you do not eat all the blueberry/cottage cheese mix with your breakfast, as it is quite filling even using half of it, eat the rest later in the day as a yummy **E** snack.

Savory Skillet Oatmeal or Quinoa – E (single serve)

This recipe is a cross between a hash brown and a seasoned oatmeal pancake. It's another great way to add even more protein to an oatmeal or quinoa breakfast.

Basic Ingredients: cooked oatmeal or quinoa ✦ egg whites ✦ sea salt and other seasonings ✦ leftover veggies

1. In a bowl, mix 1 cup cooked leftover oatmeal or quinoa with 2-3 egg whites from cracked eggs or ¼ cup 100% Liquid Egg Whites from carton.
2. Season with sea salt and pepper, or Creole for savory flavor, and leftover diced veggies.
3. Mix ingredients well. Ladle a big scoop into lightly greased nonstick skillet and brown on both sides like a pancake, or stir around until cooked through like a scramble.

If you don't want to sauté veggies in the savory version of this recipe, use the egg whites, seasonings and oatmeal. When done, top with diced tomato and a very small dollop of grated skimmed mozzarella cheese. Yum! This is a quick **E** lunch too—and cheap!

If you are at **S Helper** stage, you can enjoy a greasier "soul food" version of this recipe. Use only ¼ cup of the cooked oatmeal per serving with more egg whites or a full egg or two and go heavier on the seasoning. This way you can really "fry it up good" with a larger amount of butter or coconut oil.

Pearl chats: My daughter, Meadow makes a mouth-watering **S Helper** version of this recipe. She adds cayenne pepper for a kick and creates a delicious crisp on either side by using a little butter along with coconut oil. When eating this recipe Meadow's style, you almost feel like you are at a State Fair and are indulging in a deep fried fritter. Oh Yeah! She has a knack for taking recipes to the next level. Remember, if you are in **S Helper** stage, but don't want to halt weight loss, use no more than ⅓ cup of the oatmeal since this version is much heavier on the fats.

Coconut Porridge – S (single serve)

While this porridge is not a grain, it acts like one in this recipe, so we present it here with the other hot breakfast options.

Basic Ingredients: dried coconut ✦ golden flax meal ✦ eggs ✦ sea salt ✦ cinnamon ✦ vanilla ✦ sweetener ✦ water ✦ coconut oil

1. Put ¼ cup dried coconut into blender.
2. Add 2 tsp. flax meal and 1 omega-3 egg.
3. Throw in pinch of salt, cinnamon, vanilla, and Truvia or Nunaturals.
4. Add 1 cup water and blend until smooth.
5. Pour mixture into saucepan, bring to boil, then turn down and whisk on low for a few minutes. If you don't want to stand and whisk, place a lid on and leave for 5 minutes, but you'll have to use a hand held blender at the end to smooth it up again as the egg will set.
6. Pour into a cereal bowl. Add 1 spoonful extra virgin coconut oil and sprinkle with more cinnamon.

Not only does this porridge taste amazing, but it is a full body cleanse. You can fast on it (along with *Coconut Malted Nog* found at the end of this chapter) for a few days to detox and regenerate the body. It's a wonderful cleanse in the winter as it is nourishing, warming, and filling.

Cookie Bowl Oatmeal – Fuel Pull

Both of the next two recipes are fantastic breakfasts to pull out of the fridge in the morning. They must be prepared the night before which only takes a few minutes, but all you have to do the next morning is grab from the fridge and dig in.

They're good breakfast options for the **Fuel Pull** days in our *One Week Fuel Cycle*, Chapter 28, or any time you want to include a **Fuel Pull** breakfast to do some major damage to clinging pounds. Or, you could choose to eat them simply because they are delightfully scrumptious.

Don't eat *Cookie Bowl Oatmeal* every single morning. It's delightful if you have a sweet tooth and you might feel tempted to have it every day for breakfast. Nope. It clocks in at slightly less than 160 calories. That's fine to have as your breakfast up to three times per week, or as a snack any time. However, if you eat it for breakfast every day, your body might think you are starving it and lower your metabolism. Throw some of our other higher calorie breakfasts into your weekly mix to keep your body's furnace hot.

Pearl chats: This recipe gets its title because I think it tastes similar to *No Baked Cookies*. Hey, it has similar ingredients like oats, cocoa, and peanut butter so why not? My husband has always detested oatmeal yet his favorite cookie has always been the *No Baked Cookies*. I finally figured a way to make an oatmeal breakfast that he actually likes, (no, loves!) by borrowing the flavors from that cookie. His grin is so huge when he eats it for breakfast.

I learned a fantastic trick from some internet bloggers about making bigger bowls of oatmeal while reducing calories at the same time. The food blogger, www.chocolatecoveredkatie.com calls this idea, "Voluminous Oatmeal." Hungry girl, (TV chef, cook book author and internet blogger) calls this "Growing Oatmeal," but they both base their oatmeal bowls on the same cool idea. Basically, you mix way less oatmeal grain with way more water than is normally called for when making oatmeal. If you leave this concoction in the refrigerator overnight, the oats swell up and create a huge bowl of oatmeal for less calories. Bottom line—get full by eating more, although you are actually eating less. I love that sort of wizardry.

I realized this would work for our pound kicking **Fuel Pull** meal style since the grain amount is very minor as it has been pulled. I set out to make our version a healthy, yet sinfully treat-like breakfast, and what do you know? It worked! Glucomannan is the final touch that binds the recipe together into a perfect spoonable consistency and chia seeds offer superfood power to help you charge through your day.

Basic Ingredients: Old Fashioned Oats ✦ water ✦ sea salt ✦ unsweetened almond milk ✦ cocoa powder ✦ sweetener ✦ defatted peanut flour or peanut butter ✦ chia seeds ✦ unsweetened milk

1. Put 1 cup water in a small saucepan and bring to a boil.
2. Add ¼ cup oats and a pinch sea salt. Simmer oats for 2 minutes.
3. While oats are simmering put ¾ cup water, ¼ cup unsweetened almond milk, 1 heaping Tbs. extra dark cocoa powder, and ½ tsp. glucomannan in a blender. Blend for 30 seconds.
4. Take oats off heat and add contents of blender to saucepan.
5. Add 4 tsp. Truvia (and a very tiny dash of Nunaturals if you like it very sweet) and 1 Tbs. defatted peanut flour or ¾-1 tsp. peanut butter. Whisk well.
6. Add ½ Tbs. chia seeds. Whisk again.
7. Pour into a large cereal bowl. Cover and refrigerate overnight.

This is perfect cold out of the fridge in the morning although stir around before eating. You could reheat if you'd rather eat it warm. If the chocolate peanut butter flavor does not appeal to you, omit and add cinnamon or vanilla.

Chia Tapioca Pudding – S, E or Fuel Pull

This is another fantastic breakfast for a "gotta get going" morning. It's also a perfect neutral snack or dessert and offers the health benefits of the super seed chia in just the right amounts. The two main ingredients, chia and unsweetened almond milk, offer a Tapioca like experience. They fall into our ultra-slimming **Fuel Pull** category rather than the starchy weight-promoting one of real Tapioca pudding.

Basic Ingredients: unsweetened almond milk ✦ chia seeds ✦ vanilla ✦ glucomannan ✦ sweetener ✦ optional berries

1. Pour 1¼ cup unsweetened almond milk into blender (or a little more if you know you'll be really hungry).
2. Add ½ tsp. glucomannan and turn blender on briefly to mix glucomannan with liquid so there are no lumps. Do not keep blending until a thickening effect occurs.
3. Transfer contents of blender to a small glass jar with lid.
4. Add ¾-1 Tbs. chia seeds.
5. Add dash of vanilla and sweetener to taste.
6. Add optional 3 strawberries cut up into small pieces, or a few raspberries.
7. Place lid on jar and shake well.
8. Place jar in fridge and shake once more before going to bed.

Breakfast Burrito – E

Basic Ingredients: plan approved wrap or tortilla ✦ egg whites ✦ leftover veggies or meats

1. Warm large sprouted tortilla, either in the microwave (Pearl's idea), or the oven (don't warm too long in the oven or it won't stay flexible). Otherwise, place tortilla over the toaster while it is on and let the heat gently warm it up. This warming makes it more flexible.
2. Fill with *Egg White Scramble* from the Egg Breakfast section using any leftover veggies, or canned sockeye salmon, gently sautéed with 1 tsp. coconut oil to heat.

Pearl chats: The salmon is Serene's idea. Although I am a salmon lover, I cannot bear the idea of eating it so early in the morning. Fish does not appeal to me at that time of the day. You could throw some lean turkey sausage in with the scramble if you have taste buds more like mine. I'd much rather smell brewing coffee and sausage than fish at 7 am. All who agree say "I."

Serene chats: I'm telling you, it is delicious. I love the bright orange color of the sock-eye variety. It is the highest food source of DMAE which studies reveal brings tone to your skin and body. My secret is to sauté it with a generous sprinkle of nutritional yeast, a little cayenne pepper, and sea salt. A "fave" of mine for sure.

Crunch Alive Granola – S Helper

This is a dehydrated recipe, but low oven temps should work.

If you limit it to one cup servings of this cereal at a time, you should stay within **S Helper** guidelines. This is possible because the sprouted buckwheat is higher in protein and lower in starch than found in most whole grains. Also, the one cup serving is not all buckwheat, but contains a lot more fiber and extra protein with the added ingredients. The cheapest way to purchase hulled buckwheat groats is online in a bulk bag.

Serene chats: You'll notice the groats need to be sprouted for this recipe. Don't freak out. Sprouting is super easy. Soak them in water overnight, drain in a colander in the morning and rinse away the slimy starch water. Leave the groats in the colander and place on a dinner plate to collect the water. Rinse again in the evening and again the next morning. It is ready when the tails emerge a little way. It does not taste good with long tangled tails, so stop sprouting before they get too long.

Basic Ingredients: sprouted buckwheat ✦ dried coconut ✦ chia or flax seeds ✦ virgin coconut oil or Louanna cooking coconut oil ✦ raw nuts or seeds ✦ vanilla, sea salt, cinnamon, and Nunaturals ✦ optional goji berries or unsweetened dried cranberries

1. Fill large mixing bowl ¾ to top with hulled, sprouted buckwheat.
2. Add 3 cups unsweetened dried coconut, 1 coffee grinder full of chia or ground flax seed, any additional raw nuts and seeds (soaked overnight in water and 1 tsp. sea salt), and an optional handful of goji berries or unsweetened dried cranberries.
3. Splash in pure vanilla, cinnamon, and sea salt to taste.

4. Add plan approved sweetener to taste, e.g. Nunaturals.
5. Drizzle enough virgin coconut oil to get ingredients wet and combined (slightly warm the jar of oil in a pan of hot water to melt it first if you need to). If you can't afford all virgin coconut oil, use half (or all) cooking coconut oil which is a lot cheaper, or use extra virgin olive oil.
6. Get your hands involved and plunge them into the mixing bowl, stirring and rubbing ingredients together very well. You don't want a mouthful of stevia or salt.
7. Place mix on dehydrator trays. Don't worry, it won't fall through holes if you do it gingerly.
8. Dehydrate until crispy, which is usually overnight. If you don't have a dehydrator, place on oven tray and dry in oven at your lowest setting.

Serene chats: This granola is a raw superfood. I don't feed it to my children who will devour it in one day and will not appreciate it as much as I do. I make homemade granola for them with Old Fashioned Oats, honey, natural peanut butter, cooking coconut oil, cinnamon, vanilla, and sea salt. I bake it at 300 for an hour or so, and they love it. I keep my special cereal for my husband and me as it is very low glycemic and more suited to our needs.

Buckwheat is technically the seed of a fruit, not a grain. After sprouting, the starch content is reduced as the protein is elevated. Due to the high fiber content of the chia, flax, and coconut and combined with the additional protein of the sprouted nuts and seeds, this granola has low impact on your blood sugar levels.

Unsprouted buckwheat is 38 percent protein by weight and sprouting naturally raises this level even higher. When you sprout and rinse the buckwheat groats, you wash a lot of the starch away in the water. Buckwheat has been proven to contain the highest naturally occurring amounts of d-chiro-inositol which affects the blood sugar in a positive way. It is an excellent blood sugar regulator and has been advised for those who struggle with insulin-resistance.

Since this is an **S Helper** recipe, not an **E,** due to the generous fats, we suggest pouring either full or low-fat kefir, Greek yogurt, or unsweetened almond milk over your granola. Combined with Greek yogurt, the flavor and texture is a match made in heaven. The tart creamy cultured dairy with the sweet crunch of the granola are divine. Using this recipe as a dessert, you could splurge and enjoy a generous swirl of undiluted cream.

This granola also makes a great sprinkle over a berry whip or on top of *Tummy Tucking Ice Cream* (*Desserts,* Chapter 23).

Satisfying Granola – S

While you may have to wait a couple of months to eat the delicious *Crunch Alive Granola* since it is in **S Helper** category, you can jump right in for this recipe.

A regular oven will do a fine job with this granola. It also makes a great topping for yogurt, or you can have some in a bowl with kefir or unsweetened almond milk, sweetened up a little with one of our plan approved sweeteners. It is also great in a snack bag when you are out and about running errands.

Basic Ingredients: nuts and seeds ✦ golden flax meal ✦ optional unsweetened cranberries or dried goji berries ✦ coconut oil ✦ vanilla ✦ sweetener

1. Pour desired amounts of your choice of the following ingredients onto a baking tray: pumpkin seeds, shredded coconut, sunflower seeds, chopped almonds or other nuts, flax and sesame seeds. You may also add a few finely chopped fresh unsweetened cranberries or a small amount of dried goji berries.
2. Add ½-1 cup ground flax to the other whole nuts and seeds (depending on quantity of ingredients). This will allow for some clumping of the ingredients which occurs with most granolas.
3. Add a generous amount of coconut oil (½-1 full cup) depending on quantity of other ingredients).
4. Add vanilla and plan approved sweetener to taste (several tsp. Truvia with a dash of NuStevia Pure White Stevia Extract Powder should suffice).
5. Bake at 300 for about an hour.

To make this granola extra superfoody, soak the nuts and seeds first before adding other ingredients and dehydrate overnight instead of baking.

Cereal if You Must – E

Almost all store-bought cereals are full of mineral leaching phytates even though you will not find the word "phytates" in the ingredients. Cereals are highly processed even if they say "organic" or whole grain. Usually, they are very high in sugars and carbohydrates. It would probably be about as healthy to eat the cardboard box they come in as to eat the actual cereal.

However, there are some exceptions. The first and healthiest alternative is a cereal made from the same company which makes the delicious plan approved Ezekiel bread and sprouted tortillas. As it is sprouted, this cereal has no phytates. It is completely unprocessed at very low temperatures (200 degrees).

While this is a perfect cereal for your health, we do not want you to splurge and eat large bowls of it frequently just because it is plan approved. Remember, even a perfect grain in large quantities will spike your insulin. Have a medium-sized bowl instead. Sprinkle the cereal with berries if you desire. Since cereal is **E**, this is one of the exceptions we make where you may have a little low-fat milk, but not more than half a cup for a bowl of cereal. If you don't mind the taste of kefir with cereal, low-fat kefir is a better option. Unsweetened almond milk is another good option, too.

When eating an **E**, it is always best to get as much protein as you can to blunt insulin spikes. A good way to do this is to add half a scoop of whey protein powder to your unsweetened almond milk, skimmed milk, or kefir.

Ezekiel cereal is usually only found at natural food stores and can be a little pricey. If you are looking for a more accessible and cheaper alternative, you can find Uncle Sam's cereal at Walmart, Kroger, and just about any other supermarket. It may not be as unprocessed as Ezekiel cereal, but it is full of fiber from flax, and moderate amounts will not be as likely to spike your insulin levels as other store-bought cereals. It is pretty cheap, containing no ingredients that are too difficult to pronounce. Even though it has some flax, it is still roughly within our guidelines of an **E** cereal.

Toast Ideas

Who doesn't like toast for breakfast now and then? While grain-based toast is not a staple for us at breakfast time, we get the urge to have it every so often. If you're a mama who loves toast in the morning, you can learn to include it in a way that still allows you to have good control over your weight. We don't suggest making a habit of eating toast with jelly (even all fruit jelly) every morning. It's important to keep in mind that high protein breakfasts help control carb cravings for the remainder of the day and help you start your day with stable blood sugar. Research proves over and over again that those who eat high protein for breakfast, such as eggs, get better weight loss results and think less about their upcoming meal or snack.

The following recipes are ways to eat whole grain toast with balance. Remember to not eat more than two pieces of toast in one sitting. That would not be **E** for energizing. It would be **O** for overindulgence or **F** for failure. Sorry, we are only being cruel to be kind. Even when eating an occasional **Crossover** meal, if you have a high metabolism and need to live mostly on **Crossovers**, you should never eat more than two pieces of bread at a time. If two pieces of grain toast don't fill you up, add a whey protein smoothie **E** style with glucomannan or a half cup of Greek style low-fat yogurt. You'll get further "full" mileage.

If grain-based toast is the basis of your breakfast, you can't eat a lot of fat with it. Don't pile the butter on your toast! But, don't worry, we have plenty of creative and yummy options to put on your grain toast.

When you are up **S Helper** stage, you can have a generous amount of butter if you are only eating one piece of sprouted or sourdough bread. Of course, you can use any of our **S** bread recipes provided in the lunch section with lots of butter.

Cottage Style Toast – E

Basic Ingredients: plan approved bread ✦ low-fat cottage cheese or skim ricotta ✦ sea salt and other seasonings ✦ tomato or cucumber ✦ herbs

1. Toast 2 pieces bread (sprouted, dark rye, or homemade sourdough).
2. Spread generous amount low-fat cottage cheese or skim ricotta on top and season with salt and pepper.
3. Optional: layer thinly sliced tomato or cucumber and fresh or dried herbs on top of cottage or ricotta cheese.

Mozzarella and Turkey Toast – E

Basic Ingredients: plan approved bread ✦ skim mozzarella cheese ✦ lean turkey deli meat ✦ sea salt and other seasonings

1. Sprinkle a small amount of grated reduced fat mozzarella cheese on 2 pieces bread (sprouted dark rye or whole grain sourdough).
2. Layer with lean turkey deli meat or Canadian bacon.
3. Sprinkle with Italian herbs and black pepper.
4. Bake on tray in the oven, or toaster oven, until cheese bubbles and melts.

Sliced tomato could be used in place of, or alongside turkey, for this recipe.

Sprouted French Toast – E

Basic Ingredients: egg whites ✦ plan approved bread ✦ cinnamon ✦ vanilla ✦ sweetener ✦ optional milk

1. Break 2 egg whites into a bowl and whisk.
2. Add cinnamon, sweetener, and vanilla to egg whites. Whisk again. Optional: add 2 Tbs. skim milk or unsweetened almond milk.

turate two slices sprouted dark rye or whole grain sourdough bread into egg white ix.

4 Brown gently in nonstick pan with a smear of butter or cooking coconut oil.

Accompany with a small slice of cantaloupe and a half cup of cottage cheese or a side of lean Canadian bacon. The sides we suggest will add a little more protein to protect against sugar spikes. You can pour plan approved sugar-free syrup on the French toast if desired, or better still, use *Slim Belly Jelly*, Chapter 25. This homemade jelly, containing the miracle wonders of glucomannan, helps blunt the carb count of your toast.

Smoothies

Now that you are eating **S** and **E**, you will no longer make smoothies for yourself with regular milk since it is a liquid carb. Nor will you use bananas as a base. Don't panic smoothie lovers. We have even better alternatives.

Milk made smoothies (especially raw milk) are wonderful for your growing children with higher metabolic needs. Unless you are a super high metabolism type who struggles to maintain enough weight, you will now choose from bases of whey protein powder, kefir, coconut kefir, Greek yogurt, unsweetened almond milk, or dilutions made from small amounts of canned coconut milk (either liquid or frozen into cubes), or small amounts of heavy cream mixed with water. We promise that you won't miss regular milk or bananas. These options make awesome smoothies! We do not advise making smoothies from rice or soy milks.

Smoothie recipes are in this section since they only take a couple of minutes to make—perfectly suitable if you do not like to slave over the stove in the morning. However, these smoothies are also wonderful for desserts, snacks, a quick lunch, or an on-the-go meal. You can even drink them while driving, but please keep your eyes on the road. Do not close them in bliss from the sips of your smoothie!

Whey to Go Smoothies

If you aren't already using it, we hope you'll soon welcome whey protein into your diet for its health promoting and slimming effects. These smoothies are the best way to make that happen.

Fat Stripping Frappa – S, E or Fuel Pull

We're so excited about this recipe. You'll soon realize why it deserves first place in our smoothie recipes. This creamy, icy, chocolately drink may change your life. Begin drinking *Fat Stripping Frappa* and it's doubtful you'll ever crave a sugar-laden frap again.

An almost miraculous reaction takes place between the primary ingredients of whey powder, glucomannan, and ice. Blended together, they create a creamy cold fluff. You'll feel you are drinking oodles of fat and calories, but the opposite is true. The best news of all is that you can drink it to your heart's content. One serving makes more than a quart, if you can drink that much. If not, put some back in the fridge to save for later.

This Frappa is perfect if you need to rely on a **Fuel Pull** arsenal to attack stubborn pounds. Since it is low in carbs, fat, and calories, be careful drinking it too often as a full meal if you're already at goal weight. You could fat strip your way to too skinny! However, saying that makes us hypocrites. We are at goal weight, but find it hard to stop drinking this stuff! It makes a great filling breakfast, but also a perfect afternoon snack, especially in the summer when icy drinks are just the ticket.

Basic Ingredients: unsweetened almond milk ✦ water ✦ ice ✦ glucomannan powder ✦ vanilla ✦ sea salt ✦ sweetener ✦ cocoa powder ✦ whey protein powder ✦ optional frozen strawberries or frozen coffee cubes

1. Place in blender ½ cup of unsweetened almond milk and ½ of cup water.
2. Add 1 heaped Tbs. cocoa powder, scant ½ tsp. glucomannan powder, two pinches of sea salt, few sprinkles of NuStevia Pure White Stevia Extract Powder or Truvia to taste, and dash of vanilla.
3. Blend well before adding 1¼ trays of ice cubes (our trays hold 16 ice cubes).
4. Blend on high using a handy wooden spoon to help stir the thick mixture. Don't get it too close to the blades. Void this step if using a Vitamix or other high end blender.
5. Add 1 scoop whey protein powder (we use Swanson Premium Brand whey protein) and blend again for a little longer watching the fluff magic take place. Taste again to see if more sweetener is needed before pouring into quart glass jar.

Oops! We just realized that you most probably have a fridge with an ice-maker that actually works! Both of ours broke years ago. To equal tray amounts, use 22 large ice cubes. If you are not sure if your cubes are large enough, you can gauge by the numbers on your blender. Once you have enough ice, your liquid should reach the 2½ cup mark, the ice jutting above to reach close to the 4½ cup mark.

Use the full scoop of whey if this frappa is your complete meal, such as a breakfast. You need only use ½ or even a ¼ scoop of whey if this is part of a snack or meal that includes another protein source. Even with ½ a scoop it is still creamy. Alternatively, you can make the smoothie with the full scoop of whey and share it with a family member. Trust us, your children will beg for it once they've had a taste. Sharing with someone else will give you two cups each—still plenty.

For variety, you can make a strawberry or coffee version of this frappa which are both equally as yummy. For strawberry, omit the cocoa. Use only 1 full tray of ice cubes instead of the 1¼ trays and include a handful of frozen strawberries to make up for the missing ¼ tray of ice cubes. For coffee flavor, replace the ½ cup of water with an extra strong ½ cup of cold brewed coffee.

Pearl chats: My daughter, Meadow has a knack for taking things to the next level. She makes a strong brewed coffee version of this frappa and blends it up normally with a full scoop of whey. At the end she adds ⅓ oz. of 85% dark chocolate. She roughly chops it and then throws it into the blender for just a few seconds more. The result is to die for! Little pieces of dark chocolate floating in a sweet, thick, creamy coffee drink. She splits this with me for a post meal desert sometimes and I am one grateful mama. Meadow likes things very sweet. She uses 5 teaspoons of Truvia to make her concoction but it would only take a sprinkle or two of Nunaturals to obtain that very sweet taste people like her and my husband crave.

This little bit of chocolate still allows the frappa to stay in **Fuel Pull** mode since it is split between two people and while it creates a fun chocolate crunch, there is not much chocolate involved.

Big Boy Smoothie – S, E or Fuel Pull

Basic Ingredients: unsweetened almond milk ✦ ice ✦ sweetener ✦ sea salt ✦ whey protein powder ✦ frozen strawberries ✦ optional vanilla

Serene chats: This makes another huge weight stripping smoothie. I frequently make this recipe for my husband for breakfast. He's 6' 5", large frame, and yet this one smoothie satisfies him completely even though his job entails physical labor. He loves it, and sometimes wants it again for lunch.

I have never told him that it is a **Fuel Pull**. Actually, he's never even heard the term. You are now aware of our food science, but my husband doesn't know any of the terminology. If I told him it was slimming or "light" he'd have nothing to do with it! He would think I was trying to put him on a diet.

1. Pour unsweetened almond milk into your blender to reach perfectly to 1 cup line.
2. Add ice to 2 cup line.
3. Add a generous handful of frozen strawberries.

4. Sprinkle a few dashes of NuStevia Pure White Stevia Extract Powder to taste or use Truvia to taste.
5. Add pinch of sea salt and optional vanilla. Sea salt is important to achieve the right flavor.
6. Add 1 scoop of whey protein powder (we use Swanson Premium Brand Whey Protein).
7. Blend on high using a handy wooden spoon to help stir the thick mixture. Don't get it too close to the blades. Void this step if using a Vitamix or other high end blender.

Basic Whey Smoothie – S

The next couple of smoothies make a more manageable large cup amount if you don't want to get too full with the above whey recipes. This one includes coconut oil to help you with energy levels. It's a great post workout protein replenisher.

Basic Ingredients: whey protein ✦ water ✦ coconut oil ✦ optional coconut milk cubes ✦ optional egg yolk

1. Put 1 scoop whey protein powder (any flavor) into blender.
2. Add ¾ cup water.
3. Add I Tbs. extra virgin coconut oil for quick energy burst.
4. Add Truvia or Nunaturals if whey is unsweetened.
5. Turn on blender and while running add ¼ cup boiling (or very hot) water. This emulsifies the coconut oil beautifully into the rest of the liquid without allowing coconut oil globules to separate and rise to the top. That's annoying.
6. Add generous ice or coconut milk ice cubes and blend more.

This is your basic recipe. If you want to make a chocolate flavor, add cocoa powder, splash of vanilla, and pinch of sea salt.

Basic Whey Smoothie – E or Fuel Pull

Depending on the type of fruit you add, this can be either **E** or **Fuel Pull**. Frozen or fresh fruit such as peach, mango, or cherries may be added to make this an **E** style smoothie. A **Fuel Pull** can include small amounts of frozen berries, the best being strawberries or raspberries. Or, make it a **Fuel Pull** without any fruit or berries. You can also add cocoa powder for a delicious chocolate strawberry smoothie.

Note: If your whey protein smoothie is accompanying another food that contains a good amount of protein, you do not need to use a full scoop of whey. If you desire an **E** or **Fuel Pull** breakfast of scrambled egg whites, and want a smoothie on the side, only use half a scoop of whey. The smoothie will still be thick and delicious, your whey protein will last longer, and you won't overdue a macronutrient. Remember that suggestion for snacks also.

Basic Ingredients: whey protein ✦ water ✦ unsweetened almond milk, Greek yogurt, or light coconut milk ice cubes ✦ fruit or berries ✦ optional cocoa powder

1. Place ½-1 scoop whey protein into blender (depending on whether it is a solo snack, a meal, or an addition to another protein food like egg whites).
2. Add one of the following—½ cup unsweetened almond milk, ¼ cup 0% Greek yogurt, or 1-2 light coconut milk ice cubes.
3. Add ½ cup water if using unsweetened almond milk, or ¾ cup if using Greek yogurt or light coconut milk cubes.
4. Add frozen fruit or berries.
5. Add Truvia or Nunaturals if whey is unsweetened.
6. Add an optional 1 Tbs. cocoa powder.
7. Add additional ice cubes.
8. Blend well and enjoy.

Kefir Smoothies

If you want to learn to make your own kefir, look up Serene's kefir recipe in *Cultured Recipes*, Chapter 26. As we outlined in *Foundation Foods*, Chapter 17, Kefir is a healing drink for the body and offers beneficial bacteria to your intestinal tract.

Kefir smoothies are categorized as **S**. This is because goat's milk kefir is naturally high in healthy saturated fats and we add 1 Tbs. of coconut oil and optional egg yolks to the basic recipe. Full-fat cow's milk kefir would also be an **S**.

Note: To make these **E,** you may use raw skimmed cow's milk kefir. While goat's milk does not separate cream from liquid, cow's milk does. Therefore, you can have lower fat kefir by scooping the cream off the top before making it. Or, buy unsweetened low-fat kefir from the store (readily available). Another option for a probiotic based smoothie if you don't have kefir is to use a base of 0% Greek yogurt and water. That would be suitable for **S**, **E** and **Fuel Pull** purposes.

For **E** kefir smoothies, you do not have to stick to frozen berries. You could add other fruits like frozen peaches and cherries, etc. Remember not to add oils or egg yolks to **E** smoothies.

The following recipes can also be made with *Coconut Kefir* (*Cultured Recipes*, Chapter 26) if you have dairy allergies, or just prefer it. Smoothies made with coconut are considered **S**.

Kickin' Kefir Elixir – S (try to say this one five times really fast)!

This is the skeleton recipe for a kefir smoothie, but you can dress it up as much as you like.

Basic Ingredients: kefir ✦ coconut oil ✦ golden flax or chia ✦ sweetener

1. Pour 1 cup goat's milk kefir, or any unsweetened homemade or store-bought full-fat kefir into blender.
2. Add 1 heaped Tbs. raw virgin coconut oil.
3. Add 1 heaped tsp. golden flax or chia.
4. Add plan approved sweetener to taste.
5. Blend well and enjoy.

The following are variations on the above skeleton recipe.

Berry Bonanza – S

Basic Ingredients: KKE (*Kickin' Kefir Elixir*) ingredients ✦ berries ✦ optional coconut milk cubes ✦ optional whey protein powder ✦ optional egg yolk

1. Add ½ cup of our favorite frozen berries to KKE.
2. Add optional frozen coconut milk cubes for a creamier fluffy texture.
3. Add optional vanilla or chocolate whey protein powder (omit sweetener if using this since the whey powder is already sweetened).
4. Add optional omega-3 egg yolk.

Chocolate Decadence – S

Basic Ingredients: KKE ingredients ✦ cocoa powder ✦ sea salt ✦ vanilla ✦ ✦ optional coconut cubes ✦ optional egg yolk ✦optional peanut butter

1. To KKE, add 1 Tbs. cocoa powder, or raw cocoa nibs if you prefer.
2. Add 1 scoop chocolate whey protein powder (use sweetener but slightly less than KKE since you are adding cocoa which has bitterness).
3. Add pinch of sea salt.

4. Add dash of vanilla.
5. Add optional frozen coconut cubes.
6. Add optional egg yolks.
7. Add optional 1 tsp. peanut butter.

Vanilla Dream – S

Basic Ingredients: KKE ingredients ✦ vanilla ✦ optional vanilla whey protein ✦ optional coconut cubes ✦ optional egg yolk ✦ nutmeg or cinnamon

1. To KKE add dash of pure vanilla.
2. Add 1 scoop vanilla whey protein powder (omit sweetener if using sweetened whey).
3. Add optional frozen coconut cubes.
4. Add optional egg yolk.
5. Add a sprinkle of nutmeg or cinnamon on top of smoothie.

Superfood Toss – S (When you have superfoods a plenty)!

Basic Ingredients: KKE ingredients ✦ Barley Green ✦ hemp seeds ✦ hemp oil ✦ maca powder ✦ cocoa ✦ optional whey protein

1. To KKE add 1 Tbs. Barley Green powder.
2. Add 1 handful hemp seeds.
3. Add 1 heavy squirt of hemp oil.
4. Add 1 tsp. maca powder.
5. Add 1 tsp. cocoa.
6. Add optional chocolate whey protein powder.

Serene chats: This superfood toss may sound gross, but it tastes like heaven to me. Maybe I'm crazy, but I love the earthy tastes of greens and hemp together.

Green Purity – S

Basic Ingredients: KKE ingredients ✦ greens ✦ optional egg yolk or protein powder

1. To KKE add 2-3 huge handfuls of greens, preferably from your garden during season, or organic store-bought, e.g., spinach, romaine, parsley, or cilantro.
2. Add optional egg yolk or protein powder.

Note. Greens, like kale and collards, are too bitter for this smoothie and are best steamed or sautéed for complete nutrient absorption.

Budget Smoothie Ideas

Pearl chats: Enough with the kefir! If you're like me, the last thing you want to do at 6.00 am is go outside to milk goats! Or, if you're not inclined to seek out a source for raw goat's or cow's milk, kefir smoothies may never be on your food radar. Nah, I'm just giving Serene a hard time here since the kefir smoothies are her recipes. You can always buy plain kefir at the store if you want to try them out.

But, what if you don't have the money to buy kefir or whey protein or even unsweetened almond milk? Must smoothies be removed from your diet? No way! You can still have delicious healthy smoothies with the following options.

By far the most affordable way to make an on plan smoothie is to use a coconut milk or heavy cream dilution. All you do is use 2-3 Tbs. of liquid coconut milk from a can or 2-3 Tbs. of heavy cream and dilute these options with water. You may also freeze the coconut milk in ice cube trays and use 2-3 of these cubes with added water. It's important not to pour half a cup of heavy cream in your smoothie. That's consuming needless calories—2-3 Tbs. will do the job nicely.

These smoothies can be made either more "liquidy" like a shake, or almost like a whip or soft serve ice cream by adding less liquid and more frozen ingredients. Whips have even better texture when made in the food processor. Glucomannan helps out, too.

Most of the following recipes are considered **S** in their original recipe state. They can easily be made **E** by replacing the full-fat cream or coconut milk with a little light coconut milk straight from the can, or pre-made frozen cubes, and including frozen or fresh fruit. Light coconut milk usually has between 60-80 percent less fat. **E** smoothies could then utilize fruits other than berries.

Can we remind you again to please steer clear of bananas, or use only half a banana in an **E** smoothie? Feed whole ones to your growing children. We offer only **S** or **E** choices here for these budget smoothies. **Fuel Pull** smoothies are better left to whey powder since it offers more protein which is nice when you're pulling out your primary fuels.

Berritastic – S or E

Basic Ingredients: coconut milk in cubes or liquid, or heavy cream ✦ water ✦ berries ✦ lemon juice ✦ flax or chia ✦ sweetener ✦ optional glucomannan

1. Place 2-3 Tbs. liquid coconut milk or heavy cream into blender, or use 2-3 frozen cubes coconut milk.
2. Add 1-1½ cups water.
3. Add handful frozen berries.
4. Add optional juice of ½ a lemon, or a squeeze of lemon concentrate.
5. Add 1 tsp. ground flax or chia seed.
6. Add Nunaturals or Truvia to taste.
7. Add optional ¼-½ tsp. glucomannan while blender is running.

Chocomocho – S

Basic Ingredients: brewed coffee ✦ heavy cream ✦ cocoa ✦ sweetener ✦ water ✦ ice ✦ optional whey protein ✦ optional glucomannan

1. Put into blender 1 cup of cold coffee with heavy cream. This is in place of regular coconut/cream dilution. If making smoothie more whip like, use creamed coffee ice cubes.
2. Add ice.
3. Add 2 tsp. unsweetened cocoa.
4. Add optional egg yolk.
5. Add optional scoop of chocolate whey protein powder.
6. Add NuStevia Pure White Stevia Extract Powder or Truvia to taste, less will be needed if using pre-sweetened whey protein.
7. Add more water if desired.
8. Add optional ¼-½ tsp. glucomannan while blender is running.

Vanilla Sip – S

Basic Ingredients: coconut milk as liquid or frozen cubes, or heavy cream ✦ water ✦ ice ✦ vanilla ✦ sweetener ✦ flax or chia ✦ optional egg yolk ✦ optional vanilla whey protein ✦ nutmeg or cinnamon

1. Place into blender 2-3 Tbs. coconut milk, heavy cream, or 2-3 frozen cubes coconut milk.
2. Add 1-1½ cups water and extra ice cubes.
3. Add dash of pure vanilla.
4. Add 1 tsp. ground flax or chia seed.
5. Add optional egg yolk.
6. Add optional scoop of vanilla whey protein powder.
7. Add Nunaturals or Truvia to taste (adjust when using pre-sweetened whey protein).
8. Add sprinkle of nutmeg or cinnamon on top.

Cream and Greens – S

Basic Ingredients: coconut milk as liquid or frozen cubes, or heavy cream ✦ water ✦ ice ✦ greens ✦ sweetener ✦ egg yolk

1. Place in blender 2-3 Tbs. coconut milk or cream, or 2-3 frozen cubes of coconut milk.
2. Add 1-1½ cups of water.
3. Add ice.
4. Add 3 handfuls garden greens.
5. Add 1 egg yolk.
6. Add Truvia or Nunaturals to taste.
7. Optional scoop of whey protein.

Greek Yogurt Breakfast Swirls

Plain Greek yogurt makes a great breakfast since it has a lot of protein. It's quick and easy for the days when you don't have time to make eggs, oatmeal, or even a smoothie. If you're one who doesn't like to fuss over breakfast, plain Greek yogurt might be just the right idea for you to have frequently. Besides, it's downright yummy and adds good bacteria and live enzymes to your digestive tract.

If yogurt is going to be your sole breakfast, it is important to use Greek style to get enough protein to start your morning. Regular yogurt won't offer you enough of this important macronutrient unless you mix it with cottage cheese. The creamy consistency of Greek style is also suited to these breakfast swirls. These ideas can also be used as day and evening snacks, or even desserts.

The 0% Greek yogurt works great for either **S** or **E** breakfasts, which makes things simple. It may be fat free but it still has a very creamy texture. Zero fat Greek yogurt usually has nine grams of carbs for a full cup. Add some fruit like a chopped apple, without adding a lot of fat (like too many nuts), and you're in **E** meal territory. On another morning, include some nuts and berries with your yogurt, or a big spoon full of almond butter, and you are fine for **S** mode. That means it is also perfect as a **Fuel Pull** breakfast if paired with berries. It is so versatile since it does not contain too many carbs for a full **S** breakfast and it does not have too much fat to prevent it from being the perfect **E**. However, if you're having an **S** dessert of Greek yogurt after a fat laden **S** meal (a supper for example), we suggest you keep it to only half a cup.

While we love Truvia for a sweetener, if you don't want a crunchy feel to your smooth yogurt, you'll need to grind it in your coffee grinder first. Sprinkling in some Nunaturals may be less fuss, it works better in yogurt since the powder is finer. Liquid stevias also work great for yogurt (KAL and Swanson are both good tasting brands).

Apple Cinammon – E

Basic Ingredients: Greek yogurt ✦ apple ✦ sweetener ✦ cinnamon ✦ peanut butter or nuts

1. Dice 1 apple into small pieces.
2. Put 1 cup 0% plain Greek yogurt in a bowl and add diced apple.
3. Add Truvia, Nunaturals, or liquid stevia to taste.
4. Add a good sprinkle of cinnamon and a very small handful of chopped walnuts or 1 tsp. peanut butter.
5. Stir ingredients loosely together.

Fruity Blend – E

Basic Ingredients: Greek yogurt ✦ fruit of choice ✦ sweetener

1. Put 1 cup 0% Greek yogurt in bowl.
2. Add sliced peaches (fresh or canned in own juice), or you may use a little (¼) cup diced pineapple canned in its own juice, but strain fruit from juice as we don't want you to consume pure liquid carbs.
3. Add Truvia, Nunaturals, or liquid stevia if you require more sweetness.

Greek Pudding – S, E or Fuel Pull

This can be used as a neutral breakfast or snack since it does not contain a primary fuel of either fats or glucose. It can also be used as an addition to some **E** fruit or **S** breakfast sausage.

Basic Ingredients: Greek yogurt ✦ whey protein ✦ optional sweetener (if using unsweetened whey) ✦ optional cocoa powder

1. Put 1 cup 0% Greek yogurt in bowl.
2. Add 1 scoop whey protein and stir well.

Light Vanilla Greek Treat – S, E or Fuel Pull

Basic Ingredients: Greek yogurt ✦ unsweetened almond milk ✦ whey protein ✦ optional sweetener (if using unsweetened whey) ✦ vanilla

1. Put 1 cup 0% Greek yogurt in a bowl.
2. Add 1 scoop whey protein and stir well.
3. Add ¼ cup unsweetened almond milk or a dash more if you desire a thinner consistency.
4. Add optional sweetener and stir well until lumps disappear.

Pina Colada with Nuts – S

Basic Ingredients: Greek yogurt ✦ pina colada whey protein ✦ walnuts ✦ Dried coconut

1. Put 1 cup of 2% or 0% yogurt in a bowl.
2. Add pina colada whey protein and stir.
3. Add handful of chopped walnuts and a sprinkle of dried coconut.

Almond Raspberry Swirl – S or Fuel Pull

Depending on how much nut butter you use, this can be either **S** or **Fuel Pull**. Keep to no more than 1 tsp. if desiring a **Fuel Pull**, anything more and you're heading into **S** territory.

Basic Ingredients: Greek yogurt ✦ almond or peanut butter ✦ vanilla ✦ raspberries ✦ sweetener

1. Put 1 cup 0% Greek yogurt in bowl.
2. Add 1 tsp.-1 Tbs. almond butter or peanut butter.
3. Add dash of vanilla and some thawed raspberries.
4. Add Truvia, Nunaturals, or liquid stevia to taste.

Jelly Style – S, E or Fuel Pull

Basic Ingredients: Greek yogurt ✦ Polaner All-Fruit Jam with Fiber

This recipe is very quick, but fantastic. It makes a great snack, too. If you want to keep it as a **Fuel Pull** appropriate snack sometime, make sure to use only 1 tsp. of jelly. Or, if it is to be eaten after an **S** meal, stick to 1 tsp. of jelly and use only a ½ cup of yogurt. That way you could add a little peanut butter too if desired. You can always sweeten the yogurt up further with our approved sweeteners if only 1 tsp. of jelly does not bring enough sweetness.

The brand of jelly that we recommend is Polaner All-Fruit Jam with Fiber. It has seven net grams of carbs for 1 Tbs. which is fine for E. However, if you have *Slim Belly Jelly* in the fridge, it is even better.

1. Put 1 cup 0% yogurt in bowl.
2. Add 1 tsp.-1Tbs. Polaner All-Fruit Jam with Fiber and swirl in with yogurt.

Hemp Delight – S

Basic Ingredients: Greek yogurt ✦ hemp protein ✦ raspberries ✦ sweetener

1. Put 1 cup 2% or 0% Greek yogurt in bowl.
2. Add scoop Hemp Pro 70.
3. Add thawed red raspberries.
4. Add Truvia or Nunaturals to taste and an optional sprinkle of hemp seeds.

Serene chats: One of my favorite yogurt breakfast swirls is plain Greek yogurt with a generous sprinkle of dried organic unsweetened coconut. I don't know why it is so spectacular to me, but I am addicted to its tart simplicity with the understated natural sweet nuttiness of the coconut. It may be my own quirk, but you may become a fan, too.

Coconut Malted Nog – S

This is a smooth and hearty beverage, especially good in the winter, but a fine addition to any smaller **S** breakfast to fill you up a little more. This recipe makes a large supply so it's a good drink to pull out of the refrigerator in the morning and heat up to have alongside an **S** style Greek yogurt swirl or a fried egg or two. It gives a lot more mileage if you have an active morning ahead of you. If you are not a morning coffee drinker, this may be the perfect warming morning beverage for you.

Basic Ingredients: light coconut milk ✦ water ✦ cinnamon ✦ vanilla ✦ sweetener ✦ sea salt ✦ optional gelatin ✦ golden flax meal ✦ cream or coconut oil

1. Pour 1 can light coconut milk (365 or Kroger brands work great) into blender or Vitamix and fill rest of blender up with water.
2. Add cinnamon, vanilla, and enough NuStevia Pure White Stevia Extract Powder or Truvia to sweeten to taste.
3. Add enough sea salt to the mix to create a more caramel like flavor (about ¼ tsp.).
4. Blend well.
5. Store this dilution in an empty mason jar in the fridge. When ready to drink, shake, and pour a good coffee mug's portion into saucepan.
6. This next step is optional, but makes the drink even more super nutritious—good for muscle growth, benefits joints and ligaments, soothes the GI tract, and great for

those with IBS type problems. Add 1 rounded tsp. gelatin (Bernard Jenson's brand ordered online is best since it is made without pork and is not processed with high heat, but even plain Knox gelatin will be of benefit). Stir gelatin in before heating milk and let sit for a minute.

7 Heat on medium while stirring, bringing to nice hot coffee temperature, and pour into drinking mug.
8 Add 1 flat tsp. golden flax meal, a spot of cream, or 1 tsp. virgin coconut oil.
9 Stir for 15 seconds to let flax dissolve—and enjoy.

You can leave the flax out if you want a thinner consistency, but it gives a heartier drink which we like.

Chapter 19

Muffins, Breads, and Pizza Crusts

Muffins

Regular muffins are a fats and carbs combo. They do not make a trim waistline as they create a tandem fuel response in the body. First, your body must burn the glucose from the starch and sugar. Next (if your body can actually complete that first task), it must get around to burning any fat in your muffin. That's not likely to happen since muffins are usually high glucose spikers since they contain flours. Your insulin will be overproduced because it has to put in overtime hours to clean up the glucose mess.

Muffin lovers, breathe a sigh of relief. We would not deprive you of such wonderful fare. We think muffins bring joy and delight to life! Women and muffins have a special deep connection. Let's not deny ourselves that relationship.

The next few recipes are our tried and true muffin recipes. They are all **S**, with the exception of *Muffin in a Bowl*, so if you want to indulge in a pat of butter on top, you may. Greek yogurt is also a fantastic topping for muffins and it is naturally lower in calories.

Muffin in a Mug – S

This recipe will be Drive Thru Sue's best friend, and if you have anything in common with her, you'll love it too. It can be another of our magic tricks to keep you on plan. Who could ever feel deprived eating a decadent chocolate muffin that can be cooked in one minute? It's a perfect breakfast with a cup of coffee, or it makes a quick afternoon snack. A coffee mug becomes your muffin tin—so cute!

But, even if you're an expert in the kitchen, try out this muffin because it is super delicious and healthy. The only people who may want to skip this recipe will be those (like Serene) who don't believe in microwaves. They can go directly to the muffin recipes which are oven baked.

Just make sure you don't use a plastic cup when making this muffin. Use a ceramic mug as plastics in the microwave may leech chemicals into your food.

Walmart and most grocery stores have all the following ingredients, including golden flax meal and almond flour.

Chocolate Version:

Basic Ingredients: golden flax meal ✦ almond flour ✦ egg ✦ unsweetened cocoa powder ✦ sweetener ✦ baking powder ✦ coconut oil

1. Crack 1 egg into coffee cup and whisk it well with a fork.
2. Add 1½ Tbs. golden flax meal.
3. Add 1½ Tbs. almond flour (or grind your own).
4. Add 1 heaping Tbs. unsweetened cocoa powder.
5. Add 2-4 tsp. Truvia depending on desired sweetness or a few shakes of Nunaturals, depending on desired sweetness.
6. Add ½ tsp. aluminum free baking powder.
7. Add 1 flat Tbs. coconut oil, either extra virgin or cooking style like Louanna brand. It doesn't matter if coconut oil is solid from being cold.
8. Stir vigorously (a mini workout for your right arm).
9. Microwave for 1 minute.

The muffin should easily plop out of the mug when turned upside down and thumped a little. Dump it out on a plate. Cut it in half and smear each half with a little pat of butter, or if you prefer, top it with Greek yogurt. Mmmmm!

We suggest 2-4 tsp. Truvia, but determine your own sweetness. Start with 3 tsp. and see if that is about right for you. You may only like 2 tsp., but "newbies" switching over from a high sugar lifestyle might need 4 tsp. to get their sweet fix. To save on Truvia, you can use a combination of 1-2 tsp. Truvia and a tiny pinch of NuStevia Pure White Stevia Extract Powder if further sweetness is desired.

This muffin may be made with other flavors if you do not desire chocolate. The recipe requires a total of 4 Tbs. dry flour. In the chocolate version, 1 Tbs. comes from cocoa powder. That's why we only do 1½ Tbs. each of flax and almond flour to make up the other three.

If you would like to try a *Banana Nut* version, use 2 Tbs. each of flax and almond flour, add chopped nuts and banana extract.

A cinnamon version may be made using 2 tsp. cinnamon, 2 Tbs. flax and 1 Tbs. plus 1 tsp. almond flour. The cinnamon version goes great with a quick icing topping made from one pat butter, one pat cream cheese, squirt of lemon, and ground Truvia or Nunaturals to taste. While speaking of icings, the chocolate muffin goes great with a raspberry version of the same—1 pat butter, 1 pat cream cheese, a few thawed raspberries, and ground Truvia or Nunaturals.

If you cannot afford almond flour, or even almonds to grind up yourself, you can make this muffin with only golden flax meal which is friendlier to budgeters. Use 3 Tbs. flax and 1 Tbs. cocoa for the chocolate version. It is still a pretty great muffin that way. In fact, we like flax meal slightly more than almond flour for **S** baking when it comes to weight loss. It has less net carbs and slightly less calories. You may want to start out using both almond flour and flax meal together since that produces a more "flour" like muffin. However, you'll find that as you get used to it, you can reduce the almond flour.

Another fantastic way of making this muffin is to use 2 scant Tbs. of flax along with 2 larger Tbs. of extra dark cocoa powder. If you add berries for extra moisture content, or add 1 Tbs. of water you can make what we like to call a Volcano Mud Slide muffin. Don't cook it until it's completely done. That means without berries, you will only microwave for 40 seconds instead of one minute. If using berries, you'll need the full minute or slightly more, but don't go all the way. The muffin should be slightly gooey in the center.

My, oh my, what a dark, deeply mysterious, fantastically oozy, and chocolaty muffin this makes. It's actually a bit lower calorie too, since cocoa (which is very low-calorie) takes half the flour load. If you want to make this muffin a complete little meal, add a little swirl of heavy cream and a couple of heaping huge tablespoons of Greek yogurt. Stir around and you have a fantastic dark muffiny pudding that is rather filling. Hard to describe, but good! That's Pearl's current favorite style, but she makes all kinds for variety.

If you like the idea of having this muffin for a quick breakfast when you're pressed for time, it's a great idea to take about ten minutes one evening and make up individual baggies of the dry ingredients. Then all you need to do in the morning is take one of the baggies, pour contents into a mug, add the egg and oil, and devour. Makes quick even quicker.

Be sure to check out the other Mug recipes coming up. One is the plain version of this muffin called *Bread in a Mug*. It can be used to make a yummy grilled cheese sandwich or pizza base. Another is *Cake in a Mug*, (*Desserts*, Chapter 23).

Pearl chats: Sometimes when I sit down and savor this chocolate muffin, so moist, dark, and rich with a nice pat of butter or Greek yogurt on top, and a cup of creamy coffee steaming beside me, I become overwhelmed at how blessed I am. I grin foolishly and shake my head because I am eating a truly decadent chocolate muffin and yet a slimming and healthy food! It's almost unbelievable. I feel sorry for every other person in the world who cannot enjoy this same deliciousness without the guilt.

I should mention that I only use two teaspoons of Truvia for my chocolate muffin. I also add a little dash of Nunaturals extract. This sweetens it up further and I don't have to burn through my Truvia quite as quickly. I use that trick a lot in my baking.

Muffin in a Bowl – S, E or Fuel Pull

The previous recipe, *Muffin in a Mug* should either be a breakfast or a filling snack. Eaten in those settings it is perfect, but don't tag it on as a dessert after a big ol' **S** meal. While that muffin fits in with **S** fuels, you'll add too many needless calories eating it as an after dinner treat. However, *Muffin in a Bowl* is perfect to eat after an **S**, **E** or **Fuel Pull** meal since it has been stripped of both fats and carbs and is therefore vastly lower in calories. It is well under 70 calories if you're interested in the numbers, yet surprisingly tastes delectable and has a moist texture. This is due to the addition of magical glucomannan.

Although we've tweaked this muffin, it did not originate with us. One of the very creative forum members at www.lowcarbfriends.com (Ouizoid) came up with the idea and has given us permission to share it with you. She also originated the **Fuel Pull** friendly *Egg White Wraps* coming up soon in this chapter so be sure to check those out too.

This muffin requires oat fiber which is available inexpensively from www.netrition.com. Don't get this confused with oat bran. It is a completely different substance. Oat fiber is a "flour like" powder. While it does not have a gritty texture, it is pure fiber and contains no carbs or fat. Acting as your flour, this oat fiber, along with cocoa powder (which also has negligible carbs and fat), enables you to eat a big chocolate muffin without heading anywhere near calorie abuse. It's not as nutritious as the above *Muffin in a Mug* which nourishes you more with the inclusion of a full egg and coconut oil. The sole purpose of *Muffin in a Bowl* is to offer you chocolatey indulgence without adding extra calories.

Pearl chats: This muffin cooks best in a ceramic cereal type bowl rather than a mug. It looks more like a small cake than a muffin. You don't need to get it out of the bowl. Eat as is—less dishes to wash. Once again, this muffin uses 4 Tbs. flour. If desired, you can play around with it, remove 1 Tbs. oat fiber or cocoa and replace with 1 Tbs. defatted peanut flour to give a peanut butter taste.

Basic Ingredients: oat fiber ✦ cocoa powder ✦ optional defatted peanut flour ✦ glucomannan ✦ baking powder ✦ water ✦ carton egg whites ✦ sweetener

1. Put 2 Tbs. oat fiber in a microwave safe cereal bowl.
2. Add 2 Tbs. cocoa powder.
3. Add ¾ tsp. glucomannan and ½ tsp. baking powder.
4. Add 3 tsp. Truvia and a dash of Nunaturals. More sweetener is required in this muffin because glucomannan tends to mask sweetness. If you don't have Nunaturals, you may need to use up to 5 tsp. Truvia.
5. Mix dry ingredients well with a whisk so glucomannan is not clumpy.
6. Add ⅓ cup carton egg whites.
7. Add 3 Tbs. water.
8. Microwave for 1 minute. Do not overcook which will make the texture dry. The center should still be slightly underdone. If your microwave only runs high, check at 45 seconds.

Pearl chats: This muffin goes great with a squirt or two of Fat Free Reddi Whip. This is how I serve it to my husband if I want to keep the muffin in **Fuel Pull** or **E** territory. I enjoy it myself this way, too. Plain 0% Greek yogurt works also, but Charlie prefers the Fat Free Reddi Whip as he's not a yogurt lover. Heavy cream can be used for **S,** but it takes the calorie count off course and that defeats the purpose if you want this for pound kicking **Fuel Pull** reasons. If you don't have the specialty ingredients for the above recipe, *Muffin in a Bowl*, go to www.foodiefiasco.com and try the *All for One* grain free chocolate cake. This easy recipe uses ingredients you'll be more likely to have on hand and yet fits our **Fuel Pull** category. Kelly, the owner of the site, has other great fuel pulling desserts you may also like to try.

Blueberry Coconut Muffins – S

Serene chats: Okay, out of my way with all of that microwave nonsense. These next muffins are actually cooked with something called old fashioned heat! All this business of pressing one minute buttons and squirting chemical cream out of a can! You're killing me, Pearl! Nah, I'm just venting. I'll let you and all your shortcut followers enjoy it.

Pearl's "nuker" muffins can be made in the oven in a little ramekin sized baking dish. They take a total of about eight minutes. Only seven minutes more, worth it to me. On to my own baked beauties . . .

These *Blueberry Coconut Muffins* team with middle chain fatty acids and will rev your metabolism. Can you imagine sweet blueberry muffins actually doing you a favor instead of adding on pounds? This recipe batch makes twelve good muffins.

Coconut flour is becoming popular for its low glycemic baking talents, but it is pricey. We seldom use the flour in our recipes for this reason. One day we noticed most of the recipes using coconut flour also called for a shortening agent because the flour is defatted. We thought, why not make flour out of plain dried coconut, grind it fine in a quality blender, and leave out the shortening? The idea works and you get two products for one price, both the oil and the flour. It seems unwise to buy an expensive defatted flour and then have to add lots of extra virgin coconut oil or butter, when dried shredded coconut has its own naturally occurring healthy fat. This works with our mindset, because this book is about eating healthy without breaking your budget.

Dried coconut (even organic) is very cheap when purchased from the bulk bins at a natural food store. Or, it can be ordered inexpensively in bulk online. Don't buy the very large flakes as the smaller style is better for this purpose. Even if there is no need to pinch pennies, don't substitute commercial coconut flour in this recipe, or any other of our recipes calling for homemade coconut flour. You cannot interchange the two. They result in completely different textures.

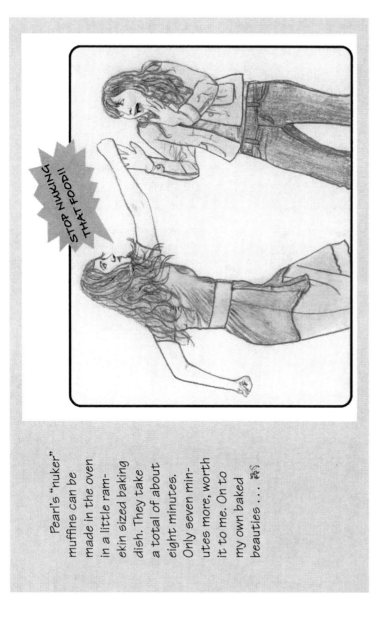

Light White Muffins further on in this section calls for store-bought coconut flour. We included it because it creates a complete different texture. Those who don't have to penny pinch, or don't want to be bothered with the first step of grinding their own coconut, may want to try that one.

If you want to store any excess homemade coconut flour, keep it in a cool dry place. Do not put it in the refrigerator unless you aren't going to use it for quite a while. The oils will cause it to harden in cold temperatures. When you take it out, you need to put it in a food processor to regain the texture of flour. We prefer to make the flour fresh each time.

Basic Ingredients: dried coconut ✦ golden flax meal ✦ baking powder ✦ xanthan gum ✦ sweetener ✦ egg whites ✦ water ✦ coconut oil ✦ blueberries

Dry Directions:

1 Pour dried coconut into blender and grind until the blades won't turn anymore.
2 Take 2½ cups of this ground fine flour and place in bowl.
3 Add ½ cup ground golden flax meal
4 Add 3 tsp. aluminum free baking powder and ¼ tsp. xanthan gum.
5 Add 8-10 tsp. Truvia or ⅛-¼ tsp. NuStevia Pure White Stevia Extract Powder.
6 Use your hands to rub all ingredients together until all lumps are gone and everything is combined to a uniform consistency (an important step).

Wet Directions:

1 Put 4 egg whites or ½ cup 100% carton egg whites into blender.
2 Add 1 cup water.
3 Add 1 scant Tbs. coconut oil.
4 Blend well.
5 Add wet ingredients to dry then throw in some frozen or fresh blueberries.
6 Bake at 350 for 35 minutes.

Serene chats: These are delicious fresh and warm from the oven. At room temperature, they should keep well for a few days. If there are any leftover after a few days (which would be surprising) you may put them in the refrigerator. Once you do that, the muffins will need to be quickly reheated in the oven. The reheating is necessary because the middle chain fatty acids of coconut harden when chilled and the muffins will be like a brick if you don't reheat them.

Easy Peazy Cinammon Muffins – S

This recipe makes 12 good sized muffins. If you don't have dried coconut lying around, hopefully you'll have some golden flax meal. If so, you've got muffins, baby!

These *Easy Peazies* look like bran muffins and make the home smell deliciously cinnamony while they are cooking. In our homes, they are gobbled up the same day (or in a few minutes), but if you have a smaller family you could freeze individual portions and reheat easily.

Be sure to drink lots of water when you eat these muffins due to the high fiber of the flax flour. Remember to drink with the *Muffin in a Mug* recipe also. Any flax muffins, plus good water intake, equals great bowel function. However, for some people, too much flax can have the opposite effect and cause some bloating, especially if you are not used to high amounts of fiber. If you are a person with a sensitive stomach, start eating only one and see how you feel over the day. They're not as big as the *Muffin in a Mug* which is large enough to be a full breakfast or a big afternoon snack. You might want to eat two of these oven muffins to get the same amount of satisfaction, if your stomach can handle all that fiber.

Basic Ingredients: eggs ✦ egg whites ✦ water ✦ coconut or olive oil ✦ vanilla ✦ flax meal ✦ baking powder ✦ baking soda ✦ cinnamon ✦ sweetener

Wet Directions:

1. Into blender put 3 eggs and 3 egg whites.
2. Add ¾ cup and 1 Tbs. water.
3. Add 3 Tbs. oil (coconut or olive).
4. Add 1 tsp. vanilla (optional).
5. Blend well for 20 seconds.

Dry Directions:

1. Put 2 cups golden flax meal into bowl (other options are 1½ cups of golden flax meal plus a ½ cup of ground dried coconut, or a ½ cup of almond meal to replace the extra ½ cup of flax. It has to add up to 2 cups).
2. Add 1 tsp. baking powder and 1 tsp. baking soda.
3. Add 4 Tbs. cinnamon (not a typo, it needs 4 Tbs. cinnamon).
4. Add 12 tsp. Truvia (if you'd like to add further sweetness to the muffin, add ⅛-¼ tsp. Nunaturals). Mix well.
5. Pour blended wet ingredients into bowl of dry ingredients and mix together well. Let mixture sit on the counter for 5 minutes to thicken a little.
6. Place into greased muffin holes and bake at 350 for 20-25 minutes.

If you have no weight issues (ectomorph body type) and would like a fattier tasting muffin, you can use five whole eggs in place of using half egg whites and yolks and increase the oil to a third of a cup. This increases calories quite a bit and makes a heavier muffin that is good to eat even without butter on top. We like butter on muffins and don't see the point of adding more calories than needed, unless you really need to put on some pounds. Flax has its own fat, so using half egg whites and just a little oil makes the perfect textured muffin for adding butter on top, some Greek yogurt, or a little whipped cream.

Pearl chats: I have tried to master flax muffins made in the oven so often during the past couple of years. I had no trouble making the *Muffin in a Mug* but all my attempts at larger batches in the oven were failures. I read about other people's success with larger batches online and tried many recipes, but there was always something wrong. The consistency was not right, they felt eggy, tasted too flaxy, didn't rise well, or they weren't sweet enough.

I threw so many muffins away and felt terrible about the waste. This recipe was a last desperate attempt, a combination of so many I had tried. I could hardly believe when they finally turned out great. They actually rose up like normal muffins and the texture and taste were perfect. Oh, the joy!

My daughter, Meadow has been my taste-test gauge for many of my strange kitchen experiments. She has tasted many terrible flax muffins and finally told me to stop trying. "Flax doesn't work for muffins in the oven, Mom." she stated emphatically. But, this recipe proved her wrong. She ate two of them fresh from the oven and gave me an enthusiastic thumbs up.

At that moment, I had to take a phone call and couldn't hear well with all the noise going on around me. I stepped out of the kitchen and when I came back, every muffin was eaten! Ten gone within a couple of minutes! The rest of my children had located the source of the good smell and chowed down enthusiastically. Needless to say, I had to make another batch because I was desperate to eat one or two myself. Now, Serene tells me I have a "muffin ministry." I bake this recipe for my mother on Mother's day, my father on Father's day, birthday presents, and baby gifts. My family and friends ask for them and want nothing else from me.

Here are some other flavor ideas:

Ginger

It is delicious in place of cinnamon. You need to use at least 3 Tbs. ginger powder for a strong enough ginger flavor. Serene actually adds a dash of cayenne pepper to her ginger muffins for added zest. A dollop of whipped cream on one of these ginger muffins is an incredible **S** dessert.

Blueberry
Add fresh or frozen blueberries to the mix and reduce cinnamon to 1 Tbs. You'll need to bake several minutes longer since the mix will be moister.

Pumpkin
Add ⅓ cup pumpkin and reduce cinnamon to 1 Tbs. Add 2½ tsp. pumpkin pie spice. Yum! You need to bake these for at least 5 minutes longer.

Cranberry Nut
Cranberries are much lower in carbs than most fruits. However, do not use the dried sweetened version. Cut fresh or thawed cranberries and throw them in the mix with pecans or walnuts. We often buy bags of cranberries when they are in season and freeze them in small baggies for later use.

Banana Nut
Omit the cinnamon, add banana flavor extract and chopped walnuts.

If you are at **S Helper** stage, you can add a few raisins to the original cinnamon version, but only a few! Cut some raisins into halves to make them go further but to give an added hint of sweetness.

Light White Muffins – S

If you want to purchase coconut flour from the store and can't be bothered grinding it yourself, this recipe is another option. The light texture of these muffins lends them to many different flavors. You could try lemon poppy seed by using lemon extract and poppy seeds. Ginger also works well. Of course, blueberries are always a popular standby. This recipe uses a food processor rather than a bowl and blender.

Basic Ingredients: store-bought coconut flour ✦ baking powder ✦ eggs ✦ sweetener ✦ coconut oil ✦ coconut milk, unsweetened almond milk, or water ✦ optional berries

1. Put ⅔ cup store-bought coconut flour into food processor.
2. Add 1 tsp. baking powder.
3. Turn food processor on for a few seconds to remove lumps and combine baking powder with flour.
4. Add 6 eggs.
5. Add Truvia or Nunaturals to taste (approximately 8-10 tsp. Truvia).
6. Add 4 Tbs. melted coconut oil and 3½ Tbs. liquid (either coconut milk, unsweetened almond milk, or even water if you don't have either of the first two options).
7. Process well until all lumps are removed and mixture is smooth.

8. Add berries if desired.
9. Pour into well-greased muffin trays and bake at 350 for 20 minutes (5 minutes longer if using berries).

Makes nine muffins.

Breads

With the exception of *Trim Healthy Pan Bread*, which is **E**, and *Egg White Wraps*, which are designed for **Fuel Pulls**, the other bread ideas in this section are all **S** style. Check out *Cultured Recipes,* Chapter 26, for Serene's **E** *Sourdough Bread* and *Cultured Mini Loaves* recipes.

Try some of these ideas. Decide what you like best and you can keep repeating your winners. There's sure to be at least one or two recipes that will hit the bread spot for you. You can then go to the next chapter for ideas for fillings.

Bread in a Mug – S

This is the plain version of *Muffin in a Mug*. This bread may also be used to make a regular **S** sandwich with mayo, lettuce, and meat of your choice.

Basic ingredients: egg ✦ golden flax meal ✦ almond flour ✦ baking powder ✦ coconut oil ✦ sea salt and other optional seasonings

1. Crack egg into coffee cup or bread sized shallow container and whisk well with fork, or use ¼ cup egg whites or Egg Beaters.
2. Add 2 Tbs. golden flax meal.
3. Add 2 Tbs. almond flour.
4. Add ½ tsp. aluminum free baking powder.
5. Add 1 tsp. coconut oil or butter.
6. Add pinch sea salt and other optional seasonings of your choice.
7. Stir vigorously.
8. Microwave for 1 minute.

In this bread version, we only use 1 tsp. of oil or butter compared to the full Tbs. we used in the muffin version. To make grilled cheese, butter the outside of the bread before placing it in the pan.

If you use the mug to make this bread, slice into six mini pieces to make three little grilled cheese sandwiches. If you slice them extra finely, you may be able to get eight pieces. Or, look around at stores or yard sales for a container that is a square or rectangle shape and would work for one large bread piece shape (make sure it is not plastic). This way you can split the bread down the middle and have two big slices.

You may multiply the ingredients by three for this recipe and then microwave for three minutes instead of one. This way you have bread for more than one meal and it allows for larger slices.

If desired, add different herbs and seasonings such as rosemary, Italian seasoning, garlic salt, or parmesan cheese. We'll leave it to your own wonderful creativity.

This basic recipe can also be used for an individual sized pizza crust. Instead of cooking it in the mug, spread mixture out on a dinner plate or over parchment paper to the size of pizza you prefer. Nuke for one minute, top with pizza sauce and toppings, and transfer to oven to broil the top until cheese is bubbly. What could be easier for a quick single serve pizza lunch?

Trim Healthy Pan Bread – E

In this recipe you may use either egg whites freshly cracked, 100% Liquid Egg Whites from a carton, or a product like Egg Beaters which is egg whites blended with salt and other savory flavors. Southwestern Egg Beaters give great flavor to these pan breads. If using whites alone, make sure to add a pinch of salt. Or, add optional flavors such as onion or garlic powder and a shake or two of hot sauce.

Basic Ingredients: Old Fashioned Oats ✦ egg whites or Egg Beaters ✦ low-fat cottage cheese ✦ baking powder ✦ sea salt and desired seasonings

1. Into blender put 1 cup Old Fashioned Oats and blend until oats turn into powder.
2. Turn off blender and add 1 cup egg whites or egg beaters and 1 cup low-fat cottage cheese (1% is best).
3. Add 2 tsp. aluminum free baking powder and pinch of salt if not using Egg Beaters.
4. Heat nonstick skillet or nonstick fry pan to medium/low temp. Spray pan or skillet with tiny bit of oil or moisten with slightest amount of butter.
5. Ladle mix onto skillet or pan in desired bread-sized shapes. You may use an egg flip to help spread shape out.
6. Once bottom of pan breads are golden browned and tops have bubbles, carefully use egg flip to free sides from sticking, then turn them to brown the other side.
7. Transfer the pan breads to a paper towel for a minute before plating.

This recipe makes 12 bread sized servings. If you make 12, you know they are about the right size. You can eat four of the pieces for one **E** serving if you wish. That makes two nice sized sandwiches that when cut in half give you four to hold. The pan bread pieces will be round, but so are some other types of sandwich bread like Panera so don't let that put you off. They make great sandwiches. Remember to keep your fillings lean—no large amounts of fat, please!

Country Biscuit – S

This is the plain version of the *Blueberry Coconut Muffins*. Without the sweetener it has a surprisingly flaky, biscuity, cornbready texture. It is the perfect addition to any **S** meal like a soup or stew.

They are delicious as is, but even better with grated cheese and a chopped jalapeño or two thrown into the mixture before baking. Or, how about curry and cheese? That's not as common here in USA, but in Downunder where we originate, cheese and curry scones are a frequent favorite. Add 1 tsp. curry powder to the mix if that appeals to you.

Basic Ingredients: dried coconut ✦ golden flax meal ✦ baking powder ✦ xanthan gum ✦ sea salt and optional curry powder ✦ egg whites ✦ water ✦ coconut oil ✦ optional cheese

Dry Directions:

1. Pour dried coconut into blender and grind until blades won't turn anymore.
2. Take 2½ cups finely ground coconut flour and place in bowl.
3. Add ½ cup golden flax meal.
4. Add 3 tsp. aluminum free baking powder and ¼ tsp. xanthan gum.
5. Add pinch of salt and optional curry powder.
6. Rub all ingredients together with your hands until all lumps are gone and everything is combined to a uniform consistency (an important step).

Wet Directions:

1. Put 4 egg whites or ½ cup 100% carton egg whites into blender.
2. Add 1 cup of water.
3. Add 1 scant Tbs. coconut oil.
4. Blend well.
5. Add wet ingredients to dry. Throw in some grated cheese at the end if desired.
6. Bake at 350 for 35 minutes.

The same applies if you put these *Country Biscuits* in the refrigerator as it does with the *Blueberry Coconut Muffins*. You'll have to reheat them so they soften up again.

Oopsie Rolls – S

Thanks and credit go to writer and humorist, Jamie VanEaton ("Cleochatra") for these great rolls. You can follow her blog at www.yourlighterside.com. It is full of great **S** style recipes that use pure ingredients, and her blog is downright funny as well.

This is our slightly adapted version of her *Oopsie Roll* recipe. It makes six large rolls. We always double this recipe, but the first time you try it you may want to start with a single batch using three eggs. Even though this recipe is basically eggs and cream cheese, give it a go. It is not eggy at all. It is more like a croissant and makes a great sandwich, while sparing your body of carbs. You can eat it with all the rich fillings you crave.

Oopsie Rolls are very versatile and a great vehicle for flavor. You can add anything to them to make different flavors. Think jalapenos, cheese, or onion. They can also be sweetened with stevia and used for desserts as you'll find out in *Desserts* (Chapter 23), or used as crusts for quick mini pizzas.

Basic Ingredients: eggs ✦ cream cheese ✦ golden flax meal ✦ sea salt ✦ sweetener ✦ xanthan gum

1. Place a metal or glass bowl in freezer for a few minutes along with the metal ends of the Egg Beaters (the cold bowl helps the egg whites become very stiff).
2. While bowl is getting cold, take out another bowl and put in 3 oz. cream cheese (⅓ less fat works great).
3. Add 1 Tbs. golden flax meal to bowl with the cream cheese.
4. Add tiny pinch of salt and ½ tsp. Truvia, or tiny sprinkle of Nunaturals, (this sweetness balances the salt).
5. Once bowl and metal ends of beater are cold from the freezer (only takes a few minutes), transfer the bowl to counter top next to other bowl.
6. Separate 3 eggs. Whites go into cold bowl, yolks into the other bowl with cream cheese.
7. Add ¼ tsp. xanthan gum to bowl with whites (this is important as it helps them remain stiff once combined with other ingredients).
8. Beat whites until you can turn bowl over and the whites don't move. They must be very stiff. This takes several minutes, but it's a fun job for the children.
9. Beat contents of other bowl with yolks and cream cheese until combined (only takes a few seconds and does not have to be perfectly smooth).
10. Spoonful by spoonful, add yolk/cream cheese mixture to the whites. Fold gently, trying not to plop the mix all on top of the whites. Stir it in from the sides. It's fine if end result stays streaky.

11. Place 6 roll type size blobs of combined mixture onto greased cookie sheet.
12. Bake for 30 minutes at 300 until golden brown.

One roll makes one side of a sandwich. These can be toasted for a few seconds if the sides become sticky. Wrap them in wax paper and put them in a loose plastic bag. They'll keep at room temperature for a few days and can then be transferred to the fridge. These are great to send to work with your husband for a sandwich.

Basic Sandwich Buns – S

We use this next recipe with permission from a very creative woman named Linda Sue. But, knowing us, we had to adapt it ever so slightly. Linda Sue is a big name in the world of carbohydrate conscious cooking. You can view her recipes at www.genaw.com. Be sure to try her *Spinach Lasagna* or some of her other casseroles; they are superb for **S** evening meals.

We like this bun recipe because it is simple, makes a great sandwich for home or brown bag purposes, and uses ingredients you should already have on hand. The best result comes from baking these buns in a muffin top pan. This is different from a muffin hole pan in that the holes in a muffin top pan are very shallow. If you don't have one, make up the bun mix and set it on the counter for up to five minutes. After the mixture thickens more, plop bun sized blobs onto a greased baking tray. They won't be as pretty, but it does the job.

You should be able to get five good sized buns from this recipe. They're not terribly high and puffy once cooked, but if you're careful, you can easily split them in half horizontally to stuff with all sorts of sandwich goodies. There should be no need to use two rolls for one sandwich if you don't rush the splitting process.

Basic Ingredients: golden flax meal ✦ eggs ✦ parmesan cheese ✦ onion powder and dried onion ✦ baking powder ✦ sweetener ✦ water ✦ oil ✦ optional glucomannan

1. Combine 1½ tsp. dried minced onion with just enough water to rehydrate and set aside.
2. Put ½ cup, plus 1 Tbs. golden flax meal into a mixing bowl.
3. Add ¼ cup, plus 2 Tbs. parmesan cheese.
4. Add 1 tsp. baking powder, 1 tsp. Truvia or sprinkle of Nunaturals, and 1½ tsp. onion powder. Combine all dry ingredients well. You may also add ¼ tsp. glucomannan or xanthan to help achieve a smoother baked result. Be sure to whisk well with other dry ingredients so no clumping occurs once wet ingredients are added.
5. Add 3 eggs.
6. Add 1½ Tbs. coconut or olive oil and 1½ Tbs. water.

7. Add rehydrated dried minced onion and stir all ingredients well.
8. Drop into 5 holes of muffin top pan and bake at 325 for 20 minutes, or drop 5 bun like shapes on greased baking tray.

Golden Flat Bread – S

This bread is Focaccia style. It can be used with as much diversity as your imagination can provide. It is easy, quick, and absolutely delicious. It is a hearty peasant-like bread that can be sweetened to make a spice or banana bread, kept savory for sandwiches, even used as a pizza base. It's great for ripping and dipping too.

We both make slightly different versions of this bread. Of course, we both think our own way is superior, so included both to keep each other happy. Take your pick.

Basic Ingredients: golden flax ✦ baking powder ✦ sea salt ✦ sweetener ✦ sea salt ✦ coconut oil ✦ eggs and egg whites ✦ water ✦ parchment paper

Dry Directions:

1. Put 2 cups golden flax meal into bowl.
2. Add 1 Tbs. aluminum free baking powder.
3. Add ¾ tsp. sea salt.
4. Add 1½ tsp. Truvia or a sprinkle of Nunaturals.

Serene's Version for Wet directions:

1. Put ¼ cup coconut oil into blender.
2. Add 7 egg whites or 1 cup 100% egg whites from carton.
3. Add ½ cup water.
4. Blend well.

Pearl's Version for Wet directions:

1. Put 2 Tbs. oil into blender or bowl (I use olive or coconut oil).
2. Add 2 whole eggs and 4 egg whites.
3. Add ¾ cup water.
4. Blend well or mix well in bowl.

Wet & Dry:

1. Add either Serene's or Pearl's wet version to dry ingredients, mix well, and let sit for 5 minutes.
2. Place parchment paper on extra large cookie sheet (9 x 15 works best) and lightly grease paper.
3. Dump dough onto middle of parchment paper and spread thinly to edges of sheet with water moistened fingers.
4. Bake at 350 for 20 minutes.
5. Cut into 10-12 pieces, or tear hunks as desired.

Pearl chats: I love to make a savory version of this bread that smells amazing while cooking. After dough is spread out, sprinkle Parmesan cheese, Italian seasoning, garlic or onion powder, and rosemary on top. It's nice to bring to the table when you have visitors. They can rip and dunk in olive oil.

If you desire a sweet bread, cut the salt quantity back, add 6-8 more teaspoons of Truvia or a ¼ tsp. NuStevia Pure White Stevia Extract Powder and make it banana nut, cinnamon, or pumpkin spice bread, depending on your mood or what flavors you have in your cupboard.

Marcy's Cheesy Rolls – S

The magic ingredient in this recipe is glucomannan. Glucomannan is one of your new best friends and wears many hats. We thank Marcy, aka (Marcea), from lowcarbfriends.com for this recipe. Marcy, who was kind enough to let us include it in this book, has a background in baking, specifically with pastries. Her health deteriorated to the point where her blood sugar surged out of control and she gained a lot of weight (pastries'll do that to ya' of course). She learned to eliminate unnecessary carbs and went "gluten-free." Recipes like this one helped get her health and weight back in line.

One batch of this recipe makes six delicious rolls. They are quite sturdy, so you can cut them in half and fill with whatever sandwich fixings you like. They are a little sturdier than *Oopsie Rolls*. While they don't work as well for desserts, they really shine for sandwiches and burgers, or as biscuits for sausage, eggs, etc. They are another great option to send as sandwiches with your husband to work. Pearl's husband really enjoys these for a brown bag lunch.

It's best to make them in an electric bowl mixer like a Bosch. Using a hand held beater can be tedious because it takes a good while to get the mix to a thick enough consistency. With a bowl mixer, you can throw in the ingredients, walk away for a while, and come back when it's ready. If you don't have an appliance like a Bosch, still give these a try. Have your children take turns holding the hand held beater. It's fun watching the ingredients transform from liquid to "glug." Once waves are forming in the dough and keep their form, you know you have your mix thick enough.

Basic Ingredients: eggs ✦ olive oil ✦ water ✦ garlic or onion salt ✦ baking powder ✦ cheese ✦ glucomannan

1. Crack four eggs into electric mixer bowl and beat until fluffy.
2. While beater is still going, add 1 Tbs. olive oil and 3 Tbs. water.
3. Add ½ tsp. garlic or onion salt and 1 Tbs. aluminum free baking powder to the bowl.
4. Slowly add 4 tsp. glucomannan (the best way to do this is put the amount in an empty salt shaker and sprinkle it in slowly while the beater is going).
5. Beat for several minutes, probably longer, depending upon the power of your appliance. Sometimes it can take ten minutes at least to get the right consistency. It should be a very thick pudding mixture which leaves waves when ready.
6. Take bowl out of beater, add 1 cup finely grated cheese to dough, and mix well with a spoon.
7. Drop 6 ball-like shapes of dough onto a well greased tray.
8. Bake at 375 for 12-15 minutes.

Spinach Bread – S

This recipe was made famous by Suzanne Somers in one of her fabulous health/diet books. It is very adaptable as it can be cut into pieces and used fresh for sandwiches, or you can freeze the pieces and pull them out as needed for quick toast. It works well for grilled cheese. We have worked on the original recipe to make it a more "classic" bread and less costly than the original.

This recipe makes one large loaf of bread. Obviously, if you fed this to your children, it would disappear very swiftly and they may not appreciate its beautiful dark green appearance, or the more adult like taste. We suggest keeping slices frozen for you and your husband's needs if the idea of spinach bread appeals to him. It's pretty much a chick recipe, but the rare husband may enjoy it.

Basic Ingredients: spinach ✦ eggs ✦ egg whites ✦ baking powder ✦ sea salt ✦ parmesan cheese ✦ golden flax meal ✦ home ground dried coconut

1. Thaw and drain 2 (16 oz.) bags frozen spinach (be sure to squeeze out all excess water from the spinach) and place in food processor.

2. Add 6 egg whites (or ¾ cup 100% carton whites), plus 2 eggs.
3. Process first 2 ingredients until spinach is broken down well, then pause processing.
4. Add 1½ tsp. aluminum free baking powder, 1 tsp. sea salt, ½ cup Parmesan cheese, ½ cup golden flax meal, and ½ cup home ground coconut meal.
5. Process all ingredients well.
6. Grease a large loaf pan.
7. Bake at 350 for 1 hour, 15 minutes.

Speedy Pesto Version – S

This is a much speedier version of the spinach bread with a pesto twist.

Basic Ingredients: pine nuts ✦ garlic ✦ basil leaves ✦ spinach ✦ eggs ✦ sea salt and other seasonings

1. Put ½ cup pine nuts, 3 cloves garlic, and 15 basil leaves in food processor and process until smooth.
2. Put pesto mix in mixing bowl and add 4 beaten eggs.
3. Add 10 oz. bag of thawed and drained frozen spinach, remembering to squeeze out all water.
4. Add salt and pepper and mix all ingredients well.
5. Pour into an 8 x 8 well-greased baking dish and bake at 400 for 15 minutes.

Nori Wraps – S

These wraps look dramatic and taste exotic. They are not only incredible health wise, but unlike pita breads that may become soggy with damp ingredients, your fillings will not seep through and will stay nicely wrapped. They are great stuffed with lettuce, avocado, tomatoes, cucumbers, sprouts, deli meats, leftover chicken, or hot and spicy or oriental flavored sautéed chicken or beef.

Nori wraps can be addictive, but that's okay because they pack a healthy punch. Seaweed, the main ingredient for this recipe is a known detox agent for the body and a rare natural source of iodine, a nutrient in which most of us are very deficient.

If you don't love sushi, don't turn your nose up at these as they do not have a fishy taste at all. They are yummilicous.

Nori sheets are readily available these days, even in the international section of Walmart, although they are smaller and will make a smaller sandwich. Bigger ones can be purchased at any Whole Foods market or oriental/international food stores.

This recipe requires a dehydrator. It yields an ample amount of Nori wraps and they store well in Ziploc bags. You won't need to make this recipe much more than once a month, even if you enjoy them frequently. Anytime you feel like a delicious wrap, they'll be ready for you. If you don't have a dehydrator, you could try drying at a very low heat in the oven.

Basic Ingredients: Nori sheets ✦ almonds ✦ sea salt and other seasonings ✦ nuts or sunflower seeds ✦ celery ✦ coconut or olive oil ✦ lemon juice

1. Soak 2 cups almonds in water and a pinch or two of sea salt the night before. If you forget to soak, don't worry and remember next time! Sunflower seeds may be used as a cheaper option.
2. Put drained nuts or sunflower seeds in food processor.
3. Add 3 stalks chopped celery into processor, along with ½ tsp. sea salt, dash of cayenne pepper, small handful of nutritional yeast, juice of ½ lemon, ½ tsp. onion powder, and a little swirl of virgin coconut oil or extra virgin olive oil.
4. Process well and taste to see if it has a slight cheesy flavor. If not, add a little more sea salt. If you like it spicy, throw in a whole jalapeno.
5. Place Nori sheets on dehydrator or oven trays before spreading the above mixture thinly on each sheet. Blob a bit of mixture in the center of each sheet and spread outward.
6. Dehydrate or oven dry to the point where they are still flexible enough to roll in half without cracking, approximately 3-4 hours depending on your dehydrator. Keep checking.

Note: Nori wraps can easily be made into crackers by dehydrating longer until they are crisp.

Egg White Wraps – Fuel Pull

These are easy and protein packed for a **Fuel Pull** breakfast, lunch, or snack. They require only two main ingredients—whole psyllium husk powder which is a pure fiber and neither an **S** or **E** fuel, and egg whites (the carton kind makes things easier). Don't purchase the fine psyllium you can buy in a pharmacy that is flavored (like orange), or that has aspartame in it. Whole psyllium husks (Now Foods brand) can be found at Trader Joe's and other health food stores or purchased online.

These wraps hold up well to lean deli meats, salad greens, and light or fat free mayos and dressings. They're great for a metabolism shake up. They throw that crazy super low-calorie **Fuel Pull** ball at your body to juggle along with regular **S** and **E** meals. Perfect, if you're in the battle against stubborn pounds. Remember the mantra we taught you earlier in the book—never adapt! Even though they're created for **Fuel Pull** use you can stuff them with **S** foods if you like. They make great tortillas for Mexican style ground beef and shredded cheese.

Basic Ingredients: egg whites ✦ psyllium powder ✦ optional seasonings like sea salt and hot pepper sauce

1. Pour 1 cup egg whites or Egg Beaters into blender.
2. Add 1/8 cup psyllium powder, pinch of sea salt, black pepper, and optional red pepper sauce.
3. Blend well and allow mix to sit and thicken for few minutes.
4. Pour wrap sized amounts onto a medium heated very lightly greased griddle or nonstick pan.
5. Turn wrap over after first side is lightly browned.

The batch should make 4 generous wraps. Two wraps stuffed with lean fillings make one serving. You can always pair the wraps with a **Fuel Pull** friendly whey protein shake using a half scoop of whey.

Pizza Crusts

The problem with pizza is not the toppings. It's the crust! A good pizza has lots of fat, cheese, meats, and olives, and it's even better drizzled with olive oil or dipped in garlic butter. What happens when you combine all that with a white flour crust? You know by now—weight disaster!

Even a whole grain crust is a problem when combined with this much fat. It's a **Crossover** for sure. It's fine for children who have open insulin receptors (try not to feed them "white" pizza too often). However, your more insulin resistant body goes into a state of high blood sugar. Plus, because of the fat on the pizza, you'll have to burn tandem fuels before you ever get the chance to burn your body fat. In other words, you WON'T burn your own body fat.

Don't worry. There are many great ways to continue eating pizza. The idea of permanently shunning pizza is the reason many a dieter decides to give it all up and head for Pizza Hut. That doesn't have to be you. You can regularly indulge, and without guilt, with our smart pizza ideas. Try some of these recipes and figure out which crust versions appeal to you most.

Maybe you will be happy using a vegetable base such as a Portobello mushroom. Crusts made from eggplant and zucchini also make great pizza bases. Top them with sauce, cheese, and pepperoni and place on an oiled cookie sheet and bake.

If you want more of a "white flour crust" feel and texture, keep in mind *Oopsie Rolls*, (*Lunches*, Chapter 20). They make personal pizzas bases, but you'll need to eat a couple of them to get your fill. And, don't forget about our *Muffin in a Mug* recipe (*Muffins, Breads, and Pizza Crusts*, Chapter 19) that can make an awesome quick little pizza base that has a more whole grain feel to it.

The important thing to remember when making pizza is to use a sauce prepared without sugar. Store bought preparations are not hard to find. Walmart's store brand Great Value pizza sauce is made without sugar. It has only three grams of carbs which is purely from the tomatoes, so that's fine. If you're more the scratch cook type, you can make your own pizza sauce from tomato paste, seasonings, and herbs.

A basic pizza sauce is 3 Tbs. tomato paste, 3 Tbs. water, and an added dash of oregano and pinch of salt. You know that Serene will make her own sauce. Our sister, Evangeline will use every ingredient grown from her own soil. No cans of anything for her when it can come from the ground. Maybe she'll have to purchase salt, although we won't put it past her to try extracting it from her rocks!

But, it doesn't matter which road you take, whether "from scratch" or from Walmart, as long as your meal arrives on your plate in a low glycemic state. Whether your sauce starts from tomatoes, tomato paste, or pizza sauce from a jar, no one is judging, so suit yourself. Remember Farm Fresh Tess? She has the mini farm and is famous for her "from scratch" cooking. She probably uses pure pepperoni from her home raised pigs, vegetables from her garden, and whole wheat freshly ground from her grain mill for her crust. However, since all her fabulous toppings are melted on grain style crust, the fat/carbs collision spreads the waistline.

For family pizza nights with a very large family, you may want to use whole grain crusts for the children. Or, a quick idea is to use whole wheat tortillas as bases for them. However, we find that our children actually prefer our lower carb crusts and have to be told "eat your own," as they try to sneak pieces. Many of these crusts are great protein sources and are a way to get hidden vegetables into fussy little eaters, if you want to make your low-carb style for everyone.

Note: If you love pineapple on pizza, you'll have to wait until you get to **S helper** stage. Even then, be very sparse with pineapple. Cut into little bits and throw here and there to give the hint of sweetness. Too much pineapple, mixed with fat, will jeopardize an otherwise perfect meal.

Fooled Ya Pizza – S

You won't believe this crust is made with cauliflower. It's delicious and actually almost indistinguishable from the real thing. This is another recipe from the food blogger, Jamie VanEaton, aka "Cleochatra." We have altered it a little to suit our purposes.

Pearl chats: The first time I made this pizza, I'll admit I was doubtful about the outcome since common cauliflower can't really make a good crust, can it? My brother was visiting and I gave him a piece fresh from the oven. He wolfed it down, trying to snatch more. I asked him if he could guess the ingredients. He thought it was made from regular flour! When I told him it was cauliflower, he could not believe me.

Once my husband got home from work, I fed it to him without telling him about the ingredients. He chowed down and kept complimenting me on the meal (we had not had pizza in a while, poor guy). I sprung the "cauliflower" word on him when he was finished and he showed as much disbelief on his face as my brother had.

This recipe amount makes one extra large pizza, completely filling a 9 x 15 cookie sheet. Double the recipe if you want more.

Basic Ingredients: cauliflower ✦ egg whites ✦ mozzarella cheese ✦ sea salt and other seasonings ✦ pizza sauce and other toppings for pizza

1. Lightly steam 1 (16 oz.) bag of frozen cauliflower.
2. Put lightly steamed cauliflower into colander and press out as much water as possible. You can do this by pressing down with a plate or using your hands to squeeze out the water. Make sure you wring out as much as possible as that allows your crust to be crispier.
3. Put cauliflower in food processor and pulse a few times, not too much. You want to end up with rice-sized pieces.
4. Add ¾ cup egg whites and pulse again for a couple of times.
5. Add 2 cups grated part skim mozzarella cheese, pinch of sea salt, dash or two of Italian seasoning, and a little onion or garlic powder to taste.
6. Mix ingredients together well with a spatula inside the food processor.
7. Line a large cookie sheet with parchment paper and grease parchment well (this is important or the crust will stick).
8. Plop entire mixture onto the middle of the tray and start spreading it outwards with a spatula or with your hands until it covers most of the sheet. Try not to have a thicker middle than sides. Keep pressing until mixture almost touches the edges of the sheet. This crust is better thin, but don't let the edges become wispy thin or they will get too dark when they cook.

9. Bake at 450 for 20 minutes. (Pearl usually turns it over after 15 minutes by flipping the pizza, including the parchment paper, then removing the parchment paper from the top. This allows the other side of the pizza to crisp on the bottom).
10. Cool crust for several minutes before topping.

Once crust has cooled you can top it with pizza sauce, a little more mozzarella (not much is needed since the crust is cheesy). Add any toppings of your choice and broil it in the oven until toppings are done.

You need to cut this pizza into smaller, rather than larger pieces. This makes it easier to hold them in your hand. Very large pieces may be slightly droopy.

Some people use three eggs in place of ¾ cup of egg whites for this crust. You can try whichever option you prefer, but since you'll have a lot of good fat and calories in your toppings, we don't see the need to put needless calories into your crust too. It's just as good with the egg whites.

If you don't have a food processor, grate the cauliflower into rice pieces or chop with a knife.

Pearl chats: Some people make a similar version of this crust with zucchini. You could give it a try. I have not had success with it, but those that have mastered it are loyal to their zucchini crusts. You grate a large zucchini and press all the water out of it before adding the eggs and cheese.

Speedy Thin Crust – S

This crust doesn't contain the cauliflower, so it is a little quicker to make without that step. It's still very good. Again, it's not our original idea. The wonderful forum, www.lowcarbfriends.com has a thread dedicated to the merits of this quick crust in the Recipe Help & Suggestions section.

Some people add 2 Tbs. golden flax meal and 2 Tbs. almond flour or coconut flour to this speedy crust to make it an even sturdier, crustier feel. Experiment for yourself.

Using skim mozzarella and cheddar cheese made with 2% milk (reduced fat) makes the crust a little crispier. But, it turns out fine with regular cheddar too.

Basic ingredients: egg ✦ egg whites ✦ mozzarella cheese ✦ cheddar cheese ✦ sea salt and other seasonings ✦ optional golden flax meal and almond flour ✦ pizza sauce and other pizza toppings

1. In a bowl, mix 1 egg with 3 egg whites, or ⅓ cup 100% carton egg whites.
2. Add 2 cups grated part skim mozzarella cheese and 1 cup 2% grated cheddar cheese.
3. Add small pinch of salt, Italian seasoning, onion or garlic powder.
4. Add optional 2 Tbs. each of flax and almond flour and mix all ingredients well.
5. Spread mixture on parchment lined, 9 x 15 cookie sheet (similar to directions in *Fooled Ya Pizza*). The mix may not spread quite to the edges, but it should fill at least ⅞ of sheet.
6. Bake at 450 for 20 minutes (turn crust at 15 minutes for an extra crispier crust feel).

Once crust has cooled, top with pizza sauce, a little more cheese and toppings, and broil to melt.

Portobello Mushroom Pizza – S or Fuel Pull

Depending on your cheese and topping choices, you can make this either **S** or **Fuel Pull** style. Use only small amounts of skim mozzarella, for **Fuel Pull** and load the top up with veggies like onions etc. Stick to small amounts of turkey pepperoni or bacon and nix the full-fat varieties. But if you want to make this **S**, go to town on all your regular toppings and indulge heartily.

Remember eggplants and zucchini work for this idea too.

Basic Ingredients: Portobello mushrooms ✦ pizza sauce and other pizza toppings

1. Scrape the gills out of Portobello mushrooms and remove stems.
2. Grill mushroom caps, stem side down, on a lightly sprayed or oiled cookie sheet under broiler for 3-4 minutes. Turn them over and grill the other side for the same amount of time.
3. Remove mushrooms from oven and spread with pizza sauce and desired toppings.
4. Return to broiler for a little longer, until cheese is bubbly.

Chicken Crust Pizza – S

This is another high protein, tasty idea that can satisfy pizza cravings. Pre-cook some chicken breasts or tenderloins by putting them in a covered baking tray and baking until tender, or poach them more quickly in a covered pot with a little water. Or, you may take the shortcut and use canned chicken breast. All options will work.

Basic Ingredients: chicken breasts or tenderloins ✦ pizza sauce and other toppings

1. Break apart cooked chicken so meat is in small pieces.
2. Spread chicken on a lightly greased cookie sheet and thin out to cover as much area as possible. This is your simple crust.
3. Cover with sugar-free pizza sauce, grated cheese, and toppings of your choice.
4. Broil in middle rack until cheese is melted and pepperoni is slightly crispy.
5. You may skip the first step of breaking chicken into smaller pieces. Keeping the pieces in tenderloin size works well, but the sauce surrounds the chicken rather than stays on top.

Tortilla Pizza – S

Basic Ingredients: low-carb tortillas ✦ pizza sauce and other pizza toppings

1. Place low-carb tortillas on oiled baking sheet (small-size Mission brand whole wheat CarbBalance, or Joseph's pitas work well).
2. Spread with sugar-free pizza sauce, cheese, and toppings.
3. Bake at 400 until bottom of tortilla crisps and cheese bubbles.
4. You may broil toppings at end of baking for 2 minutes if you want them crispier.

Note: You can do a similar thing with Joseph's pitas as the crust.

> *Pearl chats*: My daughter, Meadow makes a stuffed crust version of these low-carb tortilla pizzas. She puts sauce and toppings on one half of the tortilla, folds it over, then puts the same again on top of the folded tortilla, then bakes in the same manner. Meadow uses pineapple in small amounts in her recipe. Sometimes, I beg her to make this for me as I love pineapple on pizza and because I'm at my goal weight, why not have a little? I can't seem to make this with quite the touch she has, so I leave her to it.

Be sure to check out our *Pizza Casserole* recipe in *Evening Meals,* Chapter 21.

Joseph's Fuel Pull Pizza

Joseph's pitas make excellent thin crispy crusts that are **Fuel Pull** friendly. Depending on your appetite, you can have 2-3 of these mini pizzas and fill up nicely. Cut each one into quarters and you have a lot of hand to mouth action.

1. Cut Joseph's pitas around their seamed circumference so you can separate each one into two very thin rounds.
2. Microwave each one for 50 seconds on a paper plate or bake them in the oven until golden brown and crispy (check every minute or so as they burn easily).
3. Top crisped pitas with tomato paste and sprinkle with Italian seasoning, sea salt and pepper.
4. Add small amount of skim mozzarella then spread on some 1% cottage cheese to create a more cheesier feel without adding fat or too many calories.
5. Add turkey pepperoni or bacon, and any veggies you desire (green peppers and onions work well).
6. Place under broiler until toppings bubble.

Chapter 20

Lunches

Sandwiches, soups, and all your speedy lunchtime favorites are included here. We start with salmon. In the same manner we gave eggs their esteemed first position in the breakfast section, salmon is placed first for lunchtime because it's such an incredible superfood. Don't get the wrong impression that salmon is time consuming or expensive. A delicious salmon lunch can be quick, budget friendly, and, best of all, highly slimming.

If you have not yet found a taste for salmon, hopefully we can change your pre-conceived notions. If, despite our nagging, you simply can't stomach salmon, there are good white fish alternatives. Wild caught mahi mahi is an easy fish to work with. It has a wonderful steak-like thickness and can be used as a substitute in all the following recipes. Wild whiting and tilapia are also mild-flavored and when individually wrapped, can be a quick tasty lunch in place of salmon.

For quick lunches, frozen fish fillets are the best way to buy fish, especially if you live in a landlocked region. It's much cheaper this way. Most times, they are immediately frozen on the vessel where they were caught and stay fresher tasting.

If the best you can do is farm-raised, some of the health benefits of your fish will be diminished, but you will receive a high protein source that is a thousand times better lunch option than your typical grilled cheese sandwich on wheat bread. Dr. Perricone, author of *Ageless Skin, Ageless Mind* recommends farm-raised tilapia as a safe and healthy fish option.

When you don't have time to cook your lunch from scratch, you may like to try Gorton's Grilled Tilapia which can be bought at most supermarkets. It's wonderfully seasoned and non-fishy tasting. All you have to do is heat it, pair with some veggies or a quick salad, and you'll have a great lunch. Since it is lean, it is appropriate for all three fuel categories.

If you simply dislike fish, we ask you to throw away your usual likes and dislikes, and for health's sake try one or two of these recipes. Still can't do it? Okay, we've got plenty of non-fish lunch ideas, you'll be fine. Make sure to take your cod liver oil supplement, though.

The following individual salmon recipes will not take more than about ten minutes to prepare, but they will fuel your nutritional needs on busy days. Your children will likely be happy with peanut butter and sugar-free jelly on whole grain bread, baby carrots, and cheese sticks, but that's not what you need. Quickly making a salmon lunch for you is one way to keep from eating "kid food." Try adding a lot of lemon juice to your cooked salmon if you despise a fishy taste, but the following recipes are seasoned well to help avoid any strong salmon flavor.

Salmon Lunches

Crispy Salmon – S

Basic Ingredients: salmon ✦ sea salt and other seasonings ✦ butter or coconut oil

1. Thaw a frozen individually wrapped salmon fillet in bowl of warm water shortly before cooking (or place in fridge the night before).
2. Season one side of salmon. Seasoning ideas are sea salt, black pepper, and chili flakes; sesame seeds, dark sesame oil, and tamari; nutritional yeast, black pepper, sea salt, onion and garlic powder; or blacken with lots of chili powder and Creole seasonings.
3. Heat 1-2 Tbs. butter, coconut oil or red palm oil in a pan and place seasoned side of fillet in fat.
4. While bottom side is crisping, season top side, then flip the fillet and crisp other side.

This salmon is delicious with a large salad. Since it is **S**, you can make the dressing as decadent as you like by going creamy, or heavier with olive oil. You can also add luscious toppings such as soft goat's cheese medallions, feta cheese, pine nuts, walnuts, or half an avocado.

If you're not in the mood for salad, dice some quick-cook non-starchy veggies such as zucchini or summer squash. If diced small enough, they'll sauté up in butter in a couple of minutes and make a succulent bed for the salmon.

Pepper Crusted Salmon – S

This recipe uses a pepper blend called Hot Shot by McCormick. It's an easy way to crust your salmon and tasty, too.

Basic Ingredients: salmon ✦ sea salt and Hot Shot seasoning ✦ butter or coconut oil

1. Sprinkle a little sea salt on each side of thawed salmon fillet.
2. Liberally cover the upwards facing side of the salmon fillet with Hot Shot.
3. Place peppered side down into fry pan with hot butter or coconut oil.
4. While peppered side is browning, cover the other upward facing side with the pepper blend.
5. Turn filet over and crisp other side.

Consider using same sides as *Crispy Salmon*.

Grilled Salmon – S, E or Fuel Pull

Basic Ingredients: salmon ✦ seasonings

1. Season a thawed fillet of salmon with seasonings of your choice.
2. Place on a lightly greased oven tray and place under broiler, turning to brown both sides.

If you desire an **E** salmon lunch, it may be accompanied by salad with a light vinaigrette and ¾ cup of pre-cooked brown rice or quinoa. Alternatively, you could throw some garbanzo beans in your salad or place the grilled salmon on a piece or two of plan approved bread. Another option is a sweet potato with only 1 tsp. coconut oil on it and either Bragg Liquid Aminos and cayenne for a savory flavor, or Truvia and cinnamon to make it sweet.

Quick Poached Salmon – S, E or Fuel Pull

Basic Ingredients: salmon ✦ water ✦ soy sauce ✦ sea salt and other seasonings ✦ olive oil ✦ Balsamic vinegar

1. Place thawed fillet of salmon in small saucepan with water and a little soy sauce (enough liquid to almost cover the fish). This is only the broth in which to cook the salmon, so if you don't have soy sauce, you can season water with sea salt, onion or garlic powder, and nutritional yeast.

2 Cover with lid and bring to boil, turn to low and simmer until salmon is soft and tender.
3 Drain all liquid from saucepan and add a sprinkle of nutritional yeast and a generous drizzle of balsamic vinegar. If you desire an **E** lunch, drizzle on 1 tsp. olive oil. If you'd rather have **S**, drizzle the olive oil more liberally.
4 Flake the salmon with a fork and season with sea salt and black pepper.

You may toss this poached salmon in with a lightly dressed salad for **E**, including some beans or quinoa, or have it on a couple of pieces of plan approved toast. For an **S** meal you could add olives and a little avocado to your salad.

> *Serene chats:* I am a salmon freak and have tried it so many ways, but poaching has become my favorite. I can eat it in any fuel style and the poaching water brings great flavor and tenderness.

Southwestern Salmon/Chicken – S, E or Fuel Pull

Basic Ingredients: salmon or chicken tenderloins ◆ green salsa ◆ cream cheese or Greek yogurt

While this recipe works for a quick salmon lunch, the idea can also be used for chicken tenderloins. You can make a family meal using a full bag of chicken tenderloins.

Using cream cheese makes this recipe an **S**. But, if you grill or poach the salmon, and use 0% Greek yogurt instead of cream cheese, you could eat it with non-starchy veggies for a **Fuel Pull**, or as an **E** with sides like rice or quinoa.

1 Sauté, poach, or grill salmon or chicken tenderloins.
2 While salmon or tenderloins are cooking, mix equal parts of green salsa with ⅓ reduced fat cream cheese, or Greek yogurt in a bowl.
3 Put cream cheese or Greek yogurt/salsa mixture on top of the salmon or tenderloins at the very end of cooking so it heats up as a creamy topping.

> *Pearl chats:* I buy ⅓ reduced fat Philadelphia cream cheese from Walmart for all my cream cheese needs. Philadelphia is not riddled with fillers like other brands. It is not as dense as the high fat version, can be stirred more easily, and is still every bit as creamy in my opinion.

Lemon Dijon Salmon/Chicken – S

Here's another recipe that works for both salmon and chicken tenderloins.

Basic Ingredients: salmon or chicken tenderloins ✦ butter or coconut oil ✦ sea salt and other seasonings ✦ lemon juice ✦ Dijon mustard ✦ heavy cream or full-fat coconut milk

1. Season salmon fillet or chicken tenderloins with salt and pepper.
2. Sauté fish or chicken in pan with heated butter or coconut oil until cooked through.
3. To the pan, add juice of ½-1 lemon according to taste, another pat of butter, squirt of Dijon mustard, and a swirl of heavy cream or full-fat coconut milk. You may leave out the mustard if it is not your favorite flavor.
4. Let salmon or chicken bubble in sauce for a minute or two.

This dish is delicious over leftover pre-cooked Dreamfields pasta or konjac noodles. It is also great on a bed of *Cauliflower Rice* (*Evening Meals*, Chapter 21).

Succlulent Citrus Fish Bake – S, E or Fuel Pull

This easy lunch idea is excellent made with flaky white fish, but salmon works well also. It can be made with an orange for **E**, lemons for **Fuel Pull** or **S**. Any non-starchy veggies work well, but spinach or tomatoes blend well into the bake and further soften up the fish.

As is, this recipe does not include a fat, so if you want to add a nice pat of butter or coconut oil you will be in **S** territory.

Basic Ingredients: white fish or salmon ✦ lemon or orange ✦ spinach or other non-starchy veggies of choice ✦ sea salt and other seasonings

1. Lightly grease an extra small baking dish (preferably one that has a lid).
2. Put plenty of fresh or frozen spinach leaves at bottom of dish.
3. Season thawed fish fillet well with sea salt and black pepper (or other spices of choice) and place on spinach.
4. Peel skin off a lemon or orange (depending on what fuel type you desire for your meal).
5. Slice lemon or orange into rounds, remove any seeds, then squeeze a little of the juice onto the fillet of fish. Layer rounds on top of fillet and spinach.
6. Cover baking dish with lid or foil.
7. Bake at 375 for 15 minutes (baking time could be a little longer if using frozen spinach leaves).

Quick Blended Salmon Soups – S

The soups in this category are quick enough to be used for lunch. Remember, we don't like to spend more than about ten minutes preparing lunch.

These salmon soups use a small saucepan and a blender. They make 1-2 servings depending on how hungry you are. They are perfect if your children are eating whole grain macaroni and cheese and you want something quick, but more suited to your nutritional and metabolic needs. They are a good way to eat salmon if you are not a big fish lover as they are not fishy tasting at all.

If you do not have salmon fillets handy, you may use canned salmon. Either way these soups are chock full of protein and are great for the times in the year when your garden is loaded. We advise you to use raw virgin oils in these soup recipes. Since you will not be cooking these oils, they make their medicinal magic in your body.

Exotic Green Curry – S

Basic Ingredients: water ✦ salmon ✦ kale or other greens ✦ red palm or coconut oil ✦ tomato paste ✦ sea salt and other seasonings ✦ optional coconut milk

1. Put ½-¾ cup of water in small saucepan with one thawed fillet of salmon (if using canned salmon, only put water in pan).
2. Add 3 huge handfuls of kale, chard, or collard greens to the saucepan.
3. Cover saucepan and bring to boil (will happen quickly), turn to low and steam until fish is cooked through and greens are wilted.
4. While saucepan ingredients are simmering, place into blender 1 heaping Tbs. red palm oil or virgin coconut oil, 1 tsp. tomato paste, generous pinch sea salt, 1 Tbs. nutritional yeast, ½ tsp. curry powder, cayenne pepper to taste, and an optional 2-3 Tbs. of coconut milk. If using canned salmon now add only ⅓ drained can of salmon to blender.
5. Add steaming contents of saucepan to blender and blend all together until smooth and intensely green. If after blending, soup is not hot enough, return to saucepan to bring to desired temperature. If too thick, thin with a little water to desired consistency.

The Vitamix, or other high end blender works well for this recipe as this soup is best when greens are completely broken down to a smooth texture. It is a superfood soup and for those who love ethnic foods, you'll feel like you've been to the Taj Mahal for lunch. In larger quantities, it can also be used for a family evening meal.

Harvest Salmon Bisque – S

Basic Ingredients: salmon ✦ butternut squash ✦ water ✦ red palm oil or coconut oil ✦ sea salt and other seasonings ✦ coconut milk

1. Put ½-¾ cup of water and thawed salmon fillet in saucepan.
2. Add ¾ cup of small cubes of butternut squash to saucepan.
3. Cover saucepan and bring to boil (will happen quickly), turn to low and steam until butternut is soft.
4. While contents of saucepan are cooking, add 1 heaped Tbs. red palm oil or extra virgin coconut oil to a blender.
5. Add black pepper and sea salt to taste, 1 Tbs. nutritional yeast, and an additional dollop of canned coconut milk to blender.
6. Add the steaming contents of saucepan to blender and blend until all is smooth and creamy.

The soup will have a lovely golden hue to it, especially if red palm oil is used. It is hearty and warming.

Tuscany in a Bowl – S

Basic Ingredients: salmon ✦ water ✦ summer squash ✦ coconut oil ✦ sea salt and other seasonings ✦ tomato paste

1. Put ½-¾ cup of water and thawed salmon fillet in saucepan.
2. Add 1 small to medium diced summer squash to the saucepan.
3. Cover saucepan and bring to boil (will happen quickly), then turn to low and steam until squash is soft.
4. While contents of saucepan are cooking, add 1 heaped Tbs. of extra virgin coconut oil to blender.
5. Add a small handful of nutritional yeast, black pepper and sea salt to taste, 1 Tbs. organic tomato paste, and a sprinkle of Italian seasoning or fresh basil from the garden. You can also add chili flakes if desired.
6. Add steaming contents of saucepan to blender and pulse for a few seconds so contents are not completely blended.

You could easily make this soup an **E** by using only 1 tsp. instead of 1 Tbs. of virgin coconut oil. You may then add a handful of pre-cooked brown rice or quinoa to it while cooking.

Summer's Cup (no salmon) – S

This last blended soup is made in the same blender style, but has no salmon. Unlike the salmon blended soups which can be a whole meal since they are so well rounded, *Summer's Cup* needs to be accompanied by a protein source. This is because it is based solely on veggies and fats.

It tastes great topped with grated cheese. On the side, enjoy a *Country Biscuit*, some *Golden Flat Bread*, or *Bread in a Mug*. These options will give you more protein. Or, drop in a big plop of Greek yogurt once it's in your bowl which will also increase protein content.

This soup can also replace a salad, or a vegetable side, if you use it for a nighttime meal. It is a yummy way to get vegetables into children when cooked on a larger scale. Times up the ingredients by four to six times or more for your evening meal. Children can enjoy this soup with whole grain toast and butter.

Quick single serving version for Mom:

Basic Ingredients: zucchini ✦ spinach ✦ water ✦ coconut oil ✦ sea salt and other seasonings

1. Slice a medium-sized zucchini into saucepan with ½-¾ cup of water, or use 3 large handfuls of spinach in place of zucchini.
2. Cover saucepan and bring to boil (will happen quickly), turn to low and steam until zucchini is soft or spinach is wilted.
3. Place steaming contents in blender with 1 heaping Tbs. virgin coconut oil, sea salt and black pepper to taste, and optional sprinkle of nutritional yeast.
4. Blend until a smooth and lovely summery light green.

This can easily be made **E** by using only 1 tsp. coconut oil and adding garbanzo beans or any other cooked beans you may have on hand. Remember to put your dollop of 0% Greek yogurt on top.

> *Serene chats:* I like to cook up a whole pot of garbanzo beans and put them in **E** size baggies in the freezer. They thaw very quickly for use in a pinch. Or, you could use canned garbanzos.

Around the World in 80 Seconds Soups – S

Okay, they may take a little longer than 80 seconds, but what can we say? We're having fun with titles. To be honest, they take more like 180 seconds, but that didn't sound as good. Regardless, they are super speedy.

In need of a power lunch? These dish up. They are a single serving, superfood meals for frazzled mommies in need of a nutritional boost. After whipping up tuna and mayo whole wheat pitas for your children, take a few minutes to sit down and savor the flavors of West Africa or Thailand.

The following three recipes are from Serene, and are more superfoody! They are quick lunch versions, but we have included family sized recipes using some of the same ideas in *Evening Meals*, Chapter 21.

Taste of Thailand – S

Basic Ingredients: coconut milk ✦ leftover chicken, turkey, or canned salmon ✦ sea salt and other seasonings ✦ water ✦ coconut oil or red palm oil ✦ optional lemon juice, sweetener, basil, and ginger

1. Stir or shake can of full-fat coconut milk to distribute contents evenly (use BPA free brand with 1 carb or less such as 365 from Whole Foods or Kroger).
2. Pour about ½ cup or so of the can (you don't have to be exact) into saucepan.
3. Add leftover chicken, turkey, or canned salmon to saucepan.
4. Add 1 Tbs. nutritional yeast, sea salt or cayenne to taste, and a dash of fish sauce. If you would like a fuller Thai experience, add a squeeze of lemon or lemon concentrate, pinch of Truvia or Nunaturals, and chopped fresh basil with a dash of ginger.
5. Add water to desired soup consistency and heat.
6. Optional: when soup is heated, add 1-2 tsp. virgin coconut oil or red palm oil.

Serene chats: I eat this soup regularly for lunch and usually use the first few spices as it is quick and still tastes great. You can also buy a jar of green or red curry paste in the international section of your supermarket and add a tad of that to your liking, a dash of fish sauce, and a pinch of stevia.

Palm Butter Powerhouse – S

To obtain the ingredients for this soup, you will need to locate an African food store in your area.

Serene chats: By "in your area," I mean anything within two hour's distance. I travel about that distance to my closest African market and load up approximately three times a year with all my palm oil and palm butter needs.

Basic Ingredients: palm butter ✦ cooked chicken or turkey, or canned salmon ✦ sea salt and other seasonings ✦ water

1. Place 2 generous Tbs. canned palm butter (a firm packed variety is best, e.g., Ghana's Best) into saucepan with a portion of any leftover or canned chicken or turkey. Canned salmon is delicious also.
2. Add 1 Tbs. nutritional yeast, sea salt and cayenne pepper to taste, dash of Bragg Liquid Aminos or tamari, and a little optional curry powder.
3. For stew consistency, add a little water, or for soup consistency, thin down further with a little more water.
4. Heat, stir, and you're done.

If you are not using all your canned palm butter for other recipes within a few days, freeze what is leftover in ice cube trays for later use. Use three ice cubes for this recipe next time. This stew is great over *Cauli Rice* (*Vegetable Sides*, Chapter 22).

East African Curry – S

Serene chats: This is more stew consistency than soup. It whips up quickly, although it takes a little longer than the other two recipes. I include it in this category since it sends your taste buds to foreign shores. This meal is super high in calcium, due to the large amount of dark leafy greens and the canned salmon that includes skin and bones. You can use any canned salmon. My favorite is red sockeye, which is also highest in DMAE, but a little pricier.

Basic Ingredients: canned salmon ✦ dark leafy greens ✦ water ✦ red palm oil ✦ optional palm butter ✦ sea salt and other seasonings

1. Tear up a few large handfuls of any dark green leafy vegetable like spinach, kale, or collards (mustard greens would be too bitter) and place in food processor, not blender.
2. Pulse for a few seconds and then process until completely fine.
3. Transfer greens to skillet with just enough water to dampen them, about 2 Tbs. (too much water will ruin consistency).
4. Turn stove-top to high. As soon as greens start to bubble, cover skillet and turn heat to low, so greens can steam in their own juices until very dark green and wilted.

5. Uncover skillet and add ½ cup canned salmon, 2 heaping Tbs. red palm oil and an optional Tbs. palm butter.
6. Season with sea salt, cayenne pepper, curry powder or paste, and nutritional yeast to taste.
7. Smash everything in your skillet with a fork and turn up the heat until it is all piping hot.

Serene chats: I whip this up frequently for my own personal lunch if my children are having more "kid food" type sandwiches. This recipe also works well for a full family evening meal and is a family favorite around my house. I do it on a much larger scale with three cans of salmon and some bunches of greens (you have to process the greens in stages when making this for a whole family, but it is still a quick meal).

Quick Comfort Soups

Pearl now offers you some great alternatives to the comfort food soups, which you may not want to give up, like a good old Cream of Tomato Soup.

Just Like Campbell's Tomato Soup – S

Basic Ingredients: tomato sauce ✦ water or chicken broth ✦ heavy cream ✦ sea salt and other seasonings ✦ sweetener ✦ optional grated cheese

1. Pour 1 (8 oz.) can tomato sauce into small saucepan.
2. Add almost 1 cup of water or chicken broth (about ⅞ of cup) and 2-4 Tbs. heavy cream.
3. Add 1 tsp. Truvia or a sprinkle of Nunaturals, sea salt, and black pepper to taste and optional cayenne pepper.
4. Heat through and top with grated cheese.

This soup is ready in a jiffy and nice on a chilly winter's day. You can enjoy, knowing you won't be ingesting all the needless carbs and sugar that regular canned Cream of Tomato Soup contains. But, it tastes just as delish and chock full of lycopene from the cooked tomatoes, one of the most potent anti-cancer weapons God has provided. If you are a Drive Thru Sue, it's another easy one for you!

You can omit sweetener in this recipe and, instead, opt for a more savory flavored version. Use Creole seasoning, add a little dash of nutritional yeast, and it's a whole different sort of yummy.

Pearl chats: Sunday night is usually my "night off" cooking a big evening meal. This soup is great Sunday night fare for the whole family. Use a couple of very large cans of tomato sauce and multiply the other ingredients accordingly. I usually add some leftover chicken breast to it and whatever veggies I have in the fridge, (canned chicken breast also works fine for the added protein quota). In less than five minutes soup is ready for the whole family. Whoever is not a fan of this soup in our family has to fend for themselves.

Light Tomato Soup – E or Fuel Pull

Our niece, Rashida (Evangeline's oldest daughter and who cooks for their whole family) makes this soup a lot. Here's an individual lunch version, but it can be multiplied to feed a full family.

1. Pour 1 (8 oz.) can tomato sauce into small saucepan.
2. Add 1 cup of water or chicken broth.
3. Add ⅓ cup of low or non-fat yogurt, either Greek style or regular.
4. Add 1 tsp. Truvia, sea salt, and black pepper to taste and optional cayenne pepper.
5. Heat through.

You could eat some plan approved toast with a bowl of this soup if you want an **E** lunch. However do not use more than 1 tsp. of butter on your toast. A very small amount of skim mozzarella may also be used to top the soup.

Chicken Broth Anything Soup – S, E or Fuel Pull

Broth based soups are very slimming! They're great for weight loss because they fill you up with liquid.

Basically, if you have a can of chicken broth in your cupboard, you have the making of a quick meal. Add whatever leftovers you desire from your fridge. Heat up, spice up, and lunch is ready.

Leftover chicken breast diced up and added to the pot, or a little canned chicken breast does the job as the protein for an **E** or a **Fuel Pull**. You can also add leftover rice or quinoa for an **E**, but if you need to nudge some stubborn pounds, leave out the grain and keep to pure **Fuel Pull** mode of only protein and non-starchy veggies. Leftover beef or sausage will add some fat if you're seeking an **S** style soup.

Spinach leaves are the perfect veggie to add because they wilt and cook in very quickly, even from a frozen state. Leftover veggies such as cauliflower or broccoli are fine, too.

Basic Ingredients: chicken broth ✦ leftover diced meats ✦ spinach or leftover veggies ✦ sea salt and other seasonings

1. Pour 1 can fat-free chicken broth into a saucepan.
2. Add small amounts of leftover diced meats and leftover veggies (frozen or fresh spinach) to saucepan.
3. Season with salt and pepper, nutritional yeast, Bragg Liquid Aminos, and a little cayenne pepper if you like hot.
4. Heat and enjoy.

If you're making this soup as **S** style, top with grated cheese. Omit that completely for **E** or **Fuel Pull**, or use only a very small amount of grated skim mozzarella and use fat free chicken broth.

Zest of Southwest – S or E

Basic ingredients: chicken broth ✦ leftover chicken or canned chicken ✦ salsa or canned green chilies and tomatoes ✦ grated cheese ✦ sour cream ✦ optional *Joseph's Crackers*

1. Put 1 can fat-free chicken broth in saucepan.
2. Add leftover pieces of chicken to pot or use some canned chicken breast.
3. Add 2 Tbs. of salsa, or the same amount of canned diced green chilies and tomatoes.
4. Once heated through, top with shredded cheese, a dollop of sour cream, and crumble a few *Joseph's Crackers* (*Snacks,* Chapter 24) on top.

To make this **E**, you can add some beans to the soup, use 0% Greek yogurt in place of the sour cream, and add a little sprinkle of low-fat mozzarella or other low-fat cheese for topping. You could also add some organic baked blue corn chips, or stick with *Joseph's Crackers.*

Loaded Fotato Soup – S, E or Fuel Pull

Cauliflower is the magic in this soup. You'll barely believe how creamy, flavorful, and satisfying this soup is and yet it contains no cream and very little fat. The idea of this soup is adopted from our *Creamless Creamy Veggies* (*Vegetable Sides,* Chapter 22), using chicken broth and light Laughing Cow or Weight Watchers cheese wedges. The added ingredients of turkey bacon bits and seasonings make it taste like a loaded baked potato soup. Superb!

This recipe is specified as a one person serving so it works for a quick mama's lunch. Of course, you can multiply the recipe and feed it to your whole family who will likely appreciate it.

It is a **Fuel Pull** recipe at its core. Eat it alone, or pair it with a salad with a very light dressing, and you'll stay in that mode. Top it with grated cheese and you'll be in **S** style. Have a piece of toast with it and you'll be heading into **E** territory. The choice is up to you and your own needs, but as a **Fuel Pull** it will be the greatest pound destroyer.

Note: To make this soup a quick process, pull out a bag of frozen cauliflower at breakfast time, take out half the contents to defrost to reduce your lunch cooking time. But, if you forget, frozen cauliflower takes only a few minutes to become tender.

Pearl chats: This is my favorite of all the soups I have contributed. I'm absolutely addicted to it and continue to pat myself on the back for thinking of it. I mean, it's so deceiving. It tastes like you're eating oodles of calories, fats, and carbs. But no, just the opposite. Meadow and I often eat it together at lunch time so I double the recipe. After the first spoonful or two, I always ask, "Am I clever, or what?" She gives me that look that only teenage daughters know how to give their un-cool mothers . . . "Yes, Mom, you're very clever."

Basic Ingredients: cauliflower ✦ chicken broth ✦ light Laughing Cow or Weight Watchers cheese wedges ✦ turkey bacon bits ✦ glucomannan or xanthan gum ✦ sea salt and other seasonings ✦ optional green onion

1. Put ½ the contents of a 12 oz. bag of frozen or thawed cauliflower into small saucepan.
2. Add 2 cups fat free chicken broth.
3. Bring to boil then simmer cauliflower in broth until tender.
4. Scoop cooked cauliflower out and place in blender. Blend until smooth and return to saucepan.
5. Add 1 light Laughing Cow or Weight Watchers cheese wedge to saucepan. Heat to melt cheese, dispersing it with a whisk.
6. Season with sea salt, black pepper, optional Bragg Liquid Aminos, garlic or onion powder, a sprinkle of nutritional yeast and dash of cayenne pepper.
7. Add 2 tsp. turkey bacon bits.
8. Thicken soup to desired consistency by sprinkling in glucomannan or xanthan gum from a salt shaker little by little, and whisking briskly. This soup should be a thick consistency to resemble a potato based soup.
9. Garnish with optional green onion.

If you're the sort who likes to get a very full tummy, add more water and seasonings to the soup and thicken with more glucomannan. It's still great that way, and you are eating more volume, but no more calories.

Sandwiches, Wraps, and Roll Ups

You know by now that we are not going to deprive you of a sandwich at lunchtime. If you're more conventional in your eating style, you may be thinking, "I don't want exotic soups with spinach and salmon for lunch every day. C'mon now! Just give me a turkey sandwich!" That's fine, we are doing our best to encourage you to eat more salmon, but you can go ahead and eat your turkey sandwich and still stay on plan.

Depending upon the content of your sandwich, you will use appropriate casings. For sandwiches that contain **S** type fillings with higher fat like mayo, avocado, and cheese, you can use Romaine, Boston, or even head lettuce as roll ups. Those are delicious if you've never tried them. But, of course, make use of all our **S** bread type recipes like *Bread in a Mug*, *Oopsie Rolls*, *Basic Sandwich Buns*, *Spinach Bread*, *Nori Wraps*, *Golden Flat Bread* and *Marcy's Cheesy Rolls.* Store-bought Joseph's pita bread/lavish works fine for **S** too.

On the **E** sandwich side, you have grain-based breads like sprouted Trader Joe's and Ezekiel, sprouted wraps, homemade sourdough bread, or *Trim Healthy Pan Bread*. Joseph's also works fine for **E** or **Fuel Pull**. Lots of options.

If you miss the constant addition of regular bread in your diet after all these options, we might find a little name for you that you don't like. It might start with "spoiled" and end with "brat!" Pearl thinks we should soften that statement up a little by saying, "Ha-ha" at the end to let you know we are joking. Serene thinks we should not. She likes it just as it is. If you have come this far in the book with us, you might as well join our sisterhood shenanigans where we are not afraid to say what's really on our minds.

We are not totally removing real bread from your diet. We only want to demote it from king to servant. Keeping grain-based breads to **E** meals, and no more than two pieces at a time, naturally puts bread in a more waist friendly place where it no longer rules.

We give you a few unique sandwich recipes here first and further on remind you of your **S** and **E** options.

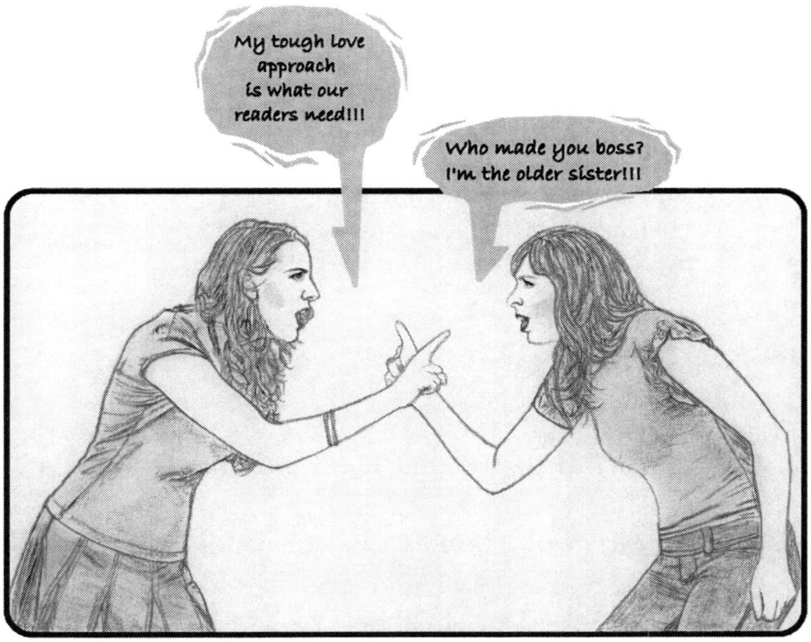

Lettuce Wraps – S, E or Fuel Pull

Basic Ingredients: lettuce leaves ✦ mayo, mustard, dijonaise or horseradish sauce ✦ meat ✦ cheese

1. Put 6 large lettuce leaves on a couple of dinner plates.
2. Spread each one with mayo and mustard or horseradish sauce (mayo can be either light or full-fat depending on **S, E** or **Fuel Pull**).
3. Add small pieces of any meat like sausage, bacon, chicken, or beef. Use only lean meats if making wraps **E** or **Fuel Pull** style.
4. Add finely diced tomato and onion if desired. (For **E**, you can add some quinoa or beans, or a little pineapple).
5. Add some grated or thin sliced cheese for **S.** For **E** or **Fuel Pull** don't use any cheese at all, or include a little skim mozzarella.
6. Roll each leaf up around the fillings, securing with a toothpick so they don't unravel on your plate.
7. Transfer all your lettuce wraps to one plate and enjoy your slimming lunch.

Scrumptilicious Sammie (Eggplant) – S

Pearl chats: My daughter, Meadow and I often love to make these for lunch. They are surprisingly quick to make. You won't be able to hold the sandwich in your hand, but will have to eat it with a knife and fork, but the yummy factor is worth it.

You can make these lots of different ways. Try turkey deli meat with cheese and tomato or onion—excellent all melty and scrumptilicious. Or, a more Italian style of tomato paste with leftover chicken and parmesan cheese.

Basic Ingredients: egg plant ✦ cheeses ✦ meats ✦ optional tomato paste ✦ sea salt and other seasonings ✦ butter or coconut oil

1. Peel an eggplant and slice it into roughly ¼ inch thick round slices (these are your bread casings).
2. Season eggplant slices with a little sea salt and black pepper.
3. Layer with cheeses, veggies, meats, and optional tomato paste.
4. Season eggplant sandwich fillings with sea salt and other seasonings of your choice.
5. Brown both top and bottom of eggplant sandwich in a generous amount of butter or olive oil until cheese inside the sandwich is melted.

You'll need to eat a couple of these sandwiches to get satisfied. You could cut the eggplant lengthwise, instead of into rounds, for one extra large sandwich.

Warm Chicken Sprouted Sandwich – E

Basic Ingredients: sprouted bread ✦ chicken breast ✦ light mayo ✦ mustard ✦ tomato ✦ sea salt and other seasonings ✦ optional turkey or Canadian bacon

1. Heat precooked seasoned chicken breast in a lightly sprayed or oiled nonstick pan.
2. Toast 2 slices sprouted Trader Joe's or Ezekiel bread.
3. Spread thin layer of light mayo on toast and add as much mustard as you desire.
4. Put slices of tomato on toast and season with sea salt and pepper.
5. Ladle on hot chicken, then slice your sandwich in half with a sharp knife.

Note: One slice of turkey or Canadian bacon on this sandwich makes it even more superb. It goes great with any **E** or **Fuel Pull** smoothie like our *Fat Stripping Frappa* (*Morning Meals*,

Chapter 18) made with a half scoop of whey. The sandwich and smoothie combo is both highly delicious and energizing.

Deli Meat Roll Ups – S, E or Fuel Pull

Basic Ingredients: lean deli meat ✦ mayonnaise ✦ mustard ✦ optional horseradish sauce ✦ cheese ✦ green pepper or celery

1. Take slices of natural, lean deli meat and pat them dry with a paper towel.
2. Spread with mayo and mustard if desired (keep to light mayo or use only mustard or horseradish for **E** or **Fuel Pull**).
3. Add pencil size (julienne cut) strips of cheese (use only very thin slices of skim mozzarella for **E** or **Fuel Pull**).
4. Add pencil size (julienne cut) strips of green pepper or celery.
5. Roll up and secure with toothpick.

If you want to make these roll ups **E** style, you can include finely chopped fresh/canned pineapple or fresh mango (so delicious)! That little sweet taste in every bite is perfect.

Three of these roll ups make a great afternoon snack with a whey protein smoothie made with half a scoop of whey. You'll need something more to help fill you up for a lunch meal. What about cottage cheese with fruit for **E**? Or, even yummier, make a *Waldorf Cottage Cheese Salad* (*Lunches,* Chapter 20).

Ideas for S Sandwiches and Wraps

Aside from our *Muffin in a Mug* or Joseph's pitas which are ready in a jiffy, we don't want you to attempt to make any bread recipes right before lunch time when you're hungry. Your breads should be a pull out item that are quick and ready for a 5-10 minute prep lunch. The other **S** breads that require full baking times, and items like Nori Wraps that need to be dehydrated for hours, can be made on a baking day or an afternoon where you have some spare time. If desired, you can bake huge batches for a two month supply, to freeze and pull out as needed.

Here's a starter list of **S** sandwich/wrap ideas:

- Chicken salad made with mayo, celery, and chopped walnuts
- Natural deli meats with lettuce, mayo, and cheese
- Egg salad (simply eggs and mayo)
- Tuna salad (simply tuna and mayo)
- Bacon, lettuce, and tomato with mayo
- Burgers of either beef, chicken, or turkey with "fixin's"

- Grilled cheese and tomato
- Fried egg sandwich
- Natural peanut butter and with stevia-sweetened homemade berry-reduction or sugar-free jelly
- Sautéed leftover chicken with sesame seeds, sesame oil, lettuce, cayenne pepper, and mayo

Let your imagination take over. Add a decadent side salad to these **S** sandwiches/wraps if you haven't already used many garden vegetables in your sandwich. Or, an **S** snack can be enjoyed as a side such as *Crunchy Kale Chips*, *Crunchy Cheese Crisps*, *Spicy Nuts,* or any of our cracker recipes from *Snacks,* Chapter 24.

You also substitute the above mentioned sides for a small **S** smoothie from *Morning Meals*, Chapter 18, which can top off a sandwich lunch nicely.

Ideas for E Sandwiches and Wraps

There are not as many options when it comes to **E** fillings, but the following are reliable.

- Lean deli meats or chicken breast with light mayo, mustard or horseradish sauce, lettuce, tomato and onion, and optional small amounts of skim mozzarella cheese
- Light packed tuna with light mayo and chopped celery

Sides to **E** sandwiches/wraps could be cottage cheese and fruit, a side salad with light dressing, *Waldorf Cottage Cheese Salad*, or an **E** or **Fuel Pull** smoothie.

Large Lunch Salads

The following can be lovely lunch meals on their own, or they can accompany other foods as smaller sides. While a side salad can be as easy as ripping up some organic romaine lettuce leaves, throwing them on a plate and pouring on the dressing, these next recipes require a little more effort, but the few minutes are worth it for a fabulous, complete lunch.

Waldorf Cottage Cheese Salad – E

Basic Ingredients: apple ✦ lemon juice ✦ low-fat cottage cheese ✦ celery ✦ toasted nuts ✦ sea salt and other seasonings

1. Dice one apple, place the pieces in a bowl, and add a couple good squeezes of lemon juice (either fresh or from concentrate).

2 Add 1 cup low-fat cottage cheese into the bowl.
3 Add 2 stalks chopped celery and a very small handful of toasted chopped walnuts or other nuts (check out *Spicy Nuts* (*Snacks,* Chapter 24).
4 Add dash of sea salt, black pepper, and shake in some chili flakes.
5 Combine ingredients with a fork or spoon.

Simple, yet incredible. Although it's **E**, it tends to be quite filling due to the ample protein from the cottage cheese. Go easy on the nuts if you want to keep it **E** and weight loss promoting. We make the nuts very spicy for this recipe and chop them very small so a small amount tossed throughout the salad makes a lot of flavor. You can double or triple the recipe for a larger family.

The Fuel Pull Salad

Pearl chats: Eat this salad a few times a week for lunch and watch stubborn pounds surrender to the power of the **Fuel Pull**! The trick with this salad is to make it huge. I've eaten this recipe out of a casserole dish a time or two! Regrettably, eating too many **Fuel Pull** main meals makes me lose weight, so even though it is a tasty salad, I've had to scale **Fuel Pulls** back and now usually include fat or carbs in my salad. I often send this salad with Charlie to work in a gigantic bowl because he eats way more calories than I do. It's a good balancing lunch for him a couple of times a week.

If you have stubborn weight issues, it will be wise to get close and friendly with this salad. You'll get your full eating it and may even have to put some back in the fridge, but it's perfectly fine if you eat every last morsel. Finish your meal with a version of our *Choco Pudding* and who could ask for anything more?

If you're the Drive Thru Sue type and don't want to fuss with pre-making your own chicken breast, this is when Tyson Grilled and Ready chicken and steak strips can come in handy. Half a bag's worth is 3 oz. of nicely seasoned meat protein. That's the limit on how much meat you should use in this salad. If you're preparing your own, this is equivalent to about two chicken tenderloins or half a chicken breast.

Making sure the dressing fits the salad correctly is extremely important for this **Fuel Pull** lunch. You can make your own vinaigrette, but be very sure to only use 1 tsp. of oil for your entire salad. You can use Balsamic or any other vinegar to make up the rest of it or try our *Hip Trim Honey Mustard* recipe. Zero calorie dressings like Green Valley Ranch or Walden Farms brand work well, as do very low-cal dressings like Wish-bone Spritzers. Most dressings termed "light" won't work for this salad. They are still too fuel heavy for this to be the big gun, fat-busting salad it is designed to be.

Basic Ingredients: lettuce ✦ other non-starchy salad veggies of choice such as baby tomatoes, green pepper, onion, cucumber ✦ chicken breast or extra lean steak ✦ cottage cheese ✦ appropriate dressing ✦ sea salt and other seasonings like chili flakes ✦ optional turkey bacon bits

1. Chop or rip up one large heart of romaine or use 4 cups of any other type of lettuce and place in bowl.
2. Add other non-starchy salad veggies such as ½ chopped green pepper, 2 chopped celery stalks, handful of baby tomatoes, ⅛ finely sliced onion, ¼ seeded and chopped cucumber.
3. Dress your salad with half the allotted dressing, e.g., if using Wishbone Spritzer, spray 10 times (you'll use the other 10 later). Toss salad veggies well in dressing.
4. Sprinkle with sea salt, black pepper, and cayenne pepper if desired, and toss veggies once again.
5. Chop 3 oz. of pre-cooked chicken breast or extra lean steak and add to salad.
6. Now add the rest of your dressing to coat both chicken and veggies thoroughly.
7. Top with 2 heaping Tbs. of 1% cottage cheese and an optional sprinkle of turkey bacon bits and chili flakes.

Mexican Cottage Cheese Salad – Fuel Pull

Here's another **Fuel Pull** salad. This one uses beans, but only ⅓ of a cup which is not enough to put you in **E** territory. If you want to make it an **E**, go ahead and add another ⅓ cup of beans or add some fruit like a little diced mango or pineapple, the flavors blend well.

If either of the next two salads do not fill you up enough (they're not quite as huge as *The Fuel Pull Salad*), then pair them with our *Fat Stripping Frappa* made with a half scoop of whey (*Morning Meals,* Chapter 18). You'll stay in **Fuel Pull** mode and feel highly satisfied.

Basic Ingredients: low-fat cottage cheese ✦ black beans (or any beans) ✦ salsa ✦ salad greens

1. Put ¾ cup 1% cottage cheese into a bowl.
2. Add ⅓ cup black beans.
3. Add ⅓ cup salsa.
4. Mix well and either dump onto a bed of salad greens or toss with 2-3 cups of salad greens.

Cajun Cottage Cheese Salad – Fuel Pull

This is a variation on the above recipe.

Basic Ingredients: low-fat cottage cheese ✦ black beans ✦ seasoning ✦ chicken breast ✦ salad greens

1. Put ¾ cup 1% cottage cheese into a bowl.
2. Add ¼ cup black beans.
3. Add ¼ cup diced chicken breast.
4. Sprinkle with Creole seasoning.
5. Place all these ingredients onto a bed of greens.

Tabouleh – S or S Helper (makes several servings)

This salad takes a little longer to prepare than the others included here, due to all the slicing and chopping. It's a great idea to make up a large quantity of *Tabouleh* when you have time one afternoon. It can then be pulled out of the fridge for a quick lunch with *Hummus* (*Snacks,* Chapter 24), and a piece of *Golden Flat Bread* or some Joseph's lavish. *Tabouleh* tastes better once the flavors have had a chance to marinate for a few hours.

It's always a great side to an evening meal too, or perfect with Quiche, or any meat item. Chicken and satay sauce with *Tabouleh* on the side, what could be better?

If you don't have any pre-made *Tabouleh* at lunch time, you can make the prep time faster by using a food processor, making sure to pulse rather than puree. You want to end up with chopped parsley, not parsley liquid! Even if your quick prep *Tabouleh* has not had time to sit and enhance in the refrigerator, it'll still be good.

You can keep to pure **S** by using *Cauli Rice* (*Vegetable Sides*, Chapter 22) as the grain replacement. Or, feel free to use quinoa, making this recipe an **S Helper** once you're at that stage. Tabouleh is traditionally made with a grain called bulgur, which is much harder on your blood sugar than quinoa, and quinoa is by far more nutritionally superior. And in our minds, even better tasting.

Basic ingredients: parsley ✦ cucumbers ✦ tomatoes ✦ quinoa or *Cauli Rice* ✦ olives ✦ sea salt and other seasonings ✦ olive oil ✦ lemon juice

1. Finely chop 1-2 bunches of parsley and place in a bowl.
2. Add 1-2 diced cucumbers.
3. Add 1-2 dices tomatoes.
4. Add 1-1½ cups pre-cooked quinoa or *Cauli Rice.*

5. Add optional sliced or whole black olives, and diced onion, or green onion.
6. Season with sea salt, black pepper, and optional mint leaves and cilantro.
7. Add ¼-½ cup olive oil and the juice of 1-2 lemons.
8. Toss well.

Nicey Ricey Salad – E

Basic Ingredients: romaine lettuce ✦ optional cucumbers or tomatoes ✦ brown rice or quinoa ✦ lean deli meat ✦ coconut oil ✦ light vinaigrette

1. Place a bunch of ripped romaine lettuce on a dinner plate.
2. Optional: Add other veggies like cucumbers or tomatoes if you have time.
3. Heat up ¾ cup pre-cooked brown rice, or ¾ cup quinoa with some diced lean deli meat in a pan with 1 tsp. coconut oil and spices of your choice.
4. Dump the hot rice/quinoa and meat on the salad.
5. Dress with a light vinaigrette.

The deli meat can be substituted with chicken breast strips or tuna. This is where your individual frozen baggies of rice or quinoa come in handy. Take one out in the morning to thaw.

Better than Chef Salad – E

Basic Ingredients: salad greens and other veggies ✦ beans ✦ fruit ✦ lean meats ✦ balsamic vinegar ✦ olive oil ✦ sea salt and black pepper

1. Put your favorite salad greens and veggies such as sliced cucumber, tomato, and onion into your favorite bowl.
2. Add a generous handful of garbanzo beans (or any beans) and a small amount of sliced fruit of your choice such as mango, apple, pineapple, or a smattering of goji berries.
3. Add diced lean deli meats or leftover/canned chicken breast.
4. Dress with generous drizzles of balsamic vinegar, a light splash of extra virgin olive oil, black pepper and sea salt.

Better than Chef Salad – S

Basic Ingredients: salad greens and other veggies ✦ meats ✦ cheese ✦ dressing

1. Put your favorite salad greens and veggies like sliced cucumber, tomato, and onion into your favorite bowl.
2. Add whatever meats you desire (even pieces of fresh rotisserie chicken with skin on), or leftover steak or beef brisket.
3. Add any of the following: cheese (goat, feta, or hard cheeses cubed or grated), olives, spicy nuts or seeds, half an avocado, etc.

Generously dress salad with your favorite homemade olive oil based dressing, or use your favorite store bought dressing as long as it is not more than two grams of carbs, one gram is better. Remember our idea of thinning store-bought creamy dressings with water?

Serene chats: I don't like to use any dressing made from soybean or canola oil unless I have no other choice. I prefer homemade dressings. If I am eating out, I stick with balsamic vinegar and olive oil. Pearl told me to be nice and not freak out our regular mamas with my purist idealism. She thinks I might turn folks away from a weight loss plan that will be healthy for them, regardless of a little "not so perfect" dressing. Our debate found a meeting ground by agreeing that the most important thing is to watch for hidden sugars in your dressings if you buy them from the store. I guess I will have to overlook that Hidden Valley ranch some may have slipped into their shopping cart!

Pearl chats: Sometimes, just saving time wins out for people like me who don't want to constantly make everything from scratch. We don't want to live with so many rules and regulations that we feel like throwing it all in and feasting on potato chips. I'll admit to using store-bought Ranch dressing, but not all the time, and I always water it down a little. Ken's ranch is my go-to, because it only has one carb. But, I often make my own homemade dressings when I have more time, or want to be healthier. I like to switch it around about 50/50.

For **E** Dressings, I sometimes buy Newman's Own "Light Balsamic" and use it when I'm in a hurry. It tastes great, is low in sugar, and does not have too much fat for **E** purposes. But, I know that since it has soybean oil in it, I shouldn't rely on it. Therefore, many times, like Serene, I drizzle balsamic and a little olive oil for **E**, or a lot of olive oil for **S**, and know I'm doing my body a better favor.

BLT Salad – S

Basic Ingredients: tomato ✦ bacon ✦ mayonnaise ✦ chili flakes ✦ lettuce

1. Dice large tomato and place in bowl, juice and all.
2. Cook up some bacon (turkey or beef bacon work too), cut bacon into bite sized pieces and add to bowl.
3. Add mayonnaise, a sprinkle of chili flakes, and stir all contents together.
4. Pour over bed of lettuce.

Odds and Ends Lunches

Luv My Sweet Potato Lunch – E

Basic Ingredients: sweet potato ✦ coconut oil or butter ✦ optional sweetener or sea salt and other seasonings ✦ fresh veggies ✦ light vinaigrette ✦ tuna or low-fat cottage cheese

1. Bake a sweet potato until it's nice and soft.
2. Top with 1 tsp. extra virgin coconut oil or butter.
3. If you prefer a sweet version, add Truvia or Nunaturals and optional cinnamon. Drizzle on Bragg Liquid Aminos or Tamari (or sea salt, pepper, and cayenne pepper) for a savory version.
4. Add fresh veggies to your plate such as cucumbers and tomatoes, or lettuce drizzled with balsamic vinegar or a store-bought light vinaigrette.
5. Top veggies or lettuce with small can of water-packed tuna or some low-fat cottage cheese.

Quick Tuna Medley – S, E or Fuel Pull

Basic Ingredients: tuna ✦ optional mayonnaise ✦ low-fat cottage cheese ✦ tomatoes and cucumbers ✦ olive oil ✦ balsamic vinegar ✦ *Joseph's Crackers* ✦ optional fruit

1. Drain can of tuna and put contents in a mound on a dinner plate (you can add mayo to the tuna if making an **S** lunch).
2. Put ½-¾ cup 1% cottage cheese in another mound on a separate part of the plate.

3. Place another mound of diced tomatoes and cucumbers, dressed liberally with olive oil (for **S** style only) and balsamic vinegar on plate.
4. Add pile of *Joseph's Crackers* to plate.
5. Add optional fruit if desiring an **E** meal.

Pearl chats: This meal sounds simple, but I love it. You can use it with any of our cracker recipes. I like to quickly nuke some *Joseph's Crackers* and put forkfuls of each mound on the crackers. This lunch can be **E, S** or **Fuel Pull**, depending upon how much fat you use or if you add fruit. For **S**, you can add mayo to the tuna if desired, or even use tuna packed in olive oil.

For **E**, use water packed tuna, leave out the mayo (or use a low-fat version) and go easy with the olive oil on the raw veggies, or don't use it at all. For an **E**, a little mound of fruit added to the plate such as half a diced mango is so refreshing. For a **Fuel Pull**, leave out any full-fat mayo, oil, or fruit, but add some berries instead. I use 1% cottage cheese for this recipe which works for **S, E** and **Fuel Pull**.

Quesedillas – S

This recipe is not in the superfood category as it uses low-carb, store-bought tortillas. You know Serene did not come up with this one. But, it is quick and delicious and fills the space inside that just craves a cheese quesadilla.

Basic Ingredients: low-carb tortillas ✦ cheese ✦ tomatoes ✦ meat ✦ sea salt and other seasonings ✦ coconut oil ✦ optional sour cream and salsa

1. Layer grated cheese on a tortilla and add any other goodies to your liking such as tomatoes, chicken, ground beef, jalapenos, etc.
2. Season with salt and pepper and add hot sauce if you like it hot.
3. Top with another low-carb tortilla and fry until brown in a skillet with some coconut oil.
4. Accompany with salsa and sour cream if desired.

Pearl chats: I like using Mission brand small size, whole grain low-carb tortillas for my quesadillas. We sometimes have quesadillas for evening meals for the whole family. I use regular whole wheat tortillas for the younger children. Charlie, Meadow, and I enjoy the low-carb variety. My husband and I actually think they taste better than regular ones.

Chapter 21

Evening Meals

Here come your comforting and hearty favorites. We've divided this chapter into methods of cooking—crockpots, oven dishes, stove top, and yes, we have also thrown in some Mexican and pasta dishes since they're supper time favorites.

Clever Crock Meals

We know there are many recipe books full of slow cooker recipes. However, have you noticed that many of the recipes are very involved and the preparation time consuming? Also, many of the ingredients would sabotage your healthy new lifestyle.

We think crockpots should be used for their original intention—slow healthy heat all day to preserve nutrients and protect protein molecules in your meats while saving you time. The most tender and succulent meat is formed by the many hours of moist heating provided by the crockpot. It's by far the healthiest way to eat meat.

Have you ever noticed when 5 pm arrives that everything goes wrong? An otherwise orderly day can turn to mayhem. The baby is screaming, the toddler needs help on the potty, the older children are fighting, hungry, and can't to wait to eat, and you are exhausted. This is when the crockpot shines.

While a delicious aroma fills your home all day, it's a reminder that your usual "crazy hour" won't be nearly as crazy. All you have to do is dish up, and at the most, prepare a fresh salad and some pre-cooked brown rice for the children to make their soup heartier. Phew! On days when you may be out of the home running errands and will be home late, the crockpot will save you a lot of mental stress. For larger families, it might be a good idea to purchase one of the extra large crockpots if you do not already have one.

Enjoy these plan approved crockpot recipes. The majority are labeled **S** as crock-cooked meat is usually created with creamy sauces or red meat. Choose a side that will not be high in carbs, such as a yummy decadent salad, a crusty *Country Biscuit (Lunches,* Chapter 20), or a non-starchy vegetable created **S** style if you have time for a little more work.

We normally cook up big pots of brown rice for the children to use as a base for their meals. There's always enough rice to spread into a couple of meals. The children can eat it with their evening crockpot meal, and then again for lunch with eggs the next day. This gives them the carbs they love and need for growing, and allows the crockpot dish to be extended which makes these meals less costly. When making the occasional **E** crockpot recipe, you can enjoy an appropriate portion of brown rice, along with the children, to accompany your meal.

The main object is to keep additional prep very simple. If brown rice is not handy, you may want to add whole grain bread and butter for the children. And, what about a bag of raw sugar snap peas? The children love these. If you use very lean meats, like chicken breast, and want to make some of these **E** recipes, you could have a slice or two of plan approved bread also. Remember to use no more than one teaspoon of butter for your bread if you're still on the journey to weight management.

Don't forget that chili is a great meal for the crockpot. We have included chili recipes further on in the *Stove Top Tummy Warmers* section of this chapter but we often make chili in the crockpot too. Check out our on plan chili recipes. All you'll have to do in the morning is brown the beef and onions, put them into the crockpot with the other ingredients and simmer all day. Flavors are amazing this way.

Tender Beef Stew – S

This recipe is perfect for cheaper, tougher cuts of meat, as the crockpot magically tenderizes them. You can buy a frozen box full of cheap steaks at bulk stores like Costco much less expensively than fresh. Aldi has good prices for them, too. In a perfect world, grass fed meat is optimum. Wives who are lucky enough to have hunters for husbands could use venison cuts. What could be healthier than venison stew?

Basic Ingredients: beef or venison cuts ✦ veggies ✦ tomato paste ✦ sea salt and other seasonings ✦ water ✦ optional heavy cream or tahini

1. In the crockpot, place enough cuts of thawed meat such as sirloin, venison, or grass fed beef to feed the whole family.
2. Add large pieces of green or red peppers, onions, 2" long cut celery and carrots (the carrots are for your children, unless you are going to use only a few as an **S helper**). You may also add chunks of cabbage, but that will be too soft unless you add in just a few hours before meal time.
3. Depending on how large your family, add 2-3 (6 oz.) cans tomato paste. For a spicier flavor, add an optional jar of salsa (containing no sugar or corn syrup).
4. Season with a generous amount of sea salt, a few squirts of Bragg Liquid Aminos or Tamari/soy sauce, onion powder, lots of black pepper, and optional cayenne pepper or hot sauce to taste.
5. Add 1 cup water for each can of tomato paste and turn crockpot to high and cook all day.
6. Before serving, add a swirl of cream, or a dollop of tahini to the stew. This cuts the acidity of the tomatoes, mellows sharp flavors, and brings out the depth of the meaty undertones.

When ready, the meat should be extremely fork tender and falling of the bones (if there are bones). You may add more water if needed, or if you prefer a very thick stew, leave the water out of the original recipe, or thicken with a little xanthan gum or glucomannan.

Frozen cuts of meat may be used if you put them in the crock the night before and cook on low rather than high all night through until the next evening.

Serene chats: Sometimes, I use ground beef for this recipe, and because I mostly use grass fed beef (we split a cow with other families which makes it a cheaper way of purchasing this superfood), there is very minimal grease and you do not have to brown or drain it. The ground beef becomes soft and tender instead of the usual firmer crumbles. My family adores it.

Pot Roast – S

Basic Ingredients: beef roast ✦ water ✦ sea salt and other seasonings

1. Place one large beef roast in crockpot.
2. Completely cover with water.

3. Season with salt, pepper, and onion powder.
4. Simmer all day on high.
5. Once ready, place on a serving dish and separate meat with a fork. Squirt Bragg Liquid Aminos over the fork pulled beef, or add a little more salt and pepper.

This recipe can either be started the night before and cooked on low all night and the following day, or cooked on high all day, turned on first thing in the morning.

Pearl chats: This is my husband's favorite meal. I make it for his birthday, or when I want to especially please him. You can add vegetables such as onions and celery to the crockpot a few hours before serving so they don't get too mushy being cooked all day. I often add a small side salad.

All Day Lentil or Chana Dahl Soup – E

This meal is cheap, cheap, cheap! But, tasty too, not to mention fantastic for your health.

Soaking both chana dahl and lentils is best, but if you forget, lentils are one legume where it doesn't matter as much. Chana dahl, on the other hand, is always best soaked. A little Indian secret is to add ¼-¾ teaspoon of baking soda to your soak water (depending on dahl amounts). This softens the hard surface of the dahl and helps it cook up softer and mushier. Pour off the water used for soaking first and add fresh before cooking.

If you have pre-diabetes, a challenging case of insulin resistance, or full blown Type 2 diabetes, it will be best for you to use chana dahl for this recipe. While lentils contain a good amount of resistant starch, chana dahl is safer for your body since this soup is tasty, and you'll probably want to eat a couple of bowls full. Chana dahl makes a lovely, creamy, thick soup. You just want to stare with awe at the creamy, golden color.

Basic Ingredients: lentils or chana dahl ✦ water or chicken stock/broth ✦ onions ✦ celery ✦ sea salt and other seasonings like turmeric, or curry if using chana dahl ✦ optional chicken breast and spinach leaves

1. Put soaked lentils or chana dahl in large crockpot with 6 cups of water or chicken stock/broth for each pound of legumes. Since we have big families we use 1½-2 lbs. of legumes. It's cheaper to use water, but using chicken broth as some of the liquid gives a fuller flavor to the soup.
2. Add diced onions and celery.
3. Season with lots of sea salt, pepper, cayenne pepper, onion powder, handful of nutritional yeast, and Bragg Liquid Aminos. If you do not have Bragg Liquid Aminos,

you will need to be pretty heavy with sea salt. Chana dahl lends itself well to curry flavors so you could also add a little curry paste or turmeric powder.

4. Cook all day, adding more liquid if needed.
5. To increase the protein content, you may add diced chicken breast and spinach leaves (which will wilt nicely) in the last hour before serving. These additions give another dimension to the soup, but are not necessary.

You can also top this soup with a little skim mozzarella cheese or non-fat Greek yogurt if desired, which increases the protein count. You may include one piece of plan approved toast without spiking your blood sugar. Or, you could choose to have a small piece of fruit for dessert. Children will want lots of grated cheese and whole wheat toast and butter with their soup.

Cabbage Rolls – S

Cabbage is the perfect low-carb vegetable. It is versatile, too.

Basic Ingredients: cabbage ✦ ground beef ✦ eggs ✦ onion ✦ green pepper ✦ sea salt and other seasonings ✦ tomato sauce or diced tomatoes ✦ Worcester sauce

1. Blanch 14 large cabbage leaves in boiling water for 5 minutes to soften.
2. In a bowl, mix 2 lbs. ground beef with 2 eggs, 1 finely cut onion, and 1 finely diced green pepper.
3. Season beef filling mix with desired seasonings—salt, pepper, chili powder, and onion powder work well.
4. Plop a little filling in the middle of each cabbage leaf and roll it up, tucking the sides in as you roll so you end up with an enclosed cylindrical shape.
5. Put rolls in crockpot and cover with 1 (8 oz.) can of tomato sauce, or 1 can diced or crushed tomatoes seasoned with Worcester sauce, sea salt, and pepper.
6. Cook on med/high in crockpot for 7-9 hours.

Once you're in **S helper** stage, you may add some quinoa to the meat/egg mix.

Corned Beef and Cabbage – S

Basic Ingredients: corned beef ✦ water ✦ cabbage ✦ seasonings

1. Place side of corned beef in crockpot, along with contents of the seasonings packet it may come with, or use your own seasonings.
2. Add as much cabbage on top of corned beef as your crockpot can hold.

3 Add water to almost cover and cook on low all day.

Alternate method: add cabbage two hours before serving and squish it down to immerse in some water so it cooks more quickly.

Moist Chicken Breast Slow Cooker Ideas

Chicken breasts can often be dry and unappealing. The crockpot changes all that. All moisture is retained, and the slow way of cooking helps marinate seasonings and flavors into the meat. Depending on the sauce accompanying the chicken breasts, they can be easily morphed into either **E** or **S** category since the breast of chicken is very lean.

Frozen tenderloins can be placed in the crockpot in the morning and they'll be soft and ready by evening. Regular sized chicken breast sizes should be thawed first or started on low the night before. You can leave the tenderloins or breasts whole. By evening, when they're ready, they will easily pull apart into much smaller pieces by using a couple of forks.

E Crockpot Chicken Ideas

Chicken breasts can still be succulent, even crockpot **E** style by the addition of chicken broth and lots of high water content vegetables such as tomatoes and onions etc. Adding 1-2 Tbs. cream, tahini, or coconut milk to the whole recipe (big enough for a large family to eat) once it is cooked, will not destroy the **E** factor, but give just enough fat to aid digestion and bring a more rounded flavor to the palette. Or, you can add 1 Tbs. coconut oil or butter.

Since the following ideas are **E**, if quinoa or brown rice are not included in the recipe itself, they will usually be a perfect accompaniment. Alternatively, you could dunk crusty whole grain sourdough bread into these **E** dishes. Remember, no more than 2 slices, even with **E**.

Any of the following recipes that do not include a starch like quinoa, rice, or beans in the actual recipe could be used for a **Fuel Pull** meal. However **Fuel Pull** meals are the only ones where we like you to keep to smaller amounts of lean meat protein e.g. 3 oz. servings. The following crockpot chicken ideas are designed to be eaten liberally, so it's probably a better idea to simply enjoy them as **E's** and not worry too much about portion size. There are plenty of other **Fuel Pulls** recipes that automatically keep your meat protein pulled back.

- **E Italian style**: Along with chicken breasts, throw in canned tomatoes, onions, long string beans, a little chicken broth, sea salt, black pepper, and Italian seasoning. Add in uncooked quinoa or brown rice, or throw in some pre-cooked or canned beans or chick peas at the end.
- **Light Coconut Curry**: Along with chicken breasts, throw in contents of one can of light coconut milk with additional water (any amount to make the meal go further).

Add onions, broccoli or cauliflower florets (or both), bamboo shoots, etc., red or green curry paste, sea salt, and black pepper. Thicken with glucomannan if curry sauce is too thin at the end. Serve over quinoa or brown rice in appropriate **E** sized portions.

- **Spinach lovers:** Along with chicken breasts, pour in 1-1½ cups of chicken stock or broth (either homemade or store-bought free range). Add sea salt, black pepper, and any other seasonings of your choice. A couple of hours before serving, add lots of bunches of fresh spinach (or 1-2 packets of frozen spinach) and let wilt and simmer with chicken for a while. To kick this up to superfood status, at the end you can add 1 Tbs. virgin coconut oil and 2 Tbs. Bernard Jensen's gelatin flakes, or even Knox gelatin if you have not made your own chicken stock. The gelatin, whether formed through homemade chicken stock, or added as powdered gelatin, soothes the digestive tract and repairs the body's joints, bones, and cartilage. Take out some of the broth from the crock-pot, put it in a cup, mix in the gelatin and return to the pot.
- **Spinach Lovers Italiano:** This is basically the same idea as the above recipe but with a couple of added ingredients. Cut up 2-3 onions into rounds and place these at the bottom of the crock before placing in the chicken breasts. Include the contents of one small can of tomato paste, Italian seasoning, onion powder, and a couple of generous swirls of balsamic vinegar. Add 1 Tbs. of coconut oil or butter at the end.
- **E Mexican style:** Along with chicken breasts, add 1 can of black beans, 1-2 jars of salsa, a little chicken broth (maybe ½ cup), onion, peppers, canned tomatoes, sea salt, and black pepper. You could accompany this meal with 0% Greek yogurt in place of sour cream, or you may use low-fat sour cream (not quite as healthy). You could sprinkle a little grated, skim mozzarella on top of your dish and even dunk in a few baked blue corn chips. Make sure the chips are baked, not fried, as fried chips cause a **Crossover** effect.
- **Spaghetti Sauce Chicken:** Along with chicken breasts, add a jar or two of "no added sugar" tomato based pasta sauce, or make your own. Ragu has one that is appropriate and available in most supermarkets. Make sure the pasta sauce is low-fat. You can enjoy this chicken over **E** appropriate amounts of quinoa or rice.

S Crockpot Chicken Ideas:

Use breast meat with the following ideas, but boneless skinless thighs work well also. Any cuts of chicken, even with bones may be used.

- **Creamy Cheesy Chicken:** Along with chicken, add 1 packet of ⅓ less fat Philadelphia cream cheese, sea salt, and black pepper. Cream cheese turns into the perfect white, creamy sauce in the crockpot as it merges with the natural juices from the chicken. Eat as a basic creamy white sauce, or you could add salsa (cream cheese and salsa are a perfect combination). Other ideas include dry white wine and a little chicken broth/stock. Or, 1 can of green chilies and/or jalapenos. Or, if you'd rather, how about chicken broth/stock, nutritional yeast, and parmesan cheese? All these combinations are delicious, and any of them can be thickened up at the end with glucomannan if they are too thin for your liking.

- **Alfredo chicken**: Along with chicken, add homemade or store-bought Alfredo sauce (you know the store-bought idea does not come from Serene). Make sure the store-bought sauce has no more than two carbs. Homemade Alfredo can be easily made with mozzarella cheese, heavy cream, mushrooms, sea salt, black pepper, and a little garlic powder all thrown into the crockpot with the chicken. These ingredients join together slowly and perfectly in the crockpot. This recipe can be eaten over Dreamfields or konjac noodles, spaghetti squash, cabbage noodles, cauliflower rice, or poured over steamed broccoli or cauliflower. join
- **S Italian style:** Along with chicken, add 1-2 cups of homemade Italian style dressing and 1-2 cups of chicken broth. Or, use a healthy store-bought jar of Italian style dressing along with the chicken broth. Try to purchase brands that don't use soybean or canola oils. But, hey, if you don't care about soy bean oil in your diet now and then, Ken's Italian dressing works great because it has only 1 carb. If you want to make your own, olive oil based dressings would be okay as heat temperatures remain lower with a crockpot. Optimally, you could make your homemade Italian style dressing with coconut oil as you won't be eating this dish cold and don't have to worry about the oil firming up. At the end of the day, you can mix in some sour cream or Greek yogurt and ¼-½ cup of Parmesan cheese. This dish is great with any of our **S** approved noodle options.
- **S Mexican Style:** Pour in 1 jar of salsa or green chilies and tomatoes to cook all day with the chicken breasts. At evening, when it's ready, top with full-fat sour cream, plenty of cheese, and sliced black olives. Please, no corn chips. However, you could try our low-carb *Joseph's Crackers/Chips* (*Snacks,* Chapter 24). You could also use ground beef in place of chicken.
- **S Style Chicken Curry:** Along with chicken, throw in contents of 1-2 cans of full-fat coconut milk, red or green Thai curry paste or curry powder, sea salt, black pepper, and lots of non-starchy veggies like broccoli and cauliflower florets, onion, cabbage, and red peppers.

Hearty Oven Dishes

Fantastic Meat Loaf – S (Serene's version)

Basic Ingredients: ground meat ✦ eggs ✦ onion ✦ celery ✦ plan approved bread crumbs or oats ✦ sea salt and other seasonings ✦ tomato paste ✦ water

1. Put 3 lbs. thawed ground meat (choose either/or combination of lamb, beef, turkey) in a bowl.
2. Add 2-3 eggs.
3. Sauté one diced onion and 2-3 large diced stalks of celery and add to bowl.
4. Blend, or food process ½ measuring cup of plan approved bread/tortillas, or ½ cup oats. These amounts, when used in this full recipe, do not even amount to an **S helper**.
5. Add sea salt, black pepper, cayenne pepper, splashes of hot sauce, tamari or Bragg Liquid Aminos, onion and/or garlic powder.
6. Mix well and put in baking dish, forming a nice loaf shape with your hands. Leave a space for a canal/moat around the outside of meat loaf.
7. Ice top of loaf with one 6 oz. can of tomato paste, then sprinkle with sea salt, black pepper, and Italian seasonings.
8. Pour ¾ cup water into canal to keep loaf moist.
9. Bake at 350 for approximately 1 hour. Check to see if done at 45 minutes.

Cooking time can be reduced by putting mixture in muffin tins. These look fun on the plate and are easily pulled out of the fridge as leftovers for the next day.

This recipe is perfect with homemade *Cauliflower Mashed Potatoes,* (*Vegetable Sides*, Chapter 22). Children, with their greater need for carbs, can enjoy sides of brown rice or real mashed potatoes, and a glass of preferably raw milk.

Serene chats: I like to use grass fed or organic beef when I can afford it for this recipe as I do not like to eat regular store-bought kind when I am not draining off the grease. Sometimes I use ground lamb. It is absolutely delicious in meat loaf and since it is not mass marketed in USA, it comes from smaller farms and is usually pastured or grass fed. You can find a cheaper source for lamb by locating an international market where Middle Eastern people purchase their special halal killed meat. These nationalities live on lamb and goat and, as it is not a specialty item to them, it can be bought without hurting your pocket too much. At one such store, they grind it up freshly in front of me and I usually ask for organ meats, like heart or liver, to be ground up with it. The organ meats are very healthy and when included in this loaf, you would never suspect it.

Easy (and fantastic) Meat Loaf – S (Pearl's version)

Pearl chats: Serene's version of meatloaf received the title "fantastic," while my version called *Easy Meatloaf* is pretty depictive of our different approaches. Hopefully, Serene doesn't find out, but I went back and sneaked the word "fantastic" into my title, too. Why should she have all the glory, huh? Nevertheless, this recipe gets lots of praise in our home. Honestly, I haven't had the budget for grass fed meat so I usually make this loaf with whatever is on sale at one of my three favorite grocery stores.

The size of this loaf, which uses 3 lbs. of beef, is just right for the seven in our family, but my boys are huuuuuuuuge eaters! They love this meal, not only because they think the meat loaf is good, but they know I usually make creamy mashed potatoes to go with it and they're crazy about "mashies." I sauté long string beans for Charlie and myself to enjoy instead of the mashed potatoes, although, if it's **Crossover** time for me, I'll also have a small helping of "mashies."

For smaller families with only two to three children, this meatloaf would be enough for two meal's worth. You could freeze half of it after cooking to save you prep time for another evening meal. Or, the next day, send some in a sandwich on an **S** approved bread with your husband to work. Rarely do we have leftovers, but on the rare occasion, my husband really enjoys a meatloaf sandwich the next day. If you have a larger family, double the recipe.

Basic Ingredients: ground beef ✦ salsa ✦ sour cream ✦ eggs ✦ optional Joseph's pita bread ground into crumbs ✦ sea salt, fajita seasoning and other seasonings

1. Put 3 lbs. thawed ground beef into a bowl.
2. Add 1-½ cups salsa (medium or hot depending on tastes).
3. Add ½ cup sour cream.
4. Add 3 beaten eggs.
5. Optional: Add ½ cup ground Joseph's crumbs, although I don't usually add the crumbs.
6. Add ½ packet of fajita or taco seasoning, 1 tsp. chili powder, plus a little extra salt and several dashes of pepper.
7. Mix all ingredients well.
8. Bake in one extra large casserole dish or two smaller ones at 350 for 60 minutes.
9. Five minutes before baking time is up, take meat loaf out of oven and pour out most of the excess grease and fluid that is created while cooking. This is pretty easy because the meat loaf separates from the sides of the casserole dish. Hold the loaf with a spatula so it doesn't fall out while pouring.

10. Broil for 5 more minutes to brown top of loaf. Alternatively, mix more salsa with grated cheese and top the meatloaf to melt 5 minutes before end of cooking.

Note: Most Taco and Fajita seasonings contain some sugar and other junky fillers. Look out for a brand called *Wick Fowler's Famous Taco Seasoning*. It is a much healthier alternative, with less carbs, too. If you can't get this brand, using only half a packet of regular taco seasoning is not too terrible for the full recipe.

Mini Meat Loaves – E or Fuel Pull

The wonderful spices give a lot of flavor to these lean mini loaves and the added veggies make them moist. They might end up as your favorite, even though it would be overkill to add the word "fantastic" to this title, too. Eat loaves with only a salad with a light dressing for a **Fuel Pull,** or make our *Creamless Creamy Veggies* as a side. For **E**, they could be eaten with a side of rice, quinoa, or *Waldorf Cottage Cheese Salad.* (*Lunches*, Chapter 20).The amount of quinoa already in the recipe is minimal and allows the loaves to stay in **Fuel Pull** territory**.**

You can freeze any that are leftover and pull one out for a quick reheatable **Fuel Pull** lunch with a salad. If you want to make this into a loaf, add 15 minutes to the cooking time.

Basic Ingredients: extra lean ground turkey ✦ 0% Greek yogurt ✦ pre-cooked quinoa ✦ onions ✦ celery ✦ tomatoes ✦ hot sauce ✦ pickled jalapenos ✦ sea salt and other seasonings ✦ Hunt's Garlic and Herb tomato paste

1. Put 3 lbs. extra lean ground turkey (96-99% lean) in a bowl.
2. Add 1 cup egg whites. Carton kind is fine, or 7 home separated whites.
3. Add ½ cup 0% Greek yogurt and ½ cup pre-cooked quinoa.
4. In a pan, sauté 2-3 diced tomatoes, 4 finely sliced stalks of celery, and 2 finely diced onions. No oil is needed due to juice from the tomatoes. Add veggies to bowl once they are very tender.
5. Add 1 tsp. sea salt, generous shakes of black pepper, an optional dash of cayenne pepper, onion powder, and garlic powder to taste.
6. Add several generous splashes of hot sauce and some diced, pickled jalapenos.
7. Mix all ingredients very well. Fill up lightly greased muffin tins with mixture.
8. Ice the top of mini loaves with tomato paste (garlic and herb works well).
9. Bake for 45 minutes at 350.

Basic Quiche – S

You won't miss the crust on this quiche. If you do, a quick basic crust can be made by whizzing up one cup of almonds in a blender (or using almond flour) and mixing it with one egg white. Spread the mix out on your greased baking dish and par-bake for 10 minutes before adding quiche ingredients on top. An even shorter version is to simply sprinkle ground nuts with a little salt and pepper on the bottom of the well greased baking dish before pouring in the quiche mixture. This gives the hint of a crust without actually being a full crust.

Basic Ingredients: eggs ✦ grated cheese ✦ sea salt and other seasonings

1. Crack 12 eggs into bowl and whisk thoroughly.
2. Add 2 cups grated cheese.
3. Add sea salt and black pepper to taste.
4. Bake at 350 for 30-45 minutes.

From this basic foundation, you can create many high protein quiche dishes for your evening meal by adding any of the following ideas to your skeleton recipe.

- Chopped spinach and bacon bits.
- Turkey or chicken sausage with finely cut green onion and green peppers.
- Canned salmon and spinach (omit cheese for this one).
- Ground beef and drained small can of green chilies and tomatoes.
- Sliced natural deli meats, olives, and mushrooms.
- Any leftovers such as baked or pulled chicken, broccoli, and finely diced onion.

The above quiches ideas are made even more delicious by finely slicing tomatoes and placing them in a single layer on top. Season the tomatoes generously with sea salt, black and red pepper, and Italian seasonings. The tomatoes crisp nicely for an added gourmet texture. However, we only do this when we have time on our hands or want to impress visitors!

Roast Lamb – S

Growing up in New Zealand, this was a weekly staple in our home. New Zealand has a sheep population of about 40 million compared to less than four and a half million people. Therefore, lamb is king of roasts Downunder. Now, due to expense, we usually only have lamb for Thanksgiving, Christmas, and other special occasions. It is our absolute favorite celebratory meal, and the aroma of it cooking brings back many great childhood memories. At Christmas time, when our whole family gets together, it is as much about smelling the lamb as it is about singing carols.

Forgive our pride for a minute, but many of us born in New Zealand think we are the only ones who know how to cook lamb properly. Long and slow is the key, which our mother taught us. To cook lamb in under four hours would be a travesty (although we don't usual cook lamb, but rather hogget or mutton).

Basic Ingredients: lamb ✦ sea salt and other seasonings including dried rosemary, thyme, or sage ✦ water

1. Season stringed roast, or leg of lamb generously with sea salt, black pepper, cayenne pepper and dried rosemary (rosemary is very important to enhance flavor and the aroma of the lamb during cooking).
2. Place in baking dish and pour in about half an inch of water.
3. Cover loosely with foil or bake in a Dutch oven (iron baking dish with lid).
4. Bake at 250 for 4-6 hours, depending on size of lamb roast.
5. Fifteen minutes before serving, remove foil or lid and either turn baking temperature up, or broil until edges are crispy.
6. Transfer roast to serving tray to carve.
7. Spoon some of the cooking juices over the meat and add squirts of Bragg Liquid Aminos, or a little more sea salt and pepper.

Make gravy by using the leftover juices in the pan, according to our *Basic Gravy* (*Gravies, Sauces, and Condiment*s, Chapter 25. This recipe also works great with lamb chops also, but less cooking time is needed.

Get Together Salmon – S

This next recipe is great when cooking fish for the entire family, or taking to a pot-luck party. It is always popular and there are no leftovers to take home or pack away. The real secret to the success of this dish is using a fresh (not previously frozen) large tray sized fillet of salmon. At "bring a dish" events everyone raves over it. You might even get the award for best dish!

Due to the expense of buying fresh fish, we make this recipe with farm raised salmon. If you have the money, then splurge on an Alaskan wild caught "melt in your mouth" fillet.

Serene chats: I make a wild caught frozen variety regularly for my family as an evening meal. It is still divine although not as incredibly sublime.

Basic Ingredients: large salmon fillet ✦ sea salt and other seasonings ✦ butter ✦ lemon ✦ red wine or balsamic vinegar

1. Place salmon fillet on large piece of foil and rub down with sea salt, black pepper, and optional onion and garlic powder. Sprinkle generously with dried dill and a few optional capers.
2. Slice thin pats of butter and lemon slices and arrange over fillet.
3. Generously drizzle with red wine or balsamic vinegar.
4. Wrap fish tightly in the foil. This makes a pouch for the salmon to steam in the wine. If using a frozen fillet, you could thinly slice a whole large onion and layer this on top of the salmon to keep the texture super moist.
5. Bake at 350 until fish flakes perfectly, about 25-30 minutes.

Whole Baked Chickens – S

Basic Ingredients: whole chickens ✦ sea salt and other seasonings ✦ mustard

1. Generously season 2-3 thawed chickens with sea salt, black pepper, nutritional yeast, and onion powder.
2. Drizzle your favorite prepared mustard in zigzags all over the chicken. The mustard is optional, but creates a gourmet effect for the eyes, as well as the palette.
3. Place chickens in oven uncovered in the early afternoon. Bake slow and easy at 225 all afternoon, basting with juices several times.

The slow baking in the oven is the key to ultimate succulent baked chicken. You can turn the oven temperature up 15 minutes before serving to give an extra crisp to the skin. Remember, chicken skin is not your enemy with **S** meals. It's actually a very healthy fat, especially if using free range chickens.

Serene chats: If there is any meat left after the meal is over, I fill little baggies of single meal portion sizes with the leaner white meat in some and the darker, higher fat meat in others. I place some in the freezer, and a few in the fridge, for quick and easy **S** or **E** protein additions for lunches. These work well for me when my children are having a lunch that's not appropriate for me. When I have taken a little extra thought to fill sandwich size baggies with appropriate sized portions of protein or **E** carbs, I am always prepared and never desperate enough to make impulsive wrong choices.

Baked Chicken Thighs – S

This chicken comes out very moist and tender, yet crispy on top. Thighs are an inexpensive part of the chicken to purchase in frozen bags. Take the bag out in the morning to thaw, or defrost in fridge overnight. If you do any defrosting in the microwave, take the chicken out of the plastic bag and put on a microwave safe plate or tray. Plastics that leach into foods from microwave heating can become xenoestrogens (harmful compounds that mimic estrogen) in the body.

These chicken pieces need to be started by 2:30–3:00 pm in the afternoon to be ready for the evening meal.

Basic Ingredients: chicken thighs ✦ Creole seasoning and optional cayenne pepper

1. Place thawed chicken thighs on a baking tray and sprinkle liberally with Creole seasoning (and cayenne pepper if you like it spicy and hot).
2. Bake, covered with foil or lid, at 275 for at least 3 hours until very tender.
3. Uncover 15 minutes before serving and broil until skin is crispy.

Coconut Crusted Chicken (or Salmon) – S

Basic Ingredients: chicken tenderloins ✦ eggs or optional mayonnaise ✦ dried coconut ✦ sea salt and other seasonings

1. Dip fresh or thawed chicken tenderloins or salmon fillets into a couple of whisked eggs, or rub pieces with mayonnaise with your hands.
2. To make breading, place the following ingredients into blender: 1 cup dried coconut flakes, salt and pepper, parsley flakes, onion and/or garlic powder, and optional cayenne pepper. Blend until fine and pour breading mix onto large dinner plate.
3. Coat chicken pieces generously with faux breading by laying each side of chicken or salmon in the crumbs.
4. Grease baking dish or two well and lay tenderloins singularly on tray and bake at 350 until meat is tender and breading is crispy, approximately 30 minutes.

Easy Chicken Yogurt Bake – S, E or Fuel Pull

Basic Ingredients: chicken breasts or tenderloins ✦ Greek yogurt ✦ sea salt and other seasonings

1. Place fresh or thawed chicken breasts or tenderloins on large baking tray.

2. In a bowl mix 2-3 cups 0% Greek yogurt with sea salt, black pepper, garlic powder, and optional dried rosemary.
3. Cover chicken with yogurt mix.
4. Bake uncovered at 350 for 45 minutes to1 hour.

For **E** style, eat with ¾ cup quinoa or rice and a side salad with a light dressing. As an **S** dish, this goes great with *Tabouleh (Lunches,* Chapter 20). If using for **Fuel Pull**, keep to only two tenderloins or half a breast.

Spicy Chicken Wings – S

This recipe should make any husband happy.

Basic Ingredients: chicken wings ✦ sea salt ✦ butter ✦ hot sauce ✦ optional cayenne pepper

1. Layer fresh or thawed drummettes, or any chicken pieces, on baking trays.
2. Sprinkle lightly with sea salt.
3. In a bowl, mix 1 cup Frank's wing sauce with ½ cup melted butter. Add cayenne pepper if you like wings spicy, because Frank's sauce does not have a lot of heat.
4. Arrange wings single layer on baking tray. Pour on sauce and mix wings well with the sauce, using your hands.
5. Bake on multiple racks if needed at 450 for about 45 minutes to1 hour, turning wings once. At the end of baking, broil the top sides until wings reach desired crispiness.

We mentioned Frank's sauce because it doesn't have carbs. Chicken wings have a lot of fat, so please don't pour on sauce with sugar which would be certain to make the fat from the wings stick to you. Unfortunately, many store-bought wings have quite a few carbs as they use sauces with sugars or coat the wings in flour first. You can use any brand of hot sauce of your choice as long as it only has 1 carb or less.

Pearl chats: We are a chicken wing loving family and when I make these I really make them. I use two full 4 lb. bags of wing sections. This way everybody in the family can eat as much as they like, and there are even leftovers for the next day for hungry family members to grab out of the fridge. Charlie and I eat a plateful of these wings, with a side of celery and sour cream in which to dip the celery. I offer a whole grain carb side to the children, but mostly we all hoe into wings. I buy the frozen bags from Aldi and pay just over $15 for the two bags. I know that is a little pricey, but we only treat ourselves to these once or twice a month.

I don't find Frank's sauce spicy enough, so I add more cayenne pepper. Charlie and I and the older children enjoy the wings very spicy. I make one tray of spicier wings for ourselves and another tray for the younger ones without the added cayenne pepper.

We are a football loving family due to my husband's influence. These are fun to make for game nights, or afternoons when we all gather around to watch the game, and either cheer or be disgusted.

Boneless Wings – S

This is another variation on hot wings.

Basic Ingredients: chicken tenderloins ✦ Parmesan cheese ✦ Frank's hot sauce ✦ sea salt ✦ butter ✦ optional lemon juice or vinegar

1. Cut thawed chicken tenderloins into smaller pieces.
2. Toss in parmesan cheese and a little sea salt.
3. Broil on well-oiled tray for 20 minutes, turning once.
4. While wings are cooking, heat up sauce in saucepan consisting of 2 Tbs. butter, 1 cup Frank's hot sauce, and 1 optional Tbs. lemon juice or vinegar.
5. Pour over chicken and broil 5 more minutes.

Balsamic Chicken – E

Basic Ingredients: chicken breasts or tenderloins ✦ tomatoes ✦ onions ✦ tomato paste ✦ balsamic vinegar ✦ sweetener ✦ chicken broth/stock or water ✦ sea salt and other seasonings

1. Place family size amount of frozen chicken breasts or tenderloins, single layer, on large baking tray.
2. Cover with diced tomatoes and onions.
3. Blend 1 (6 oz.) can tomato paste with a few generous splashes of balsamic vinegar, 2 tsp. Truvia or a tiny dash of Nunaturals, 1 cup chicken broth/stock or 1 cup water, handful of nutritional yeast, 1 tsp. sea salt, and fresh or dried Italian herbs.
4. Pour blended sauce mixture on top of chicken and vegetables.

5. Bake uncovered at 350 until chicken is tender and sauce is reduced a little, about 45 minutes.
6. Serve over **E** appropriate amounts of quinoa or brown rice.

Children can have a pat of butter with their chicken to make sure they get adequate amounts of primary fuels.

Peanut Crusted Chicken – S

The credit for this delicious recipe goes to our sister-in-law, Monique. She created it when she had chicken, a jar of peanut butter, and not much else. It works fantastically with boneless chicken thigh tenderloins, but breast tenderloins are fine also.

Basic Ingredients: boneless chicken breasts or thighs ✦ sugar-free peanut butter ✦ water ✦ coconut oil ✦ sea salt and other seasonings including lots of black pepper

1. Pre-cook chicken boneless breasts or thighs by poaching in a pot with water, or bake in a covered tray until nearly tender.
2. In a small bowl, mix 1 cup peanut butter with ¼ cup water using a whisk.
3. To the bowl add Bragg Liquid Aminos, 2 Tbs. coconut oil, red pepper, sea salt, lots of black pepper (much more than you think you should), and onion powder. Mix all sauce ingredients together.
4. Place cooked chicken pieces on large dinner plate and pour peanut sauce on top. Using your hands, toss chicken around in the sauce, making sure all pieces are well covered. Messy, but fun.
5. Place coated chicken on oiled cookie sheet.
6. Broil on middle rack, turning chicken a couple of times so both sides become nicely browned and very crispy.

An alternative way to make this recipe is to use uncooked breast tenderloins, coat them in the sauce, and fry them in coconut oil. Still yummy, but takes longer for those with large families, as you'll have to do multiple batches.

Chile Relleno Casserole – S

Basic Ingredients: chicken breasts or tenderloins ✦ eggs ✦ cans of diced chilies and tomatoes ✦ grated cheese ✦ sea salt and other seasonings

1. Poach or bake bag of chicken breasts or tenderloins to cook quickly.

2. Once chicken is cooked through, dice into bite size pieces and set aside.
3. Beat seven eggs in bowl.
4. Drain 2 (15 oz.) cans Rotel style diced chilies and tomatoes, or 3 small cans diced green chilies and to bowl.
5. Grate 2 (8 oz.) blocks cheddar or Monterrey Jack cheese and add to bowl.
6. Add diced cooked chicken to bowl.
7. Season with a little salt and pepper and mix ingredients well.
8. Pour into greased baking or casserole dish and bake at 350 for 45 minutes.

Cheeseburger Pie – S

This is a memorable treat for a meal. On a whole, the male species love this one. It's high fat, which is fine, as high fat meals are welcome on our plan. However, you might want to leave out any **S Helpers** when eating this recipe. It's that decadent.

There are many versions of this basic recipe floating around. That's because we all have our own ideas of what a perfect cheeseburger should be like. Basically, anyway you like your cheeseburger can apply to this pie. You could include a layer of finely diced sautéed onions, dill pickles, jalapeños, or even a layer of tomatoes. Our children love to top this pie with a little mustard and lots of ketchup. If topping with ketchup, make sure you use a homemade one without sugar, or a store-bought sugar-free version.

Basic Ingredients: ground beef ✦ sea salt and other seasonings including onion powder or onion soup mix ✦ grated cheese ✦ eggs ✦ mayonnaise ✦ heavy cream ✦optional onions, pickles, jalapeños or tomatoes

1. Brown 2 lbs. beef and drain fat if it is not grass fed.
2. Add 3 tsp. onion powder and 1 tsp. salt. Alternatively, use 1 packet onion soup mix instead of onion powder and salt. It makes it taste fantastic, but is not as healthy and has a couple of carbs, but Pearl says she still likes to use it now and then for pleasure's sake!
3. Place beef mixture in casserole dish and stir in 6 oz. grated cheese.
4. Place layer of any optional mentioned ingredients over beef and cheese combination, or skip this step for a more basic pie.
5. In another bowl beat 2 eggs, ½ cup mayo, ½ cup heavy cream, sea salt, and black pepper.
6. Pour mix over beef and top with another 6 oz. cheese.

7 Bake at 350 for 35 minutes.

Serve with either, or both, a side salad and steamed buttery vegetables.

Pizza Casserole – S

Basic Ingredients: ground beef ✦ plan approved pizza sauce ✦ green peppers ✦ olives ✦ onions ✦ grated mozzarella cheese ✦ pepperoni

1. Brown 2 lbs. ground beef and drain off fat if it is not grass fed.
2. Spread layer of ground beef at bottom of large casserole dish.
3. Spread thin layer of no added sugar pizza or pasta sauce over meat.
4. Add layer of finely chopped green peppers, olives, and onions (or other veggies you like with pizza).
5. Add layer of grated mozzarella cheese.
6. Add layer of pepperoni (we use turkey).
7. Add another layer of ground beef.
8. Add another very thin layer of pizza or pasta sauce.
9. Top with more grated cheese and scattered pepperoni.
10. Bake at 400 for 20 minutes, or until cheese is bubbly and toppings are crisping. You may broil at the end for a crispier topping.

Stove Top Tummy Warmers— (Chili, Curries, Stews & Soups)

Chili and hot soups—the ultimate in comfort foods. They bring the family together and you'll be glad to know you can still enjoy them on plan.

Regarding chili, if you're just starting out toward weight loss, it is best to eat chili without too many beans. One can of beans in a large pot of chili, big enough to feed a whole family, would still be in **S** category. Beans are slow to raise blood sugar, and a few of them won't hinder weight loss too much in an **S** meal. But, chili is high in tomatoes, both paste and diced tomatoes, which are slightly more carby than most non-starchy veggies. If you add more beans than one can on top of all the tomato products, you are easily at **S helper** status. Adding in further amounts of beans would put you in **Crossover** mode.

We, as sisters, have quite different approaches to chili. Pearl's is short-cut inspired and more practical. Serene cuts no corners for health and purity's sake.

Pearl's Chili – S or S Helper (feeds large family)

Pearl chats: My chili is famous around these parts. Just honking my own horn—somebody's got to do it!

Basic Ingredients: ground beef ✦ onion ✦ cans of diced green chilies and tomatoes ✦ tomato sauce ✦ beans ✦ water ✦ sea salt and other seasonings

1. Brown 3 lbs. meat in large pot and drain off excess fat.
2. Add 1 large chopped onion and cook with ground beef for a couple of minutes.
3. Add 2 cans diced Rotel green chilies and tomatoes for spicier chili, or 1 can Rotel style chilies and tomatoes and 1 can petite diced tomatoes for a milder chili.
4. Add 1 small (8 oz.) can tomato sauce.
5. Add 1-1½ drained (15 oz.) cans of any type of beans.
6. Add 1-2 empty cans of water, depending on how much broth you like.
7. Add sea salt, 1 Tbs. chili powder, 1 tsp. onion powder, good squirt or two of Bragg Liquid Aminos, and for those who like it extra spicy, some good shakes of cayenne pepper.
8. Simmer all ingredients for 45 minutes to 1 hour on stove, or cook on low in crock-pot all day.

Pearl chats: If you need the chili to go further for a big family so everyone can have seconds, put in at least two cans of beans. If I do this, I make sure to not put as many beans in Charlie's and my bowls when I dish out. I ladle the chili into our bowls and take a few seconds to skim out extra beans and return them to the pot. This way the children get more beans in their servings to help fill them up.

If you really love more beans in your chili, think about using two or more cans of Eden's Black soy beans. We have previously discussed that they are a very low carb bean option so you won't have to worry about quantity. However, skip this soy option if you have any thyroid issues.

Serve this chili with grated cheese and optional sour cream. Along with the grated cheese, my children like to crumble whole wheat saltine crackers or organic blue corn chips on top. Charlie and I don't miss these.

Serene's Company Chili (works for S or S Helper for you, but ends up Crossover for everybody else).

This makes a huge amount of chili. Make sure you have an extra large cauldron in which to cook it.

Basic Ingredients: pinto beans ✦ apple cider vinegar ✦ ground beef ✦ onions ✦ tomato paste ✦ water ✦ sea salt and other seasonings ✦ tahini

1. Overnight soak 2 lbs. pinto beans in pot of warm water and 2 spoonfuls of apple cider vinegar to remove phytates. Leave plenty of room for beans to expand.
2. Next morning drain beans, place back in pot, and add water to an inch over beans.
3. Add generous pinch of sea salt to beans, cover, and bring to boil, then turn to med/low and simmer until beans are tender, about 2-3 hours. Once they are tender, set beans aside in fridge until it's close to supper time.
4. Later that afternoon, brown 5 lbs. ground beef (preferably grass fed). Drain fat if meat is not grass fed.
5. Add 2-3 diced onions to drained meat.
6. Add 3 small cans tomato paste and enough water to pot to allow for a consistency that is neither too gluggy, nor too brothy.
7. Add sea salt, chili powder, nutritional yeast, cayenne pepper, hot sauce, and onion and garlic powder to taste.
8. Add 1-2 heaping Tbs. tahini (sesame seed paste) which helps bring out deep meaty flavors.
9. Simmer for a while until flavors nicely mingle.
10. Close to meal time, remove your chili portion from pot (maybe more for second helpings, or for a quick reheatable lunch for the next day).
11. Add very small portion of beans to your chili, then pour rest of beans into the pot with the rest of ingredients.
12. Taste, and add more flavors if necessary since the addition of the beans will neutralize some of the original flavor of the chili.

Serene chats: This is a wonderful meal that is always enjoyed and drained to the bottom of the pot by a large crowd. I make it for birthday parties for the main course where up to 20 or more people may be digging in. They also top up with blue corn chips, salsa, and lots of grated cheese. I also make this large batch for an evening meal and heat the leftovers for the children for lunch the next day. I enjoy it with cheese and salsa only. However, if you really miss the crunch, appropriate chips and cracker recipes can be found in *Snacks*, Chapter 24.

Lighter Side of Chili – E

Basic Ingredients: extra lean ground turkey or pulled chicken breast ✦ onion ✦ can of diced tomatoes and green chilies ✦ green or red peppers ✦ chicken broth/stock or water ✦ nutritional yeast ✦ tomato paste ✦ beans ✦ sea salt and other seasonings ✦ optional 0% Greek yogurt

1. Brown 2 lbs. extra lean ground turkey or use pulled white chicken meat and set aside.
2. Cook 1 large diced onion with 1 (15 oz.) can of diced tomatoes and green chilies. You could also use fresh diced tomatoes and 2 diced jalapenos from your garden.
3. Add sliced green or red peppers, or a mixture of the rainbow pepper colors. They are a yummy addition and make the dish look beautiful.
4. Add a combination of homemade chicken stock (fat skimmed off) or store-bought fat-free chicken broth and water. You can also use water and a large handful of nutritional yeast for a quick stock alternative. Use enough liquid to make perfect soupy consistency.
5. Add 1small can tomato paste and season your simmering meal with sea salt, black pepper, Bragg Liquid Aminos, chili powder, onion and garlic powder, and hot sauce to taste. Be careful when salting your chili if using chicken broth that has already been salted.
6. Add 2-3 cans of your favorite beans (white, navy, northern). Baby lima beans look lovely in this dish, as they are white and match this chili's leaner meat choice. You can also use beans you have cooked from scratch.
7. Simmer until all flavors mingle nicely.
8. Serve topped with 0% Greek yogurt, or in a pinch, low-fat sour cream.

You may use baked blue corn chips (not fried) as dunkers, or use homemade baked healthy chips, using plan approved sprouted tortillas, crisped in the oven, and broken into wedges. You may also use a small amount of grated skimmed mozzarella cheese, or an alternative reduced fat cheese to garnish your chili.

Kai Si Ming – S (feeds large family)

We grew up with this recipe as a weekly staple in our home. Now it is comfort food for our families on chilly evenings. Cabbage is a very inexpensive vegetable that goes a long way and has high nutritional value. Don't worry about keeping the cabbage raw and crisp. It is one vegetable that needs to be cooked well to be digested without gas trouble.

This one-pot meal is delicious served alone, or with one of our **S** bread options such as sliced *Bread in a Mug, Golden Flat Bread, Country Biscuit*, or store-bought Joseph's pita or lavish bread. We enjoy adding extra cayenne pepper to our bowls. Children love it with brown rice, or whole grain buttered bread or pitas.

Basic Ingredients: ground beef ✦ cabbage ✦ onions ✦ sea salt and other seasonings ✦ water and optional stock/broth

1. Brown 3 lbs. ground beef in large pot.
2. While meat is browning, slice 1½ half large cabbages thinly (keeping strands long).
3. Slice 2 large onions thinly.
4. Drain most of grease from the meat, but leave a little for flavor.
5. Add cabbage and onion to meat. Put lid on pot and let cabbage wilt down a little for a few minutes.
6. Add 1 tsp. sea salt and lots of black pepper, 2-3 Tbs. nutritional yeast, a dash or two of cayenne pepper, onion powder, and some generous splashes of soy sauce or Bragg Liquid Aminos.
7. Add 4 cups water, or 2 cups of water and 2 cups of stock/broth.
8. Cover pot with lid and simmer slowly, stirring now and then until cabbage is soft and well cooked, about 30 to 45 minutes.

Golden Palm Butter Soup/Stew – S

This is the larger, family style version of the single serve lunch recipe by the same name.

Basic Ingredients: palm butter ✦ water ✦ onions ✦ peppers ✦ veggies of choice ✦ cans of salmon or pulled chicken ✦ sea salt and other seasonings

1. Place contents of 2 large cans of palm butter in large pot.
2. Use 1 empty can to add 3 cans of water.

3. Add two sliced onions, 4-6 whole peppers (habanera for the hard core heat lovers) and other vegetables of your choice, e.g., broccoli, cauliflower, etc.
4. Add either 2-3 drained cans of wild caught salmon, or pre-cooked sliced or pulled chicken.
5. Season with 2 Tbs. nutritional yeast, onion and garlic powder, sea salt, black pepper, Bragg Liquid Aminos/tamari and an optional 1-2 tsp. curry powder according to your taste. Go easy with curry powder and taste as you add.
6. Simmer all ingredients until onions are soft and clear and flavors have united.
7. Once dish is ready, squash peppers with a spoon against the side of the pot to release their heat. Taste to see if spicy enough, and if so, remove them.

Children enjoy this over brown rice. We enjoy it alone with an optional sprinkle of hemp seeds to garnish on top. A plate of lime wedges on the table for people to squeeze into their bowl makes this dish even better. You can use a ¼ cup of brown rice in your bowl if you are at **S Helper** stage, or use ⅓-½ cup of quinoa. *Cauli Rice* is always a great option, too.

Taste of Thailand – S

This recipe is another large scale version from the quick style lunch options. This makes plenty, so if your family is smaller, you'll have plenty to freeze for another meal.

Basic Ingredients: coconut milk ✦ chicken broth or water ✦ nutritional yeast ✦ chicken or canned salmon ✦ veggies of choice ✦ sea salt and other seasonings, including curry paste ✦ optional red palm oil

1. Pour contents of 3 cans of full-fat coconut milk into large pot (make sure it is a brand with 1 or less carbs per serving).
2. Add 3 cans of water, or the same amount of homemade or store-bought chicken broth (free range is best), or a combination of both. If using only water, include nutritional yeast as a seasoning.
3. Add any amount of sliced or pulled pre-cooked chicken, or 3 cans of wild caught salmon (if using salmon, only use water, not chicken broth).
4. Add non-starchy vegetables of your choice, e.g., broccoli, cauliflower, baby corn (surprisingly low-carb) and/or water chestnuts.
5. One way of seasoning this dish is to use 3 heaped tsp. Red Thai curry paste, 1½ tsp. Truvia, or a dash of NuStevia Pure White Stevia Extract Powder and a little fish sauce. The alternative, more involved way is to use the following spices to taste: onion and garlic powder, sea salt, fish sauce, cayenne pepper, 1½ tsp. Truvia or a

dash of NuStevia Pure White Stevia Extract Powder, ½ tsp. ginger powder, and a squeeze or so of fresh concentrated lemon or lime juice.

6 If you have access to fresh basil leaves, tear some up and throw them in the pot for the last minutes of cooking. Or, if you have fresh red peppers, use in place of cayenne pepper, in the same manner as squashed peppers in *Golden Palm Butter Soup/Stew*. Red pepper flakes can also be used instead of cayenne or floating whole peppers.

7 Simmer to combine flavors and tenderize vegetables and meat. Optional: in the last few minutes of cooking you can add 2 heaped Tbs. red palm oil which gives a beautiful hue to the soup as well as additional health benefits.

Serving suggestions are the same as the preceding *Golden Palm Butter Soup/Stew*.

Serene chats: If you're the type who loves the idea of scratch/whole food cooking, you can try the following to make a nutritious chicken stock for the above recipe. Our sister, Evangeline was the originator of this Thai coconut soup recipe and, being the personality that she is, she made everything from scratch, including the broth. Pearl loved the soup, but never wanted to make broth—too time consuming for her quick and easy food philosophy. I came up with the quick version and she enjoys this recipe in her household now, too. Using homemade stock brings something extra to the recipe, not to mention the incredible health benefits from the natural gelatin in the stock.

Homemade Stock

Basic Ingredients: chicken ✦ onions ✦ parsley ✦ garlic ✦ celery ✦ ginger ✦ apple cider vinegar ✦ water

1 Place whole free range chicken in large stock pot with a few cut onions, parsley, bulb of peeled garlic cloves, a few sticks of celery, and a wedge of ginger.

2 Add 2 Tbs. apple cider vinegar to the pot (this pulls minerals from the bones of the chicken).

3 Cover with 2-3 quarts of pure water and bring to a boil (remove bubbly scum that may rise on the top after it starts to boil).

4 Turn to low and cover. Simmer gently for the entire day (start this procedure in the morning).

5 At dinner preparation time, remove chicken and pull meat from the bones. Drain veggies from liquid. All the minerals and electrolytes will already be drawn out of the vegetables into the stock so you can discard them or feed them to pets.

6. This liquid can now be used as the stock for your soup. Freeze excess portions for future recipes.

Hearty Red Soup – S (large scale for big family and company, or two meal's worth)

Basic Ingredients: ground beef ✦ onions ✦ cabbage ✦ frozen green beans ✦ parsley ✦ water ✦ tomato paste sea salt and other seasonings, including nutritional yeast ✦ optional cream or tahini

1. Brown 5 lbs. ground beef in large pot and drain, if not using grass fed beef.
2. Add 3 sliced onions and a whole sliced cabbage, 1 frozen package of long green beans, and 1 whole bunch of parsley, finely chopped.
3. Add enough water to the pot to cook vegetables (you do not necessarily need to cover veggies with water as they will sink down and wilt as they cook).
4. Add 3 small (6 oz.) cans of tomato paste.
5. Add following spices to taste: sea salt, lots of black pepper, Bragg Liquid Aminos/tamari, onion and garlic powder, nutritional yeast, and optional chili flakes.
6. Add more water as needed to obtain desired soup consistency. It does not need to be extremely brothy.
7. Once vegetables are tender and soup flavors have mingled, add a dollop or so of cream or tahini to cut the acidity of the soup and bring out the depth of flavors.

This may be served with warmed and buttered whole wheat pita bread for growing children. You may enjoy a coconut dinner roll with this meal, or choose any of our **S** cracker recipe options. Since this soup makes a large batch, you can freeze leftovers to be reheated for "no brainer" nights.

Hearty Green Soup – E (large scale for big family and company, or two meal's worth)

Basic Ingredients: green split peas ✦ apple cider vinegar ✦ cabbage ✦ carrots ✦ parsley water or chicken stock/broth ✦ sea salt and other seasonings including nutritional yeast ✦ heavy cream

1. Soak 2 lbs. green split peas overnight or during the day for about 7 hours. Use ample water for soaking and 2 Tbs. of apple cider vinegar to remove phytates.

2 In mid afternoon, drain water and add fresh water to slightly cover split peas. Add 3 diced onions, 4 large stalks of celery, and chopped peeled garlic cloves.

3 Bring to boil, turn heat to low, and cover with lid.

4 Simmer slowly until split peas turn to mush.

5 Check contents of pot. Stir occasionally to make sure split peas do not stick and burn at the bottom of the pot.

6 Once split peas are soft, add one whole cut cabbage, a few diced carrots, a bunch of parsley finely diced, and enough water or chicken broth to cook vegetables effectively and achieve the right soup consistency.

7 Season with sea salt, black pepper, Bragg Liquid Aminos, nutritional yeast, and onion powder.

8 Keep simmering until new vegetables are tender.

9 Toward the end of cooking, add 3 Tbs. of cream to help unify the flavors and give a touch of fat. There is no other fat in these ingredients so this amount of cream in such a big soup stays within **E** guidelines.

This may be served with warmed and buttered whole wheat pita bread for the growing children and a glass of milk, preferably raw. You could have a piece of sprouted or homemade sour dough toast or some of our approved crackers. Of course, a wonderful accompaniment to any soup meal is a lovely fresh salad.

Serene chats: I have a large family, and in order to feed all of us and stay on a budget, we often eat homemade soups for our evening meal. We eat these last two soups so often during winter that my children have often asked at the table, "Which one tonight, Mom, red or green?" If you have a small family, freeze extra for future evening meals.

Creamy Broccoli and Cheese Soup – S

This soup can be the makings of a full evening meal if your family is smaller. If you have a larger family, double the recipe and throw in a little diced cooked chicken breast at the end to increase the protein content, or use some from a can.

Basic Ingredients: broccoli ✦ water ✦ chicken broth ✦ cream cheese ✦ heavy cream ✦ optional glucomannan ✦ sea salt and other seasonings ✦ grated cheese

1 Steam 2 frozen (12 oz.) packages of broccoli, or a couple of heads of fresh broccoli.

2. Put steamed broccoli into blender in batches with just enough water to enable it to blend smoothly. You may keep some broccoli aside if you want some chunkiness to the soup.
3. Pour blended broccoli into a pot with 4 cups of chicken broth, or 2 cups of chicken broth and 2 cups of water.
4. Add 1 (8 oz.) package of ⅓ less fat cream cheese and ⅓ cup of heavy cream.
5. Season generously with sea salt, pepper, and optional cayenne pepper.
6. Add more water to create a soupy consistency. Thicken with a little glucomannan if too thin for your liking. Simmer for a few minutes.

Grated cheese on top is the perfect way to enjoy this soup. Not only is it healthy for you as it is filled with greens and vitamins, but broccoli lowers harmful aggressive estrogens in the body. Your husband will benefit as it is common for estrogen to rise in men as they grow older. That is not a good thing—think libido loss, brain fog and depression! Including broccoli, or other cruciferous veggies like cauliflower, Brussels sprouts, and cabbage in several meals each week helps to keep a safe and healthy estrogen ratio in the body, known as the 2/16 ratio. Broccoli is the best known food to enhance this ratio, and therefore reduces breast cancer risk. Some people hate eating broccoli on its own, but they like a cheesy broccoli soup. Whichever way works for you and yours, make it happen.

This blending idea can turn any non-starchy vegetable into a creamy soup. Cauliflower and squash work great as well. It's even more amazing if you pre-bake them with butter rather than steam before blending. If you don't want to use cream cheese, use more chicken broth and add regular grated cheese into the soup.

Chicken Satay Soup – S (feeds a large family)

Basic Ingredients: chicken breasts or tenderloins ✦ sugar-free peanut butter ✦ hot peppers ✦ sea salt and other seasonings, including nutritional yeast ✦ water or chicken stock/broth ✦ xanthan gum or glucomannan ✦ broccoli ✦ cabbage ✦ snow peas ✦ string green beans ✦ optional basil leaves, chili flakes, and coconut milk

1. Poach or bake a large bag of chicken breasts or tenderloins, or use leftover cooked chicken if you have any available.
2. In blender combine ½ (16 oz.) jar of all natural sugar-free peanut butter, a couple of hot peppers (leave out if you are not a spice loving family and use black pepper or a little cayenne pepper), sea salt, Bragg Liquid Aminos/soy sauce, nutritional yeast, onion and garlic powder, and a tiny dash of NuStevia Pure White Stevia Extract Powder or 1½ tsp. Truvia.

3. Add 2 cups water or chicken stock/broth, and ½ tsp. xanthan gum or glucomannan. Blend until smooth.
4. Put contents of blender and diced chicken into large pot. Add more water while heating to create a thick soup consistency.
5. Add broccoli florets (frozen are fine) and optional cabbage wedges, snow peas, string green beans, etc.
6. Simmer until all vegetables are tender. During the last few minutes of cooking, add a few torn up fresh basil leaves, red chili pepper flakes, and an optional swirl of coconut milk for extra creaminess.

This is great over brown rice for the children. For you it is perfect with a yummy side salad, if you didn't already have fresh vegetables for your lunch meal.

Peanut Sauce Night – S

Pearl chats: While Serene makes her Chicken Satay in one big pot, I keep the sauce separate from the chicken and broccoli. For some reason, my children prefer it when I make the sauce separately and pour it over the other ingredients at the end. They call this evening meal, "Peanut Sauce Night." We all enjoy our chicken, satay sauce, and broccoli over Dreamfields noodles. You could also use konjac noodles which would be an even healthier option. This is great with a side of *Tabouleh* (*Lunches*, Chapter 20).

Basic Ingredients: chicken tenderloins ✦ coconut oil or butter ✦ sugar-free peanut butter ✦ water ✦ sea salt and other seasonings, including Bragg Liquid Aminos ✦ sweetener ✦ glucomannan

1. Put contents of 1 bag of frozen chicken tenderloins in baking tray, season with sea salt and black pepper, add butter or coconut oil and bake in the oven.
2. While chicken is baking, put ¾ cup of smooth sugar-free peanut butter in a medium-sized saucepan.
3. Turn stove to medium and add 3 cups water, sea salt, black pepper, lots of chili powder, onion powder, a few good squirts of Bragg Liquid Aminos, and some generous shakes of cayenne pepper. You may add an optional ½ tsp. Truvia or the tiniest pinch of NuStevia Pure White Stevia Extract Powder. Don't overdo the sweetener! Too much, and this sauce becomes bitter for some reason.

4. As sauce is heating, whisk well until the sauce is smooth. Put some glucomannan in a salt shaker and start shaking and whisking like crazy until sauce is at desired thickness. You can always add more water and seasonings if it becomes too thick.
5. While sauce is simmering and chicken is baking, steam a bag or two or broccoli florets. Once they're ready, toss them in a little butter and a sprinkle of sea salt.
6. At meal time, place noodles in bowls first, followed by chicken pieces, followed by broccoli florets and ladle lots of sauce on top.

Pearl chats: Traditional satay sauce is made from peanut paste and coconut milk. Sometimes I add a swirl of coconut milk at the end, but we usually have our satay sauce predominantly peanut based. Feel free to experiment with adding coconut milk to yours.

Skillet Stuff

Sponge Bob's Crabby Patties – S (feeds large family)

Basic Ingredients: canned salmon ✦ eggs ✦ Joseph's bread crumbs or oats ✦ all purpose seasoning, or other sea food seasoning of your choice ✦ coconut oil ✦ optional parsley and sesame seeds

1. Depending on how large your family drain 2-3 cans of wild caught salmon and put contents in a large mixing bowl.
2. Mash the salmon well with a fork, bones and all.
3. Add 2-3 eggs, 1 for each can.
4. Make ½ cup bread crumbs from Joseph's pitas by whizzing them up in your coffee grinder, then add to bowl. If you don't have Joseph's, throw in ⅓ cup of oats. Spread throughout the whole recipe, the oats should not even put you in **S Helper** territory.
5. Add ½ a small finely diced onion.
6. Add a very light sprinkle of Lawry's Seasoned Salt (MSG free). Be careful not to add too much seasoning because canned salmon already has a salty flavor.
7. Mix all ingredients well with a fork.
8. Heat generous amount of coconut oil in a skillet. Place large spoonfuls of patty mix (burger size) into skillet and fry until browned on both sides.

Pearl chats: These are my children's favorite burgers. Maybe they don't beat beef burgers, but they are, none the less, well liked. We have them about once a week and while they are not made from crab, the children labeled them "crabby patties" after the Sponge Bob cartoon that spends so much time obsessing about seafood patties. Charlie and I enjoy the patties as much as the children. They are perfect with a salad and a side of buttery broccoli. Or, place them in a whole wheat bun for your children. For a change, you can substitute tuna for the salmon.

I've been making these for years, but Serene has only recently started making this recipe. I have to say that hers taste even better than my original version so I've started to copy her. She adds finely diced parsley, sesame seeds, and a toss or two of nutritional yeast to the recipe, and wow, they taste gourmet! I shortcut the parsley and buy dried parsley flakes which still works great.

Bean or Chana Dahl Burgers – E

Use home-soaked, cooked, and drained beans of any kind. Or, use drained canned beans if you're not the "from scratch" type. For the safest blood sugar effect, chana dahl is your best choice. Remember to soak it overnight for at least 7 hours with ¼-¾ tsp. of baking soda to soften it up nicely.

Basic Ingredients: beans or Chana dahl ✦ egg whites ✦ oats or plan approved bread crumbs ✦ onion ✦ sea salt and other seasonings

1. Put contents of 2 drained (15 oz.) cans of beans into a bowl or use 3 generous cups of home-cooked chana dahl or beans.
2. Add 4 egg whites or ½ cup 100% carton whites.
3. Add ½ cup oats, sprouted bread crumbs, or sourdough bread crumbs. Grind in coffee grinder.
4. Add an optional finely diced ½ onion.
5. Add sea salt, black pepper, and onion powder.
6. Form into patties and bake on oiled tray at 350 for 20-30 minutes.

Beef Burger Night – S

You just gotta have a juicy beef burger now and then. Go ahead! Grass fed beef or bison will make it a superfood meal. However, if you don't have access to grass fed beef, you can still enjoy delicious beef burgers without gaining weight, if you do it the way we suggest. Pearl uses 3 lbs. of ground beef for her family. Serene uses 5 lbs.

Basic Ingredients: ground beef ✦ sea salt and other seasonings, including dried rosemary

1. Put thawed ground beef or bison in bowl. Add a sprinkle of dried rosemary, Creole, black pepper, sea salt, and onion powder. If desired, add very finely diced onion and jalapenos.
2. Place palm-sized burgers in hot skillet, brown on both sides, or cook on outside grill.

Burgers can be sandwiched between whole wheat rolls or bread for your growing children and fixings of their choice. You can have them between *Oopsie Rolls*, in a split Joseph's pita, or even encased in large lettuce leaves. Throw on the works—mayo, mustard, cheese, pickles, lettuce (if not using for casing), tomato, sautéed mushrooms, and avocado. The sky is the limit.

Pearl chats: Here's a tip. I try to add rosemary whenever I prepare charred or darkly browned meat. Rosemary is a potent antioxidant. It combats the carcinogens (HCA's) that are formed when meat is browned or gets charred and crusty. It's a great idea to add rosemary any time you are trying to get a good crisp on meat, but especially important when char grilling.

Rosemary adds a great taste and it's a wonderful anti-inflammatory aid for the body. Drinking a small glass of dry red wine or a mug of green tea after a meal that includes crispy meat will go even further to prevent damage.

One of my favorite ways to have beef burgers is bun-less. I lay them naked on a plate and top them with a little mayonnaise and mustard, pile on sautéed onions, and top with sliced tomatoes that are sprinkled with salt and pepper. This way, I have to eat with a knife and fork. When I get the urge to hold something in my hands, I put the burgers in Joseph's pitas and load up with every fixin' I can think of. That gives me more of a real burger fix, and I'm good and satisfied.

Alfredo Beef and Broccoli – S

This is a quick meal idea for nights when you don't want to get complicated. It is also delicious and filling.

Basic Ingredients: ground beef ✦ sea salt and other seasonings ✦ broccoli ✦ Alfredo sauce ✦ optional cayenne pepper and Creole seasoning

1. Brown 3 lbs. ground beef in a large skillet and drain off fat if not using grass fed beef.
2. Season beef with salt and pepper or Creole seasoning.
3. Add 2 packets frozen broccoli florets to cooked beef.

4. Put lid on skillet and let steam broccoli until almost tender, stirring every now and then. If you thaw broccoli before placing in skillet, it will only take about 5 minutes.
5. Once broccoli is on its way to tender, add 1½ jars of Alfredo sauce, or the same amount of homemade Alfredo sauce, plus 1 cup of water.
6. Stir water and sauce into other ingredients and heat, but don't cook so long that the broccoli is over cooked.
7. For spice lovers, add cayenne pepper and Creole seasoning to give a wonderful kick.

Your children can eat this one-pot meal over rice. You can have it over *Cauli Rice* or on its own. Sprinkle each plated meal with Parmesan cheese.

Pearl chats: If you use store-bought Alfredo sauce, which I do, the meal is not exactly on Serene's superfood list. But, let's look at its merits. It's chock full of health-benefiting broccoli and a no-brainer to whip up, which is less stress. It will be kind to your waistline, despite its heartiness. I had to include this recipe for these reasons.

You could add mushrooms and onions while you are sautéing the beef, but my children prefer it with broccoli only. Try to find Alfredo sauce with two grams of carbs or less. This means it is not loaded with fillers and does not contain any sugar.

For smaller families, this recipe amount should give you leftovers to be heated up for a yummy lunch. It would be great folded into *Crepes* (*Morning Meals*, Chapter 18). But, at our home, there is never a morsel left, and the children who want third helpings get told, "Sorry."

Sweet and Spicy Asian Stir Fry – Fuel Pull or E

If you are afflicted with tough pounds that resist being shed, this is a great stir fry to incorporate into your evenings once you are already adept at implementing the core of our **S** and **E** plan. We don't have a lot of **Fuel Pull** evening meals since we think it is best if supper can be shared with the whole family. Although designed to be a **Fuel Pull**, this particular recipe can work for everyone since it is both delicious and versatile.

For serious weight reducing purposes, eat this stir fry with konjac noodles as a **Fuel Pull**. It is a body fat destroyer this way. The smartest thing to do is to set aside a packet of konjac noodles for you, and the rest of the family can enjoy it with rice or another type of noodle. Of course, if you find yourself all alone on a rare evening, reduce the amount of ingredients and make yourself a single serve. That works for a lunch too. If you do not need more serious help with weight, enjoy it with ¾ cup of rice or quinoa for yourself for **E** style.

Basic Ingredients: fat free chicken broth ✦ frozen stir fry veggies ✦ chicken breasts or optional extra lean steak ✦ peanut flour or peanut butter ✦ soy sauce ✦ cayenne pepper and onion powder ✦ chili flakes ✦ optional sugar-free pancake syrup ✦ sweetener ✦ glucomannan ✦ konjac noodles or rice or quinoa

1. Prebake or poach bag of chicken tenderloins.
2. Put 1 cup fat free chicken broth in large skillet.
3. Add 1-2 (12 oz.) packets of frozen stir fry veggies (depending on size of family).
4. Once veggies are nearly tender, add 4 Tbs. peanut flour or 4 flat tsp. peanut butter and whisk well.
5. Add optional 4 Tbs. sugar-free pancake syrup, and/or several drops Swanson stevia drops (depending on desired sweetness), ¼-½ cup soy sauce, cayenne pepper, and onion powder to taste. We use stevia drops because they seem to taste best in this sauce, but Truvia and Nunaturals work well too. Try 1-2 Tbs. Truvia and adjust to taste.
6. Add 1-2 more cups of chicken broth, then thicken sauce by moving the veggies to one side of the skillet so you can have better access to the liquid. Shake in glucomannan from a salt shaker a little at a time and whisking until desired thickness is achieved. Taste to see if more sweetener, spice, or soy sauce is needed for your preference.
7. Dice chicken breasts, season with salt and pepper and add to vegetables and sauce.
8. Serve with konjac noodles, rice, or quinoa and top with chili flakes if desired.

Note: If making this in single serve size, use half a packet (3 oz.) of Tyson Grilled and Ready chicken breasts or lean steak strips. This eliminates the need for prebaking chicken breasts. Make sure to use only 1 Tbs. peanut flour or 1 tsp. peanut butter so you'll stay within **Fuel Pull** fat perimeters. Don't overdo the peanut butter by using a big old heaping teaspoon. It is only to hint at flavor and our recommended amount does the job well. Remember also that **Fuel Pulls** are the only time we ask you to go easy on your meat protein. Even if you're eating this dish along with the rest of your family, if you want to stay in **Fuel Pull** mode, use only about 3 oz of the meat in your serving. That equals about 2 chicken tenderloins or half a breast.

Basic Chicken and Vegetable Stir Fry – S (feeds medium to large family)

You can use the fresh veggies suggested for this recipe, but if you want to shortcut, use two bags of frozen stir fry veggies. If you opt for frozen, allow a few minutes extra cooking time. You can also use pre-cooked chicken in this recipe to make it quicker. There are no hard and fast rules. This is more of a skeleton recipe for you to flesh out with your own imagination.

Basic Ingredients: chicken breasts, tenderloins or boneless thighs✦ sesame oil ✦ garlic ✦ ginger ✦ non-starchy veggies such as pea pods, baby corn, broccoli, celery, and green onion ✦ soy sauce ✦ glucomannan or xanthan gum

1. Cut up 2 lbs. boneless and skinless chicken breasts, tenderloins, or boneless thighs into chunks and set aside.
2. Heat 2 Tbs. coconut oil and 1 Tbs. sesame oil in a large skillet over medium/high temperature.
3. Add 2-3 cloves minced garlic and 2 Tbs. fresh minced ginger to oil.
4. Cook garlic and ginger for about 1 minute.
5. Add chicken chunks and cook 4-5 minutes, stirring constantly as they brown.
6. Remove chicken and keep warm.
7. Add 2 more Tbs. sesame oil to skillet and add following vegetables: 3 cups of pea pods, 2 drained 15 oz. cans of baby corn, 4 cups of broccoli florets, 2 cups of loosely cut celery, and one bunch of cut green onions.
8. Stir fry veggies for 2-3 minutes.
9. Add ⅓ cup Soy/Tamari sauce.
10. In a separate bowl, whisk in ½ tsp. glucomannan or xanthan into 2 cups of chicken broth by sprinkling it from a salt shaker to prevent clumping. Add to skillet with other ingredients and cook a few minutes more until vegetables are still crisp tender and sauce is thickened.
11. Return chicken to skillet to warm up shortly before serving.

This recipe will extend a lot further for a big family if your children eat it over brown rice. You can enjoy it alone, or with *Cauli Rice*, or an **S Helper** serving of rice or quinoa (those little pre-made baggies come in handy again).

Speedy Chinese Broccoli and Beef – S

Basic Ingredients: deli style roast beef ✦ broccoli ✦ onion ✦ hot chili sauce ✦ sweetener ✦ soy sauce and black pepper ✦ glucomannan or xanthan gum ✦ water or chicken broth

1. Depending on family size, cut up 1-2 packages of natural deli style roast beef into strips (or use any other stir fry suitable beef).
2. Toss beef in a small amount of oil in skillet to brown edges slightly and then remove meat from pan.

3. Add fresh broccoli florets and optional large pieces of onion to pan and stir fry in a little more oil.
4. Make up sauce in a bowl by combining hot chili sauce, soy sauce to taste (about ¼ cup), a little Truvia (about 2 tsp.) or a dash of Nunaturals (a tiny pinch) and black pepper. Add 1-1½ cups of water or chicken broth and then sprinkle in ½ tsp. glucomannan or xanthan gum from a salt shaker and whisk briskly.
5. Transfer meat back to skillet with the vegetables and pour sauce over all.
6. Heat and simmer sauce with meat and vegetables for a few minutes. If it seems too thin, shake in more glucomannan or xanthan gum and whisk quickly. If too thick, add more water or broth.

This dish can be as mild, or as hot and spicy as you prefer, according to the amount of hot chili sauce you add. Be sure to purchase one with only one carb. Huy Fong Foods brand is suitable and available at most grocery stores in the international food aisle.

As a stir fry, you can enjoy this with either *Cauli Rice,* konjac, or Dreamfields noodles, but it's absolutely great on its own. The flavors and textures offer so much that it doesn't need a lot of dressing up.

This is another recipe you could make **E** by using chicken breast in place of the beef and pull back oil to a minimum. The sauce is not high in fat so there is not a lot to change around. If **E**, enjoy with ¾ cup of brown rice or quinoa.

Fried Breaded Fish – S

Thinner style white fish fillets, like tilapia or whiting, are best suited to this recipe. Wild caught flounder is inexpensive if bought frozen, and works well too. About two hours before meal prep time, thaw your frozen fish fillets in a big bowl of room temperature water, and they'll be ready to go.

We use a combination of oat flour and Joseph's bread crumbs as the main breading. It is a thin coating on the fish, not dredged or double coated, and the grain is barely enough to consider it being an **S Helper**. But, if you need to stay carefully on plan, use only Joseph's pita crumbs, it's just as good.

Basic Ingredients: white fish fillets ✦ oats ✦ Joseph's pita ✦ sea salt and other seasonings ✦ coconut oil ✦ butter

1. Grind up ½ cup of oats in blender or coffee grinder and ½ cup Joseph's pita crumbs (this coats about 10 good sized fillets, so less flour would be needed for smaller amounts of fish).

2. Place flour on a large dinner plate and add 1 tsp. salt, ½ tsp. black pepper, and 2 heaped tsp. onion powder. Mix well with a fork.
3. Rinse off thawed white fish fillets under water and press each side into the flour mixture (the moisture from the water allows enough coating to stay on the fish).
4. Lightly brown fish on both sides in a mixture of coconut oil and butter. You may have to do 3-4 batches for a large family. Keep cooked fillets warm in oven while the other batches are frying.

Pearl chats: I chuckle a lot when I serve my children this meal as I receive so many compliments. They love these breaded fillets with lots of ketchup and usually say, "Mom, you are the best fish cooker in the world." That strikes me as funny, because this recipe is so simple that even someone completely clueless in the kitchen could probably manage it extremely well.

I make a tartar sauce out of mayonnaise, finely chopped pickles, and a little stevia sweetener. Charlie and I prefer the tartar sauce better than ketchup. I make *Pea Salad* (*Vegetable Sides*, Chapter 22) for Charlie and myself, but the children enjoy the fish with seasoned, fried brown rice.

Chicken Tenders – S

Basic Ingredients: chicken breasts or tenderloins ✦ mayonnaise ✦ Joseph's pita ✦ sea salt and other seasonings ✦ coconut oil

1. Poach or pre-bake 1 bag of frozen chicken breasts or tenderloins.
2. Slice cooked breasts into strips or cubes.
3. Put 1 Tbs. mayonnaise onto chicken pieces and work with your hands to make sure each piece has a thin covering.
4. Grind 1 Joseph's pita bread in coffee grinder or blender. Season ground crumbs with generous amounts of salt, pepper, and onion and/or garlic powder.
5. Roll chicken pieces in bread crumbs until they have a good coating and fry in coconut oil until nicely browned.

If you don't have Joseph's pitas, or you are like Serene and take a more pure foods approach, you may roll the mayonnaise covered chicken pieces in store-bought coconut flour (homemade coconut flour will not work for this purpose), season with above mentioned seasonings, and then fry.

These chicken tenders are scrumptious dipped into our homemade *Honey Mustard Dressing* or *Ketchup* (*Gravies, Sauces, and Condiments,* Chapter 25).

Mexican Meals

Fajitas – S

Basic Ingredients: steak or chicken ✦ taco or fajita seasoning ✦ green peppers ✦ onions ✦ optional tomatoes ✦ optional coconut oil ✦ lettuce ✦ grated cheese ✦ salsa ✦ sour cream

1. Sauté fajita suitable steak, or chicken pieces in skillet with fajita or taco seasoning (*Rick Fowler's* Taco seasoning is best).
2. While meat is cooking, slice 2-3 green or red peppers and 2-3 onions. Add optional sliced tomatoes.
3. Once meat is ready, transfer it to plate. Stir fry vegetables in the pan in which the meat was cooked and add more seasoning and coconut oil if the meat was lean and did not leave enough grease.
4. Put meat back in the pan with the vegetables once they are ready (veggies should be a little browned and crispy in places) and toss ingredients together.
5. Add sides such as chopped lettuce, tomato, grated cheese, salsa, and sour cream, which work perfectly with fajitas. We don't miss the flour tortillas.

You can make an **E** version by using chicken breast as the meat, cooked in a scant amount of oil. Top with low-fat Greek yogurt or low-fat sour cream, and small amounts of reduced fat cheese. You could also add some fat-free refried beans or brown rice as a side.

Tostadas – S

Basic Ingredients: ground beef or turkey ✦ taco seasoning ✦ cheddar cheese ✦ sour cream ✦ lettuce ✦ salsa

1. Sauté ground beef, ground turkey, or chicken in a skillet with taco or fajita style seasonings (Wick Fowler's brand is best).
2. Using the process outlined in *Crunchy Cheese Crisps* (*Snacks*, Chapter 24) make up large round cheese crisps for your tostada bases, about the size of a regular Mexican style corn tostada. Cook a few at a time in the oven, or one at a time in the microwave. Always use parchment paper.

3. Smear the crunchy cheese tostadas generously with sour cream and add shredded lettuce (layering the lettuce first on the sour cream helps it to stay put).
4. Add a layer of cooked ground beef, turkey, or shredded chicken. Add diced tomatoes and a little more shredded cheese.
5. Top with salsa.

The same idea can be used for Tacos, but when you make taco shells, cook the cheese half way until it's bendable, fold it over into a taco shape, then finish cooking until it gets crispy. These are also great for a lunch idea.

Taco Salad – S (feeds large family)

Basic Ingredients: ground beef or turkey ✦ taco seasoning ✦ lettuce ✦ grated cheese ✦ olives, onions and tomatoes ✦ sour cream ✦ salsa

1. Brown 3 lbs. ground beef or turkey in skillet.
2. Drain meat and add taco seasoning like Wick Fowler's.
3. Slice up romaine lettuce thinly to fill a big bowl.
4. Grate a block or two of cheese and slice up other salad toppings like olives, onions, and tomatoes and place in bowls.
5. Layer lettuce, beef, cheese, and other fixings and top with sour cream and salsa.

Your children will likely want a few corn chips on the top of their salad. Yours will taste great as is, or crumble a few of our **S** approved crackers or chips on top.

Mexican Noodles – S

Pearl chats: My son, Bowen gave the name to this recipe. It's one of his favorites. He likes it because he thinks the sauce has a Mexican flavor to it, yet he prefers it over noodles which are not Mexican cuisine. Strange combination, but it makes him and all my other children happy. Charlie and I have it with either *Cauli Rice* (*Vegetable Sides*, Chapter 22), a bed of lettuce leaves, or on its own in a bowl with a couple of sliced and buttered pieces of Joseph's lavish or pita on the side (my favorite way). If you want to keep to the theme of the title, it also works pretty well over konjac or Dreamfields noodles.

Note: To make this dish spread further for a large family, and to increase the nutritional content, add one finely sliced cabbage. The cabbage wilts nicely and is barely noticeable, but creates larger volume for the meal. It is not exactly a Mexican vegetable, but works great regardless.

Basic Ingredients: ground beef or turkey ✦ canned diced chilies and tomatoes ✦ cream cheese ✦ water ✦ grated cheese

1. Brown 3 lbs. ground beef or turkey in large skillet and drain fat if necessary.
2. Add 2 cans Rotel style diced chili and tomatoes, either mild, medium, or hot depending on your tolerance for spice, and an optional finely sliced cabbage.
3. Add 1½ packets of ⅓ less fat Philadelphia cream cheese, ½ cup of water, and one cup of grated cheese.
4. Combine all ingredients well. Simmer for a while with a lid on until everything is cooked.

Pasta Ideas

All of the following ideas go well with either Dreamfields pasta, zucchini, or spaghetti squash noodles. Konjac noodles can be used in more Asian style dishes, like satays. Check *Vegetable Sides,* Chapter 22 for zucchini and spaghetti squash noodles.

Remember, even when eating a lower carb style of pasta like Dreamfields, don't go "hog wild." Take a smaller portion of pasta and a larger portion of sauce. Try not to eat more than 1/5 of a box of Dreamfields pasta as a serving at one time. You can go more "hog wild" with konjac noodles, if you get the urge, since they cannot raise blood sugar. Eat them to your heart's content!

We don't recommend you use whole grain pastas made from wheat or spelt with a low-fat sauce as a full **E** meal option. You could consider using a little whole grain pasta with a lean sauce as a side to an **E** meal. A full plate of whole grain pasta causes too high a glycemic response, even though the fiber is still in the grain. The quantity is just too much.

> *Pearl chats:* I once tested my blood sugar after a meal of whole grain pasta and sauce. This was two hours after my meal and my level was 157! Blood sugar should not be over 120 two hours after a meal, and for optimum health, it should be lower. Spiking my glucose level that high was enough for me to swear off a big bowl of whole grain spaghetti forever. You can be assured I have never done it again.

The following pasta sauce ideas will not spike your blood sugar and you will leave the table feeling satisfied, due to the fat content involved in the sauces. All the following ideas are **S**.

1. **Alfredo sauce** with chicken or beef, (either store-bought with 2 carbs or less per serving, or homemade).
2. **Bolognese sauce**. Do not use store-bought sauces that have sugar or corn in their ingredients, Use sugar-free preparations, or check out our recipe below.
3. **White sauce** made from white wine, heavy cream, parmesan cheese, sea salt, garlic powder and black pepper, thickened with a little glucomannan or xanthan gum.
4. **Satay sauce** can be quick and easy by combining peanut butter, coconut milk, water, ¼-½ tsp. glucomannan or xanthan gum, onion and garlic powder, chili powder, cayenne pepper or a whole hot pepper, sea salt, Bragg Liquid Aminos and nutritional yeast (optional) into blender. Blend all, transfer to saucepan and heat. Perfect over chicken, canned wild salmon and vegetables, and, of course, appropriate pasta.
5. **Simple** plan approved pasta can be tossed with extra virgin olive oil or coconut oil, sea salt, pepper, and a little nutritional yeast or Parmesan cheese. Konjac noodles are fabulous tossed with sesame oil and the other seasonings listed.
6. **Lasagna** can be made with Dreamfields lasagna noodles. Remember to avoid spaghetti sauces that use sugar if you use store-bought versions in your recipe. Check out our next lasagna recipe using eggplant, or try Linda Sue's famous Spinach Lasagna found at www.genaw.com.

Eggplant Lasagna – S

If you've never made lasagna from scratch before, don't be intimidated. This is Pearl's recipe which is stripped down to basics, but still tastes great. It may seem like there are a lot of steps, but they are all easy. It makes a really huge lasagna for a big family, or two meal's worth for a smaller family. It's not too time consuming and is perfectly paired with only a side salad.

Basic ingredients: eggplants ✦ ground beef ✦ tomato sauce ✦ ricotta cheese ✦ mozzarella cheese ✦ eggs ✦ sea salt and other seasonings

1. Peel 2 eggplants and slice vertically to make large lasagna type noodles of about ⅛ inch thick.
2. Season eggplant "noodles" with sea salt and black pepper and place on 2 large oiled cookie sheets.
3. Rub coconut oil over tops of eggplant noodles with your fingers and bake in oven for 20 minutes at 400.

4. While eggplant noodles are baking, brown 1½ lbs. ground beef and drain fat if not using grass fed.
5. Pour 3 (8 oz.) cans tomato sauce into a mixing bowl, leaving about 2 Tbs. of sauce in one of the cans for further use.
6. Add cooked ground beef to the bowl and season the beef/sauce mixture with sea salt, black pepper, onion powder, cayenne pepper, and Italian seasoning. Mix well.
7. Put 15 oz. ricotta cheese in separate bowl (Kraft brand skim ricotta works well and saves on calorie excess).
8. Add 4 eggs to bowl with ricotta and mix well.
9. Find a super large baking tray (or two medium casserole dishes) and spread leftover tomato sauce thinly on bottom of tray.
10. Layer on all cooked eggplant noodles so entire bottom of tray is covered fully.
11. Spread ricotta/egg mix over noodles.
12. Layer 8 oz. grated mozzarella cheese over ricotta/egg mix.
13. Spread beef/sauce mix over layer of cheese as evenly as possible.
14. Layer another 8 oz. grated mozzarella cheese on top.
15. Bake at 350 for 35 minutes.

Spaghetti Bolognese – S

Here's a "go to" sauce that is a regular pasta favorite in both our homes.

Basic Ingredients: ground beef ✦ onion and optional garlic ✦ tomato paste ✦ canned petite diced tomatoes ✦ mushrooms ✦ water ✦ sea salt and other seasonings ✦ parmesan cheese

1. Brown 3 lbs. ground beef. Pour off any grease (if not using grass fed beef).
2. Add 1 large finely chopped onion and optional finely cut garlic to cook with meat for a few minutes.
3. Add 2 (6 oz.) cans tomato paste, 1can petite diced tomatoes, optional sliced mushrooms and enough water to make correct saucy consistency.
4. Add Bragg Liquid Aminos, sea salt, onion powder, chili powder, and cayenne pepper (we use lots of cayenne).
5. Simmer for 30 minutes to 1 hour, or until onions are soft and translucent.
6. Cook Dreamfields noodles toward end. You'll need two boxes of the spaghetti kind if you are making it for a large family. Make sure you boil the pasta for no longer than 9 minutes.

7. Put noodles in bowls, pour on sauce, and add parmesan cheese on top.

Creamy Mushroom Pasta – S

Basic Ingredients: onions ✦ mushrooms ✦ squash or zucchini ✦ pre-cooked beef or chicken ✦ coconut oil and butter ✦ sea salt and other seasonings ✦ heavy cream ✦ optional water and glucomannan ✦ parmesan cheese

1. Slice 1-2 onions in chunky pieces and sauté in coconut oil and butter in large skillet.
2. Add 1 large container of sliced button mushrooms to pan.
3. Add 2 diced summer squash or zucchini.
4. Add sliced or diced roast beef, deli meat, or pre-cooked steak or chicken pieces.
5. Toss vegetables and meat in butter and oil and season with sea salt, pepper, Cajun seasoning, Bragg Liquid Aminos, and cayenne pepper.
6. Once vegetables are just tender, add a few small swirls of heavy cream and simmer for a few more minutes. You may add water if you want more sauce and thicken with glucomannan by shaking and whisking.
7. Pour sauce over pasta and add parmesan cheese.

This recipe works with any of the noodles we advise, including konjac noodles.

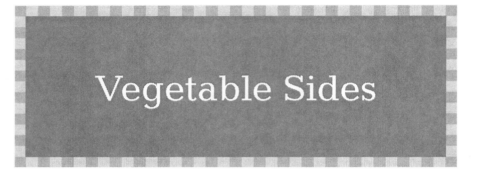

Chapter 22

Vegetable Sides

Fresh vegetables picked straight from the garden are the optimal choices to use in the following recipes. If you do not have access to a garden, don't feel too bad about using frozen vegetables. They are picked at the height of freshness and usually snap frozen to preserve freshness and nutrients. They're a great second choice to home grown, and often preferable to vegetables from a supermarket that may have may have been sitting around for days and weeks, losing much of their fresh vitality.

Note. When using frozen broccoli and cauliflower, buy packets that contain only the florets. The florets of these vegetables are lower carb than the stalks (which are not the yummiest part of those vegetables anyway).

With the exception of the first recipe and our *Tuna Stuffed Tomatoes* recipe, all others are **S** only. Non-starchy veggies paired with fats are the perfect duo.

Creamless Creamy Veggies – S, E or Fuel Pull

Adopting this recipe will enable you to fully enjoy cooked vegetables with your **E** meals if that is what you crave. It is also the perfect recipe for **Fuel Pull** days outlined in the *One Week Fuel Cycle*, Chapter 28, if you have stubborn weight to lose or anytime you feel ready to include a **Fuel Pull**. This basic low-fat cream sauce idea also works great with konjac noodles for an extremely weight reducing **Fuel Pull** meal.

If you have the strictest of purist mindsets like Serene, this recipe may not appeal to you since it uses Laughing Cow light cheese, which is a European cheese found in most supermarkets. Thankfully, it is without dyes and other harmful ingredients, but it contains two preservatives. These are not the worst preservatives you could ingest (less hazardous than what most store-bought salad dressings contain), but we thought we should let you know. Weight Watchers cheese wedges (a similar product) also work for this recipe and are a little more budget friendly.

Basic Ingredients: fat free chicken broth ✦ any non-starchy veggies of choice ✦ Laughing Cow or Weight Watchers cheese wedges✦ sea salt and other seasonings ✦ parmesan cheese ✦ optional glucomannan

1. Put veggies in a saucepan with ¼-½ cup of fat free chicken broth to simmer. Any veggies will work, but angel hair shredded cabbage is your fastest veggie to cook. Broccoli and cauliflower florets will take a little longer. They should be cut to smaller size for optimum appeal.
2. Once vegetables are tender, add 1-2 wedges of Laughing Cow light cheese (depending on amount of veggies) and melt in naturally. Use no more than 1 wedge per person.
3. Add generous shake or two of sea salt and lots of black pepper, along with optional Bragg Liquid Aminos, cayenne pepper, or garlic and/or onion powder. This sauce tastes a lot better well seasoned.
4. Add 1 Tbs. parmesan cheese and stir in to rest of ingredients.
5. You can leave recipe as is, or decide to make more sauce. You will do this by adding more chicken broth to the pan and thickening the extra fluid to sauce consistency by shaking in glucomannan from a salt shaker and whisking it in briskly with the broth. Adjust seasonings if needed after adding more fluid to the recipe as glucomannan can sometimes mask flavor.
6. Serve with a small sprinkle of parmesan cheese on top.

Baked Eggplant Rounds – S

These are a more like mini pizzas.

Basic Ingredients: egg plant ✦ tomato paste ✦ sea salt and other seasonings, including nutritional yeast ✦ coconut oil

1. Cut eggplant in ¼-½ inch rounds and place on greased baking tray.
2. Ice each eggplant round with tomato paste.
3. Sprinkle with sea salt, black pepper, onion and garlic powder, and nutritional yeast. You can replace nutritional yeast with parmesan or mozzarella cheese for more of an eggplant parmesan style recipe.
4. Drizzle a little coconut oil (or olive oil) onto each round.
5. Bake at 350 until eggplant is cooked through and a little crispy, approximately 20 minutes.

Simple Steamed Broccoli or Cauliflower – S

Basic Ingredients: broccoli ✦ butter, sea salt, and other seasonings ✦ grated cheese

1. Steam frozen bags of broccoli or cauliflower florets until tender.
2. Drain water and return broccoli to pot.
3. Add a few generous dollops of butter.
4. Season with sea salt and pepper.
5. Grate cheddar cheese on top and let melt.
6. Toss all together gently.

Roasted Vegetable Medley – S

Basic Ingredients: broccoli ✦ cauliflower ✦ cabbage ✦ onions ✦ coconut oil ✦ sea salt and other seasonings, including nutritional yeast or parmesan cheese

1. Place broccoli and cauliflower florets, thin wedges of cabbage, and sliced onions in large roasting pan.
2. Add generous amounts of coconut oil, sea salt, black pepper, onion and garlic powder, nutritional yeast (if you don't have the yeast, use parmesan cheese) and cayenne pepper.
3. Toss all ingredients together and assemble into as much of a single layer as possible.
4. Bake at 350 until veggies are crispy on the outside and very tender on the inside, tossing occasionally, approximately 45 minutes.

Vangi's Parmesan Zucchini – S

Basic Ingredients: butter ✦ zucchini ✦ parmesan cheese ✦ sea salt and other seasonings

1. Melt butter in a fry pan.
2. Add 2-3 sliced zucchinis to pan.
3. Shake in generous amounts of parmesan cheese and salt and pepper to taste.
4. Toss until browned.

Our sister, Evangeline has the green thumb in our family and has passed her gift on to most of her ten children, many of whom have their own gardens. Her oldest son, Zadok is now a market gardener, known as Zadok the Natural Farmer. Vangi always has an abundant harvest and is kind enough to give her two inferior gardener sisters plenty. We especially love her zucchini. Her garden is spectacular every year. By spectacular, think extremely large scale, all organic, picturesque, and flourishing.

Serene chats: I have always shared the love of gardening with my sister, Evangeline, but lacked the gifting that turns simple dirt and seeds into paradise and overflowing harvests. I love to dig and do the hard work, but then forget to plant. I spend three weeks double digging with a spade and hours of sweat and toil under the hot Tennessee sun preparing my chert rock yard into workable soil. But, the buck stops there, and each year I end up with empty beds that soon overgrow with weeds. Well, I do manage to plant herbs and stevia plants.

Evangeline enjoys every aspect of gardening and relishes being in her garden so much that she wants to put a day bed in it to rest and drink in the fragrant breezes after a day of toil. It is amazing how three sisters can be so different. Pearl, on the other hand, detests the entire thought of gardening. She does not like getting dirt under her fingernails or the thought of seeing a spider, or being bitten by a bug. She doesn't like to be either too hot or cold either, so toiling outside doesn't suit her "princess" personality.

Pearl chats: Sounds like I'm a pampered brat, but I have to admit what she said is all true. But, I thankfully receive Evangeline's gifts of cucumbers, tomatoes and other delicious veggies she bestows on me every year, My mother has a great garden also, so I get extra blessed every summer and fall by both their bountiful harvests, and I don't even have to pull one weed. Am I lucky or what? I obviously don't deserve them since I am Mrs. Prima Donna.

Spaghetti Squash Noodles – S

If you love gardening, plant plenty of spaghetti squash this growing season! You'll use them all up making oodles of noodles. Grow heaps, cook heaps, and freeze heaps for the entire year.

If using spaghetti squash for yourself only, there will likely be some leftover and you can bag it in individual portions. Children are usually happy with whole wheat noodles on pasta nights. However, if you have plenty from your garden, feed it to everyone in the family. It's an awesome and delicious food.

Basic Ingredients: spaghetti squash

1. Pierce holes in 1 spaghetti squash as you would for a potato before baking.
2. Cut squash lengthwise in half and remove seeds.
3. Place cut sides down on a lightly greased baking tray.
4. Bake at 350 for 30 minutes or until it feels tender to a fork.
5. Using a fork, pull apart the squash flesh which will string into long, angel hair type noodles. Place noodles into bowl and cover with your favorite pasta sauce, either white and creamy, or red and meaty. Or, drizzle with sesame oil, sea salt, chili flakes, and parmesan cheese.

Zucchini Noodles – S

These noodles cook up very quickly and are great with everything from fried eggs to spaghetti sauce to salmon.

Basic Ingredients: zucchini or yellow squash ✦ coconut oil ✦ sea salt and other seasonings

1. Use a potato peeler to cut very thin strips or slices from zucchinis or yellow squash, rotating the vegetable as you peel.
2. Use as much of the zucchini or squash as possible. You may have to discard the very center.
3. Heat a little coconut oil in skillet and toss noodles in batches, adding salt and pepper while they are cooking
4. It only takes a few minutes in the skillet until they are ready.

Zucchini Fries – S

Basic Ingredients: zucchini ✦ mayonnaise or egg wash (egg with water) ✦ parmesan cheese ✦ Creole seasoning ✦ coconut or palm oil

1. Cut zucchini into strips the length of regular home fries.
2. Use your hands to rub about 2 Tbs. mayonnaise onto zucchini (messy, but fun), or dip zucchini strips in an egg wash.
3. Mix parmesan cheese with a little Cajun seasoning or seasoning of your choice and sprinkle over mayo covered fries. Get your hands in the bowl again and mix well. If you don't like getting your hands messy, throw all ingredients into a plastic bag and shake well.
4. Fry until nicely browned in coconut or palm oil, or oven bake on well greased tray.

Green Fries – S

Basic Ingredients: string green beans ✦ coconut oil and butter, or olive oil ✦ parmesan cheese ✦ sea salt and other seasonings

1. Pour 1 packet of frozen string green beans onto baking tray.
2. Drizzle with olive oil, or butter and coconut oil.
3. Sprinkle generously with parmesan cheese, black pepper, sea salt, and onion or garlic powder.
4. Bake at 350 for 30 minutes.

Serene chats: You'll need two or three full trays for larger families. These green fries do a magical disappearing act with children. ✣S

Sauteed String Green Beans – S

The final result of this recipe is similar to *Green Fries*, but if you have other things in the oven taking up space, you can easily prepare them in a skillet.

Basic Ingredients: frozen string green beans ✦ sea salt and other seasonings ✦ parmesan cheese ✦ coconut oil

1. Pour 1 frozen thawed bag of string green beans (or fresh from garden) into a hot skillet with 2-3 heaped Tbs. melted coconut oil.
2. Add seasonings like sea salt, black pepper, cayenne pepper, and Bragg Liquid Aminos.
3. Toss beans well every few minutes (frozen beans may need to start with the lid on skillet to get them thawed).
4. A couple of minutes before serving, coat bens well with shakes of parmesan cheese.

Cauli Rice – S

Basic Ingredients: cauliflower ✦ sea salt and other seasonings ✦ olive oil

1. Lightly steam cauliflower (either fresh or frozen).
2. Place on chopping board and chop into small rice sized pieces (doesn't matter if some are slightly bigger). Or, use food processor to obtain correct size. Don't over process or you'll have mashed cauliflower.
3. Add butter or a swirl of extra virgin olive oil and salt and pepper to taste.

Pearl chats: My husband dislikes rice in any form, but quite enjoys this. We have it under so many dishes so I make large batches of it to store in the freezer. If you don't like the above version, lightly sauté *Cauli Rice* in a pan to make it a little crispier, but I don't find that necessary.

Spinach Casserole or (Green Bean Casserole) – S

Basic Ingredients: frozen spinach or green beans ✦ water ✦ heavy cream ✦ butter ✦ sea salt and other seasonings ✦ glucomannan ✦ skim mozzarella cheese

1. Lightly steam 2 (16 oz.) bags of frozen spinach until wilted (or thaw them naturally).
2. Put spinach in colander and squeeze all water out by grabbing handfuls and squeezing into the sink, or pressing down with a plate until every bit of liquid runs out. Make sure it is squeezed out well.
3. Transfer squeezed out spinach to greased casserole dish.
4. Put 1 ⅔ cup of water into blender.
5. Add ⅓ cup heavy cream and 2 level Tbs. butter to blender.
6. Add 1 tsp. sea salt, generous sprinkles of black pepper, and onion and garlic powder to taste.

7. Add 1 tsp. glucomannan and blend well until mixture is thick and gluggy.
8. Pour blended mix over spinach and mix together well with your hands (messy, but fun).
9. Grate 1 cup skim mozzarella. Add ½ cup to spinach and mix around. Sprinkle other ½ cup on top of casserole.
10. Bake at 350 for 20 minutes.

Serene chats: This is one of my husband's favorites as he's fond of casseroles. I make this same recipe using lightly steamed string beans. It's much healthier than regular *Green Bean Casserole* but still tastes incredible.

Macafoni and Cheese – S

Basic Ingredients: cauliflower ✦ cream cheese ✦ heavy cream ✦ unsweetened almond milk ✦ water ✦ sea salt and other seasonings, including Dijon mustard ✦ grated cheese ✦ optional glucomannan

1. Steam either 2 bags frozen cauliflower, or 1 large fresh cauliflower until ½ way to tender.
2. Cut 6 oz. ⅓ less fat cream cheese into small pieces and set aside.
3. Heat ¼ cup heavy cream, ¾ cup unsweetened almond milk, and 1 cup water in saucepan.
4. Once liquid begins to simmer, whisk in 1 tsp. Dijon mustard and add sea salt and pepper to taste.
5. Add cut up cream cheese to saucepan, along with 2 cups of shredded or grated cheddar cheese.
6. Add cauliflower pieces to sauce and simmer until pieces are fully tender and cheese sauce is nice and bubbly. (If sauce is not thick enough for your liking, sprinkle in some glucomannan from a salt shaker and whisk vigorously until your desired thickness).

This cheese sauce can also be used over Dreamfields pasta, but we like the whole food approach of using cauliflower as a more frequent option.

Baked Cauliflower – S

Basic Ingredients: cauliflower ✦ coconut oil and butter ✦ sea salt and other seasonings

1. Empty 1-2 frozen bags of cauliflower, or cut up fresh head of cauliflower and place in baking dish.
2. Add some coconut oil, butter, sea salt and black pepper
3. Bake at 375-400 for 30 minutes.

Stuffed Cauli or Broccoli – S

Basic Ingredients: cauliflower or broccoli ✦ onion or green onion ✦ sour cream or cream cheese ✦ grated cheese ✦ bacon bits ✦ sea salt and other seasonings

1. Empty frozen bags of cauliflower and broccoli florets into baking dish (or use fresh).
2. Add diced onion or chopped green onion, and a few dollops of sour cream or cream cheese.
3. Add grated cheddar cheese, bacon bits (we use turkey bacon bits), and season with salt and pepper.
4. Cover and bake covered at 400 for about 30 minutes. Halfway through cooking time, toss ingredients well and return to oven to finish.

Stir Fry Veggies Deluxe – S

Basic Ingredients: stir fry veggies ✦ coconut oil ✦ sea salt and other seasonings ✦ optional sesame oil

1. Heat 2-3 Tbs. coconut oil in large fry pan.
2. Add 1-2 packets frozen stir fry veggies.
3. Season with Bragg Liquid Aminos or soy sauce, a little sea salt, black pepper, and a dash of cayenne pepper.
4. Toss and simmer until veggies are ready, but still slightly crunchy.
5. You may like to add a few drops of sesame oil once veggies are ready.

Cauliflower Mashed Potatoes – S

If you do these the right way, you can barely tell the difference between this dish and real mashed potatoes. The secret is the food processor.

Basic Ingredients: cauliflower ✦ butter ✦ sea salt and other seasonings ✦optional heavy cream

1. Steam 2 bags of frozen cauliflower until tender, or steam a fresh head of cauliflower.
2. Place florets in food processor and add a good dollop or two of butter, sea salt, and black pepper. You may also add 1 Tbs. cream if you desire.
3. Process on high until creamy.

White Bean Mashies – E

Why are we including *White Bean Mashies* in a chapter for vegetable dishes? Because, if no one sees you cooking it, they might not believe these "mashies" are not real mashed potatoes. "Mashies" are delectable with *Basic Gravy* made **E** style and drizzled on top. A family favorite.

Basic Ingredients: any white beans ✦ sea salt and black pepper ✦ optional 1-2 tsp. butter

1. Soak white beans overnight. Our favorite is baby limas as they are ultra creamy when cooked.
2. Pour off water, add fresh water and cook until over-tender.
3. Pour beans through colander to drain water.
4. Place in food processor and process until creamy and smooth. If you are feeding a big family, do it in batches.
5. Add sea salt and black pepper to taste
6. Add optional butter. The tiny amount you will eat in your serving will not affect your **E** fat limit.

Make with chana dahl if you want to really "dig in" to this dish, although you would now have "golden mashies." Chana dahl has very little effect on insulin levels.

Creamed Spinach – S

Basic Ingredients: spinach ✦ water ✦ sea salt and other seasonings ✦ cream cheese ✦ parmesan cheese

1. Place 1 bag of frozen loose leaf spinach in saucepan (or use several bunches of fresh spinach).
2. Add a little water and cover until spinach is wilted and tender, stirring occasionally.
3. Season with sea salt and pepper.
4. Add 4 oz. ⅓ less fat Philadelphia cream cheese and ¼ cup parmesan cheese and stir.
5. Simmer for a couple more minutes until all ingredients have mingled nicely together.

Twice Baked Zucchini – S

Basic Ingredients: zucchini ✦ tomatoes ✦ cheese ✦ green onion ✦ bacon bits ✦ optional ground beef

1. Cut zucchinis lengthwise and scoop out seedy middle part.
2. Par-bake in oven at 400 for around 10 minutes.
3. Take zucchinis out and stuff centers with diced tomatoes, cheese, green onions, and bacon bits (we use turkey bacon bits). Or, to make this side dish into a main course, add leftover cooked ground beef.
4. Bake for another 10-15 minutes at 400.

Baked Brussel Sprouts – S

Basic Ingredients: Brussels sprouts ✦ coconut oil and butter ✦ sea salt and other seasonings, including nutritional yeast and/or parmesan cheese

1. Empty 1-2 frozen bags of Brussels sprouts into baking dish.
2. Add coconut oil and a little butter and lots of Bragg Liquid Aminos, or sea salt, black pepper, and sprinkle of cayenne pepper. Adding1-2 Tbs. nutritional yeast or a sprinkle of parmesan cheese adds further flavor to this recipe.
3. Bake uncovered until nicely browned (but not too soft and shriveled) for about 30-45 minutes. Turn once during baking.

Stuffed Peppers – S

Basic Ingredients: peppers ✦ cream cheese ✦ grated cheese ✦ sea salt and other seasonings ✦ optional ground beef and quinoa

1 Mix 4 oz. ⅓ less fat cream cheese with 8 oz. grated cheese.
2 Add onion or garlic powder, pepper, and sea salt.
3 Slice green or red peppers in half and fill with cheesy mixture.
4 Bake at 350 for about 20 minutes.

As is, this recipe is more of a side dish. You can make it the center of a full meal if you have lots of peppers from your garden, or purchase enough to fill the whole family. You could then add browned ground beef to the cheese mix, along with enough quinoa to give a hint of a "rice feel: to the stuffing. Or, stuff with *Mexican Noodles* (*Evening Meals,* Chapter 21).

Tuna Stuffed Tomatoes – S, E or Fuel Pull

Basic Ingredients: tomatoes ✦ tuna ✦ mayonnaise

1 Slice tomatoes in half and scoop out seeds and middle parts.
2 Fill with tuna mixed with mayonnaise.

This recipe can be made **E** or **Fuel Pull** friendly by using low-fat mayo combined with mustard, or horseradish spread. You can also stuff tomatoes with cottage cheese for an **E** or **Fuel Pull** option.

Cauli Potato Salad – S

Pearl chats: My husband is crazy about real potato salad, but he thinks this one is a pretty good second best. I make this for barbecue get-togethers in the summer months and always receive a lot of compliments. It goes great with burgers. Sometimes, instead of steaming the cauliflower as outlined below, I sauté or roast it with salt and pepper. This makes for an even more flavorful salad.

Basic Ingredients: cauliflower ✦ eggs ✦ mayonnaise ✦ onion ✦ sea salt and other seasonings

1 Lightly steam 1-2 bags frozen cauliflower or a fresh head of cauliflower (do not let cauliflower get mushy).

2. Boil 4-6 eggs and peel off shells, dice eggs, and place in a bowl.
3. Transfer cooked cauliflower to bowl and cut any big pieces to resemble the size of diced potatoes.
4. Add ½ finely diced onion.
5. Add Creole seasoning, or sea salt and black pepper.
6. Add enough mayonnaise to coat everything well. Mix all ingredients together without mashing too much.

Pea Salad – S

Peas are slightly higher in carbs than other non-starchy vegetables, but if you have made some good progress managing your weight, you may include them in your meals in moderate doses. This salad goes well as a side to salmon or white fish meals and is very quick and simple.

Basic Ingredients: peas ✦ onion ✦ cheese ✦ mayonnaise

1. Put 1-2 cans drained peas into bowl, or cook frozen or fresh peas in saucepan. Drain before adding to bowl.
2. Add ½ small onion, finely diced.
3. Cut 2-3 oz. cheddar cheese (Pepper Jack tastes good too) into small cubes and add.
4. Add enough mayo to coat well and mix all together.

Chapter 23

Desserts

Check This Information

When we mention measurements for Truvia in the following dessert recipes, this applies to store-bought or homemade, according to Lauren Benning's directions at www.healthyindulgences.net/.

As we mentioned in *Foundation Foods*, Chapter 17, NuStevia Pure White Stevia Extract Powder is extremely sweet. In an uncooked recipe, ⅛ tsp. is equal to about ¼ cup of sugar. Cooking decreases the sweetness of stevia somewhat. Therefore, in a cooked recipe, a ¼ tsp. of powder could be equal to around ¼ cup of sugar, although stevia is hard to pin down to hard numbers. Sometimes, cooked recipes need more powder to achieve sweetness, sometimes they don't. Other ingredients also play a part in how much they mask sweetness. In each of our recipes we have given the closest approximation that we can with regard to the NuStevia Pure White Stevia Extract Powder. Some of our recipes call for a dash or sprinkle of the powder. Take that to mean quite a bit less than ⅛ of a teaspoon. When we refer to Nunaturals, remember that it is the pure white Stevia extract powder that we are talking about.

Also remember, if your budget is extremely tight, you can try using Nunaturals alone since it goes a lot further.

Choco Pudding – S, E or Fuel Pull (makes two or more full cup servings)

We love this pudding, because you can make it in a jiffy, anytime. Our basic recipe uses unsweetened almond milk. We like Silk brand, only 30 calories per cup. Who's counting, right? But, it's smart to not eat more calories than necessary.

We give this pudding the honor of first place dessert as it matches all **S**, **E** and **Fuel Pull** foods since it is both low in carbs and does not have a lot of fat. It gives a great chocolate fix and while we called it *Choco Pudding*, you can put any flavor you desire in front of the word "pudding." Let your imagination fly.

Pearl's favorite is banana nut, using defatted peanut flour and banana extract to match **Fuel Pull** or **E**, or adding a big spoonful of unsweetened peanut butter for an indulgent **S**. Serene's favorite flavor is plain vanilla. You may even like to try chocolate mint by adding a couple of drops of mint essence to the basic cocoa recipe. Or, add strawberries for chocolate strawberry. Or, omit the cocoa and use vanilla, lemon, or banana extract.

Some of our other dessert recipes are higher in fat and calories. That's fine if kept in **S** settings, but this pudding is great whenever you feel the chocolate itch. Scratch it with this pudding without splurging on excess fat and calories. You don't have to worry which category of meal you just ate, whether it is **S** or **E**. If the munchies come on, eat this pudding (heaps of it), and without guilt. You can even make it with half almond milk and half water to if you are determined to further reduce calories. It still tastes great, but that's not really necessary.

There's no need to make your own almond milk. The result is less smooth and a lot more caloric. Silk brand uses natural vegetable thickeners like locust bean gum and sunflower lecithin (extremely healthy) that thicken and give a creamy mouth taste without the use of so many nuts.

If you don't have unsweetened almond milk handy (it's not overly cheap), you can use whatever plan approved liquid you like, but make sure you categorize the pudding into its appropriate meal category. You can use a mixture of water with a dollop or two of heavy whipping cream. Or, combine water with some full-fat coconut milk from the can for a real creamy taste. Or, use a mixture of water and light coconut milk. You can even use leftover morning coffee and add some cream for a Frappuccino type pudding. Delish! All of these creamy options would be **S**.

This recipe makes two or more servings. Triple, quadruple, or expand this recipe for the whole family. Our children love it.

Basic Ingredients: unsweetened almond milk ✦ sweetener ✦ cocoa powder ✦ sea salt ✦ vanilla

1 Pour 2 cups unsweetened almond milk into blender.

2. Add 4 rounded tsp. Truvia and an extra pinch of Nunaturals to sweeten further. If you don't have Nunaturals, add another 2 tsp. Truvia.
3. Add 2 heaped Tbs. cocoa powder.
4. Add tiny pinch of salt and dash of vanilla.
5. Start blender. While it is running, slowly add 1½ tsp. glucomannan. Blend for a couple of minutes. Stop blender and let contents rest for half a minute. Restart blender and whip again until pudding thickens. You will know when the pudding consistency is achieved when blender begins to make "chug, glug-a-glug" noises.
6. Transfer to bowl or container with lid (like quart sized preserving jar or yogurt container) and put in refrigerator. *Choco Pudding* will thicken up further, and in our opinion, and tastes better chilled. But, if you're hungry, go ahead and eat some straight away.

Glucomannan tips: The longer you blend, the thicker your pudding will become. Therefore, if you want to save money, see how little gluc you can get away with by blending up a storm. Some find they need only a ½ tsp. to thicken one cup of liquid to pudding consistency. If you're frugal, experiment.

If you like a hot pudding, glucomannan thickens even faster with heat. Hence, you could use even less glucomannan and make the pudding in a saucepan using a whisk and sprinkle in the gluc from a salt shaker.

Lemon Mousse – S, E or Fuel Pull (makes 2 or more full cup servings)

This is another variation on the above pudding recipe, except in place of unsweetened almond milk it uses Greek yogurt or light coconut milk and water as the base. It is a light and refreshing bowl of deliciousness. Again, you can eat lots of it because, thanks to glucomannan doing such a fine job of thickening the yogurt/coconut milk, water, and lemon juice into spoonable food, you get lots of mousse for very little ingredients and calories. This is the reason we affectionately call these glucomannan desserts "slick tricks." You think you're eating quite a lot, but you're not. It's one of our secret tips (well, no secret any longer). We share it to help you slim down further while still keeping deliciousness in your life. Keep some of it constantly handy in your fridge (if you can as children love it, too). It's a great bed time snack, or anytime filler, when you want a sweet, tangy taste.

Due to the inclusion of the full lemon, this mousse offers incredible superfood qualities, including all the bioflavonoids from the white of the lemon. Bioflavonoids are essential for blood vessel health and help to reduce free radical damage in the body. Given that both lemon and glucomannan are both super alkalizes, this mousse is the perfect balancing dessert after a meat meal, as meat leaves a more acidic ash after digestion.

If you don't have a whole lemon handy, use lemon concentrate (from the yellow, lemon like looking container at your supermarket). It is not a superfood approach, but has the right taste, the same slimming effect, and gets the job done with ease.

Basic Ingredients: lemon ✦ Greek yogurt or light coconut milk ✦ water ✦ sweetener ✦ glucomannan

1. Peel only yellow rind off a lemon, leaving as much of the white as you can. Cut lemon up into chunks, removing any seeds that are visible.
2. Put all lemon pieces and juice into blender, or use several good squirts of lemon juice concentrate.
3. Add 4 Tbs. 0% Greek yogurt, or ¼ cup light coconut milk.
4. Add 2 cups water.
5. Add 4 rounded tsp. Truvia. If you prefer a more sweet taste, add dash of Nunaturals.
6. While blender is running, slowly add 2 tsp. glucomannan. Blend for a couple of minutes. Stop blender and let contents rest for a couple more minutes. Restart blender and whip again until mousse is starting to thicken well.

If you are not partial to lemon flavor, this same mousse idea can be made with vanilla or berry flavors. You can also use Hansen's Natural Fruit Stix. Add contents of one pack to make a zesty berry flavored mousse in place of the lemon. Or, you can use real berries for added antioxidant and nutritional value. Serene makes a yummy version of this "slick trick" idea using blueberries and cinnamon to flavor.

Tummy Tucking Ice Cream – S, E or Fuel Pull

Now you do not have to feel guilty while eating ice cream. This treat supports vibrant health rather than degrading it. And it's good, good, good! This recipe makes one generous serving, but it's easy to multiply the ingredients if you want to feed others in the family, or freeze leftovers. It works better, however, to only process one batch at a time. One batch produces one large single bowl of goodness.

If you want to make up several batches at a time so you have extra ice cream to put in the freezer, you will need to add vegetable glycerin. This is available at most health stores. The glycerin prevents a hard freeze occurring so you can still dip and serve. Rather than doing this, we usually keep lots of frozen cubes ready in the freezer. Once again, baggies come in handy. You can put one serving's worth of frozen cubes into each baggie. Whenever you feel like ice cream, pull a baggie from the freezer and you can make up ice cream in a few minutes.

Pearl chats: Serene came up with this recipe, first using light coconut milk as the base. We enjoyed it frequently as an **S**. I tried it once with unsweetened almond milk. It was every bit as good, possibly better and much more flexible for the plan since it can be eaten as a dessert after an **E**, **S** or **Fuel Pull** meal at any time. Now, we both only use unsweetened almond milk for this recipe.

The example recipe below is vanilla flavored, but you can create any flavor to suit your cravings. Peanut butter flavor is good using 1 Tbs. defatted peanut flour, or 1 tsp. peanut butter to keep within **E** and **Fuel Pull** guidelines. Adding cocoa powder makes for great chocolate flavor—chocolate mint is good. Or, try frozen strawberries. A nice delicacy is to drizzle our *Skinny Chocolate* (warmed up to room temperature) over the ice cream for a magic shell type ice cream treat, but always keep that in **S** setting.

In addition to the almond milk in this recipe, we call for 1 tsp. of either heavy cream, peanut butter, or tahini. This truly helps to make the ice cream creamier, but still allows you to stay in **Fuel Pull** or **E** mode. Without this little bit of fat, the consistency is a little more sherbet like in texture, but still good. However, adding this tiny amount of fat makes it more like real homemade ice cream. (Pearl's husband thinks it tastes just like the homemade ice cream he ate every summer as a child in Oklahoma). Tahini works great for this purpose in any of your flavor options. It gives a creamy consistency and goes well with cocoa for a chocolate flavor. Serene always uses tahini while Pearl sticks to heavy cream. You'll find your own favorite preference after trying out the options.

Basic Ingredients: unsweetened almond milk ✦ sweetener ✦ glucomannan✦ vanilla✦ heavy cream or tahini or peanut butter ✦ optional vegetable glycerin

Step A:

1 Pour 1 cup unsweetened almond milk into blender.

2 Add 3-4 tsp. Truvia (and a tiny dash of Nunaturals if you like very sweet ice cream).

3 Add 1tsp. vanilla and ¼ tsp. glucomannan or xanthan gum.

4 Blend for 30 seconds to 1 minute then pour this liquid into 1½ ice cube trays and freeze. If you only use 1 ice cube tray, the frozen cubes will be too big for your food processor to handle.

Step B:

5 When you are ready to eat your ice cream, take frozen cubes from freezer and place in food processor or high end blender like a Vitamix (a cheap blender will not likely

do the job). Add a few drops of vegetable glycerin if you want to return any leftover ice cream to freezer.

6 Process or blend until a powdery consistency is reached (like dry snow).

7 Stop processing. Add about 2-4 more Tbs. unsweetened almond milk and 1 tsp. heavy cream, tahini, or peanut butter. Process, or blend again for a few minutes until an ice cream/soft serve texture forms and the consistency is no longer like powdery snow, but holds together.

Serene chats: I like to add a ¼ scoop of whey protein powder to the food processor right before processing. It gives more protein and I think makes the texture even better. Pearl prefers it without this addition.

Mouth Watering Meringues – S, E or Fuel Pull

These are a great treat to eat between meals if you are unsure of your next meal's fuel style. Like the above recipes, they won't force you to eat either **E** or **S** since they fit easily into either meal style. They're an extremely low-calorie dessert even though they melt in your mouth. If you want to eat something sweet, but don't need to overdo more calories, think of these. They'll also be useful if you are trying the *One Week Fuel Cycle*, Chapter 28 and want a cookie type treat on the two toughest full **Fuel Pull** days.

And the best thing, they're cheap! Only four egg whites and some sweetener for oodles of cookies. Way to go, meringues!

Basic Ingredients: egg whites ✦ sweetener ✦ vanilla ✦ xanthan gum

1 Place glass or metal bowl, along with metal ends of your electric beater, to chill in freezer.

2 While cooling down in freezer, grind 7 tsp. Truvia in your coffee grinder. The grinding creates a smoother feel to the meringue.

3 Once bowl and metal ends are cool (only takes a few minutes), take them out and place on counter.

4 Crack 4 eggs and drop only whites into cold bowl. You must use fresh egg whites for this recipe as the carton kind will not work.

5 Add 2 tsp. vanilla and ¼ tsp. xanthan gum.

6 Start beating, slowly adding ground Truvia a little at a time. Optional: add ⅛ tsp. Nunaturals to further sweeten meringues.

7 Continue beating until whites are so stiff that you can turn the bowl upside down and the peaks will not fall out. Takes up to 10 minutes, but it's fun watching it change.

8. Place small cookie-sized amounts on a baking tray lined with parchment paper. Or, if you want to get fancy, put mix in a quart-sized Ziploc bag, cut a hole in the corner end, and squeeze out pretty shapes.
9. Bake at 300 for 20-25 minutes. Turn off oven and let meringues oven dry for another 2 hours. (You're supposed to leave the oven door open to dry meringues, but we think that is dangerous when you have little ones running around).

You can use other flavors like ginger, cinnamon, nutmeg, or even add ¼ cup cocoa powder for a chocolate flavor.

Skinny Chocolate – S

This chocolate is so easy, so delish, and so slimming as long as it is eaten in an **S** setting. But, don't eat it with a bunch of carbs at the same time unless you want to fatten up.

Many who have tasted this recipe say it tastes similar to the Almond J*oy* candy bar. It is a good way to get in your servings of virgin coconut oil. However, if your budget does not allow you to indulge in too much virgin coconut oil, it can be made with plain coconut oil. We buy Louanna brand from Walmart for cooking purposes. While it doesn't have the same superfood and medicinal values, it contains the healthy, medium chain fatty acids and ALA's, and tastes great in this chocolate, but less Almond Joyish.

Basic Ingredients: cocoa powder ✦ coconut oil ✦ sweetener

1. Put ¼ cup cocoa powder into small bowl.
2. Add ½ cup coconut oil (if it is in solid form due to cooler weather, heat jar for a few seconds in a small saucepan until it liquefies, but don't let jar get too hot).
3. Add 3-4 tsp. Truvia (ground in coffee grinder) depending on desired sweetness, or Nunaturals to taste.
4. Stir all ingredients together with fork.
5. Line plastic plate with wax paper or foil and pour liquid chocolate on top.
6. Freeze until solidified.

The chocolate may be transferred to the refrigerator if you like it slightly softer. We like it straight out of the freezer as it melts in your mouth. Snap pieces off and enjoy.

You can add nuts, unsweetened dried coconut, and other flavors like coffee or vanilla to this basic recipe. You can also dip chilled strawberries into this chocolate if you heat it to melting point. When the chocolate cools, it hardens on cold food, just like that unhealthy, but yummy *Magic Chocolate Shell* that you can purchase. The difference being that this chocolate promotes health while the other detracts from it. You can try this with our *Tummy Tucking Ice Cream* or Breyers low-carb ice cream variety from the store. You'll be amazed!

Chocolate Nut Slab – S

Basic Ingredients: unsweetened baker's chocolate ✦ sweetener ✦ heavy cream ✦ vanilla ✦ peanuts or chopped nuts of choice

1. Place 2 (1 oz.) unsweetened squares of baking chocolate in microwave safe bowl and heat in microwave for approximately 1 minute, 20 seconds.
2. In coffee grinder, grind 4-5 tsp. Truvia, or 2 tsp. Truvia and a dash of Nunaturals to further sweeten.
3. Add sweetener to the bowl of melted chocolate, plus dash of vanilla.
4. Add approximately ⅓ cup of cream to bowl (more or less, depending upon how light or dark you like your chocolate), and stir vigorously.
5. Add peanuts or chopped almonds to chocolate mixture and stir in.

For slab type chocolate, pour mixture onto wax paper, place in freezer and break pieces off when set. For small size chocolate pieces, spoon blobs onto wax paper, pulling from bottom to top with spoon to make Chocolate *Kisses* type shapes.

Pearl chats: You should have seen Serene's scowl and heard her huffs just now as I dared to write the word "microwave" again. I'm sure she can't wait to get her more noble little fingers back to the keyboard to sway you back to her purist notions.

But, this is how I do this recipe, so quick and easy, and it has kept my husband from constantly eating sugar laden desserts as he used to. He enjoys it when I alternate between the *Skinny Chocolate* recipe and this one. Sometimes, I mix things up and combine the two, using cream and coconut oil with cocoa powder and unsweetened cooking chocolate squares. It always turns out yummy, no matter what.

My daughter, Meadow likes to make this chocolate and adds natural flavors like mint or orange essence. On a couple of occasions, I have made the above recipe into "Reeses" type candy by mixing peanut butter, a little cream, and more sweetener. I spread it on top of the chocolate after it has been in the freezer for a while and then return it to chill again. Or, to save time, dollop a little peanut butter into each piece if making blobs, a great combination. This chocolate is very rich so you don't need a lot to feel satisfied.

Serene chats: I'll just say that you can easily melt the unsweetened chocolate squares in a saucepan on low heat, or with a double boiler.

Basic Cheesecake – S

Basic Ingredients: cream cheese ✦ eggs ✦ sweetener ✦ vanilla ✦ lemon juice ✦ optional glucomannan

1. Empty contents of 2 (8 oz.) packages ⅓ less fat cream cheese into mixing bowl.
2. Add 2 eggs, 10 tsp. Truvia, splash of vanilla, and juice from ½ a lemon or 2 squirts lemon concentrate.
3. Optional: add ¼ tsp. glucomannan or xanthan gum (tends to make the end result smoother, but works fine without).
4. Beat well with electric beater for 3-5 minutes.
5. Pour mix into small greased baking dish. Place this dish in a bigger roasting pan with some water that comes up halfway on your cheesecake pan (the water surrounds the outside of the dish in which you are baking your cheesecake). This is a water bath and will stop your cheesecake from sinking in the middle.
6. Bake at 350 for approximately 30 minutes.

This basic recipe is crustless. Surprisingly, you will probably not miss the crust, but if you do, simply throw some finely chopped nuts or ground almond meal on the well greased baking dish before pouring in the cheesecake mixture. Or, you can make a more real crust by par-baking 1 cup of almond flour mixed with 1 egg white and 2 tsp. Truvia for 10 minutes. Once it has cooled somewhat from the oven, top it with the cheese cake mix and bake the full amount of time. Berries can be added to the cheesecake if you desire.

You can also make mini cheesecakes from this mixture by putting the mix in well greased muffin pans. The mini cheesecakes do sink in the middle, but that becomes a perfect space for adding homemade berry sauce and whipped cream, or some chocolate sauce (try our melted down *Chocolate Nut Slab* without the nuts).

Tip: Mini cheesecakes are a nice idea for a quick breakfast for husbands who have a sweet tooth. If your husband leaves early for work and you can't get out of bed to make him breakfast, let him know he can grab one or two mini cheesecakes out of the fridge in the morning for a delicious, on the go, first meal. They'll help him trim down if he has a weight problem, but he'll feel like he's eating a "naughty" breakfast, if he's the type who likes being naughty!

Cheesecake Berry Crunch – S

If you love the taste of cheesecake, you will love this super simple but scrumptious dessert. It is almost like a crumbly cheesecake and will fulfill a craving for the real thing, along with scratching your crunch itch. It's great if you only have a little time to prepare since there is no cooking involved.

Basic Ingredients: berries ✦ dry roasted almonds ✦ vanilla ✦ cream cheese ✦ lemon juice

1. Fill a food processor halfway with frozen berries (a medley such as blackberries, blueberries, and raspberries is delicious. Strawberries are too big unless you halve them first).
2. Add 2 generous handfuls of lightly salted dry roasted almonds. You can use unsalted or raw almonds if you add a pinch or two of salt, but the raw almonds will miss the ultimate crunch.
3. Add splash of vanilla and almond essence, dash of Nunaturals or Truvia to taste, and 2-3 heaped Tbs. ⅓ less fat cream cheese. Add an optional squeeze of lemon for a tart burst amidst the sweetness.
4. Pulse the food processor just a little until the mixture is nice and crumbly and the almonds are no longer whole. Do not pulse until ingredients are smooth or mushy. This recipe needs to be crunchy, but all ingredients combined nicely.

Serene chats: My husband often asks me to make this recipe for his breakfast and I think it is a super healthy way for him to start the day. When I take this to parties or potlucks, it is more enjoyed and appreciated than recipes I spend hours preparing. This little quickie shines like a star. Remember, if you want to make a huge batch, just repeat the recipe again and again. It is yummy eaten fresh, but if you are taking it to a party, put it in the freezer, and take it out half an hour before serving and fluff it up a bit. Bon appétit!

Chunky Cream Pops – S

Oh my! You are going to love us for giving you this little frozen treat idea. It's not the quickest of our dessert recipes, but once you have made a full batch, you'll have enough treats for a week or so (providing your children don't gobble them all). Keeping Ziploc baggies of these stored in your freezer will help keep you away from ever wanting to cheat on a quart of *Häagen-Dazs* again. They are so insanely good!

Your freezer is filling up with all sorts of baggies now, huh? We are encouraging you to freeze and bag almost everything, but it's a habit that works to make eating on plan more efficient.

You cannot wolf these pops down. They take a while to eat since they're frozen, but it's fun because each creamy pop is on its own little stick. When you eat a couple of pops it feels like you are eating much more than you really are and this helps with portion control. It's still not a good idea to go overboard and stuff yourself as the pops are not exactly low-calorie like our puddings and mousses made with glucomannan.

Your children will love them. They are reasonably cheap to make and the mixture goes a long way. You can feel good about the whole family enjoying pops together as a healthy dessert. But, you'll just have to make more. That's okay, because it's a fun recipe.

Basic Ingredients: cream cheese ✦ *Skinny Chocolate* ✦ sweetener ✦ vanilla ✦ peanut butter ✦ toothpicks

1. Make up a batch of *Skinny Chocolate* and place it in the freezer to harden.
2. Put 2 (8 oz.) blocks ⅓ less fat cream cheese into bowl.
3. Add 10 tsp. Truvia and dash or two of vanilla.
4. Beat ingredients until fluffy with an electric egg beater (2-4 minutes).
5. Cut up ¾ of batch of *Skinny Chocolate* into small pieces. Add to cream cheese mix.
6. Add 2 heaped Tbs. natural sugar-free peanut butter into cream cheese mix.
7. Loosely combine all ingredients with a fork so chocolate chunks and peanut butter are still in bits.
8. Place wax paper or aluminum foil on a cookie sheet and dump bite size spoonfuls of mix onto the wax paper. Make sure you get chunks and swirls of peanut butter and chocolate in every spoonful. You should get about 24-28 pops from mix.
9. Put a toothpick into the middle of each one to be used as mini ice cream stick. For children, use toothpicks where one end is blunt, and insert sharp end into pops.
10. Transfer to freezer.
11. After about an hour, pull pops off wax paper or foil (don't pull on the toothpick, it might come out) and transfer to Ziploc baggies for easy access.

Chocolate Dipped Cream Pops – S

This is a similar recipe to the one above with a couple of alterations.

Basic ingredients: *Cream Pop* mixture ✦ *Skinny Chocolate* ✦ toothpicks

1. Make plain *Cream Pop* mixture (without peanut butter and chocolate) and freeze pops with toothpicks in them.
2. Make *Skinny Chocolate* recipe, but keep it at room temperature or above so it stays in liquid form.

3 Once *Cream Pops* are frozen, hold on to toothpick and twice dip each one into liquid chocolate, then place back on foil to return to freezer.

4 Transfer pops to Ziploc baggies once chocolate has set.

Best Macaroon Cookies – S

Pearl chats: Serene created this recipe but I came up with the title. We couldn't call them the name we use between ourselves. You're curious? Please don't be offended, although I am sure you're used to us by now. We call them "poop cookies." Don't let that put you off because they're super delicious. They are so fiber filled that when you eat them, you'll have a better experience on the "potty" the next morning.

This will likely be the healthiest cookie you have ever eaten, but, they require a lot of chewing. You get a workout for your mouth, but they're worth it.

Basic Ingredients: egg whites ✦ sea salt ✦ sweetener ✦ cocoa powder ✦ vanilla

1 Put 6 egg whites or ¾ cup from a carton of 100% carton egg whites in bowl and add 3 small pinches sea salt.

2 Beat whites with an electric beater until stiff peaks form.

3 Add ⅛ tsp. Nunaturals or 6 tsp. Truvia, 4 Tbs. cocoa powder, and dash of vanilla.

4 Beat in added ingredients for about 30 seconds until they have combined well with egg whites.

5 Add 2½ cups unsweetened dried coconut (from bulk bins at a health store) and 1 cup walnuts, either halved or loosely chopped.

6 Add 1 Tbs. coconut oil in liquid form.

7 Combine new ingredients with beaten ingredients, using a spoon.

8 Using slightly oiled fingers, take dropfuls of mix about cookie size and gently press into balls. Place on oiled cookie sheet and press down slightly to spread out a little.

9 Bake on middle rack, 15-20 minutes, (20 minutes gives a crispier feel and the walnuts get a deeper flavor and crunch).

Frozen Yogurt – S, E or Fuel Pull (single serve)

This is a light refreshing dessert or snack and since it is neutral, you can have it after an **S** or **E** meal.

Basic Ingredients: 0% Greek yogurt ✦ frozen strawberries ✦ sweetener ✦ vanilla ✦ optional maca powder

1. Put ¾ cup yogurt and 6 frozen strawberries in food processor.
2. Add 2-3 tsp. Truvia and dash of vanilla.
3. Add 1 optional tsp. maca powder.
4. Process well and enjoy

Frozen Yogurt Pops – S, E or Fuel Pull

Basic Ingredients: 0% Greek yogurt ✦ sweetener ✦ flavorings like Hansen's Fruit Stix or berries ✦ optional toothpicks

1. Put 1-2 cups Greek yogurt into quart sized Ziploc bag.
2. Add sugar-free drink flavoring of choice, or berries, and ground Truvia or Nunaturals to taste.
3. Mix all together and push yogurt mix tightly down to one corner of bag.
4. Snip a hole in corner end of bag and squeeze out small dollops onto foil lined tray.
5. Put toothpick in each one, or leave as they are, then freeze.

Peanut Squares – S

Basic Ingredients: ground almonds or store-bought almond flour ✦ dry roasted peanuts ✦ butter ✦ sweetener ✦ cream cheese ✦ peanut butter ✦ cream

1. Put 1 cup ground almonds or almond flour in bowl.
2. Add ½ cup finely chopped dry roasted peanuts, ¼ cup melted butter, and 2 tsp. Truvia and mix together well.
3. Press mixed ingredients into baking tray and bake for 10-15 minutes at 350.
4. While crust is baking, put 1½ packets ⅓ less fat cream cheese and 10 tsp. Truvia into bowl and beat until light and fluffy.
5. Add ⅔ cup peanut butter and beat some more.
6. In separate bowl, beat ¾ cup cream and fold in to rest of mixture.
7. Top cooled crust with mixture and place dessert in refrigerator to chill.

Ricotta Creme – S, E or Fuel Pull (makes one serving)

This quick little protein rich dessert can be enjoyed after an **S** or **E** meal as it is made with skim ricotta cheese. It was made popular by the author of *The South Beach Diet*, Dr. Arthur Agatston. However, he suggested using Splenda, but we like to use healthier stevia based sweeteners.

Basic Ingredients: skim ricotta ✦ vanilla ✦ sweetener

1. Put ⅓-½ cup skim ricotta cheese into bowl (*Kraft* brand tastes great, is very creamy, and has less carbs than most ricotta cheeses).
2. Add dash vanilla, and 1½ tsp. ground Truvia (you wouldn't want to crunch on large Truvia grains) or a tiny dash of Nunaturals.
3. Stir and enjoy.

This can be made chocolate flavored by adding cocoa powder, or use any other flavor you desire such as almond extract or natural strawberry essence.

Pearl chats: I send this recipe to work with my husband quite often. I find it hard to send other desserts with him (other than puddings) as they either have to be frozen, or have the "squish factor" if not carefully handled. You can whip this dessert up in less than one minute, put it in a little container with a lid, and he'll have a little something sweet after his lunch. I send him ¼-½ cup's worth, a little sweet ending to his meal.

Stawberry Ricotta Parfait – S, E or Fuel Pull

Ricotta Crème gets all dressed up in this easy recipe.

Basic Ingredients: strawberries ✦ sweetener ✦ skim ricotta ✦ almond extract ✦ almond flakes

1. Cut up strawberries and toss them with a little Truvia. Let it for a few minutes.
2. Whisk ¾ cup skim ricotta with 1½ tsp. ground Truvia, or dash of Nunaturals and dash of almond extract.
3. Layer the strawberries and ricotta in a parfait glass using a couple of layers of each.
4. Top with almond flakes.

Cottage Berry Whip – S or E or Fuel Pull

Basic Ingredients: low-fat cottage cheese ✦ berries ✦ sweetener ✦ vanilla

1. Put ½ cup low-fat cottage cheese and ½ cup frozen berries in blender.
2. Add Truvia or Nunaturals to taste, dash of vanilla, and blend well.
3. Place in a parfait glass and enjoy.

Baked Grapefruit – E

Basic Ingredients: grapefruit ✦ sweetener ✦ vanilla

1. Cut grapefruit in half.
2. Sprinkle with Truvia or Nunaturals and drizzle with vanilla.
3. Broil on high until the tops of grapefruit caramelize a little.

Enjoy this easy dessert by using a spoon to dig into the bursting pockets of goodness. Baking the grapefruit really brings out the sweetness and if you haven't liked this fruit before, you might find yourself changing your mind.

Baked Apples – E

Basic Ingredients: apples ✦ sweetener ✦ cinnamon

1. Remove cores from apples with coring tool.
2. Sprinkle Truvia or Nunaturals and cinnamon inside core and over top of apples.
3. Place apples on a lightly greased baking tray and bake at 350 for 45 minutes.

These are delicious with 0% Greek yogurt, sweetened with stevia or Truvia. Your children can enjoy them with regular heavy cream poured over top. The ultimate treat, when your weight is managed to the point of **Crossovers**, is to enjoy these baked apples with heavy cream.

Cake in a Mug – S

This recipe is part of our *Mug* recipe series. It is a close relation to *Muffin in a Mug* and *Bread in a Mug*. However, this one is completely flourless so it's richer and more cake like. It is decadent and feels very sinful, the way a good chocolate cake should taste when you take a bite. It makes a quick one person serving or to share with your spouse. As with our other *Mug* recipes, it takes only one minute in the microwave.

Basic Ingredients: egg ✦ cocoa powder ✦ sweetener ✦ baking powder ✦ vanilla ✦ water ✦ coconut oil

1. Crack one egg into a mug and whisk well with a fork.
2. Add 2 heaping Tbs. cocoa powder.
3. Add 3-4 tsp. Truvia or a few shakes of Nunaturals, depending on desired sweetness.
4. Add ½ tsp. aluminum free baking powder.
5. Add dash of vanilla.
6. Add 1 Tbs. water.
7. Add 1 level Tbs. coconut oil, either extra virgin or cooking style like Louanna brand (it doesn't matter if coconut oil is solid from being cold).
8. Stir vigorously (a mini workout for your right arm).
9. Microwave for 1 minute.

Pearl chats: Everyone in my family loves this cake. My 12 year old son, Rocky is an expert at this recipe and has it memorized. He uses honey in place of Truvia as his sweetener. He's a lean wiry boy so he easily burns the glucose from the honey. He's got a real sweet tooth so I'm all too glad to remind him to make *Cake in a Mug* when he's begging for something sweet. It's a far better option for his health than most sweets children eat.

I saw the idea for the original recipe of this cake on the lowcarbfriends website. This is my own version with a few tweaks. When this cake comes out of the mug, all warm and steaming, I cut it into two, and either top it with Greek yogurt, Fat Free Reddi Whip, or pour a little heavy cream over top. You can also make a very yummy raspberry frosting out of 1 tsp. butter, 1 Tbs. cream cheese, a few thawed raspberries, and ground Truvia to taste. It's amazing with this cake!

Our good friend, Amelia, who lost 30 pounds eating on our plan, ate this cake everyday for two weeks until she couldn't look at chocolate any more, yet she still lost weight. She told me recently that she ate this cake so often at the beginning of the plan, she can barely think about eating it now.

But before you do the same I should make a caution. Amelia is in her twenties and has a very healthy metabolism. Some of you may have to be slightly more cautious with *Cake in a Mug*. It can be eaten after an **S** meal for dessert if you are seeing a steady direction toward a healthier weight. Since it *does* not contain any nut flours, it is more "after dinner" calorie friendly than our *Muffin in a Mug* which we advise you keep solely for breakfast or snack use. If however, you have very stubborn weight, opt for the lighter *Muffin in a Bowl* (*Muffins, Breads, and Pizza Crusts*, Chapter 19) as a more frequent after dinner treat. Enjoy this as dessert now and then but not several times a week since it does have the higher calories of the full egg and the coconut oil. It is welcome as perfect **S** afternoon snack anytime. Remember, while the *Muffin in a Bowl* can also be eaten after **E** foods since it is a **Fuel Pull**, this cake must stay with **S** friendly foods, due to the inclusion of the coconut oil.

Serene chats: Pearl, someone once wanted to give me a really nice microwave and I flat out declined. If you keep it up, I might have to put a warning about you on the front of the book, like "Beware of the Microwave Queen. She may nuke you!" Seriously, Pearl, can't you come up with a healthy "bake in the oven version" for "dot the i and cross the t" health perfectionists like me? I tell you what. Let's try an oven version for me and all my other health nut friends. We want decadent chocolate cake, too!

5 long years...
I need a vacation
from this book!!
I need a vacation
from her!

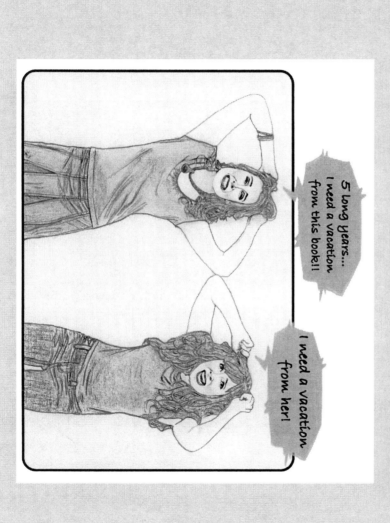

Mini Chocolate Cakes for Purists – S

Okay, it took a couple of tries, but here we are several days later with chocolate cakes in the oven now. They are still quick to make, only 12-15 minutes baking time. You'll get your rich chocolate fix in no time. They are in perfect muffin size individual portions and this recipe makes six muffins. We discovered they dry out in the oven a little more than in the microwave, therefore the addition of sour cream. You could use Greek yogurt in place of the sour cream if desired.

Pearl chats: I am actually partial to making these in the oven now and my poor microwave is getting less use. Is Serene brainwashing me? The trouble with making these in the oven is that my children beg to have one and they are gobbled before I can almost turn my head.

Basic Ingredients: eggs ✦ cocoa powder ✦ baking powder ✦ sweetener ✦ water ✦ sour cream or Greek yogurt ✦ coconut oil

1. Crack 3 eggs into a bowl and whisk.
2. Add 6 heaping Tbs. unsweetened cocoa powder.
3. Add 1½ tsp. baking powder.
4. Add 3 Tbs. water.
5. Add 3 heaping Tbs. 0% Greek yogurt or sour cream.
6. Add 3 Tbs. coconut oil.
7. Add 10 tsp. Truvia (this amount only gives a semisweet taste, therefore add ⅛ tsp. of NuStevia Pure White Stevia Extract Powder if you need further sweetness).
8. Whisk ingredients well and pour into a muffin tin with 6 sprayed or greased holes.
9. Bake for 12-15 minutes at 350 or until tops are just done (don't overcook).

These are a great dessert to serve to visitors. Adorn with cut strawberries and a squirt of Fat Free Reddi Whip if you're not a purist, or more decadently drizzled with heavy whipping cream. Very impressive! Or, try the raspberry/cream cheese frosting. No one would know they were eating a dessert that is not making them gain several pounds.

Special Agent Brownie Cake – S

One of the high points about this brownie cake with all its variations is that it is really inexpensive. We make it often in both our homes, but use honey as the sweetener for the children's versions. They even love to make their own. It's so easy—all ingredients are simply dumped into a food processor. They don't know it's so healthy for them; they just know they like it. We use Truvia and Nunaturals to sweeten our versions.

What's the secret agent? Drum roll . . . BEANS!

Don't think for a minute that this cake ends up tasting like beans. You cannot taste any beaniness, only a lovely flavor and texture. It's moist and delicious and put together in a jiffy. Variations of this bean cake have been flying around books and internet sites for many years, but the South Beach diet people made it most famous. They cannot take full acclaim though as Japanese cuisine used beans as a base to their desserts for thousands of years.

You may wonder how we can use beans and still call this an **S** recipe. Beans are a slow burning carbohydrate and full of resistant starch, which actually hinders blood sugar from spiking. Using the recipe outlined below, and cutting the cake into nine generous servings, will make each piece about 6 net carbs. We don't want you to be worried about carb counting, but this puts your mind at ease. This recipe is well within **S** limits. Because we count **S helpers** at around 15 carbs, a serving of this recipe is less than half the limit.

To bring the carb count even lower, some like to use black soy beans instead of regular beans in this recipe. Black soy beans have only 1 net carb per serving. You can find dry or canned black soy beans in most health food stores under Eden's Organic brand. We are not keen on a lot of soy, but having a non-processed source of soy like beans now and then is probably fine for most people.

Another option is to use chana dahl as the bean source for this recipe. Chana dahl will not elevate blood sugar or cause a carbs/fat collision. And it works great. It is our favorite legume option for this cake since it has a more creamy texture than other beans.

This cake is **S** because of using two whole eggs and the two Tbs. of coconut oil. The cake itself is not loaded with fat, yet it is moist due to the texture of the beans. It suits a butter based frosting so the fat content ends up rising. Be sure to pair it with only **S** friendly foods.

Basic Ingredients: black beans or chana dahl ✦ eggs ✦ egg whites ✦ cocoa powder ✦ baking powder ✦ baking soda ✦ coconut oil or butter ✦ vanilla ✦ ricotta or cream cheese ✦ sweetener

1. Put 1 drained can of black beans or 1½ cups of soaked and cooked chana dahl or other soaked and cooked beans into blender.
2. Add 2 eggs and 4 egg whites or ⅔ cup from a carton of 100% egg whites.
3. Add 4 Tbs. cocoa powder.
4. Add 1½ tsp. baking powder and ½ tsp. baking soda.
5. Add 2 Tbs. coconut oil or butter.
6. Add 2 tsp. vanilla.
7. Add ⅓ cup ricotta or cream cheese.

8 Add 4 Tbs. Truvia and ¼ tsp. Nunaturals. (We use concentrate to save money. If you don't have concentrate you'll need to use a lot more Truvia, perhaps 2 Tbs. or more, which gets expensive if you don't make your own. As the beans tend to mask sweetness, more sweetener is required if you like a good sweet brownie.

9 Process ingredients for 3-5 minutes.

10 Pour into greased baking tray and bake at 350 for 30-35 minutes.

Pearl chats: I ice these brownies with my version of the butter icing included in the *Special Occasion Cake* recipe. Or, sometimes, I make the raspberry icing which is a combination of cream cheese, a little butter, raspberries and Truvia. The raspberry is by far my favorite icing, but my husband likes chocolate better.

I know it sounds strange to admit, but sometimes I love to eat a big piece of this cake for breakfast along with my coffee. I get full, and it's a good protein source, so why not? I'm sure there's an unspoken rule against brownies for breakfast, but I like coloring outside the lines sometimes.

You do not have to stick to chocolate flavor. My mother makes a lovely ginger/cinnamon version of this recipe using white or pinto beans. Less sweetener is needed if you make the chocolate free versions since you do not have to combat the bitterness of unsweetened cocoa.

I make a wonderful banana/walnut bread using this basic recipe (if I do say so myself)! If you are not a purist and do not mind using some banana extract, go for it. I use 2 Tbs. banana extract, less Truvia, and omit the cocoa of course. Once the ingredients have been processed, I add a large handful of chopped nuts. Charlie and the children go "nuts" over it, especially with freshly whipped cream. I love it with peanut butter on top.

Special Occasion Chocolate Cake – S

This makes a large layered, moist cake that works well for birthdays or other festive occasions. It's a bit more pricey using store-bought coconut flour and other superfood ingredients so we save it for special occasions. It's a Serene inspired recipe, so a very nourishing treat for your body, full of the best fats the earth has to offer.

Basic Ingredients: store-bought coconut flour ✦ unsweetened cocoa powder ✦ golden flax meal ✦ baking powder ✦ baking soda ✦ sweetener ✦ eggs ✦ coconut oil ✦ coconut milk ✦ vanilla

Dry Directions:

1 Place 1 cup store-bought coconut flour into mixing bowl.

2. Add ½ cup ground golden flax, ½ cup unsweetened cocoa powder, 2 tsp. baking powder, and 2 tsp. baking soda.
3. Add 3-4 Tbs. Truvia and ¼ tsp. Nunaturals. This is a large layered cake so you need quite a bit of sweetness.
4. Rub all ingredients between palms of your hands to remove lumps and combine well into a nice fine meal.

Wet Directions:

1. Crack 10 eggs into blender.
2. Add ½ cup coconut oil.
3. Add 1½ cans full-fat coconut milk.
4. Add generous dash of vanilla.
5. Blend well and pour contents of blender into dry ingredients.
6. Combine ingredients well and let sit for 5 minutes while greasing two cake or bread tins.
7. Divide mixture evenly between two cake tins and bake at 350 for 1 hour.
8. Cool cakes before trying to remove them from tins.

Icing for Cake – S (Serene's superfood option)

Basic Ingredients: coconut milk ✦ eggs ✦ vanilla ✦ cocoa powder ✦ sweetener ✦ coconut oil

1. Pour 1 can full-fat coconut milk into blender.
2. Add 2 omega-3 eggs.
3. Add 1Tbs. pure vanilla.
4. Add ½ cup cocoa powder.
5. Add enough sweetener to taste. If using only Nunaturals, use at least ⅛ tsp. If you have a real sweet tooth, you will need ¼ tsp. If using only Truvia, you'll need 8-10 tsp. You can also use a combination of the two sweeteners.
6. Add ¾ cup virgin coconut oil (use Louanna cooking coconut oil if budget is an issue, but since we're going "all out" in this recipe, virgin is best).
7. Blend well and transfer to refrigerator for mix to chill and thicken as hard as butter.

Serene chats: This icing is best pre-made and chilled in the fridge. It should harden up like butter, so remove from fridge half an hour before icing your cake. Once icing is of spreadable consistency, spread a half inch layer on one of the cakes, then place the other cake on top. The icing will be like mortar between bricks. In my opinion, a nice layer of stevia-sweetened whipped cream on the top of this cake sets it off to rival any cake found at any fine dining restaurant. If you don't want to spend the time or extra money on the above icing recipe, try the recipe below. Use it in the same fashion as the filling between the layered cake.

This cake is delicious with homemade stevia-sweetened ice cream, or our *Polar Bear Soft Serve* ice cream. If you are not of the "purist" camp and don't mind a little Splenda every now and then, you can have this cake with Breyers Carb Smart Ice Cream.

Icing for Cake – S (Pearl's quick version)

Basic Ingredients: unsalted butter ✦ unsweetened baker's chocolate or cocoa powder ✦ sweetener ✦ hot water

1. Put 1½ quarters softened unsalted butter into a mixing bowl.
2. Add 1oz. melted unsweetened chocolate square. Use 2 unsweetened chocolate squares if you like a darker chocolate taste, or the squares may be substituted with ¼ cup unsweetened cocoa powder.
3. Grind 10 tsp. Truvia in coffee grinder and add to mixing bowl, or use ¼ tsp Nunaturals
4. Beat mixture with electric beater for a few minutes.
5. Add a little hot water to thin consistency to more spreadable icing.
6. Taste for sweetness and add more ground Truvia if desired.

Rich Chocolate Fudge – S

Pearl chats: This recipe is too sweet and rich for me, but I've never been a fudge loving person. My daughter makes it for herself and Charlie every now and then and they both love it. If you like reeeeeeal rich desserts, you'll get your fix with this fudge.

Basic Ingredients: butter ✦ peanut butter ✦ cocoa powder ✦ sweetener ✦ cream cheese

1. Melt 1 stick of butter with a ½ cup of peanut butter in saucepan.
2. Take sauce pan off heat and stir in 2 oz. ⅓ less fat cream cheese. Stir well.
3. Add 4 Tbs. unsweetened cocoa powder and keep stirring.
4. Add 11 tsp. ground Truvia and combine until mix is smooth.
5. Pour into a wax paper or foil lined shallow dish.
6. Freeze for 15 minutes and cut into bite size pieces.
7. Return to freezer or refrigerator.

Peanut Butter Chocolate Cookies – S

You would not know these cookies do not contain any flour. Simple and easy, but you better watch closely if you want to eat a couple, because your children might snatch and run with them before you can turn around.

Basic Ingredients: peanut butter ✦ egg ✦ cocoa powder ✦ vanilla ✦ sweetener

1. Put 1 cup peanut butter into bowl.
2. Add 1 egg.
3. Add 2 Tbs. cocoa, 1 tsp. vanilla, 10 tsp. Truvia, and ¼ tsp. Nunaturals.
4. Mix all ingredients well and roll it all into a dough ball with your hands.
5. Press cookie size rounds onto well greased cookie sheet and bake at 350 for 10 minutes.

Oopsie Chocolate Eclairs – S

Basic Ingredients: *Oopsie Roll* batter ✦ *Chocolate Nut Slab*

1. Make a double batch of *Oopsie Roll* batter (*Muffins, Breads, and Pizza Crusts,* Chapter 19), using 6 eggs and 6 oz. cream cheese. Add 3-5 tsp. Truvia to sweeten *Oopsie* batter.
2. Grease muffin tins well and place the batter ¾ way to the top of each muffin hole.
3. Bake for 30 minutes at 300.
4. While *Oopsie* muffins are baking, make *Chocolate Nut Slab* recipe, but omit nuts and keep it warm for a spoonable consistency.

5. Once *Oopsies* are cooked and taken out of the oven, they will deflate in the centers. Fill centers with chocolate mixture and top with stevia-sweetened whipped cream.

Pearl chats: Meadow, her cousin, Rashida, and Aunt Mercy (who is more like a sister) often organize Tea Parties where they dress up in their finest and ask girls over to sip tea and eat sweet goodies. Meadow usually makes up a big batch of *Oopsie Chocolate Éclairs* and they are always a big hit.

Meadow and I have had to write this recipe out for so many of their young lady guests, who, after tasting, want to immediately take the recipe home to their families. They can barely believe it is not a fattening dessert when paired with other **S** friendly foods.

Pumpkin Treat – S

This recipe works as a basic pumpkin pie. We enjoy eating it topped with whipped cream or Greek yogurt in the fall when pumpkin treats fit the atmosphere perfectly. If you don't want to have a cheat meal for Thanksgiving Day, bring this to your gathering and you will not feel you are missing out.

Basic Ingredients: eggs ✦ egg whites ✦ sweetener ✦ pumpkin pie spice ✦ cinnamon ✦ vanilla

1. Put 3 eggs and 4 egg whites (or ½ cup from a carton of 100% whites) in a large mixing bowl.
2. Add 10 tsp. Truvia.
3. Add 1 large 15 oz. can natural unsweetened pumpkin.
4. Add 1 flat Tbs. pumpkin pie spice.
5. Add 2 tsp. cinnamon and dash of vanilla.
6. Transfer mixture to well greased baking dish.
7. Bake at 350 for approx 40 minutes.

If you miss the crust, sprinkle ground almonds or crushed nuts in the greased baking tray before pouring in mixture.

Ginger Snaps – S

While we're discussing fall type desserts, we wouldn't want to leave out *Ginger Snaps*. They are Serene's husband's favorite cookie. He loved the unhealthy kind but is just as pleased with this recipe.

Basic Ingredients: almond flour or home ground almonds ✦ egg white ✦ ground ginger ✦ cinnamon ✦ vanilla ✦ sea salt ✦ plan approved sweetener

1. Put 1 cup almond flour into bowl, or grind enough almonds to make 1 cup of almond flour.
2. Add 1 egg white.
3. Add 2-3 tsp. ground ginger, 6-8 tsp. truvia or several shakes NuNaturals Stevia, cinnamon, vanilla and a little sea salt to taste.
4. Using your hands, shape mixture into a dough ball.
5. Place ball on parchment paper covered cookie sheet.
6. Spray or rub some oil on wax paper and place it face down over rolled out dough. This prevents the rolling pin from sticking to the dough.
7. Roll the ball out thinly, making sure dough is not thicker in the middle than edges.
8. Score into squares and bake at 325 for 10-15 minutes.
9. Once cooled, snap the baked slab into scored size crackers.

These ginger snaps are delicious with stevia-sweetened whipped cream for desserts or snacks around the fall season, or just about any time. Of course, you can eat them on their own.

Coconut Whipped Cream – S

Serene chats: This is a good alternative for purists who don't have access to raw cream and do not want to use pasteurized cream. I always opt for raw unpasteurized cream and thankfully I have a wonderful raw milk source. This is a yummy healthy and such a good alternative. I love it over berries.

I'm slowly learning to not be too strict with myself, and when I am at Pearl's house, you bet I'll pour some of her Walmart cream in my coffee. Or, if I go to Starbucks, in goes the heavy cream or the half and half.

Basic Ingredients: coconut milk ✦ egg ✦ coconut oil ✦ vanilla ✦ sweetener

1. Put 1 can full-fat coconut milk in blender.
2. Add 1 whole omega-3 egg.
3. Add 3 heaped Tbs. extra virgin coconut oil.
4. Add 1-2 tsp. vanilla and blend for 1 full minute.
5. Add stevia sweetener to taste, but it's enjoyable as is.
6. Transfer to fridge in sealed container and mixture will set into a nice spoonable whipped consistency.

Chapter 24

Snacks

Kale Chips – S, E or Fuel Pull

Depending on the amount of oil you use, this can be a **Fuel Pull** snack, a nice side to an **E** sandwich, or it can pair with other **S** foods. If you use the 2-3 Tbs. of oil version, the chips must stay with other **S** foods and not be paired with a grain-based sandwich.

To keep it **Fuel Pull** or **E** friendly, spray or spritz a small amount of olive oil on your baking tray and lightly spritz your kale pieces. That will give you about one teaspoon's worth. The **S** method is to more thoroughly drench the kale with room temperature coconut oil in a Ziploc baggie. Both ways are delicious and you can choose depending upon your needs or desires.

If you want to make enough to feed the whole family, you'll have to make these in multiple batches, but they don't take long to cook so the process is easy. The recipe below is a single serving and uses about 2 cups of kale pieces.

Basic Ingredients: kale ✦ olive oil or coconut oil ✦ sea salt and other seasonings ✦ optional parmesan cheese

1. Wash and dry kale and take off stems, or use from a big bag of pre-washed kale pieces.

2. Tear kale into smaller pieces. Lay them on an olive oil spritzed baking tray for lighter version, or put them in a gallon size Ziploc baggie with 2 Tbs. coconut oil.
3. Spritz the leaves on the baking tray lightly with olive oil and sprinkle with sea salt, or add sea salt to Ziploc bag and shake or massage the bag well to evenly coat kale pieces.
4. Bake for 12-15 minutes at 400.

Don't let the name put you off these snacks. They can be as addictive as the slogan, "Bet you can't eat just one." They do a really good job of fulfilling what potato and corn chips offer, but in a much healthier manner. Great for movie nights and you don't even have to feel guilty after eating a whole baggie full. All of our children love them and what a delicious way for them to eat vegetables.

Use whatever potato chip flavors you love—salt and vinegar, ranch, chipotle, or cheese and onion, etc.

Simple Flax Crackers – S (dehydrated version)

In Serene's previous book, *Rejuvenate Your Life, Recipes for Energy*, she has recipes for gourmet style flax crackers. If you want to be adventurous with flax crackers, check out her book, only keep in mind the book places little emphasis on animal protein which we now understand is so vital.

We don't have time for recipes that are too involved. This recipe is stripped down and simple, but, surprisingly yummy. *Simple Flax Crackers* are one of our inexpensive staples. You can top them with cheese, avocado, tomato, or sprinkle with salt and pepper and dip and dunk into luscious dips.

If you don't have a dehydrator, skip to the *Oven Flax Crackers*.

Basic Ingredients: golden flax seeds ✦ golden flax meal ✦ water ✦ sea salt ✦ optional red palm oil

1. Pour whole golden flax seeds in a bowl, depending on how many you want to make. Add some golden flax meal as it helps crackers stay together. Make sure your whole flax seeds are at least three quarters of your entire flax. Serene says that using brown flax seeds makes the crackers look like dried brown " dog poop" wafers, so if you care about looks, use the golden seeds.
2. Add enough water to create a thick oatmeal consistency, sea salt to taste, and 1 optional heaped Tbs. of red palm oil to intensify color and bring a more "fat taste" to the bite.

3. Pour mixture into food processor. Do this in batches if you have made a large amount of mix. Process well. It won't break down all the seeds, but it will cut some of them down somewhat so you eat a slightly smoother cracker rather than one that consists of whole seeds only.
4. Let mixture sit for 10 minutes.
5. If mixture has thickened too much to stir or spread easily, add a little more water. Spread immediately onto dehydrator trays with parchment paper covering the whole trays. The easiest way to spread the cracker mix is to use a spatula or the back of a large spoon. If that doesn't work for you, place a bowl of water near your working area. Wet your hands in the water frequently and spread the mix with your fingers. Don't spread crackers any thicker than ⅛ of an inch.
6. Dehydrate for a few hours, then flip cracker sheets over and continue to dehydrate until they reach ultimate crispiness, approximately 12 hours total or overnight. The best way to do this is to start dehydrating in the late afternoon, flip them before you go to bed, and they'll be ready by morning.
7. Break into cracker size shapes and, once cooled, put them in Ziploc baggies. They will last for months. They can be stored in the freezer for ultimate crisp. They do not need to be thawed as they have no water.

There's hardly any work involved in these crackers, only dehydrator time. You'll have crackers galore doing this once every two to three months.

Oven Flax Crackers – S

This is a simple flax cracker recipe from a great friend of ours, named Kris. This lady is a mother of nine, a personal trainer with a fabulous figure and fit physique. We sisters come together for a day with Kris several times a year. Our children play together while we share our latest recipes and talk healthy food, exercise, and our latest inspirations. It's a great day of encouragement.

Basic Ingredients: golden flax meal ✦ parmesan cheese ✦ sea salt and other seasonings including garlic or onion powder ✦ water

1. Put 1 cup golden flax meal into a bowl.
2. Add ⅓ cup parmesan cheese.
3. Add 1½ tsp. garlic powder and ½ tsp. salt or any other seasonings you desire.
4. Add ½ cup water and mix well.
5. Spread on parchment lined cookie sheet.
6. Cover with cling wrap or wax paper.

7 Roll with jar or rolling pan until mix is spread out evenly, about ⅛ inch thick.

8 Push in the edges of the spread mix so they are not thin and wispy. Thinner edges will cook much faster and may burn.

9 Take off cling wrap or wax paper and bake at 400 for 15-18 minutes.

These crackers will stay crisp for a day or two. If they un-crisp with time, they can quickly be reheated in the oven and will crisp back up. The thinner you can spread this mix, the crispier it will stay.

Joseph's Crackers/Chips – S, E or Fuel Pull

These crackers work using either Joseph's lavish bread or pita bread, available at most Walmarts and many other grocery chains. Pearl does a quick microwave version and thinks nothing could be quicker or easier.

Basic Ingredients: Joseph's pita or lavish bread

1 Cut a Joseph's pita or lavish in half, then cut the half into triangles that are cracker size.

2 Place the pieces on a paper plate and microwave about 1-1½ minutes until nicely golden brown. If you don't have a paper plate, use a regular plate, but line it with parchment paper.

Pearl chats: That's it. These crackers are fantastic. I love them with cheese and tomato, or even peanut butter. They work well with Light Laughing Cow or Weight Watchers cheese wedges for **Fuel Pull** or **E** needs. Sometimes my brother, Rocklyn, and his wife come over on a Saturday night. We love to watch travel DVDs of Europe. He brings over camembert or brie cheese and a dry red wine. I slice tomato and cucumber, pour olives into a bowl, and we use these crackers as bases for our creations. It's pure **S** indulgence. We get to go to Europe for an evening, sample European goodies, and not gain a pound on the rich food!

You can use your oven to make bigger batches of these crackers, which Serene will approve more. Place the cracker size pieces on an oiled baking tray and bake for a few minutes at 350 until brown. There is no need to turn them, but watch carefully, as they burn easily.

To make them corn chip style, cut into triangular pieces, pat or spritz with coconut or olive oil, and shake sea salt on before nuking or baking. They make yummy nachos, topped with cheese, jalapenos, and other fixin's.

Crunchy Cheese Crackers – S

Pearl chats: Another hit around our house. Children and parents both love 'em. I use the microwave, but they can be baked in the oven on parchment paper for bigger batches. It is best to use a reduced fat (2%) sharp cheddar cheese. It makes the crispiest little crackers! Kraft makes a nice cheddar using 2% milk from cows that are not fed antibiotics. Regular cheddar works fine, but not quite as well, but if that's all you have, you'll still be impressed. I haven't had success with mozzarella as it does not crisp. These crackers are good as a crunchy side to an **S** style sandwich, but they make a nice snack on their own. In our house, we like to top them with a dollop of salsa and sour cream. My husband thinks they are best pre-seasoned with Creole seasoning and cayenne pepper.

Basic ingredients: cheese ✦ optional seasonings

1. Cut cheese into thin cracker size pieces and place on a parchment paper lined dinner plate.
2. Microwave for about a minute or until oil has been released from cheese and they turn slightly light brown and bubble.
3. Once crackers have cooled, they should snap nicely and not be bendy.

Homemade Ezekiel Crackers/Chips – E

Basic Ingredients: sprouted wraps ✦ coconut oil ✦ sea salt and other seasonings

1. Take a few sprouted store-bought Ezekiel 4:9 tortillas and rub a little coconut oil on top of each one or use a healthy oil spray. Because you will use less than 1 tsp. of oil for this entire batch, and will not eat the whole lot in one sitting, it will not really count for the allowed 1 tsp. of oil in an **E** meal.
2. Sprinkle sea salt or seasonings of your choice. They will stick, thanks to the little bit of oil.
3. Place tortillas straight onto oven rack and bake at 350 until crispy. This only takes a few minutes. Be careful. They brown quickly and they crisp even a little more after they have cooled.
4. Break into chip or cracker size pieces and serve on the side of an **E** meal.

These work great with **E** Mexican meals or *The Lighter Side of Chili* (*Evening Meals,* Chapter 21). They are also great with light packed tuna and cottage cheese.

Pearl chats: The above is Serene's version. She doesn't like the idea of putting healthy sprouted tortillas in the microwave, but they can be made the same way as *Joseph's Crackers.*

Just Like Wheat Thins – S

Basic Ingredients: golden flax meal ✦ almond flour ✦ egg whites ✦ sea salt and other seasonings, including nutritional yeast ✦ coconut oil or olive oil ✦ baking soda

1. Put ¾ cup golden flax in bowl.
2. Add ¾ cup almond flour or home ground almonds.
3. Add 2 egg whites.
4. Add 2 Tbs. nutritional yeast, 1 Tbs. parmesan cheese, ¼ tsp. sea salt, sprinkle of black pepper, onion powder, and garlic powder.
5. Add 1 Tbs. coconut or olive oil and ½ tsp. baking soda.
6. Combine ingredients well and work into a dough ball with your hands.
7. Place ball on parchment lined cookie sheet.
8. Place another sheet of wax paper or cling wrap over the top and roll out ball into a slab about the thickness of a cracker (⅛ inch or less thick). Take off top piece of paper and score slab into small squares.
9. Bake at 350 for 15-20 minutes.

The possibilities for flavorings are endless. Consider adding sesame seeds, parsley flakes, diced chives, cayenne pepper, or even chicken bouillon. You could even make these crackers out of ground chia seeds made into meal in your coffee grounder, instead of using flax meal.

Spicy Nuts – S (Pearl's version)

Basic Ingredients: nuts ✦ coconut oil ✦ sea salt and other seasonings, including cayenne pepper

1. Pour any raw nuts onto a baking tray. Pecans and walnuts work really well.
2. Add 1-2 tsp. coconut oil.

3. Season with sea salt and cayenne pepper, or use a couple of squirts of Bragg Liquid Aminos in place of sea salt.
4. Toss nuts in seasonings.
5. Broil for about 2 minutes until coconut oil melts (if it was in a solid state). Take out baking tray and stir oil around with the nuts.
6. Return to oven and broil until nuts are browning. Toss once more.
7. Be sure not to let nuts burn. Broiling time doesn't take long. Keep a good watch.

The nuts will become crunchy once they have cooled. They are delicious eaten with small cubes of cheese or thrown in salads. You might need to portion size them into little baggies if you have a tendency to overdo.

Dehydrated Nuts – S (Serene's version)

Basic Ingredients: nuts ✦ sea salt and other seasonings

1. Soak any type of nuts in pure water and a little sea salt for at least 7 hours.
2. Drain and add sea salt and spices to taste.
3. Place nuts on dehydrator sheets until crispy (usually takes 12-24 hours).

These will be lighter in feel and much easier on the digestive system than either raw or roasted nuts. It's best to make large batches every couple of months or so, store in air tight containers in the freezer, and take out to eat whenever you need them.

Roasted Crispy Garbanzos – E

Basic Ingredients: garbanzo beans ✦ olive oil ✦ sea salt and other seasonings

1. Drain 1 can garbanzo beans (chick peas). Blot beans with paper towels, or use clean dish towel to absorb all possible water. Or, use 1½ cups home-soaked garbanzos.
2. Transfer dried garbanzos to bowl and season with ¼ tsp. salt and ¼ tsp. garlic powder.
3. Add 1 tsp. olive oil and toss beans well with seasonings and oil.
4. Spread garbanzos on a nonstick cookie sheet, or slightly oiled regular cookie sheet.
5. Bake at 425 for 30 minutes. Toss beans a couple of times while cooking by gently shaking cookie sheet.

The sky is the limit for flavors. If you don't want garlic, try Creole, or a hotter spice like cayenne. What about rosemary or mustard? Or, how about cinnamon and Truvia for a sweet version?

If you don't have garbanzos handy, you may use any beans of choice. You can fit two cans of drained beans on each cookie sheet. If you want to make this snack for a large family on a movie night, you can easily quadruple the recipe.

If you have leftovers, keep in the fridge in an air-tight sealed container. They get a little more chewy than crunchy after being refrigerated, but if you microwave them for 30 seconds, they crisp up again. Put in a baggie, they're a great snack for your toddler and yourself, when going out.

Coconut Divine Fudge Squares – S

Serene chats: These squares could have been placed in the dessert recipes, but we think they go best with the rest of the squares and balls recipes coming up. These yummy snacks not only incorporate the incredible middle chain fatty acids of coconut, but it's wonderful cleansing fiber, which has incredible intestinal detoxifying abilities. You wouldn't know you're eating a colon cleanse and healing superfats as you take bites of such a sinful tasting treat. That's why we call them divine. They contain only God's "goodness."

Coconut concentrate is the magic in this recipe. It is sometimes called other names, but it is actually coconut butter with the fiber included. Look for ingredients on the label that say, "100% ground coconut." It looks like thick white paste, rather like white peanut butter. It can be pricey if you don't shop carefully. We found the brand, Let's Do Organic which is less than half the price of most others. It comes in packets, rather than jars, and is around $2.50 a packet. I find mine at Whole Foods markets, but you could order it in online. This recipe, using two packets, makes a lot of snacks. Overall, it's quite inexpensive.

You can make a vanilla fudge instead of chocolate by using vanilla flavored Jay Robb's protein powder and adding a splash or two of pure vanilla essence.

This fudge will not melt like other coconut oil chocolates, unless you leave it out on a sunny picnic table for several hours. It stays solid in its squares, even if you've packed it in little Ziploc bags for an "on the go" snack.

Basic Ingredients: coconut concentrate ✦ coconut oil ✦ chocolate whey protein ✦ cocoa powder ✦ sweetener

1 Put 2 packets of Let's Do Organic coconut concentrate in a bowl of warm water to soften for several minutes. Keep the plastic on for this step.

2. Empty contents of packets into food processor.
3. Add 2 heaped Tbs. virgin coconut oil.
4. Add 1½ scoops of Jay Robb's chocolate whey protein powder. If you only have unsweetened whey protein, add a little more Truvia or Nunaturals for extra sweetening.
5. Add 4 Tbs. unsweetened cocoa powder.
6. Add small amount of Truvia or Nunaturals to taste. Not too much will be required since Jay Robb's is already sweetened.
7. Process well.
8. Pour into flexible container and place in freezer for 10-20 minutes until set.
9. Manipulate container so fudge slips out in one block onto large plate.
10. Score and cut into squares.
11. Keep squares in fridge in little baggies.

To take this fudge to a more interesting level, add therapeutic grade essential oils to the mix. I like to add a few drops of Thieves from Young Living Oils. This adds an exotic deep flavor and aroma and brings even more superfoodiness to the recipe.

Island Fresh Fudge Squares – S

This recipe is a little cheaper than the above fudge squares because we use one fresh brown coconut as a base instead of coconut concentrate packets. Be careful in choosing your coconut. Check for moldy spots and leaking eyes. Shake the coconut to make sure there is plenty of water as this is a sign of freshness. The older the coconut, the less water.

Basic Ingredients: fresh brown coconut ✦ virgin coconut oil ✦ sweetener ✦ vanilla ✦ sea salt ✦ cocoa powder ✦ golden flax meal ✦ optional protein powder

1. Open brown coconut by first puncturing softest of the three coconut eyes with a sharp knife edge to initiate opening process. Insert a single chop stick into hole. Replace it with a straw and let one of the children drink the sweet juice. Or, pour into jar to later culture with water grains. Google if this idea interests you.
2. With a hammer, crack the coconut at mid-center point. Now coconut is opened, press into coconut flesh with end of knife and flick bite-sized chunks out of shell onto counter.
3. Don't peel off the brown outer layer of coconut meat as it is filled with nutrients and since you'll be turning it into chocolate fudge, it will not affect the end result. If you

get a "baddie," you may have to peel off the outer layer if it is discolored or slightly moldy in places.

4 Place coconut chunks from entire coconut in food processor and process as smoothly as possible.

5 Add Nunaturals to taste. Just a pinch or two is all you need. We put a little on the end of knife. Or, if you purchase the shaker bottle, adjust to smallest hole-size and shake a few times.

6 Add dash of sea salt and vanilla to taste and 4 heaping Tbs. unsweetened cocoa powder.

7 Add 4 heaping Tbs. virgin coconut oil.

8 Add two generous tsp. flax meal (if you don't have any on hand, it doesn't matter).

9 Add optional scoop or two of whey protein powder. Further option—superfood such as maca powder.

10 Process until well combined. Place in square plastic container and press down. Place in fridge and when set hard, score into squares, or roll mixture into balls.

11 If you don't think you can eat them all in a week, use the "freezer to fridge" trick, where you put a portion in the fridge and the remainder in the freezer. When first batch is eaten, refill your fridge stash.

Serene chats: In the last few weeks of my pregnancy with Haven Rest and my "baby-moon" afterwards I was addicted to *Island Fresh Fudge Squares.* Not only are the middle chain fatty acids found in coconut extremely healthy, but it makes the environment of the womb even more protective with its anti-viral, anti-bacterial, and immune supporting properties. The more extra virgin coconut oil you consume the more protective your milk for your baby.

Basic Treat Squares – S

Treat squares/balls are great little "pick me ups." As long as you know you have some treat squares in the fridge or freezer, you don't have to worry about caving in and eating that leftover piece of Domino's pizza friends brought over, because you sure didn't buy it—and if you did!

Basic Ingredients: nuts ✦ seeds ✦ protein powders or hemp powder ✦ golden flax meal or chia ✦ sweetener ✦ flavorings and extracts of choice ✦ coconut oil and/or concentrate

1 Throw a few handfuls of raw nuts, seeds, and dried or fresh coconut into food processor.

2. Add 2 or more scoops of protein powders, green food powders, or superfood powders such as maca and hemp.
3. Add ½ cup golden flax meal or chia.
4. Add Truvia or Nunaturals to taste and desired flavorings such as cocoa powder or melted squares of unsweetened chocolate. You may like to add vanilla, mint, lemon, or almond extracts, but not all at once, of course!
5. Add a few heaping Tbs. raw coconut oil, and/or coconut concentrate, and/or favorite nut butter of choice.
6. Process in food processor until combined. Taste and add more sweetener or flavors if needed.
7. If not moist enough to hold together, add more coconut oil, coconut concentrate, or nut butters. We have also used a little coconut milk at times to aid in moisture content.
8. Transfer to a flexible plastic lid or flexible plastic cutting board and form into 1 inch high loaf. Score into squares. Place in freezer for 10 minutes.
9. Remove and cut squares fully. Place in baggies and store in fridge.

We often make large batches and store half in the fridge and half in the freezer. When the fridge treats are eaten up, we place the frozen ones in the fridge.

I hope you noticed that we did not rely on dried fruits like dates, raisins, or sticky sweeteners such as honey, maple, or agave syrup to hold our recipe together. This is too fattening when combined with all the healthy fats and nuts. However, you could use a few goji berries, or unsweetened cranberries, to add bursts of chewy sweet tartness.

Each time we make these treats, they come out differently as we have different ingredients on hand. Sometimes they can be as simple as ground almonds, coconut oil, cocoa, and flavorings. Or, they can be as elaborate as a paragraph of ingredients. Use your own creativity. The combinations are endless.

Flax Seed Protein Bars – S

We're not going to take the glory for this recipe. It is found on many body building sites due to its high protein content. It's great for a quick filling snack. You can throw a few pieces in a baggie for you and your children when you go out.

Basic Ingredients: chocolate whey protein powder ✦ golden flax meal ✦ water ✦ peanut butter or almond butter ✦ sweetener

1. Put 4 scoops of chocolate whey protein powder in food processor. Make sure the brand you use is sweetened with stevia or xylitol and has 1 or less carb per serving.
2. Add ⅔ cup golden flax meal.
3. Add ⅓ cup water.
4. Add 4 Tbs. natural peanut butter or almond butter.
5. Add 2 tsp. Truvia, or a dash of Nunaturals to taste if you want the bars sweeter.
6. Process ingredients and shape into balls or larger bars. Store in plastic wrap in refrigerator. Or, freeze for longer term storage, but they need to be thawed before eating.

You may add a few goji berries for a more chewy taste. Or, go green by adding your favorite green powder such as spirulina or Barley Green. Flax meal will need to be reduced according to the amount of green powder you add to keep the correct dry/wet ratio.

Fridge Fudge – S

This high protein recipe is a much more elaborate, expensive, and superfoodish version of the skeleton *Flax Seed Protein Bars.*

Basic Ingredients: chocolate whey protein powder ✦ ground chia ✦ water ✦ coconut cream concentrate ✦ coconut oil ✦ unsweetened chocolate ✦ sweetener ✦ maca powder

1. Put 4 scoops chocolate whey protein in food processor.
2. Add ⅔ cup ground chia.
3. Add ⅔ cup water.
4. Add ¾ cup coconut cream concentrate. If you do not have this available, grind fresh coconut meal measuring ¾ cup and add 2 Tbs. coconut oil.
5. Add 4 Tbs. extra virgin coconut oil.
6. Add 4 oz. melted unsweetened chocolate.
7. Add a little NuStevia Pure White Stevia Extract Powder or ground Truvia to taste and a dash of vanilla.
8. Add ½ cup maca powder if you have it on hand.
9. Process all ingredients until smooth.
10. Spread mix ½ inch high on anything plastic and flexible such as a flexible cutting board or bendable plastic lid.
11. Place in freezer for 15 minutes.
12. Before it gets too hard, take out and cut into small squares.

13. Put half the fudge into Ziploc baggies in the fridge and store rest in freezer, as this makes a large batch.

Whip of Wonders – S Helper

Not only is this recipe creamy and delicious, but we can't think of anything more healthy. Your body will be moisturized inside and out. These ingredients are good for your skin, brain, and endocrine system. It's fine to add more blueberries to this recipe, but that puts you further into the **S Helper** range. Using wild blueberries (available at Walmart) keeps the carbs lower as wild berries are naturally lower in sugar then cultivated berries. If you want to try this recipe, but are not yet in **S Helper** stage, pull the blueberry content back to a ½ cup.

Basic Ingredients: avocado ✦ blueberries ✦ chocolate whey protein powder ✦ cocoa powder ✦ vanilla ✦ sweetener

1. Put ½ large Haas avocado in food processor.
2. Add ¾ cup frozen blueberries.
3. Add ½ scoop of chocolate Jay Robb's whey protein powder.
4. Add 2 heaped tsp. unsweetened cocoa powder, dash of vanilla, and a small amount of Truvia or Nunaturals to taste.
5. Add 1 optional tsp. store-bought coconut flour, but not necessary.
6. Pulse until the mixture starts good movement, then process until completely whipped and smoothed.
7. Enjoy immediately or keep chilled.

Dips

You will want some dips to enjoy with all the cracker/chip recipes we have included. Another dipping option to consider is a vegetable called jicama. It has a nice crunch when cut into chip-like slices. It has a neutral flavor and is low carb.

Party Salmon Dip – S (makes many servings)

This is a party favorite. You can arrange a bunch of *Joseph's Crackers* (*Snacks,* Chapter 24) around a bowl of this dip. It's quite likely you'll be asked for the recipe which often happens to us. Don't want to party? This is a tasty, healthy dip to eat at home anytime. As it makes a large dip, you can easily halve or quarter this recipe.

Basic Ingredients: canned salmon ✦ cream cheese ✦ lemon juice ✦ hickory smoke sauce ✦ green onion ✦ chili flakes

1. Drain 2 cans wild caught salmon and empty contents into bowl or food processor.
2. Add 2 (8 oz.) packets ⅓ less fat cream cheese.
3. Add 3 Tbs. lemon concentrate or juice of 1 lemon, and 1 tsp. hickory smoke sauce.
4. Beat ingredients until smooth with electric beater or food processor.
5. Add chopped green onions or chives and generous sprinkle of chili pepper flakes. Stir in with spoon or fork.
6. Place dip in bowl and sprinkle more chili flakes on top as a garnish.

Rustic Eggplant Dip – S

Basic Ingredients: eggplant ✦ basil ✦ raw almonds ✦ sea salt and other seasonings ✦ coconut oil ✦ tomato paste ✦ balsamic vinegar ✦optional garlic cloves

1. Prick large eggplant all over and bake at 350 until wrinkled and soft.
2. Scrape flesh of eggplant into food processor.
3. Add large handful of chopped fresh basil and handful of raw almonds.
4. Add black pepper, sea salt, and onion powder to taste.
5. Add 2 generous Tbs. virgin coconut oil, 2 generous Tbs. tomato paste, and 2 good splashes of balsamic vinegar. Garlic lovers could roast some garlic cloves alongside the eggplant and add to mix.
6. Process well.

This is great with any **S** friendly crackers or raw vegetables. It also goes well as a side to *Tabouleh* (*Lunches*, Chapter 20).

Greek Onion Dip – S, E or Fuel Pull

Basic ingredients: onion ✦ Greek yogurt ✦ sea salt and other seasonings

1. Bake onion in oven with skin on until flesh is completely softened and slightly caramelized.
2. Peel skin off onion and place in food processor.
3. Add 1 cup 0% Greek yogurt.

4. Add sea salt, black pepper to taste, and extra onion powder if stronger flavor is desired.
5. Pulse until desired texture. It's okay to keep some of the onion chunky.

Depending on your meal type, it can be used with either **S** or **E** crackers for a couple of different snacks. *Joseph's Crackers,* (*Snacks,* Chapter 24) will work for all three fuel styles including **Fuel Pull**. Or, to make this only **E**, choose *Homemade Ezekiel Crackers* (*Snacks,* Chapter 24).

Hummus Dip – S or S helper (makes several servings)

We use chana dahl to keep this recipe **S** friendly. A ¼-½ cup serving will allow you to stay in **S** mode. If you want to use garbanzo beans, you'll be in **S Helper** territory from the start. No problem if you're up to that stage.

Hummus goes perfectly with *Tabouleh.* Check the recipe in *Lunches,* Chapter 20, which uses quinoa or *Cauli Rice* to replace the more traditional bulgur grain. The two dishes together will put you into **S Helper** mode if you use the version of *Tabouleh* with quinoa instead of *Cauli Rice,* but that's fine for when you are up to that stage. They're both incredibly healthy, and combining these two recipes offers a duo of superstar superfoods.

Basic Ingredients: chana dahl ✦ tahini ✦ sea salt and other seasonings ✦ lemon juice

1. Put 2 cups cooked chana dahl in food processor (make sure it has cooled since cooking).
2. Add ½ cup tahini (sesame seed paste).
3. Add 1 tsp. sea salt, garlic powder to taste, lemon juice to taste (approximately 2 lemon's worth or similar amount of concentrate), and an optional 1 tsp. each of cumin and coriander powder.
4. Process well. A little water may be added to arrive at desired consistency. The dip can stay very thick, but is also fine to be thinner with added water.
5. Taste and re-season if needed by adding more salt, garlic powder, or lemon juice to satisfaction.
6. Transfer to plastic tub with lid. Before covering, drizzle with extra virgin olive oil, sprinkle with paprika powder, and add a sprig of parsley for garnish (if desired). Place lid on and refrigerate.

This dip is hearty and full of protein. Your children can dip in pieces of whole wheat warmed pita pieces. You could use Joseph's pitas, *Golden Flat Bread* (*Muffins, Breads, and Pizza Crusts,* Chapter 19), or vegetable crudités.

Remember to keep to reasonable portions of this dip to keep it in **S** or **S Helper** setting. You wouldn't want to sit down and eat half the bowl. If so, you'd be heading right past **S Helper** territory into **Crossover** land. However, if you are in need of a **Crossover** meal, dig in. You could even enjoy it with some homemade or store-bought sourdough or sprouted bread, but don't go over the two piece threshold.

Australian Guacomole – S

Basic Ingredients: avocado ✦ Greek yogurt ✦ sea salt and other seasonings

1. Mash 1 avocado in bowl.
2. Add 1 cup Greek yogurt (any fat percent is fine).
3. Add sea salt, black pepper, and optional garlic or onion powder.
4. Combine well with fork.

This adds protein to traditional guacamole and makes a lovely light olive green color. This is the way guacamole is made in Australia, except sour cream is used. The Greek yogurt is higher in protein and packs a healthier punch, not to mention all the beneficial probiotics. Use sour cream if you prefer.

Try this dip with either our dehydrated or oven *Flax Cracker* recipes, *Joseph's Crackers*, or even *Crunchy Cheese Crisps*. Please don't use any chips made from corn with this dip unless you're trying to fatten up.

Energizing Yogurt Dip – S, E or Fuel Pull

Basic Ingredients: turkey or Canadian bacon✦ Greek yogurt ✦ cottage cheese ✦ sea salt and other seasonings

1. Cook 3 strips of turkey or Canadian bacon, drain on paper towel, and crumble into bowl.
2. Add 2 cups 0% Greek yogurt (regular non-fat yogurt will be fine if you only use this dip for **E** purposes).
3. Add 1 cup 1% cottage cheese.
4. Season with sea salt and pepper to taste and combine ingredients well.

This dip works well with baked corn chips for an **E** snack or with either of our two **S** Flax Cracker recipes. Or, scoop the seeds out of halved cucumbers, cut them into two inch strips and fill with this dip for a refreshing **Fuel Pull** hors d'oeuvre. If you do decide to use regular non-fat yogurt rather than Greek, don't use this dip with **S** crackers or chips that include fat, like the pre-mentioned flax crackers, if weight loss is desired.

I'm Hungry Snack Ideas

Here's a basic list of snack options in case you get hungry for a snack and your brain is blank for ideas. A blank brain is not good, because if there is a bag of chips or a candy bar anywhere in reaching, walking or driving distance, you may find yourself falling for their seduction.

This is your support list, with all the options ready for an "at a glance" idea. We don't want you to reach at the back of your cupboard for that packet of Doritos when you can quickly come up with something on this list. Promise us—if you are in between meals, the munchies are happening, and you don't want to spend time thinking about what to eat—give this list a scan. It'll prompt you back in the right direction. And if you ever find yourself in an extreme "food now!" frenzy, opt for any of snack ideas on the list which fall into the **Fuel Pull** category as that will eliminate any meal matching worries.

Please put this exhaustive list on your refrigerator with a super strong magnet. Don't use those magnet numbers and letters you put there for your preschoolers to learn their alphabet. You know those don't hold much weight and soon our darling list will be on the floor and lost in that crack between your refrigerator and your cupboards. That space is a black hole, right?

1. Either of our "slick trick" slimming desserts that you have our permission to overdo, *Choco Pudding* or *Lemon Mousse* (*Desserts,* Chapter 23) – **S, E or Fuel Pull**
2. *Fat Stripping Frappa* or any of our smoothies (*Morning Meals,* Chapter 18) – **S, E or Fuel Pull**
3. *Greek Yogurt Swirls* (*Morning Meals,* Chapter 18) – **S, E or Fuel Pull**
4. Celery and peanut butter – **S**
5. Plan approved **S, E or Fuel Pull** crackers and their appropriate fuel matching dips – **S, E or Fuel Pull**
6. Plan approved **S, E or Fuel Pull** crackers smeared with Light Laughing Cow or Weight Watchers cheese wedges (store-bought Ryvita crackers are fine too) – **S, E or Fuel Pull**
7. **S** friendly crackers and your favorite sliced cheese – **S**
8. **S** friendly crackers and peanut butter – **S**
9. **S** friendly crackers with tuna and full-fat mayo – **S**
10. **E or Fuel Pull** friendly crackers with tuna mixed with light mayo or light vinaigrette – **E or Fuel Pull**
11. *Melt in your Mouth Meringues* (*Desserts,* Chapter 23) – **S, E or Fuel Pull**
12. *Tummy Tucking Ice Cream* (*Desserts,* Chapter 23) – **S, E or Fuel Pull**
13. *Ricotta Crème* (*Desserts,* Chapter 23) – **S, E or Fuel Pull**

14. Low-fat cottage cheese with fruit – **E**
15. Low-fat cottage cheese with berries – **S, E or Fuel Pull**
16. Seeded cucumber boats with low-fat cottage cheese – **S, E or Fuel Pull**
17. Any % cottage cheese mixed with *Spicy Nuts* (*Snacks,* Chapter 24) – **S**
18. Cubes of cheese and *Spicy Nuts (Snacks*, Chapter 24) – **S**
19. *Kale chips* (*Snacks,* Chapter 24) – **S, E or Fuel Pull**
20. *Roasted Garbanzos* (*Snacks,* Chapter 24) – **E**
21. Four to five cups of popcorn (using a scant amount of fat) – **E**
22. One or two *Trim Healthy Pancakes* (*Morning Meals*, Chapter 18) rolled up with skim ricotta and 1 Tbs. of Polaner All-Fruit Jam with Fiber – **E**
23. *Muffin in a Mug* (*Muffins, Breads, and Pizza Crusts*, Chapter 19) – **S**
24. *Cake in a Mug* (*Desserts*, Chapter 23) – **S**
25. *Muffin in a Bowl* (*Muffins, Breads, and Pizza Crusts,* Chapter 19) – **S, E or Fuel Pull**
26. Either a *Blueberry Coconut Muffin* or two, or an *Easy Peazy Cinnamon Muffin* or two (*Muffins, Breads, and Pizza Crusts*, Chapter 19) – **S**
27. One apple and one teaspoon of peanut butter – **E**
28. Greek yogurt or full-fat kefir topped with *Crunch Alive Granola* or *Low Impact Granola* (*Morning Meals,* Chapter 18) – **S** or **S Helper**
29. Fresh tomato or cucumber slices with thin slices of your favorite cheese on top – **S**
30. Fresh tomato or cucumber slices smeared with Light Laughing Cow or Weight Watchers cheese wedges – **S, E or Fuel Pull**
31. Piece of *Basic Cheesecake* (*Desserts,* Chapter 23) and a cup of coffee – **S**
32. Fresh or thawed berries and heavy cream – **S**
33. Fresh or thawed berries and Fat Free Reddi Whip – **S, E or Fuel Pull**
34. One or two boiled eggs sprinkled with salt and pepper – **S**
35. Any of our protein bars or fudge square recipes (*Snacks*, Chapter 24) – **S**
36. *Deli Meat Roll Ups* (*Lunches*, Chapter 20) – **S, E or Fuel Pull**
37. A chunk or two of *Skinny Chocolate* (*Desserts,* Chapter 23) and a cup of coffee – **S**
38. A couple of pieces of Lucienne's chocolate or regular store-bought 85% chocolate with green tea or coffee – **S**
39. Leftover reheated sweet potato with cinnamon, Truvia, sea salt, and 1 tsp. coconut oil – **E**
40. Cold strawberries from the fridge dunked into melted *Skinny Chocolate* so they form a shell – **S**
41. Choice of 1 peach, 2 plums, 2 mandarins, small bowl of cherries, 1 orange or 1 grapefruit with either 8 almonds or a very small handful of other favorite nuts to help blunt glycemic response – **E**

42. *Chia Tapioca Pudding* or *Cookie Bowl Oatmeal* (*Morning Meals*, Chapter 18) – **S, E or Fuel Pull**
43. Half to one whole red or green pepper, stuffed with cream cheese and a few spicy nuts – **S**
44. Half to one whole red or green pepper, stuffed with tuna mixed with low-fat mayo or vinaigrette – **S, E or Fuel Pull**
45. Any leftover meal in a snack sized portion, heated up – **S, E or Fuel Pull**

Chapter 25

Gravies, Sauces, and Condiments

Basic Gravy – S, E or Fuel Pull

Basic Ingredients: meat juice or broth/stock ✦ sea salt and other seasonings, including nutritional yeast and Bragg Liquid Aminos ✦ water ✦ glucomannan or xanthan gum

1. Pour 1 cup of either meat juice from roasting pan (omit when making **E** or **Fuel Pull**), chicken or beef broth/stock (homemade or store-bought), or plain water into saucepan.
2. Turn element to medium and add generous shakes of onion powder, sea salt, black pepper, red pepper, 1-2 Tbs. nutritional yeast, and generous squirts of Bragg Liquid Aminos.
3. Add 1-2 cups water or chicken broth.
4. Once gravy liquid is hot, shake in glucomannan or xanthan gum from empty salt shaker (or a combination of both) and stir like crazy with a whisk.
5. Keep shaking and stirring until gravy starts to thicken. Do not let thickening form blobs. If this happens, it would be better to add the glucomannan or xanthan to a separate ½ cup of water to dissolve in first then add to the hot gravy.

6. Simmer gravy for several minutes, stirring every so often. Taste for final seasoning adjustments.

If you don't have stock or meat juice for this gravy and you are using water for liquid, adding nutritional yeast is a must. It is not as necessary to add it when using stock, but it makes the gravy extra delicious.

It usually takes between ¾-1½ tsp. of glucomannan to thicken 3-4 cups of liquid to a gravy consistency.

Slim Belly Jelly – S, E or Fuel Pull

Basic Ingredients: frozen berries ✦ water ✦ lemon juice ✦ glucomannan ✦ sweetener

1. In blender put 2 cups water, 3 tsp. glucomannan, 1 cup frozen berries, and ¼ cup lemon juice concentrate and blend well. If making **Fuel Pull**, keep berries to only strawberries and/or raspberries.
2. Pour mixture into saucepan and add about 2-3 cups whole frozen berries and stir while bringing to boil. When bubbles appear, simmer until berries are heated through and a nice gel has formed. You may need to add more water to thin, or alternatively, carefully sprinkle in a little more glucomannan if not thick enough. Never dump glucomannan in saucepan. Carefully sprinkle only ¼ tsp. at a time and quickly stir. Glucomannan clumps are a choking hazard.
3. Sweeten to taste with Nunaturals or Truvia and stir vigorously again.

Enjoy *Slim Belly Jelly* hot or chilled. Delicious swirled over Greek yogurt, *Trim Healthy Pancakes*, or any of our muffins or breads.

Ketchup – S, E or Fuel Pull

Basic Ingredients: tomato paste ✦ water ✦ balsamic or red wine vinegar ✦ sea salt and other seasonings ✦ sweetener

1. Empty 6 oz. can tomato paste into bowl.
2. Add 6 oz. water.
3. Add 2 Tbs. Balsamic or Red Wine Vinegar.
4. Add 1 tsp. sea salt, ½ tsp. onion powder, and 4 tsp. Truvia ground fine in coffee grinder or a few shakes of Nunaturals.
5. Whisk together well, place in covered jar or squeeze bottle, and keep refrigerated.

Honey Mustard Dip or Dressing – S

Basic Ingredients: mayonnaise ✦ mustard ✦ sweetener

1. Mix ¼ cup mayo and ¼ cup mustard in bowl.
2. Add 2 tsp. ground Truvia or a dash of Nunaturals.
3. Whisk well.

This mix can be thinned down with a little water if it is to be used as a dressing for salad.

Hip Trim Honey Mustard – S, E Or Fuel Pull

Basic Ingredients:water ✦ Dijon mustard ✦ sea salt and other seasonings ✦ apple cider vinegar ✦ red palm oil ✦ sweetener ✦ glucomannan

1. Put 1 cup water in blender.
2. Add 2 tsp. Dijon mustard, 1 tsp. sea salt, dash of onion powder and sprinkle of black pepper.
3. Add ¼ cup apple cider vinegar (raw is best) and 1 tsp. red palm oil.
4. Sprinkle in some Nunaturals to taste or add 1-2 tsp. Truvia.
5. Blend on high. While blending add generous ½ tsp. glucomannan (almost ¾ tsp.).
6. Keep blending and drizzle in ¼ cup boiling water. This will emulsify palm oil so it does not sit on top. Blend until creamy consistency is achieved.
7. Pour dressing into a squeeze bottle e.g. empty mustard bottle and refrigerate.

This dressing is great for all salads and also works as a topping or dip for grilled or sautéed chicken. You could use the basic skeleton of this recipe and make other flavors. Omit the mustard and add Italian seasonings for Italian style. Use almond milk in place of water and add an MSG free ranch flavoring packet for Ranch style.

Tartare Sauce – S, E or Fuel Pull

If you want to use this sauce in only an **S** setting, you can use full-fat mayonnaise. The Greek yogurt will work for all three fuel styles.

Basic Ingredients: mayonnaise or 0% Greek yogurt✦ unsweetened pickles or pickle relish ✦ sweetener

1. Put ¼ cup mayonnaise or 0% Greek yogurt in bowl.
2. Finely chop some unsweetened pickles and add to bowl, or add 1 Tbs. unsweetened pickle relish.
3. Sweeten with ground Truvia to taste (about 1-2 tsp.), or add dash of Nunaturals.

Mayonnaise – S

This recipe is for the "scratch purists" who would rather not buy mayonnaise from the store.

Basic Ingredients: eggs ✦ lemon juice ✦ sea salt and other seasonings ✦ coconut oil ✦ olive oil

1. Put 1 egg and 2 egg yolks in blender.
2. Add 1 Tbs. lemon juice.
3. Add ½ tsp. sea salt, dash of pepper, and optional dash of onion powder if desired.
4. Blend well.
5. While blender is still running, slowly add ½ cup expeller pressed coconut oil and ½ cup extra virgin olive oil.
6. Chill before serving.
7. You may also add 1 Tbs. Dijon mustard if you like a little kick.

Chapter 26

Cultured Recipes

by Serene Allison

I spent seven years eating only raw foods. I never touched any food heated above 105 degrees to my lips. I kept to this extreme diet to preserve a high enzyme count in my body.

It has been established that cooking can destroy food enzymes and the raw-food mania holds up the importance of enzymes for health as its banner. What I, and many "raw food converts" failed to realize, is that many foods need to be cooked for proper absorption and digestion. There are also some foods that actually become more nutritious the longer they are heated, such as tomatoes and mushrooms.

As far as enzymes are concerned, eating a balanced raw and cooked whole foods diet, with the inclusion of cultured foods, is far more enzyme rich than a raw diet alone. Cultured foods leave regular raw foods in the dust. They are teeming with enzymes and millions of wonderful bacteria to help preserve the ecology of the body.

What are cultured foods? They are fermented foods. Some examples of cultured dairy are yogurt, kefir, and raw cheeses. Examples of cultured vegetables are sauerkraut and kimchi. Actually, there are many foods that are suited to fermentation. Coconut milk makes an excellent kefir. Grains that are allowed to sprout or ferment are many times more nutritious than regular grains. Sourdough bread is a wonderful fermented food that is a staple for my growing children.

The following are some of my favorite cultured recipes. Don't be intimidated by the thought of making these artisan food creations. I will give you easy instructions. Nothing complicated. I don't have time for unnecessary slaving in the kitchen, even for ultimate superfoods.

Pearl chats: Good, because the idea of culturing anything has always felt too intimidating and overwhelming to me. But, I love the taste of these foods you make, Serene, and I want the health benefits.

Raw Goat's or Cow's Milk Kefir – S or E

My favorite is kefir made from goat's milk. It is smoother, has a better texture, and a more pleasing flavor than cow's milk. However, I enjoy kefir from raw cow's milk when goat's milk is unavailable. If you don't have a milking animal, or cannot find the "gold" of raw milk, you can still make kefir with good quality store-bought milk.

Remember, while we consider milk a no-no for weight control, culturing the milk eats the lactose which is the milk sugar, and renders it a much lower glycemic beverage. If you use goat's milk, your kefir will always be **S**, because goat's milk cream will not separate. You can, however, make a lower fat **E** approved kefir by using cow's milk that has the cream skimmed from the top, or a low-fat milk from the store.

Amish farms that surround many cities are inexpensive raw milk sources. There are also raw-milk co-ops in many cities which you can research online, or contact your local Farmers Market for information. You can also look up *Weston A. Price Foundation* in your search engine to discover local sources of free range milk, eggs, and meat.

You may be the type who doesn't want the bother of finding and collecting raw milk. Your adventurous spirit will be satisfied by making kefir from scratch at home with store-bought milk. This is still good for you and will cost much less than the already fermented counterpart at your health food market. Store-bought pasteurized milk, when cultured, comes back to life. Even though it may not be as nutritious as raw sources, it is still an anti-aging superfood when revived.

You can obtain kefir grains, which you will need to ferment the milk, online. Or, you may be able to obtain them from a friend. Those who make kefir have loads of grains to give away and usually don't charge for the favor. Kefir grains grow and grow and grow, and soon you will be looking for people to give them to also.

Basic Ingredients: kefir grains ✦ milk

1. Place approximately a ½ cup of kefir grains in a sterilized quart glass jar.
2. Fill 2 inches from the top with your milk of choice. The fermentation process usually needs room to expand, so don't fill all the way.
3. Screw on plastic lid. If using regular metal lid, line it with plastic wrap. You do not want any metal in contact with your kefir grains as it will kill them.
4. Ferment kefir in a dark cupboard for 12-24 hours. How long depends upon your personal taste. The longer the culturing time, the more tart the taste.
5. Once you are ready to harvest your kefir, shake the jar, and pour it into a bowl through a plastic colander that has small holes. Use a plastic or wooden spoon to help the kefir drain through the colander. Remember, anything metal that touches the grains is a sure way to kill your culturing success. The kefir itself, once fermented, is fine in a metal container, but don't let the grains near it!
6. Place your harvested kefir in the fridge and place the kefir grains back in the same glass jar. Fill up with fresh milk to be placed back in your dark cupboard.

That's it! Not too difficult.

There is no need to clean your jar every time. Leaving your jar with the kefir residue inside helps to culture a new growth of kefir grains. This is a healthy culturing practice for one week, after which you will want to exchange it with a fresh sterilized jar. At this time, if there has been enough growth of your kefir grains to be noticeable, remove them to store, give away, fertilize your garden, or feed them to your pets. Some people love to give them to their children as little pro-biotic chews. Sadly, my children don't fall for that treat. You may want to place them in a larger glass jar to start culturing greater amounts of kefir.

If you are in a hurry, it has been 24 hours, and you don't have the time to deal with straining your kefir, don't worry. Place it in the fridge and this will slow down the culturing process and give you more time. You wouldn't want to leave it more than another day as it will become sourer, albeit more slowly in the fridge. Kefir thickens in the fridge and I often use this trick as I enjoy the taste and texture even more.

What if you are leaving town and won't be home to look after your kefir? You can't find a kefir baby sitter and you wish they would go to sleep for a while like good little grains. Guess what? They can. Kefir grains are fun easy pets. They will nap for you and wake up with no grouchiness if you treat them kindly. To make them go to sleep, drain kefir as usual and run the colander of grains under cold clear water until the water runs clear out the bottom of the colander. Place the grains in a sterilized plastic container, cover with clean water, and freeze. Once you are ready to use them again, thaw, and use as normal. It might take at least one ferment cycle for them to become active again. The first renewed kefir is still healthy, only not quite as thick or tart.

If your break from making kefir is not going to be long enough to warrant freezing the grains, place your sterilized plastic jar filled with grains in the refrigerator, but not for more than a week. What if your week is up and you change your mind? You still don't feel like waking the pets, but you don't know if you want to freeze them yet either. She'll be right mate! Just add 1 Tbs. of any milk, per day, to the grains. This will feed them a little food to live on so they won't starve or die.

Coconut Kefir – S

If you are lactose intolerant, you may still be able to enjoy goat's milk kefir, as the lactose content is not as high to begin with and the culturing process eats up the rest. But, if you are one who cannot even tolerated fermented dairy, or you are out of a good milk source for a season, you can still enjoy kefir by using coconut milk. You will also receive the added benefits of all the middle chain fatty acids that coconut milk provides. Follow the same directions for regular kefir, using pure coconut milk from a can that has no preservatives (remember to use a canned brand that is BPA free). Make sure you use the full-fat coconut milk variety. The light coconut version does not work as well since it has more water content and less natural carbs to feed the fermentation process.

Once the coconut kefir has been fermented, it will be thick like Greek yogurt. Straining it through a colander is a little harder than with milk kefir because of the thickness. Add some more water as you drain by pouring a little water in the jar you kefired in and add splashes of it to the colander to help the coconut kefir flow through. Once you return your kefir to the fridge, it will thicken up again.

Use it thick for topping berries, or put it in the blender with more water as a 2:1 water to coconut kefir ratio to make it drinkable. This way you will have a lot more kefir for smoothies and it will make the end product not too "rich" tasting. At this point, you can add a little stevia sweetener or flavors if you so desire.

Adding a spoonful or two of chocolate whey protein powder to the thickened kefir makes a delicious pro-biotic mousse.

Raw Neufchatel Cultured Cheese – S or E (depending on whether using goat's milk or skim cow's milk)

This is a spectacular cheese, probably one of my favorite foods. I like the distinctive flavor of goat's milk for this recipe, but raw cow's milk works fine if you remove the cream from the top first. Leaving the cream in doesn't work because it rises to the top during fermentation and affects the final texture. Using skim cow's milk for this recipe enables it to be used for both **S** and **E** situations but goat's milk will only be **S**.

Basic Ingredients: milk ✦ kefir or buttermilk ✦ rennet ✦ water ✦ sea salt and other seasonings

1. Place a 1 gallon bottle of raw milk in a sink full of hot water. You can use store-bought if that is your only option.
2. Leave this for a while and let the water warm the milk to room temperature. I like this method better than stirring milk over the stove until the right temperature is achieved as some people do.
3. Once the milk is warmed, remove it from the sink of water and pour it into a large sterilized stainless steel pot.
4. Add ¼ cup kefir, or ¼ cup cultured buttermilk (store-bought is fine for either, or use your own).
5. Dissolve ¼ tablet of rennet in ¼ cup of water and add this to the pot. I use Junket rennet tablets purchased from Walmart.
6. Stir milk thoroughly, cover, and let sit overnight undisturbed at room temperature. If it is winter and your house gets very cold overnight, place the pot in an ice chest (without ice of course) to stop it from chilling.
7. In the morning, the whey (liquid) should be separated from the curd. You will see a solid white mass with cloudy looking water around it. Slice the curd into cubes while in the pot. In other words, you slice the block of curd with a knife into several smaller pieces.
8. Carefully pour the contents of the pot into a colander that has been lined with an opened fine mesh bag (so the contents actually go into the bag). Go to any good paint store to purchase inexpensive paint strainers. These nylon mesh bags have been my best friends for yogurt straining and cheese making for many years. I can't be bothered with messy layers of cheese cloths. Artisan cooks may not have lots of children running around the house playing super heroes in the kitchen. They have to fold the cheese cloth multiple times and gingerly tie up the corners before the curd slips away with the whey. Oh, what a mess to put in the washing machine.
9. Make sure your colander is over a pot that can collect the whey as it can be used for adding to your oatmeal soaking water, or to inoculate your cultured vegetables with the good bacteria for fermentation. You can also throw it on the garden, give it to your pets, or better yet, to your children if they'll accept the lemony tart flavor. It is filled with minerals and living enzymes, but don't drink it if you're seeking weight loss as it has not been fermented long enough and still holds carbs.

10. After your first drain, grab the top of the mesh bag and give the bag a good shake a few times. Knead it a little with your hands to help get out extra liquid.
11. Put the bag of cheese back in the colander. Place a small plate on top of your cheese bag then weigh it down with a large can of beans or a heavy rock. This ensures there is enough pressure to keep the draining process going. Place this weighted colander in the fridge with a large dinner plate underneath to collect the extra whey and let drain for another 12 hours.
12. Once the whey has been drained, take your soft cheese and flavor to the creative whim of your imagination. I like to add a high quality finely ground Celtic sea salt. You could also divide your cheese and make different flavor combinations. I like to use red pepper flakes, fresh herbs like dill or chives, or garlic.
13. Mould your flavored cheese into a round mound with your hands and cover with cling wrap.

This cheese is simple to make. It is a whole lot easier than it sounds. Many directions sound complicated at first such as setting up a Port-a-Crib. So many different diagrams and complicated explanations, when all it takes really is a one, two, three—Bing, Bang, Boom!

Simple Sauerkraut – S, E or Fuel Pull

Cultured vegetables are a wonderful addition to any **S** or **E** meal. Because they teem with enzymes, you can sit down to your steak dinner and feel even better about yourself than the raw foodists who are dutifully working their way through a tub of "plant only" salad.

Basic Ingredients: cabbage ✦ water ✦ sea salt ✦ whey water

1. Slice a few organic cabbages finely or shred them in the food processor.
2. Fill as many sterilized glass quart jars as needed to use up your sliced cabbage. Fill jars ¾ of the way to the top only and make sure you pack cabbage down hard.
3. Fill the jars with enough pure water to cover the cabbage.
4. Add 1 flat Tbs. of good grade sea salt to each jar and 2 Tbs. of whey water from your cheese making. If you do not have whey, add another ½ Tbs. salt. For those liking a less salty flavor, you can reduce the amount, or leave it out altogether, providing you use whey. Whey inoculates your kraut with the right kind of bacteria to start the fermentation process on the right track. The good bacterium proliferates and leaves no room for any "bad guy" bacteria. If you don't have whey, using enough salt will inhibit the bad guys so only the good guys can grow.

5 Make sure you leave at least 2 inches of room at the top before securing the lid as jars could overflow from the fermentation.

6 Leave for three days and then transfer all jars to the refrigerator.

Your sauerkraut is now ready, but will only get better with time, just like fine aged wine. It can keep for years in the refrigerator and the flavors will only mature and deepen. You could store jars in a root cellar as an alternative to the fridge.

The above is the basic skeleton for culturing vegetables. You can add any other vegetables or spices. You can even culture fresh salsa. The flavor of cultured salsa is zingy and wonderful—a superfood way of enjoying this common condiment.

Sourdough Bread – E

This recipe does not use conventional yeast. You get to make your own starter and watch the forces of nature activate your bread to rise rather than relying on packaged yeast. It's a remarkable process and will take you back to how bread was healthfully made for millenniums. I'm going to teach you how to "catch a starter," but if for some reason you don't succeed (in some places the wild yeast may not be as prolific), you can order one on line.

This bread is made with two grains, primarily rye and a little spelt. My reason for choosing these grains is as follows. Rye is the cheapest grain to purchase in bulk which is a plus for big families on a tight budget. Rye also boasts the most fiber of any other grain which makes it super colon friendly. Rye, being so high in fiber, makes the glycemic index of this bread less than other grain breads.

My reason for choosing spelt is because it is high in protein and a non-hybridized ancient grain. It also gives the mixture a nice spongy texture. This recipe is centered on these two grains and their proportions. It took a whole summer (several years ago) of experimenting to come up with this mix.

Try it first with these particular grains in the exact measurements I have listed. If you would prefer to use all wheat, or other grains, feel free to experiment. You may have to change the proportions of water to flour, or the wetness of the mixture. The key to this recipe is to make a very wet dough. If you achieve this, you will reap super soft loaves, not hard bricks.

First, here's how to make your starter.

Basic Ingredients: water ✦ rye flour

1 In a sterilized bowl (pour boiling water over it to sterilize) add one cup of rye flour and one cup of pure water. Keep it on your counter top and cover with a breathable cloth. Every day for seven days swap it to a new clean sterilized bowl and add one

extra cup of rye flour and one extra cup of water. You swap bowls to make sure you do not catch bad bacteria while catching your wild yeast from the air.

2. After seven days your starter should be bubbly and spongy and should smell good and sour. If this is what yours looks like, congratulations, you have caught your yeast. Put your new starter into a clean home—a plastic or glass bowl that will hold three quarts of liquid. Never use metal. There is no need to switch bowls any more.

Now, here's how to make your bread. This recipe makes five loaves. If you don't need that many, you could halve the recipe.

Basic Ingredients: sour dough starter ✦ rye flour ✦ spelt flour ✦ sea salt ✦ water

1. Put 2 quarts of your starter in a large pot or bowl.
2. Add 6 ½ cups rye flour and 6 ½ cups of spelt flour (freshly ground if possible).
3. Add 2 ½ Tbs. sea salt and 1 ½ quarts water—more or less may be needed.
4. Knead with a big wooden rolling pin (or wooden spoon or some other device) by pulling the pin towards you and pushing it away from you—about five minutes, or 10 minutes for those who want extra toned arms. You can even get your hands into the gooey mixture and kneed. You cannot knead this mixture poured out on a counter. It is meant to look and feel like goo. Seek a texture that is wet, gooey, and similar to oatmeal porridge consistency. Adjust with either more flour or water if necessary. Test for consistency midway kneading, rather than at the beginning as the dough will get thicker when the gluten fibers start coming together after a few minutes.
5. Put in lightly greased tins to rise. To transfer this gooey mixture into your tins, wet a cereal bowl, dip it into the dough and flop it into your pans. Each tin should be a generous half full. Wet your hands and flatten the bread with the slap of a wet palm.
6. I raise my bread for at least **seven** hours for a good rise. Sometimes you will get the height you want after only four hours but the phytates will not be removed until at least seven hours. I either make the bread in the morning and bake for evening dinner or make it in the evening, leave overnight to rise, and bake for breakfast.
7. Bake at 350 for 1 hour.

If you want to go all the way, put a pan of water on the bottom rack of your oven, underneath the rack where your bread is cooking. This will steam your bread at the same time as baking, giving it a wonderful chewy texture.

Helpful Starter Hints

1. You can think of your starter as another family pet. Take it out and clean its home once a month. Feed it one cup of flour and one cup of water every day. Cover with

a breathable cloth—I use a nylon mesh bag from the painting store. These are fantastic as they allow air in and keep insects out.

2. When you feed your starter and stir it around, only use plastic or wooden utensils. No metal please, or you will kill your new pet.
3. Don't use up your entire starter when baking your bread. Try to leave at least one full cup over to begin growing your starter for the next batch. If for some reason you don't have a cupful of starter left, but only a spoonful, feed it one spoonful of flour and one spoonful of water. In a few hours, feed it two spoonfuls of each. A few hours later, feed it four of each until you have your cup—and then you can continue as usual.
4. Sometimes you will want to bake sooner than your starter will grow. In this case, if you have a quart of starter, you can feed it a quart of flour and a quart of water each day. The key is not to feed more food to your starter than the volume of your starter. You will dilute it too much and it will die.
5. My mother and I have kept our pet alive for over five years from when I first made the starter. A good idea is to share some of your starter with a friend. If you go away, or forget to keep it going, you may be able to get some back from her. Mom has come to my rescue on a number of occasions.

Chewy Sprouted Mini Loaves – E

A hearty chunk of one of these rolls is one of my favorite **E** meals. I love it toasted with 1 tsp. of virgin coconut oil and some savory shredded chicken breast with balsamic vinegar. These rolls are moist and chewy on the inside and satisfyingly crunchy on the outside—a perfect combination.

I make lots of these rolls when I make this recipe and store most of them in the freezer to thaw out for later use. I use organic spelt berries, kamut, or even regular organic wheat berries.

There are two parts to this recipe. You have to sprout the berries first, but it's not a big deal.

Basic Ingredients: wheat, kamut or spelt berries ✦ sea salt

Sprouting Directions:

1. Soak a substantial amount (5 or 6 coffee mugs) of grain in a pot of water overnight.
2. In the morning, drain soaked grain through a very large colander or use two of the largest colanders you can find.

3. Rinse grain berries while in the colander with a kitchen spray attachment or use your regular kitchen tap. Use your hands to swirl the water around the berries.
4. Once rinsed, set the colander on a plate, cover lightly with a kitchen towel and keep on kitchen counter. Rinse grain berries again before going to bed and continue to rinse morning and night until sprouts appear and grow a nice little tail, about ¾-1 cm. long. This takes approximately two days. Rinsing only takes a minute or so, less work than brushing your teeth.
5. Now you are ready to make your bread, but start when sprouts are not freshly rinsed and logged with water. They need to be a little dry.

Baking Directions:

1. Fill food processor (not blender) with sprouts.
2. Add generous pinch or two of course gray Celtic sea salt and process until a dough has formed and all sprouts are broken down.
3. Transfer the first batch of dough to a large bowl and repeat the processing procedure (adding salt each time), until you have used up all sprouts and have a large bowl of dough in front of you. Never, at any time, add any water or liquid to this recipe.
4. Grease baking trays with coconut oil or butter. For a softer crust, line baking trays with parchment paper. For a very chewy crust, forego the paper.
5. Moisten your hands with water, grab a bit of dough and form into 1-1½ inch high loaves, roughly the length and width of your hand. For extra chewiness, keep them the same height and length, but make them only two inches wide.
6. Place trays in oven (you can use multiple racks). On the bottom rack, place a small Pyrex dish filled with water in order for the bread to steam as it slowly bakes.
7. Bake superfood loaves slowly at 250 for 2½-3 hours. If you want to keep baking beyond this point to obtain a drier loaf, turn temperature down to 200 and bake for another couple of hours.

Isn't that easy? Only two ingredients—sprouted wheat berries and salt! Can you believe it? And you don't have to grind anything into flour with a big expensive mill. Any old food processor will do.

Pearl chats: I feel like I could almost do this one. I'm a little bit scared of all the soaking and sprouting, but the other part, I could totally do. I'll give you back to Serene and her capable hands.

As I mentioned, the sprouting is a cinch. Pearl, I know you are not the type to want to catch sour dough starters and keep them alive, but you can do this. Anyone can do it. The sprouting takes less than a minute twice a day. And just think, you're going to get so many cute loaves to put in your freezer. You won't have to do this recipe very often to keep up a good supply.

When you sprout grain, you not only remove the phytates that bind up the nutrients, but you also increase the protein content impressively. Using whole sprouted kernels instead of flour also lowers the glycemic index and is much friendlier to your blood sugar.

This bread is super healthy and delicious. Remember to keep your **S Helper** or **E** portion allowances in mind. Don't overdo a grain recipe, even though it is touted in this book. Always keep your carbohydrates within healthy blood-sugar parameters. This way, they can be enjoyed for energy, taste, and nutrition without exploding your hips, butt, and thighs!

Chapter 27

Earth Milk – S, E or Fuel Pull

by Serene Allison

A whole chapter devoted to one recipe? It deserves this solo esteem because it is the elixir of the best the earth has to offer.

This is a recipe I created after I had some dental work and couldn't chew properly, but I still wanted to keep greens in my diet. It is so delicious and, of course, nutritious, that I still use it. It guarantees a jam-packed, raw, green diet in a very absorbable way.

Most people juice to achieve what I get from this recipe. I don't have the time or money for that anymore and I hate cleaning a multi-compartment juicer. In fact, the stress of juicing may outweigh the benefits in my situation. This *Earth Milk* recipe is quicker and easier than juicing and a heck of a lot tastier than a green juice. You'll get the same cleansing benefits without all the extra fuss that juicing requires.

Earth Milk keeps, rather than discards, the cleansing properties of the green's fiber. This is important, not only for the fiber's ability to sweep toxins from the colon, but it also helps to stabilize blood sugar. But, this beverage is also creamy, hence the name, milk. Since this recipe calls for young, succulent greens, not hard fibrous ones that should be cooked anyway, it has a “smooth mouth” feel. You don’t feel like you’re chuggin’ tablespoons of Metamucil while it’s going down.

You can use this elixir to help with your weight management goals. It is just the thing to help you through our *One Week Fuel Cycle,* Chapter 28. One of my daily secrets is to often drink a small glass before one, or all of my meals, and sometimes a smaller glass before each snack. Since I’m breast feeding, I often just go to the fridge right before bed and take a good swig which helps sustain me throughout the night.

Drinking *Earth Milk* before meals ensures you get your greens before getting full on other foods. You can’t look at another salad? Fine, this is a perfect substitute. Even the best of us get “saladed” out now and then, especially on cold wintery nights when you don’t feel like chewing cold lettuce. With all its nutrients and fiber, *Earth Milk* also serves to suppress a huge appetite. The fat burning properties of Oolong or green tea in the recipe also help blast off those extra pounds by causing a significant metabolism boost.

If you already have your weight in check (hey, so do I), it can still be an integral part of your diet for further reasons. Earth Milk is a nutrient powerhouse that alkalizes the body, is anti-inflammatory, restores lost electrolytes, provides high mineral content, and hydrates and moisturizes the body from the inside out. Hello, radiant skin!

Another helpful trick is to take this sustaining drink in a “to go” bottle with you when you are out and about on errands. It stops you from getting low blood sugar at the worst possible time—when you are away from the safety of your kitchen with all its healthy choices. Often when you are out and about, the munchies hit, and it’s tempting to give in to unhealthy fast food. Earth milk can help satiate you on a cellular level and fill your tummy so you are not tempted.

You can also make this drink for your older baby or young toddler, but leave out the tea. Adding *Earth Milk* to their sippy cup ensures organic healthy raw greens in their diet. It was one of my baby’s first foods. She loves this green, creamy, slightly sweetened drink and gets excited when she sees me making it.

You will need a high end blender such as a Vitamix to ensure you get a smooth, creamy end product. A regular blender may leave tiny green bits in your drink to spoil the milk effect.

Basic Ingredients: greens ✦ sea salt ✦ coconut oil ✦ coconut milk ✦ vanilla ✦ sweetener ✦ water ✦ oolong or green tea ✦ cinnamon ✦ optional whey protein powder or cocoa powder

1 Fill a Vitamix, or other high end blender, with about 5 hefty handfuls of one, or a combination of the following greens: mixed field greens, parsley, cilantro, dark leafy romaine and spinach. Remember that spinach is best cooked, which removes oxalic acid content, but raw can be used in small amounts. I use whatever soft greens I have on hand. Sometimes it might only be two organic bunches of parsley with most of

the stalks removed—that's cheap. Other times, I may use field greens, a little parsley, and cilantro.

2 Add 2 generous pinches of gray, coarse, Celtic salt. I say coarse, because it is half the price and you are blending it anyway.

3 Add 3-4 Tbs. virgin coconut oil for an **S** version. To make it **E** or **Fuel Pull** friendly, instead use 1 Tbs. extra virgin coconut oil and a splash or two of light coconut milk. You will not be drinking this whole recipe at once so these quantities of fat keep you within bounds for **E** or **Fuel Pulls**. If you don't have the money for the virgin coconut oil, do not use the cooking kind. This is a superfood recipe. As a substitute to help make this drink creamy, add a generous splash or two of full-fat coconut milk that is BPA free.

4 Add some shakes of cinnamon powder which stabilizes the blood sugar and also tastes delicious.

5 Add drizzle of pure vanilla extract.

6 Add NuStevia Pure White Stevia Extract Powder or Truvia to taste. The idea is to not make a super sweet drink, but a neutral milk flavor like milk is itself. Use just enough to disguise a little of the deep earthy flavors of the baby greens and herbs.

7 Boil 1 cup of water in a small saucepan and add 3 tea bags of a classic green or Oolong variety and let steep 5 minutes.

8 Remove tea bags and add enough water to the saucepan until the water is no longer boiling hot, but very warm.

9 As you add this warm liquid to the blender it will emulsify the coconut oil nicely into the *Earth Milk* while blending. If you use cold water, the oil will return to the top and will not combine with the drink. Never use hot tea straight as it destroys the fresh greens. It's gotta be warm.

10 Blend all of the above on high for 2 minutes, or until smooth and creamy. If you are using a Vitamix blender, do not blend too long or the blender will heat up the drink and destroy the raw enzymes.

11 Remove from blender and pour into a 2 quart glass canning jar. Add pure, cold water until the jar is full. Put on the lid and shake well. Taste and sweeten more if needed.

12 Refrigerate and drink freely, saturating your body with superfoods and life.

You can use an optional scoop of vanilla or chocolate flavored un-denatured whey protein powder, but I usually save that more expensive item for my after workout shake. The whey protein powder does kick the yummy notch up a little, though. It provides this milk with a complete protein source which makes for complete nutrition. That's a plus when using this as an energy meal replacement while on the run. For this reason, even though the whey protein is not so friendly on my budget, I throw in a scoop from time to time. Optionally, you can also add 2 heaping Tbs. of unsweetened cocoa powder if you feel like a chocolate flavor for a change. If you use cocoa, you will need to add more sweetener as the chocolate absorbs much of the sweetness.

Using a chocolate flavor in a green drink is a lovely, harmonious combination. It's like pairing coffee and chocolate. Greens have a deep, slightly bitter, earthy flavor like coffee and compliment the base notes of dark chocolate beautifully. It is a delicious flavor arrangement. But, with all that being said, I usually enjoy the original, malty tasting *Earth Milk*. But, you know what they say, "A change is as good as a holiday." I hate ruts.

This recipe can be addicting for "green nuts" like me. I can almost overdo this stuff. There are only pros and no cons when it comes to the extreme health benefits of *Earth Milk*. However, it is a potent detoxifier and contains copious amounts of fiber. After drinking it continually for awhile, my stomach can feel bloated and gassy, and this is my cue to take a week's break. To broom out the colon is good, but not continually.

Pearl chats: You can guess that I have never made this recipe. If you think you have to make *Earth Milk* for our plan to work, stop worrying—you don't. Serene has told me about this recipe so many times and I often enjoy taking sips of her drink as she frequently takes it wherever she goes. She often forces me, "Just taste it, Pearl! You won't believe how fantastic it is. C'mon drink up!" She basically holds my face and pours it down my gullet. Well not quite, but almost.

Okay, I admit, for a green drink it's actually quite palatable. I could possible even call it yummy. It's delicious in a weird way! And now that I see it printed out in easy steps, it doesn't seem so intimidating to me.

Serene, you are so brainwashing me with your Earth Mother ways! I'm supposed to be the shortcut queen, but now I am tempted to make this fandangled drink for myself! And to make things worse, this drink is catching on like a craze in our area. I just have to shake my head as I see more and more women carrying around their *Earth Milk* wherever they go. What's the world coming to? The granola moms are taking over the planet.

Maybe I'll give it a go. I'm sure it could further enhance my health, but I can't promise I'll stick to it. It might be too much of an extra frill for my no frills approach. I guess I could take a month and use it as a once a year spring cleaning for my body. Or, include it one week per month to keep me healthy. That's something to think about.

Some will jump straight on this *Earth Milk* wagon. But, if you're not that type, relax. You can walk with me and still feel good about your own *Trim Healthy Mama* approach.

Chapter 28

One Week Fuel Cycle

Are you still struggling with stubborn weight? Do you need some structure to help you get the scale moving more? This chapter is for you.

If you are still having trouble losing weight on the **S** and **E** plan, you should check your thyroid levels. See Pearl's chapters on hormones if you are suspicious of low thyroid, or have been diagnosed with a thyroid issue. Weight management will be extremely difficult until this issue is remedied.

If you have entered menopause, or had surgery to remove any of your reproductive organs, you will experience hormonal decline. Losing your sex hormones also makes weight loss a lot more difficult. It is a good idea for you to have blood tests taken and find a doctor that can help you get back to more youthful hormone levels.

However, we have helped people with thyroid conditions and sexual hormone decline lose stubborn weight, even without the use of thyroid meds or estrogen therapy. It's harder to achieve, but it can happen.

However, what happens if you've been trying our eating plan, your thyroid and other hormones are in good working order, but you are still not getting the weight loss results you desire?

Honesty Check

First, be honest with yourself. Have you really followed the guidelines? Are you merging **E** and **S** at times by crossing over, or not waiting three hours between switches? Are you eating any refined white junk foods? What about honey? Are you adding it to your tea? Are you still baking with it? Are you still snatching food from your children's plates, or eating junk on the run, using the "just this once" excuse?

You're not drinking milk, fruit juice, or even carrot juice, are you? You're not still putting lots of bananas in your smoothies, are you? How about store-bought cereals that aren't on plan? We hope you are not using them just because they're quick and easy? What about homemade bread that is not sourdough, dark rye, or sprouted? Do you still think that dried fruit is a healthy snack? Are mashed potatoes part of your **E** meals?

Are you staying on a one meal style like **S** for too long, just because it's easier and thereby not changing your fuels and calories enough? Have you not given fat busting **Fuel Pull** breakfasts and snacks a fair go yet? Do you sleep walk to the fridge and gorge on leftover pizza? Okay, that last one was a joke, but this checklist is important before we can help you more.

Maybe you've been eating too many "franken foods." These are store-bought low-carb items that help some of us out so we don't feel too restricted, but they should not be the staples of our diet. If you are eating too many store-bought low-carb tortillas, breads, pasta, protein bars, ice cream, candy, etc. this could be your cause of halting weight loss.

Coffee with cream can sometimes be another staller. Yes, cream is fine with **S** meals and you should not have to go without, but it is so high in calories that you shouldn't constantly over do it. Have one or two creamy hot drinks per day with just a small swirl of cream or half and half, not half a mug's worth. Make sure the rest of your drinks are without milk or cream so your body is not constantly bombarded with it. Cream has a small amount of carb in the form of skim milk, unlike butter, and it is a dense calorie food. Some people will not be able to handle it as well as others.

Our **S** desserts that involve cream cheese, lots of nuts, peanut butter, or cream are usually fine in moderation for most people. However, if you're yet to see weight loss on our plan, you might need to pull them back and eat them only for special occasions. There are plenty of other desserts which do not promote stalls, namely our puddings made with glucomannan, also *Skinny Chocolate, Tummy Tucking Ice Cream, Muffin in a Bowl,* and *Melt in your Mouth Meringues* (*Desserts*, Chapter 23).

Is it possible that you're too liberal with nuts and cheese? Some people have such sluggish metabolisms that they need to pull back a little on these two foods since they're very calorie dense. You can still include some nuts and cheese in your **S** meals, but don't eat them to your heart's content. Cut your cheese slices thinner. Go easier on the nuts. Enjoy flavors but don't overdo. See what happens.

The best way to lose weight is to eat basic whole foods. The most powerful weight loss meals are very simple, like salmon and salad with an olive oil dressing for **S**. In fact, any protein source, whether leftover chicken, fish, or even fried eggs over a bed of greens with an olive oil and vinegar dressing is an excellent slimming lunch or dinner. The hot protein cooked in some fat is hearty and satisfying and the lettuce underneath fills you up and offers a lot of fork to mouth satisfaction. Maybe you've been trying to get too fancy and need to go back to simple meals like these and see what happens on the scale. Simple **E** meals such as soups made with chana dahl or lentils, lean meat salads with quinoa, *Trim Healthy Pancakes* (*Morning Meals*, Chapter 18) sweet potatoes with salad, and water packed tuna are winners for that meal style.

In fairness to those who have been doing everything right and are still struggling, don't beat yourself up. Some people are more insulin resistant than others. Some have body types that are more prone to holding onto weight. Hang in there! We have some ways to pull you out of the ditch.

Body Types

There are three different body types—Ectomorphs, Mesomorphs, and Endomorphs. We'll briefly describe each type but you could do a more in depth study on this subject if it interests you. It's quite fascinating.

Ectomorphs are the high metabolism types that find it hard to put on muscle and often have trouble keeping on enough weight. They're the people who need to eat more **Crossover**s so they don't get too skinny.

Mesomorphs are the middle group. They can easily put on muscle, are usually naturally athletic, but can more easily gain fat than Ectomorphs. Mesomorphs, when in good shape have broader shoulders, trim waists and well toned muscles, but when they're out of shape they can easily put fat on their bellies.

The last group is the endomorphic body type. If you are reading this chapter with interest, you might be in this group. Endomorphs can gain muscle, but they also gain fat much more easily than the two other body types. Endo men and women usually have larger hips, trunks, and overall heavier skeletal frames.

A lot of endos carry their weight in the bottom half of their body like thighs and buttocks. Endo women are often very curvy. When in shape, these women have the ultimate feminine figure, but it is much more difficult for them to keep the pounds from accumulating. Endos have to work harder than others, therefore the following structured cycle will help those with this body type. Not all of us are one pure body type. Some people can be a combination of two, but if you look at yourself, you will likely find you fit more predominately into one group.

Temporary Tune Up

The following method is not as practical for a long term lifestyle as the "freestyling" method we have taught you in the rest of the book. Some may grab onto these stricter rules at first because they look more like a regular diet with structure and rigidity. If you are skipping other chapters and coming here first because you just want to follow rules and do a "no think diet," please go back. We want you to learn the art of long term healthy eating and let it become as natural as breathing. We don't want this short term cycle to take over your life and squash the "freestyling" approach we have encouraged. Let it be a tool to help you over the bumps and stalls that come when the body gets grumpy about letting go of extra weight, then get back to freestyling and enjoying yourself.

This cycle can also be used periodically for a general overhaul of your metabolism. It's like going to Jiffy Lube after putting a few thousand miles on your vehicle. Anyone, regardless of weight (except pregnant and nursing mothers), is welcome to try it, just for kicks, every couple of months or so. However do not use it during pregnancy and the first few months of nursing a newborn. That is a time where every meal should provide optimal nourishment. Since this cycle pulls out your primary fuels for a full two days, it promotes more rapid weight loss and that is not advisable for those seasons of life. But, if your nursing baby is at least four to six months, it should be okay for you to try this cycle. Just make sure to keep in a lot of nutritious snacks according to the fuel of the day.

In this cycle you will actively shift between three different metabolic pathways. This will help to re-awaken your metabolism in a deeper stimulating way than "freestyling" our plan alone. Other areas in your body, aside from weight loss that are affected by the metabolism process, will be enhanced. If you're already at goal weight, but you want to try this cycle to rev your metabolism for an overall health boost, and consequently lose a few more pounds than needed, you'll have fun climbing back up to goal weight by "crossing over." Hey, you can try doing this a week or so before the holiday season so you can really enjoy turkey and stuffing.

The cycle is a seven day process. You will repeat it at least once for a total of two weeks. Please don't skip any meals on this cycle or go much longer than four hours between meals. That may have a slowing effect on the metabolism. After two fuel cycles back to back, you go back to freestyling **S** and **E**. You **don't** go back to your old eating lifestyle.

Day 1: Deep S

This is a full day of **S** alone. You will dive into **S** in the deepest way possible.

- Do not use any **S helpers**.
- Do not even have berries. No fruit, grains, or beans at all.

- Do not eat any nuts or seeds for the next three days. No avocado and NO PEANUT BUTTER! That means none of our desserts made with nuts or seeds. Nuts and seeds are usually wonderful **S** foods, but this cycle is super strict because those foods are often overdone. If you have stubborn weight, you need to pull back on some of these concentrated foods so your body can only burn the simplest of **S** foods. The two exceptions to nuts are unsweetened almond or flax milk and small amounts of light coconut milk for smoothies. Unsweetened almond and flax milks are nut and seed based, but neither are concentrated liquids so they are welcome on these deep **S** days.
- Keep all carbohydrates to leafy greens, or maybe a few cooked, buttered, non-starchy vegetables.
- Be liberal with fats like extra virgin coconut oil and butter.
- All meats and eggs are welcome, with as much salmon as possible. Grass fed beef and omega-3 eggs are best.
- Use only homemade dressings, heavy with superfood type oils. Pour on the olive oil, Mama!
- You may drink the **S** or **Fuel Pull** friendly version of *Earth Milk* (Chapter 27) today if it is something you like and make. It will help sustain you and cleanse your body.
- No kefir smoothies today since kefir has a few carbs. You can make chocolate or vanilla whey protein smoothies, using water or unsweetened almond milk, with optional added virgin coconut oil. Don't add berries to these whey smoothies.
- No yogurt (Greek or otherwise), cottage cheese, ricotta cheese, or cream cheese.
- Do not use tomato based products like paste, sauce, or ketchup.
- Eat very few onions, and no sweet peas, as these are more middle carb level veggie options.
- Avoid any store-bought pasta sauces.
- Enjoy cheese in small amounts (raw cheeses are best).
- Whey protein is most welcome.

That's a lot of "do not's," but stubborn weight is going to call for more drastic measures than the more laid back approach we take with freestyling. But, you certainly don't have to go hungry. In fact, you can eat plenty to stay well satiated. These deep **S** days will be easy if you remember to eat well from simple fats and proteins and limit carbohydrates to a minimum.

Ideas?

For breakfast, have eggs alone cooked in butter, coconut, or palm oil. Or, have eggs with organic sausage or bacon and sautéed mushrooms. Or, enjoy a large whey smoothie with added coconut oil and an egg yolk.

For lunch, have chicken or fish over salad greens, with lots of olive oil and some vinegar on your lettuce. Or, try one of Serene's superfood blended soups with salmon, greens, and coconut or red palm oil. For an afternoon snack try another smoothie with coconut oil and whey or enjoy a big glucomannan based pudding. Or, you could have some *Kale Chips* (*Snacks,* Chapter 24) for a crunchy snack, or a few lettuce roll ups with meat, mustard, or homemade mayonnaise and a small amount of cheese. Have a nice source of meat for your evening meal with some buttered, non-starchy vegetables, or another green salad heavy with oils. This might be the perfect time to splurge on a nice grass fed steak since you are cutting out other regular **S** foods and need to bless yourself a little to keep up morale.

On this day, you are flushing excess glucose from cells and switching to pure fat burning for fuel. Just on these deep **S** cycle days, we ask you to leave off even our **S** bread recipes. This day is purely about whole foods in their simplest form. Avoid all store-bought, low-carb items like Dreamfields pasta, Joseph's pitas or Mission tortillas.

Even on this more stringent fuel cycle your sweet tooth need not be denied. You can enjoy our homemade *Skinny Chocolate* in liberal quantities since it is made from coconut oil. Adding lots of coconut oil in these deep **S** days will help supply you with more energy, and boost your thermogenic temperature. Our *Melt in your Mouth Meringues, Tummy Tucking Ice Cream,* slick trick puddings and whey smoothies are also good desserts. But these are your only sweet snack and dessert options during the **S** part of the cycle. No cheesecake or other usual **S** treats.

During these three **S** fuel days, remember to keep your focus on healthy meats and fish, lots of omega-3 eggs, fats like coconut and extra virgin olive oil, abundant fresh salad greens, and just a few cooked non-starchy veggies. These foods are the nucleus of the **S** fuel style. But they are often under-eaten, replaced by **S** condiments that can be easily abused. It's very easy to overdo nuts, cheese, peanut butter, store-bought heavy cream, cream cheese, and **S** Franken foods. Let these days teach you what pure **S** looks, feels, and tastes like. Those foods will still be welcome on free-style days. Don't be sad, you're not saying goodbye to them forever.

Day 2: Deep S

This is another full **S** day. Remember the fuel of your **S** days is fat, pure and simply. It's not a time to skimp on superfood fats. We don't mean you should gorge on heavy whipping cream, but feel free to have a little swirl in your coffee. If you have access to raw grass-fed cream, you could be a little more generous in your servings as it is a healing superfood for the body. Store-bought heavy cream, while allowed on this plan, is pasteurized and does not have the same benefits. We'd rather you focus on the fats that help you shed weight and give you energy, namely extra virgin coconut oil. Extra virgin coconut oil will accelerate your weight loss on these three **S** days and will also help keep your brain from fogginess. Your glucose will dip into a lower state from constant **S** meals, and coconut oil is an excellent brain fuel source.

The healthy, immediate energy that coconut oil supplies keeps your body in an anabolic (cell repairing) state, even though your body will eat into its own fat reserves and would normally start to be in a catabolic (breaking down) state.

If your budget does not allow for extra virgin coconut oil, do not fret. Do the best you can with your cheap Walmart Louanna coconut oil.

You don't have to skimp on butter. Feel free to cook your food with it. Utilize lots of extra virgin olive oil on your salads. We want you to bathe the inside of your body with these healthy fats, because after day three of this cycle, they're going bye bye. You certainly won't be enjoying them in the same ample amounts. But, you'll be eating other fun foods, so don't worry. Even during this extreme cycle week, we want all the meals to preserve your body, not abuse it. Low-fat for too long is abusive. These three fat filled days should tide your body over well once you get to the next part of your cycle.

Day 3: Deep S

The same as day one and two. Remember to stay away from low-carb "franken foods."

Day 4: Pull the Fuels

The last three days of deep **S** have ensured you are now in a state where your muscle cells are completely empty of glucose. Your body has been burning only fats as its primary fuel. Hopefully, by now it is also dipping into your own adipose tissue and gnawing away at that. But, let's make sure of that by turning up the amps on your body's fat burning power.

How will you do this? You'll now strip away most of that dietary fat. Your body will have nothing left to turn to for fuel but its own fat stores. It will have to dig deeply into them. Normally in our plan, if we removed fat from your plate, we offer you glucose to burn instead, as we don't want you in a catabolic state. However, for the next two days, the only primary fuel you burn will be your own excess, the stuff around your belly that you hate to be able to pinch. **E** meals come later in the week. You'll only be in these **Fuel Pull** trenches for two days. And you might be surprised. We're going to make it as enjoyable as possible.

Make sure all your meals significantly pull back both **S** fuels of fat and **E** fuels of carbs. You will eat only neutral foods that are still healthy, but are not primary sources of these fuels. Calories will naturally be much lower on these next two days. It's doubtful you will go over 1000 calories for the whole day which is a good shake up for your body. It will not harm your metabolism since you won't stay in the low-calorie state for too long. Thankfully, we have a lot of trick foods to help you feel full and help you think you are eating a whole lot more than you are.

- Keep fats to the strictest of our **E** meal portions, i.e., one teaspoon of oil and no nuts or nut butters or seeds or seed butters.
- Eat lots of salads if desired but keep dressings extra light, utilizing vinegars, lemon juice, and very small amounts of extra virgin olive oil (no more than one teaspoon). Include lean proteins with your salads. Try out *The Fuel Pull Salad* (*Lunches,* Chapter 20), which is huge and delectable with our *Hip Trim Honey Mustard.* If you are not of a purist mindset, Wishbone brand of salad spritzers might be a helpful addition for these days. Or, if you don't mind a little Splenda now and then, Walden Farms brand of calorie free dressings and sauces may help you out since they have no carbs or fat. Green Valley Ranch would be a more pure choice yet still calorie free.
- Fill up on your cooked non-starchy veggies also. You won't be able to sauté them with lots of butter like you do on your regular **S** days, but there are still plenty of ways to enjoy them in neutral fuel style. How about a soup based on fat free chicken broth, laced with diced chicken breast, wilted spinach or other veggies like cauliflower and red pepper flakes? Or try our *Loaded Fotato Soup* (*Lunches,* Chapter 20). That recipe is so tasty and filling. Utilize our *Creamless, Creamy Veggies* (*Vegetable Sides,* Chapter 22). Angel hair sliced cabbage cooked in that way is a fantastic filling meal with some diced chicken breast on top.
- Glucomannan powder and foods derived from this substance can be your "oh so clever" trick to fill up. Use konjac/glucomannan noodles to fill you up since they're zero calorie, zero carb, and zero fat. They're wonderful with sauces made from chicken broth and seasonings, thickened a little with glucomannan powder. Or, try our *Sweet and Spicy Asian Stir Fry* (*Evening Meals,* Chapter 21), which is a great **Fuel Pull** and works perfectly with these noodles. Have as many of these konjac noodles as you want or can afford. You could even try a low-fat sugar-free marinara sauce over the noodles with 1 Tbs. of parmesan cheese on top.
- Tomatoes are now welcome back on your menu for the rest of the week. On the deep **S** days of this week we kept you away from tomatoes as they are slightly higher in carbs than most non-starchy vegetables and we don't want them mixing with your fat fuel. (Notice, we are not that finicky with regular **S** meals.) But, now there's basically no fat so there will be no chance of a collision. It is preferable to make your marinara sauce at home, but there are some store-bought, light style, sugar-free preparations that can work. You can find recipes for other **Fuel Pull** sauces to have over glucomannan noodles or cooked non-starchy veggies in the links provided toward the end of this chapter.
- No fruit for the next two days, except berries.
- No grains, beans, and starchy veggies. That means no sweet potatoes, but a few raw baby carrots will not be a problem.

- There are certain dairy products that will work well for your **Fuel Pull** days. Greek yogurt (0%) is back for the rest of the week. Yay! It's a good foundation, and you may also include desserts like *Frozen Yogurt* or *Frozen Yogurt Pops* (*Deserts,* Chapter 23) in moderation. Take note that Greek style yogurt is the only acceptable yogurt during this part of the cycle. Avoid regular yogurt, as it is a higher source of carbs which are a primary fuel.

  Low-fat, (1%) cottage cheese is perfectly suitable, but do not use ricotta for just these two days. We list dessert recipes like *Ricotta Crème*, as **Fuel Pull** friendly in our recipe section for general freestyling, but we are pushing you into a more extreme state in this cycle week. Although it is a rather lean dairy protein, even skim ricotta is higher in calories than Greek yogurt and 1% cottage cheese, therefore give it a pause for these couple of days.

  No kefir please, either full-fat or low-fat, as both contain a primary fuel. Parmesan cheese from the green can is fine in small amounts. It will help you out a lot with flavor while adding barely any fat or carbs. No full-fat cheeses, but very small amounts of skim mozzarella will be okay. Grate a little and sprinkle it sparsely on your salads, proteins, and use it mixed with 1% cottage cheese for a **Fuel Pull** friendly pizza which is described at the end of the *Muffins, Breads, and Pizza Crusts*, Chapter 19. Light Laughing Cow or Weight Watchers cheese wedges are both allowed.
- We want you to enjoy lean meat proteins on **Fuel Pull** days, but don't overdo them. Eat lean meats in small to moderate amounts on these trench days, no more than about 3 oz. per meal.
- Your meat proteins will be easy to remember. Referring to grains, we always say, "Whites are out!" But, in this case, whites are in—white chicken breast, white flaky fish, and extra lean ground turkey or chicken. No red meat, please.

  Fish is invited to the menu. While it won't halt progress to eat salmon for these two days, we encourage you to eat white fish because it is lower in fat. This also allows more of a fun change since salmon is the sea food we usually promote. If you're not a scratch cook, Gorton's Grilled Tilapia from the frozen seafood section of your local grocery store is a handy and tasty meat option for a **Fuel Pull** meal.
- Keeping with the white theme, egg whites will be your best friend. *Egg White Wraps* (*Muffins, Breads, and Pizza Crusts*, Chapter 19), *Egg White Omelet/Scramble*, (*Morning Meals*, Chapter 18), and egg white cookies, namely our *Melt in your Mouth Meringues* (*Desserts*, Chapter 23), are all great ideas. Don't forget about our *Light Baked Custard* (*Morning Meals*, Chapter 18). It's base is egg whites, but it tastes like a sweet treat and could be a lovely breakfast on either of these next two days.

- Don't forget about our two fabulous **Fuel Pull** friendly breakfasts (can also be used as snack options) which you prepare the night before. These are *Cookie Bowl Oatmeal* and *Chia Tapioca Pudding* (*Morning Meals,* Chapter 18). They're both filling and yummy.
- You may use Joseph's pitas if you want to make a sandwich as they are low in carbs, fat, and calories, or for a base to make a **Fuel Pull** Pizza. Keep fillings lean—mustard, Dijonaise or horseradish sauce, or a very small amount of light mayonnaise. Include lots of lettuce, very lean deli meat, and if desired, a sparse amount of grated skim mozzarella. You may also purchase Wasa crackers (no more than 2 per serving) or GG Crisp breads and top them with light toppings like Light Laughing Cow or Weight Watches cheese wedges, lean deli meats, tomatoes, and sliced cucumber.
- Unsweetened almond or flax milk, along with plan approved whey protein powder are perfect neutral foods as they do not contain a primary fuel. You won't have to feel hungry if you include our *Fat Stripping Frappa* or *Big Boy Smoothie* recipes (*Morning Meals,* Chapter 18). Don't forget you can also make your gluc puddings with a base of 0% Greek yogurt blended with water. Any of our dessert recipes that are labeled as **Fuel Pull** are fine with the only exception of those based on ricotta cheese. Don't forget our *Muffin in a Bowl* (*Muffins, Breads, and Pizza Crusts,* Chapter 19), which is the perfect treat to give you some chocolate satisfaction so you won't feel deprived in any way. Have it with a squirt or two of Fat Free Reddi Whip if you wish.
- Serene's **E** and **Fuel Pull** friendly version of *Earth Milk* is a wonderful filling, yet cleansing drink for these two days. It will help you keep nutrition high even while stripping primary fuels, due to its super vitamin, mineral and chlorophyll content.
- No full-fat cream or creamer in your coffee. Drink your coffee black, or use a little unsweetened almond milk or "plain" coconut creamer.

Day 5: Pull the Fuels

Same as day four.

Day 6: E – Refuel

Refuel day! Your body has not had to juggle the carb ball for five days. Wooaahh! Your muscle cells will be like a sponge when you offer them glucose. Let's give them what they want! However, we'll do it with safe boundaries that will still ensure you stay in body fat burning mode. We're not going to spike your sugar levels which would be a sure way to halt your fat loss progress. No carb binging—you know that! We didn't have to tell you, but couldn't help it!

It's now time for a big 360—time to force your body to burn a completely different fuel source. Bring on the glucose! This is a full **E** day.

- Do not leave lean protein out of any snack or meal (this will help blunt any possible sugar spikes and enable your body to release glucagon along with insulin to temper its effect).
- Chana dahl and quinoa are great for this **E** day. Make smart use of them since they are such wonderful sources of slow burning carbohydrates.
- Do not use more than 1 tsp. of fat with any snack or meal, but you don't have to leave it out completely (this is in addition to the natural fat in lean protein).
- Make use of our *Trim Healthy Pancakes* (*Morning Meals,* Chapter 18) with 0% Greek yogurt and berries, or make *Trim Healthy Pan Bread (Muffins, Breads, and Pizza Crusts,* Chapter 19) with appropriate sandwich fillings. If you don't feel like doing a lot of cooking, stick to our approved sprouted or sourdough breads, but no more than 2 pieces per meal
- Try to change your **E** glucose options between sweet potatoes, beans, and different grains. You could start your day with egg whites inside a sprouted wrap or with one or two pieces of sprouted toast. Lunch could be a sweet potato with salad and water packed tuna. The evening meal could be chana dahl soup with spinach and lean chicken. Snacks might include Greek yogurt with 1 Tbs. of all fruit jelly.
- Enjoy fruit if you wish. Your body will love you when you give it an apple. What a sweet treat after not eating one for several days. Remember not to overdo fruit (your liver only has a small storehouse for fructose).
- Utilize low-fat cottage cheese and ricotta, low-fat Greek and regular yogurt, egg whites, low-fat kefir, chicken breast and fish (canned tuna and salmon are fine).
- No egg yolks today.
- No homemade kefir from full-fat milks. Goat's milk is also high in fat, so avoid it today.
- No full-fat cream or creamer in your coffee—drink it black or use a little skimmed milk, unsweetened almond or flax milk, or "plain" coconut creamer.
- Serene's **E** and **Fuel Pull** friendly *Earth Milk* (Chapter 27) is welcome and encouraged.
- Any of our **E** recipes are appropriate, but we don't suggest even plan approved boxed cereal for today as we are promoting primarily whole foods for this week.

Day 7: E Refuel

Same as day six.

Repeat the Cycle

One full cycle has been completed. Congratulations!

Tomorrow, you'll start again at day one. Your metabolism has just been awakened with this first round. You'll need to do this complete cycle again if you have very stubborn weight. You can even repeat it a further time for a complete three rounds if you think you can endure it. Think of those old push lawnmowers. You had to pull the starter at least two to three times to get the motor running. That's what you're doing here. If you pull it only once, you may not get your lawn mowed!

After completing two or more rounds of this fuel cycle, go back to freestyling **S** and **E**. If you have lots of stubborn weight to lose, you may want to start the cycle again after another month has gone by. Some people have what we call "donkey weight." It needs to be pushed and cajoled all the way to the end. It is perfectly healthy for you to keep rotating fuel cycling with freestyling for as long as it takes to reach a weight where you feel great about yourself and the donkey has become a race horse. A good arrangement may be to include a full two to three week fuel cycle every other month.

In between your fuel cycles and back to freestyling **S** and **E**, you can utilize more **Fuel Pull** meals and snacks here and there, especially now that you have more experience with them. However, be sure to have plenty of fueled meals also so you don't stay too low in calories for too long and lower your metabolism.

The one week cycle pushed you into two full **Fuel Pull** days back to back. That should be the limit on how long you should ever drag out that style of eating. Any longer and your body will catch on to what you are trying to do and lower your metabolism in retaliation. Go ahead and throw a few complete **Fuel Pull** days into your freestyling, if you can make it work with the rest of your family's needs, but don't stay permanently in that mode. Or, think about incorporating some mini cycle days where your breakfast and lunch will be deep pure **S** to help empty glucose from your cells. Then make your afternoon snack and evening meal **Fuel Pull** to force your body into adipose burning.

Web Sources for Fuel Pull Days

Below, we give you the link to a forum for recipes that utilizes a diet called JUDD (The Johnson Up Day Down Day Diet). The founder of the diet, Dr. Johnson has written an intriguing book called, *Alternate Day Fasting*. It is a great read for dietary science sake.

As with other diet books, we take the positives and throw away the negatives. There are some fascinating positives to Dr. Johnson's diet, but we see some pitfalls, too. The positives are that this diet focuses on the science of caloric changes, a premise that our own **S** and **E** plan implements more loosely. The JUDD diet zigzags calories in a very extreme fashion. JUDD dieters do one high calorie day, followed by an extremely low-calorie day that is almost like a fast, and keep repeating this pattern.

The lower calorie days trick the body into thinking it's starving and the body then turns on a gene called SIRT1. This is known as the longevity gene and is a fascinating subject to research. SIRT 1 reduces inflammation in the body, reduces insulin resistance, reduces and sometimes eliminates inflammatory conditions like asthma and arthritis, and saves lean muscle while promoting a state where fat is gobbled up. There's also evidence that it can prevent Alzheimer's disease. The higher calorie days prevents the body from lowering metabolism but do not turn off the longevity gene.

Some of the more clever and knowledgeable followers of this diet have created a forum that has oodles of recipes that you can tweak in a healthy way for your **Fuel Pull** days on the cycle, or during your general freestyling. They've come up with creative muffins, crepes, pancakes, sauces, curries, and gravies for meals that support a no fuel approach for their low-calorie days, yet still include lots of protein and use mostly healthy ingredients.

But, caution. The JUDD diet itself does not take a superfood approach to eating. It does not care so much what you eat except the difference in calories between one day and the next. While this premise may enable success for long term weight loss since it doesn't allow for a lowered metabolism, it can be abused with low-calorie junk foods devoid of nourishment and non-foods laced with chemicals. Some JUDD dieters fast completely on their very low-calorie days, or eat extremely little, so they can eat whatever they want on their higher calorie days, including sugary, refined foods. Dr. Johnson, while presenting some ground-breaking and thought-provoking information, does not understand the importance of healthy saturated fats like coconut oil. His book still sweeps all fats into the "bad" category.

On the whole, if you're a busy mama in the home, we don't believe stripping your meals of their primary fuels every second day like this would flow naturally with family centered meal times, especially in the evening. Now and then during freestyling you may be able to pull off some **Fuel Pull** evening meals for yourself, but every other day could easily detract from your important focus of growing robust, healthy children.

We also don't want you to start obsessively calorie counting or weighing foods as JUDD dieters are advised to, or using a lot of chemical non-foods just because they may be low-calorie and promote "fast weight shedding." Our book is *Trim Healthy Mama*, not *Skinny* ***Unhealthy*** *Mama*. Don't get sidetracked from your important goal of healthfully nourishing your family and yourself, even if you notice a lot of weight loss success for others on this diet forum.

The helpful recipe thread we refer to is found at the site we have mentioned frequently, www.lowcarbfriends.com. On this webpage, there is also a sub forum devoted to the premise of the JUDD diet. Once you click on the JUDD forum, you will notice a sticky thread near the top of the JUDD page called *Down Days Recipes Only*. That's the one that may be a big help to you if you're interested in creating more **Fuel Pull** meals.

Not all of the recipes fit our whole food approach, but many of them will. This site has some smart people chiming in who take a more sensible approach to the JUDD diet. Most of the members at this forum understand the principles of low glycemic eating and utilize healthier low-cal foods such as the alkalizing super-root glucomannan (both powder and noodles) and oat fiber, rather than relying on packaged, devitalized, and processed low-cal foods. After reading our book, you will be able to choose recipes from this thread with more discretion.

If you are older, your children have grown, and you are no longer responsible for their nutrition, adopting a loose form of JUDD, combined with the whole foods approach of our plan may be a great idea for you to consider. Often, weight can be harder to shed after menopause. Pulling your calories down every other day, or even for three days per week, through eating lean protein and veggie rich **Fuel Pull** type meals will help shed tough weight, turn on the SIRT1 gene, and likely provide amazing health benefits. If this is something you want to do, make sure the rest of the days in your week are made up of plenty of healthful **S** and **E** and possibly even **Crossover** meals, full of the good fats and energizing carbs that God made for your health. This JUDD idea, combined with the core of our plan, would work wonderfully for anyone in senior stages of life to help fight off the diseases of inflammatory aging.

If you want to be even better armed with an array of **Fuel Pull** recipes, you may also want to visit www.hungrygirl.com. She is the author of many low-cal recipe books and is clever about making tasty filling foods, many of them without a primary fuel source. You can use some of her more healthy recipes for **Fuel Pull** meals and snacks, but please be diligent in choosing because many of her desserts use sugar and frequently include chemical laden ingredients. Don't be tempted into making all your meals her low-calorie way. That will slow your metabolism. Use them only as change ups.

Double Attack

If you don't have a good exercise program already, go to *Get Movin', Mama*, Chapter 36 to kick it into action. The metabolism rev of safe fuel cycling, combined with the extra metabolic boost of intense anaerobic exercise, is a double attack on stubborn pounds.

Drink Up

Consider teas to help melt stubborn weight. Pre-make a gallon of green tea, using 6-8 tea bags. Sweeten, it if desired, with our stevia options and a few squeezes of lemon and sip on this throughout your fuel cycle days. Sipping this tea will also keep you hydrated and help to curb needless cravings. Green tea is renowned for its ability to help weight loss. A study published in the *Journal of Clinical Nutrition* showed a significant increase in metabolism after drinking tea. The participants studied experienced an average of four percent increase in metabolic rate after drinking green tea. That's a pretty good boost.

You may also like to try Oolong tea. This is a Chinese tea that is high in poly-phenols and antioxidants. In China, where this tea is the beverage of choice, obesity rates are one of the lowest in the world. Oolong tea helps the body absorb nutrients and block accumulation of dietary fat. Research at the *US Agricultural Research Service's Diet and Human Performance laboratory* found that only one cup can help burn off an extra 67 calories, without trying. It also turbo charges metabolism by a whopping 12 percent. Imagine what sipping on a whole gallon will do for you.

Oolong can be quite pricey from your regular grocery store or health food market. However, if you visit an international store with an Asian food section, you can find Oolong tea for less than half the cost. Both of these teas are used in Serene's *Earth Milk* recipe.

Water

It's time to talk about water. It's been preached from every health pulpit. Drinking a lot of water does aid your health and will help you slim down. It helps flush away bloat, keeps you regular, is fantastic for your skin, but also helps you realize when you are truly hungry.

Constant snacking can be kept in control by drinking adequate water or tea. Perhaps you've already eaten your afternoon snack and yet still feel like eating more. Sit down to a nice cup of tea, or drink a full glass of water with a splash of lemon, and then ask yourself if you still feel snacky. It is a good way to test your true hunger.

Neither of us like to drink cold water, but there is evidence that drinking very cold water forces the body to turn up its thermostat to regulate the body. This in turn, burns more calories. We'll stick to our lukewarm water, because that's the way we like it!

Supplements to Consider

We don't believe in magic elixirs to lose weight. Pills and potions have not proved to have long lasting success. Look around at the growing obesity problem and it's easy to conclude that if there were a magic pill, there wouldn't be so many overweight people. There is no "wonder supplement" that can transform a person's physique if their diet is unwise at the core. Many so-called "weight loss supplements" have proved to be harmful since they are strong stimulants.

But, there is one supplement that has piqued our interest and shows too much promise to be dismissed. Dr. Oz promoted a supplement called Irvingia Gabonensis, or what is more commonly known as African Mango on his television show. The extract of the seed of this fruit is called IGOB131 and is touted to influence the leptin hormone. This spiked our curiosity enough to look further into this supplement since we know leptin controls human food intake and energy levels by activating receptors in the brain. Leptin is a biggie when it comes to weight control and scientists are only just beginning to understand its significance.

Leptin levels increase as a person gets fatter. Remember how we talked about that all important insulin hormone? We need insulin to deal with blood sugar but when insulin is too high it causes our cells to become desensitized to it. We become insulin resistant. Similarly, too much leptin interferes with the brain cell's abilities to receive the full signal leptin is supposed to give. It is also possible to become leptin resistant. Apparently African Mango extract helps ease this overload so we can more easily receive the, "you've had enough to eat" signal from our brains. The extract is also high in antioxidants that soothe inflammation. This is necessary because inflammation also interferes with leptin's "full" signaling.

Several studies have shown this extract to have remarkable weight reducing results that include decreased stubborn fat and waist circumference, but one study in particular is worth mentioning. In a ten week study published in 2009 in the journal, *Lipids in Health and Disease*, 102 overweight men and women were followed for ten weeks. They were split into either a placebo group or a group that received 350 mg of African Mango extract. At the end of the study, the group that received the extract lost an average of 28 pounds versus only one pound for the placebo group. Impressive and intriguing results we have to admit.

African Mango is similar to glucomannan in that it delays gastric emptying and causes you to feel full for a longer time. Like glucomannan, it is a potent source of fiber. One study showed that subjects taking African Mango in doses of 350 mg, three times a day, reduced bad cholesterol (LDL) by 46% and raised good cholesterol (HDL) by 47%. Some supplement companies are combining glucomannan, African Mango, and green tea extract as they all appear to be synergistic together. Life Extension brand sells the correct potent extract in a formula called *Integra Lean Irvingia*. It costs around $21 for one month's supply at most online vitamin stores.

Dr. Oz. recommends people take 150 mg of African Mango twice a day, half an hour before both lunch and dinner. Make sure the brand you purchase contains the potent IGOB-131extract, not just the fruit. Some companies sell extracts of the fruit less expensively but it is only the potent seed with that strange number for a name that has proven to show such amazing results.

This supplement does not increase heart rate, blood pressure, or have other negative or harmful side effects from what we have been able to research. Some people reported mild gassiness from the fiber content.

Even if you decide to purchase African Mango, we stress the importance of not relying on a capsule for your health and weight control. It may benefit your journey toward your goal weight but it cannot replace long term, healthy, low glycemic food choices.

Two more supplements that have scientific data behind their effectiveness are chromium pilonate and L Glutamine. Both of these reduce sugar cravings, help shed pounds, lower blood sugar levels, and help insulin resistance issues. You can study more online to check if they would be suitable for you.

Part IV

Our Past and Present

No sugar coating our stories.
From our mistakes we found the way
to give you hope.

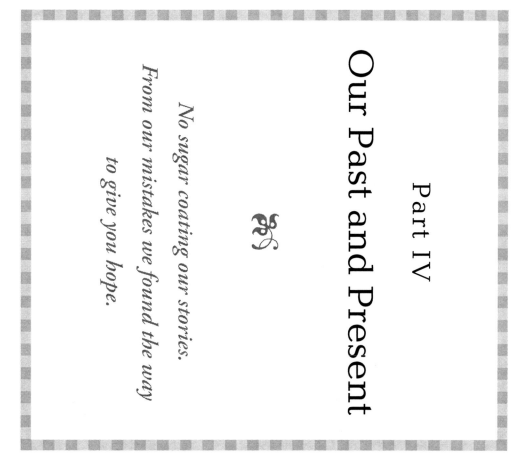

Chapter 29

Serene's Story

I am one of those strange people who have been interested in health and fitness since early childhood. Some of my earliest memories are of worrying if what I was eating was healthy. After feeling guilty from eating cake at a birthday party, I decided at seven years old, to never eat sugar again.

Even as a pre-teen, my favorite place to visit was the health food store. I felt like I was in heaven as I smelled the earthy herbs and spices permeating the air, scanned all the product labels, and read books in the corner for hours. Once I was a little older, I would ask my parents to drop me off at a health food store and pick me up after a full afternoon. My favorite present for Christmas was a good health book which I would read over and over.

As I look back on the many crazy paths I took before I found a more balanced healthy approach, I realize that the idea of healthy living may have been a bit of an obsession for me. Did I really say *may*? Who am I kidding?

There is one good point. I can surely say that I have been there and done that. I have not only tried, but lived so many different health journeys and have consequently experienced firsthand what really works and what doesn't.

I started out as a little girl being careful to only eat a whole foods diet with no "junk" whatsoever! In my early teens I became a strict vegetarian which progressed into full blown veganism by my 14th birthday. I lived this lifestyle, full of gusto, preaching it to whoever I could until the age of 22. This is when I officially became a "raw foodist."

My father-in-law was battling a horrible cancer. At the same time my husband was dealing with cancer that was growing rapidly on his back. I threw myself into the study of raw food cleansing and saw some powerful results with my family and others who were battling serious diseases. I witnessed the healing power God has placed in raw plant food. This approach is truly an incredible cleanse. I decided that if it is good enough to heal cancer, it is good for life! For me, while nursing all night, and even pregnant!

I felt so amazing in the beginning. But, raw foodism became a seven year journey, and I became trapped by my stubbornness to stick with it. Concerned friends sent me different articles and Scriptures pointing out the dangers of such an extreme diet, but I wasn't willing to listen. After all, my father-in-law's cancer growth disappeared on raw foods and nobody could convince me it wasn't the perfect diet.

My version of raw foodism was rich in organic superfoods. Yet, eventually my body began to fall apart. I ended up in a real mess. I could hardly digest a simple apple without abdominal bloating. It seemed my digestive system was beginning to shut down from so many years of never allowing it to digest anything with substance. It got lazy.

I became skinny, with muscle deterioration (even though I was an avid exerciser), and yet I had an embarrassing protruding bloated abdomen. I say embarrassing, because people would ask me if I was pregnant, when I wasn't, and that made me want to cry. Now, I know this was because I was trying to live a lifestyle fit for a cow with four stomachs. Mine couldn't handle it, and I ended up looking like a bloated goat.

My subsequent research has taught me that even cancer patients, after their initial cleanse, need to slowly add healthy, healing, clean sources of protein and animal fats such as wild salmon and raw fermented goat kefir. This helps keep up their body's strength in order to maintain the fight.

After my babies' teeth came in discolored from my raw pregnancies, I knew enough was enough! God began removing the wool from my eyes. So many Scriptures, as well as research which supported the gift of animal foods, confronted me. I started reading the Bible as a physical health book as well as my spiritual guide. My eyes were opened to receive the truth I had previously read and scoffed at in books such as *Nourishing Traditions*, *The Maker's Diet* and Dr. Schwarzbein's writings.

I switched my diet overnight and prayed for a love for the taste of healthy meat and fish. It had been almost 20 years since I had eaten flesh foods! They have now become my favorite foods and their aroma while cooking in my kitchen is a gift for the whole family.

My slouching posture straightened. My bloat completely disappeared. Nice muscle tone and strength returned. I became slim and strong all over, instead of skinny with a pooch. I started lifting heavier weights, which supported my change. I made sure to feed my two raw pregnancy children lots of healthy animal protein along with daily cod liver oil and their adult teeth came in shining white and perfect!

I am very tall, an avid exerciser with a high metabolism, so the reintroduction of animal foods did not cause too much of a noticeable weight increase. The book, *Nourishing Traditions* is an excellent read for everybody (although it is not from a Biblical perspective), and its health principles are sound, especially for growing families. However, many people I knew who followed these principles battled what I called "farm weight." They were very healthy and robust, never battling colds and flues, but were well padded on the hips, thighs, and bottom.

I knew the abundant superfoods and healthy balance of raw and cultured foods, soaked grains, and healthy animal fats and proteins was an optimum diet, but there was a missing link to beautifying the waist line.

After searching and researching, Pearl and I have come up with what we feel is that missing link. It's incredibly effective. Sometimes it works too well when you don't need it to. I stayed muscled and strong, but basically stripped the fat off my body by sticking to **S** and **E** perfectly. Once I added some **Crossover** meals for maintenance, my weight normalized.

By sticking to the **S** and **E** plan, while adding some **Crossovers** and **S Helpers**, I can have lots of creamy foods which I absolutely love and keep a perfect weight. This plan has been very effective for us. You can basically pick an ideal weight and maintain it easily. Some women don't like to be too skinny and their husbands don't like it either. They would add more **Crossover** meals. Those who like to be thin (we don't suggest the waif look), simply keep to **S** and **E** more strictly and utilize more **Fuel Pull** snacks and meals. It's that easy.

I love life, I love food, and I love the freedom of enjoying both on this program. We want you to know that as you follow this plan, Pearl and I are doing it right alongside of you. Let's embrace the best that life has, together.

If you want to know what my diet really looks like, here's a sneak peek into a week in my food life. I hardly have to think anymore about how many **E** meals versus **S** meals I should have. I usually go by what my body is telling me. If I am feeling tired, or haven't eaten enough healthy carb foods, I realize I need an **E** meal.

S meals are my favorite foods because I love the taste of luscious fat. When I think I am getting on the "skinny minny" side, I throw in a few **Crossovers**. It is so easy and becomes second nature. Sometimes I allot certain days to either **S** or **E**, but not every week. I do quite a few **Fuel Pull** snacks some weeks, and even some meals since many of them are too scrumptious to resist, but since I am at goal weight, I need to include more **Crossovers** when I do this. If you are not yet at goal weight, **Fuel Pull** snacks and meals, without the addition of **Crossovers**, will help you have consistent success. As we keep insisting, just don't stay on them permanently.

You'll notice that I repeat meals, and some of them are so simple, but this is because it works for me. I am pregnant (at this stage of writing) and on maintenance. Therefore, I include more **Crossovers** and **S Helpers** now than I normally would. If you are beginning and have weight to lose, don't follow me in this at first.

Weekly Menu

Day 1

Breakfast (about 7 a.m.): One cup cooked steel cut oats (soak first), including low-fat cottage cheese mixed with blueberries. Green tea. **E**

Mid-morning snack (3 hours later): Raw crudités like peppers and cucumbers, or a couple of *Coconut Divine Fudge* squares. **S**

Lunch (2 ½ hours later): One large sprouted tortilla filled with one single serving can of sockeye salmon, heated in a tiny bit of coconut oil and cayenne pepper, a smidgen of healthy mayo and sliced tomato, and a handful of blueberries. Chamomile tea. **E**

Afternoon Snack: One cup of raw full-fat goat kefir, with a handful of frozen raspberries stirred in with vanilla and Nunaturals. If still hungry, eat one heaped teaspoon of almond butter right off the spoon. **S**

Dinner: Grass fed *Fantastic Meatloaf* with creamy *Mashed Cauliflower*. Drizzle hemp oil all over meal. **S**

Evening snack: Swiss water decaf hazelnut coffee with plenty of raw cream and some *Skinny Chocolate*. **S**

Day 2

Breakfast: Raw goats' milk kefir superfood smoothie including whey protein, raw egg yolk, and raw coconut oil. **S**

Mid morning snack: Half a cucumber with *Hummus*, a handful of raw walnuts, and green tea. **S**

Lunch: Sautéed salmon fillet and a rich side salad with avocado and homemade *Raw Neufchatel Cultured Cheese* made from goat's milk. Green tea chai with stevia and raw cream. **S**

Afternoon snack: An organic apple with 1 tsp. peanut butter and a few strips of crisp green pepper. Mint herbal tea. **E**

Dinner: Start with ¼ cup raw homemade goat milk kefir (for added enzymes). Coconut Thai salmon soup, plus ¼ cup brown rice and ¼ cup hemp seeds. **S Helper**

Evening Snack: Swiss water decaf hazelnut coffee with plenty of raw cream and a couple of *Coconut Divine Fudge* squares. **S**

Day 3

Breakfast: Three-quarters cup of soaked and cooked steel cut oats, including 0% Greek yogurt, whey protein, small sprinkle of walnuts, and a handful of blueberries. Green tea. **E**

Mid morning snack: *Raw Neufchatel Cultured Cheese* made with goat's milk on sprouted *Ezekiel Crackers*, with sliced tomato and cracked pepper. **Crossover**

Lunch: *Zucchini Fritter* made with omega-3 eggs, drizzled with olive oil and sprinkled with nutritional yeast. Half avocado on the side. Herbal chai tea with cream and stevia**. S**

Afternoon Snack: Half an apple with 1 tsp. peanut butter and a stalk of celery. Fruity herb tea with stevia. **S** or **E** (not enough fats or carbs to lean either way)

Dinner: Sautéed hormone free chicken tenderloins with a large salad, including goat's cheese, spicy nuts, hemp oil vinaigrette, and all the works. **S**

Evening Snack: Handful of blueberries and a homemade protein ball or two. Chamomile tea. **S**

Day 4

Breakfast: Three fried omega-3 eggs in coconut oil on one small slice of homemade sourdough bread, with raw butter and *Frank's* hot sauce on top. Green tea with raw cream. **S Helper**

Mid morning snack: Half cup 0% Greek yogurt with raspberries, 1 tsp. almond butter, and dash of Nunaturals all swirled in the bowl. **E** or **S**

Lunch: Sautéed salmon in lots of virgin coconut oil and a decadent green salad with dehydrated spicy nuts, goat's cheese, and a little avocado. Green chai tea with raw cream and stevia. **S**

Afternoon snack: Chia pudding made with ½ glass of raw full-fat goat's milk kefir, 1 Tbs. chia seeds, vanilla, frozen raspberries, and stevia swirled around. Half a cucumber from my garden (can't believe they actually grew)! **S**

Dinner: Hormone free chicken and vegetable full-fat coconut curry, with ½ cup of brown rice and ¼ cup hemp seeds. One small organic apple. **Crossover**

Evening Snack: Chai tea with raw cream and some *Coconut Divine Fudge* Squares. **S**

Day 5

Breakfast: One cup soaked and then cooked steel cut oatmeal, including low-fat cottage cheese processed with blueberries. Green tea. **E**

Mid morning snack: Full-fat goat's milk kefir smoothie with hemp oil and cocoa powder. **S**

Lunch: Sprouted wrap with leftover chicken breast sautéed in 1 tsp. sesame oil and cayenne pepper. Sliced raw onion with thinly spread healthy mayo. Mint tea. **E**

Afternoon snack: Two slices of raw cheese and a handful of raw walnuts. Eat a crisp celery stalk if still hungry. Magnesium Calm tea. **S**

Dinner: Start with ¼ cup raw full-fat kefir for enzymes, baked salmon with red wine and butter, roasted eggplant, and caramelized onions. **S**

Evening Snack: Swiss water decaf coffee with raw cream and a handful of blueberries. **S**

Day 6

Breakfast: Omelet made with three omega-3 eggs and onion, drizzled with olive oil and nutritional yeast, and *Raw, Neufchatel Cultured Cheese* on the side. **S**

Mid morning snack: None! Big breakfast, too full!

Lunch: Big green salad with the works, including avocado and *Raw Neufchatel Cultured Cheese*, followed by Greek strained yogurt with almond butter swirled around. **S**

Afternoon snack: One orange and a few walnuts. Magnesium calm tea. **E**

Dinner: Ground bison with broccoli and cauliflower stir fry made with sesame seeds, tamari sauce, and dark sesame oil. Half cup full-fat kefir with vanilla and a dash of Nunaturals. **S**

Evening Snack: Green chai with cream. **S**

Day 7

Breakfast: Raw full-fat goat's kefir superfood smoothie with all the works. **S**

Snack: Couple of squares of *Fridge Fudge*. Green tea. S

Lunch: *Coconut Chicken Thai Soup* with ¾ cup quinoa and a small green salad with diced apple and hemp vinaigrette. **Crossover**

Afternoon Snack: Non-fat Greek yogurt with hemp seed protein powder and goji berries. **E**

Dinner: Two fried eggs on two slices of sourdough toast with raw butter. **Crossover**

Evening Snack: Half cup of raw kefir with blueberries. **E or S** (depending on fat content of my kefir)

Edit: It is now a year later since writing this chapter and I will fill you in on changes to my weekly menu. Toddling around my feet is a beautiful fat baby girl named *Breeze Ember* who has huge cuddly cheeks and thighs. Adorably squeezable! I believe my healthy low glycemic approach to my diet while pregnant is evident in her robust health. While she was born a lovely 8 pounds, I had no extra weight to lose and another pregnancy did no damage to my waistline. Pregnancy is never the reason for excess fat, but rather from a less-than-ideal diet and exercise choices.

I now start most of my days with a strong organic coffee with organic cream. I never sweeten it, but enjoy savoring the mysterious depth of each warming sip. Coffee time is my special time as I snuggle up on a comfy chair in the early hours. The children know to not run riot when they see a cup of "Joe" in my hand. I love this coffee ritual, not only for the sheer comfort, but because it is a wonderful bowel cleanser.

After my coffee, I often have three omega-3 eggs scrambled with virgin coconut oil. If I am still a little hungry after nursing all night I drink a glass of *Earth Milk*. I hadn't invented the *Earth Milk* recipe when I wrote up the sample week.

When I was pregnant I ate more **S Helpers** and added healthy carbs in small doses instead of eating too many **E** meals. My reason for this is because pregnancy is a time when you are slightly more insulin resistant, due to extremely high progesterone levels. I do not think having an **E** meal puts you in any danger of spiking your insulin. Nevertheless, I am a psycho when it comes to food and the science of how it works within the human body, and choose to watch my insulin levels a little closer. If I had known about the low glycemic properties of chana dahl during this last pregnancy, I would have used it more for **E** meals.

Because I'm no longer pregnant, I do more true **S** and **E** meals and less **S Helpers**. This way, I rev my metabolism with the shock of changing the fuel sources of my meals more dramatically. I usually use Saturday, and sometimes even Sundays, as my **Crossover** days. And yes, I drink a lot of *Earth Milk*.

Further Edit: It has taken nearly five years to complete this book. We keep adding more recipes, additional research, and new found tips and tricks. In my arms, as I sit doing a final check, I hold a precious gift from heaven—a new baby girl, *Haven Rest* who is two weeks old and snuggled against my breast.

It was a wonderful pregnancy and my second time using the *Trim Healthy Mama* lifestyle. I ate **S** smoothies every day—filled with raw farm fresh egg yolks, cod liver oil, coconut oil, raw cream, maca, whey protein powder, and overloaded with fresh greens. I ate salmon almost twice a day (frozen wild fillets from Walmart) and I ate gobs of virgin coconut oil.

I did, however, rev my metabolism more this pregnancy by including light **E** meals with chana dahl or quinoa. I craved cucumbers and ate them whole, skin and all, like a banana. I went through hundreds of bunches of celery and ate plenty of large green salads. I always had egg whites left over from my super fat smoothies so I made lots of egg white scrambles. I also became addicted to our **Fuel Pull** slick trick glucomannan puddings and ate them as my "before bed" snacks.

Toward the end of my pregnancy I made **Fuel Pull** noodle dinners using my favorite recipe, *Sweet and Spicy Asian Stir Fry* (*Evening Meals,* Chapter 21) for my husband. I ended up eating a few of these dinners myself as I love these Asian style noodles.

Because the end of my pregnancy was in the middle of summer, I also enjoyed a lot of **Fuel Pull** style treats like *Tummy Tucking Ice Cream* (*Desserts,* Chapter 23). The problem was that I didn't need to incorporate Uncle **Fuel Pull** so often in my pregnancy. I did not need to receive the consequences of less weight gain due to eating lighter fare. Because of these slight changes, I gained even less weight than with Breeze's pregnancy of 23 pounds. I gained only 13 pounds with Haven. I didn't purpose to have these results as I was very happy with Breeze's pregnancy weight. It happened because of my craving for glucomannan based foods like the noodles and puddings, juggling between **S** and **E**, and so many cucumbers. Immediately after Haven's birth I weighed less than my pre-pregnancy weight. Ouch!

I will have to watch carefully to not lose any more weight while nursing and even work toward gaining a few pounds back. This may be hard since I love my **S** and **E** meals so much, but they are both slimming meals. And I am in love with our *Fat Stripping Frappa* recipe. That's a dilemma because right now I don't have enough body fat to strip. **Crossover** here I come, and **Crossover** I must.

My point in sharing this testimony is for anyone who has trouble controlling weight during pregnancy, or starting heavier than you would like to begin your pregnancy. My accidental lack of weight gain could be your purposeful healthy approach if you find your scale moving up too quickly. Please feed your growing baby with wonderful superfood fat for its optimal development, but balance with some lighter fare from Uncle **Fuel Pull**. Don't indulge in excessive heavily laden **S** meals constantly or **Crossovers** too often.

I also did an intensive kettlebell pregnancy regime. I love the results and integrity of my ab muscles. I had no back aches during pregnancy and enjoyed a quick and easy birth. I credit this to the core strengthening power of kettlebells.

I should also mention that although I did not gain a whole lot of weight, I didn't look sickly like my raw pregnancies. I kept all my muscles and some, and felt strong and healthy.

P.S. From Serene's mother, final editor of this book. I have to confirm that Serene is a living testimony of the nutrition and exercise program they teach in this book. Only one week after giving birth to Haven (her seventh pregnancy), Serene's stomach was perfectly flat and muscle toned. It is perfectly doable if you are prepared to embrace this lifestyle.

Chapter 30

Pearl's Story

Growing up, junk food was rare in our home. We lived on homemade bread from freshly ground wheat, eggs from a backyard chicken coop, greens from Mom's garden, and an annual freezer full of pasture fed lamb delivered to us from our sheep shearer grandfather. This was a healthy way for our parents to raise us six children. But, I took it for granted.

As soon as I was of an age to make my own food decisions, I abandoned my dietary upbringing and gravitated to foods that had never been on our menu at home. I had never eaten much white bread and its soft texture appealed to me. Using money from various part time jobs, I indulged in fast foods, pastries, and developed a sweet tooth, desiring a candy bar every day.

All six of us children never had any weight problems growing up (by children, I mean original children—my parents adopted after we were grown and gone). That changed when I woke up on my 20th birthday and realized my nice figure had disappeared under a layer of fat. I was not terribly overweight, probably only 15 pounds or so, but I hated the new way my body wobbled when I walked. I spent most of that birthday crying. I realized my new way of eating was harming me, but after developing a taste for these new foods, the addiction was too hard to give up. The pounds slowly crept up that year.

It was my little sister, Serene, who coaxed me into changing my ways. She's always been a zealot about not putting anything "bad" into her mouth. I used to think she was crazy, but once I was 20 or so pounds past my slim figure, I was willing to listen to her extreme ideas. She told me I should adopt a vegetarian lifestyle and shoved ten books in my face to read. The books convinced me. I became a vegetarian of the strictest sort—a vegan, and promptly lost all the weight I had accumulated.

Even on my vegan diet, I was still able to eat a lot of sweets. In fact, to make up for the lack of fat and protein, I developed a strong reliance on dried fruit. Feasting on a whole box of raisins was okay in my books, and I could remain slim. Eating two or three bananas in one sitting was not unusual for me. I had no knowledge of the dangers of spiking blood sugar. Youth is forgiving. Thanks to my healthy childhood, I was not yet insulin resistant and I spent my early twenties, without problems, proud of my vegan lifestyle.

I never had any second thoughts about lack of meat or protein until I became pregnant with my first child and started to crave forbidden foods like butter and red meat. Looking back, I am thankful I gave into those cravings during my pregnancies. I know my children are healthier for it.

Following each pregnancy I returned to my vegetarian lifestyle. I loosened up a little and allowed the occasional egg, some cheese, and a little butter. Every now and then I'd have some meat, but felt guilty whenever I did. I never had enough self control to switch to a completely raw diet, even though I watched Serene flourish in her first couple of years. I was simply too lazy to do all that juicing and dehydrating. I tried several times, but swiftly gave up.

Mostly, I relied on soy products as the bases to all my meals. Salads and vegetables did not satisfy more hearty food cravings and I used soy to create the artificial meat and dairy taste. I used soy milk on my cereal and in smoothies, soy burger as meat, and soy cheese for grilled sandwiches. I even learned to make tofu into cheeses, mayonnaise, and sauces.

My husband didn't complain too much about the lack of meat I served him, but every now and then he would say, "Meat makes me feel like a man, honey! I need some." A problem developed. There was so little fat in the meals I made that my husband would finish his food and half hour later grab a bag of potato chips and dig in. He was craving fat and needed to be satisfied! This turned into a nightly habit. I had been convinced that a vegetarian diet was the healthiest, but started to second guess when my husband slowly gained a good 30 pounds and eventually developed a bad case of high blood pressure.

I was not without my own problems. After more than a decade of vegetarianism, I began to have bouts of severe fatigue. My skin became extremely dry, migraine headaches plagued me, and my periods became so heavy that they were almost unbearable. A blood test revealed I was anemic with a ferritin level of only three. That was border line in needing a blood transfusion! Further ultra sound testing revealed my uterine lining was dangerously thickened with polyps and fibroids. I spent three weeks of every month bleeding.

I could not understand why. All conventional advice said the perfect diet to avoid uterine fibroids needed to be low in saturated fats and high in fruits and vegetables. Huh? That was my diet to a tee! I had none of the other risks, like being overweight, which can lead to harmful estrogens made in fat cells.

A doctor convinced me to try six months on the pill to regulate my bleeding. I was reluctant, but desperate. Not only did it not help my condition, I became depressed for the first time in my life. I'm usually a very confident and happy person. The pill changed all that. It messed with my brain neurotransmitters and caused self loathing. This constant feeling was so drastic I had fleeting thoughts of suicide. It was a feeling of "What good am I? Why should I even be here?" My husband hardly knew this woman. I gained 10 pounds and knew the pill was not the answer. Surgery came next. That was only a temporary fix. My uterine problems soon returned.

During this time I stumbled across the book, *Nourishing Traditions* and a light bulb turned on. I learned that cholesterol is required to make hormones. For too many years I had seldom allowed cholesterol into my diet. My hormones were now off balance, some in serious decline, and I was only in my mid-thirties! After blood tests, my progesterone came back low. It could no longer counterbalance my estrogen levels from proliferating my uterus. My years of heavy soy eating were also a possible suspect. Soy has shown to have estrogenic effects in the body. By eating all that soy, I'd only been feeding the problem. No, I didn't have too much estrogen, but not enough progesterone to counter my estrogen levels.

Nourishing Traditions taught me the importance of fats and animal products. I increased these in my diet and felt a renewed strength in my body. Once back on good fats, I wondered how I had lived without them. I found a source for raw milk and cream from an Amish community within driving distance of my home. What a treat! I felt satiated and nourished. I made raw whole milk smoothies with honey and bananas, poured fresh raw cream over fruit, and enjoyed fried eggs with lots of brown rice and spinach which helped my iron levels.

I also incorporated meat back into my diet. There was just one problem. I hadn't been able to lose my 10 pound "pill" weight gain and I kept slowly gaining more weight. Only a pound or two every month or so, but it was adding up, and I could no longer fit into any of my jeans. It was a sad day for me when I had to buy clothes in a bigger size. However, I decided I would rather be heavier than anemic and in premature hormonal decline.

The weight crept up little by little and I began to get serious about finding a solution. Since I was not willing to give up my delicious new fats, I decided to try the low-carb Atkins style diet. That way I could eat all the fat I wanted! I lost a few pounds, but in a few months my body was depleted of glycogen. I could barely walk down our driveway! I was in desperate need of carbohydrates for energy.

My weight loss halted on this type of diet. The books told me goal weight on this type of plan would usually be heavier than a low-fat diet due to more protein consumption. I was not content with this answer. I could still not fit back into the jeans my husband liked. I'd get a stomach ache a few minutes after I poured myself into them. They were just too tight. He said he didn't care and was sweet and encouraging about my new size, but it wasn't for me. Although I'm tall, I have a tiny skeletal frame and was carrying more fat than it appeared. I looked an average size, but that was deceptive. Also, I could not survive the busy demands of my life with such little energy.

I kept studying, constantly discussing my ideas with Serene who was second guessing her devout raw foodism at the time, and was as intent in discovering answers as I was. Next, I tried eating like body builders, having a couple of days of very high carbs, and then dipping back into carb reduction for the rest of the week. It was the same problem—huge swings in blood sugar along with energy slumps and highs.

Suzanne Somers, whose health books I highly recommend, and who has been an incredible source of information to help with my hormone problem, has an eating plan called "Somersizing." On this plan, she recommends completely separating carbs from fats and proteins. I loved gaining knowledge from her books, but after several months of "Somersizing," her plan did not work for me either. Naked carbs, even in a whole grain state, caused my blood sugar (tested by a diabetic monitor) to spike. I found no joy in eating them without any fats and proteins either. I was basically left eating her fat/protein meals, similar to Atkins. This put me back in a low energy state. However, I still recommend her books on nutrition. They explain insulin response very well, and since our plan does have some similarities to hers, many of the recipes in her books can be used. I'm a huge fan of Suzanne Somers, because she takes a relentless pursuit to health and hormones—a true, brave pioneer!

Our **S** and **E** plan was birthed once everything else had failed. Serene and I started sharing Bible Scriptures with each other that discussed God's design for food. We realized that eliminating whole food groups was not a biblical approach. We discovered real answers to keep balanced blood sugar levels, have complete weight control, and yet eat decadent and energy promoting superfoods. We became our own lab rats, constantly discussing, testing, and honing the **S** and **E** idea until it became effortless. The results were startling.

After a few months of eating this way, I easily fitted back into my jeans! Thankfully I had not thrown them out. In fact, my husband thought I looked better in them because of the resistance training I had begun.

He finally let me take over his diet. He agreed, only after seeing how good I felt, and how tasty and yummy my foods were. He was wary though, because as you read in the Foreword, I'd taken him down so many different strange food paths. He did not want to eat bunny food or anything too weird! And, he sure didn't want to be hungry.

Within a year, he lost 35 pounds with the new food I served him. He was hooked! That, along with an herbal formulation for his blood pressure enabled him to come off his blood pressure medicine and brought it down to a normal range. I started telling everyone about the wonders of this **S** and **E** plan. Those who tried it shared the same type of success. Soon friends, family, and others came on board. We received so many phone calls, emails, and questions as word spread. It was too overwhelming and we knew there would have to be a book. It's hard to say to someone over the phone, "Just eat **S** and **E**." This approach requires explanation.

Now, I have to add a few **Crossover** meals each week. My metabolism has become a red hot furnace and I have to watch that I don't get too thin. This is not a hard issue to manage. If I notice I am too far below my ideal weight, I eat oatmeal with cream, or whole grain bread with butter and cheese, and up I go—slightly.

My uterine problem is so much better now. My periods are much improved, and I no longer bleed for most of the month. My cycles are nicely spaced apart since I introduced the hormones my body was missing. My last blood test revealed my iron levels had normalized. I keep learning how to better balance my hormones and this, along with our **S** and **E** plan, has turned my life around.

I'll give you a peek into a week of my diet, also. You'll notice that there are quite a few differences in the foods Serene and I choose, yet both styles work with this plan. I'm not the purist she is, so you won't see "homemade goat's milk kefir" in any of my meals. If I want kefir now and then, I buy it from the store. My eating style is probably a little more normal looking than hers, yet I have gained much health and my weight is perfect. If you are one who cannot see yourself making homemade sourdough bread or milking goats, don't feel left out. I am not that way either.

Day 1

Breakfast: Omelet made with two eggs, a dab or two of cream cheese, cheddar cheese, and onion. Small side of berries with ¼ cup 0% Greek yogurt. Coffee with a dash of cream. **S**

Lunch: Sautéed seasoned salmon in nonstick pan with 1 tsp. coconut oil and ¾ cup quinoa. Side salad with Newman's Own Light balsamic vinaigrette. Green Tea. **E**

Afternoon snack: Blue Diamond spicy nuts with a few pieces of cheddar cheese. Green tea**. S**

Dinner: *Baked Chicken Thighs*, broccoli with butter and sea salt, and side salad with ranch dressing. **S**

Dessert: *Basic Cheesecake*. **S**

Day 2

Breakfast: Two or three *Trim Healthy Pancakes* with blueberries, 0% Greek yogurt and a swirl of sugar-free syrup (I can't always manage three pancakes). Coffee with unsweetened almond milk. **E**

Lunch: Grilled cheese and tomato sandwich made with *Bread in a Mug* recipe. Peanut butter and celery. **S**

Afternoon snack: Leftover *Trim Healthy Pancake* with Skim Ricotta and 1 tsp. Polaner All-Fruit Jam with Fiber. Small ½ scoop chocolate whey smoothie made with light coconut cubes. **E**

Dinner: *Fooled Ya Pizza* (lots of it). **S**

Dessert: *Skinny Chocolate*. Peppermint tea. **S**

Day 3

Breakfast: Two fried eggs over one piece of Trader Joe's Sprouted bread. Coffee with a little cream. **S Helper**

Lunch: One medium baked sweet potato with 1 tsp. coconut oil, Bragg Liquid Aminos and a dash of stevia, ripped romaine lettuce as salad with a can of tuna on it and some light vinaigrette dressing. Green Tea. **E**

Afternoon snack: *Joseph's Crackers* with butter, cheese and tomato and chocolate whey protein shake. **S**

Dinner: *Spaghetti Bolognese* with Dreamfields pasta and side salad with balsamic vinegar and olive oil. Glass of dry wine. **S**

Dessert: Berries and cream. Decaf chai tea. **S**

Day 4

Breakfast: Oatmeal with cream and sliced strawberries. Green tea. **Crossover**

Lunch: Sautéed salmon with lemon butter sauce over leftover Dreamfields noodles. **S**

Afternoon Snack: Low-fat cottage cheese mixed with a little Greek yogurt and ¼ cup crushed pineapple from a can. Coffee with skim milk. **E**

Dinner: Crockpot chicken made with Alfredo sauce and spinach over *Cauli Rice* mixed with ⅓-½ cup quinoa. **S Helper**

Dessert: Breyers Carb Smart Fudge Bar. **S**

Day 5

Breakfast: 0% Greek yogurt swirled with berries, Pro Hemp powder, stevia, and peanut butter. Coffee with cream. **S**

Late Mid morning snack (3 hours after breakfast): An apple with 1 tsp. peanut butter. **E**

Lunch: Sautéed salmon over ¾ cup of quinoa and side salad with low-fat vinaigrette. **E**

Afternoon Snack: One *Trim Healthy Pancake* wrapped around 2 Tbs. ricotta cheese and 1 tsp. Polaner All-Fruit Jam with Fiber. Green Tea. **E**

Dinner: Pot roast with onions made in the crockpot with *Cauliflower Mashed Potatoes* and celery with peanut butter. **S**

Dessert: Few pieces of *Skinny Chocolate*. Peppermint tea. **S**

Day 6

Breakfast: Fried eggs and beef sausage. Coffee with cream. **S**

Lunch: Canned Tyson chicken breast sautéed with spices and layered on a bed of greens with grated cheese, olive oil, and balsamic vinegar. **S**

Afternoon Snack: Chocolate *Muffin in a Mug*. Coffee with cream. **S**

Dinner: Crockpot lentil soup (2 bowls of it) with a small amount of reduced fat cheese and side salad with low-fat vinaigrette. **E**

Dessert: Low-fat cottage cheese mixed with yogurt and ¼ cup crushed pineapple. **E**

Day 7

Breakfast: Oatmeal with a sprinkle of flax seed, 1 tsp. coconut oil, and hot water. Coffee with unsweetened almond milk. **E**

Lunch: Leftover lentil soup with a liberal amount of cheese and a few crumbled blue corn chips, plus side salad with full-fat dressing. **Crossover**

Afternoon Snack: Chocolate whey shake plus a couple hunks of cheese. **S**

Dinner: Chicken and cheese quesadillas on low-carb *Mission* brand tortillas with onion, tomato, and topped with sour cream. Glass of dry wine. **S**

Dessert: Breyers Carb Smart Fudge Bar. **S**

Edit: Over a year has passed since I wrote this sample menu. Looking back, not too much has changed, except I have more glucomannan puddings and shakes. We didn't know about glucomannan a year ago. It's made this way of eating even better for me and I'm now very addicted to those puddings and *Tummy Tucking Ice Cream*.

I also eat more **E** sandwiches made with *Trim Healthy Pan Bread*. Lately I've been having a lot of fried eggs over salad for lunch. It is quick and easy and I'm on an olive oil kick. It seems to keep headaches at bay for me due to its ibuprofen like qualities. I go through stages where I eat a lot of one recipe, give it a rest for a while, and start enjoying another.

I also have more **Crossovers** now. I actually have to take full days as **Crossovers**, or I find myself too far down on the scale.

Part V

More than Food

Eat drink and be merry.
Let's learn the "merry" part.

Chapter 31

Mama's Balancing Act
(The Ups and Downs of Hormones)

By Pearl Barrett

Serene has a nickname for me. She calls me "Horms." That's because I won't quit talking about hormones. Learning how to get them balanced in my body helped turn my negative health issues around. My own health struggles enabled me to better understand the importance of balanced hormones for vital health. In this chapter we'll look at some very common female problems that are caused by the imbalance of hormones and how these issues can be addressed from the inside out rather than band-aiding with medications.

The study of hormones and physiology has become my passionate pursuit. Their role in our bodies is fascinating and I find myself constantly spouting off my latest discovery to anyone who will, or won't listen. My husband gets to be the most frequent target for my hormone monologues. He dutifully and patiently listens, grins a little when I wait for his response then quickly changes the subject to ask what's for dinner. Well, he is a man of few words, and he likes to use them to find out what he's going to eat! To be fair to him, he's had more than his fair share of earfuls on this subject.

Dear reader, you are my latest target—brace yourself. These next five chapters are *all mine*! Serene will take over and do her own clobbering. Oh, I meant to say "encouraging," when she talks about exercise.

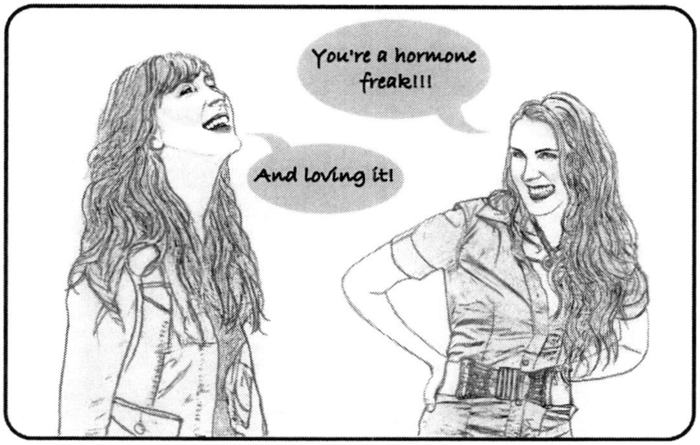
You're a hormone freak!!!
And loving it!

The Power of Hormones

As women, it is our hormones that enable us to fall in love, charge our pregnancies, fuel our lactation periods, and rule our menstrual cycles. As they decline, we are thrown into menopause where the risks of all major diseases increase. Why? Our precious hormones are no longer available to be the first line of defense to tell our bodies that we are worth saving.

For example, a woman has only a very small risk for high blood pressure or heart disease while she is still ovulating, but once a post menopausal woman loses her hormonal protection, in less than 15 years she will be at the same high risk as men of her age. By the age of 65 she is twice as likely to die from a heart attack as a man is.

Throughout the entirety of this book, we have been talking about balancing the all-important hormone, insulin. Getting better management of your insulin levels can make remarkable improvements in your life. But, when it is overly stimulated for lengths of time, the repercussions are devastating—weight gain, diabetic problems, and earlier disease, etc. But, insulin is not the only hormone we must learn to balance. All hormones must be brought into optimum range to help us enjoy a vibrant life.

It's all About Balance

Every cell in your body is controlled by hormones. In his book, *The Natural Superwoman*, Dr. Uzzi Reiss describes how hormones play the most powerful role in all our biological functions, "From how well you sleep to how easily you get up, how your skin looks when you look in the mirror in the morning to your energy level throughout the day, how well you can recall and perform the tasks you must complete each day, how you feel about the people you must interact with, how much you eat and drink, and much, much more."

You can learn to eat correctly, and you can exercise, but if your hormones are in chaos and not addressed, you will not reach optimum health. Our hormones are our protectors. Balanced hormones are our secret weapon to fight the diseases of aging. Suzanne Somers, in her book, *The Sexy Years,* calls them "our own all natural anti-aging pill."

I like the way Suzanne Somers uses the description of a seesaw effect. On one side of the seesaw is our major hormone, insulin. On the other side of the seesaw are our sex hormones—estrogen, progesterone and testosterone. If one, or all of our sex hormones go down too far, up swings insulin and the balance is lost. Alternatively, if insulin is pushed too high through a poor diet, then sex hormones, especially testosterone, is lowered. This is another reason not to constantly stimulate insulin from poor food choices. You need your sex hormones, Mama!

I am not saying that aligning your hormones perfectly will automatically bring immaculate health. Our attitudes and thoughts also have huge impacts on our physical bodies. I believe fear, bitterness, resentment, hate, anger, deep grief and other intense emotions can easily contribute to poor health. Proverbs 17:22 tells us, *"A merry heart doeth good like a medicine."* There are also diseases and health dilemmas that cannot be blamed on anything. Sometimes unfair grave and terminal diseases occur, and I don't pretend to have all the answers as to why.

However, I do believe hormones play a greater role in our health than we give them credit. A few women appear to sail through menopause. They are often the body types who never had high estrogen levels even in their youth. Even though the hormone loss will still likely contribute to bone loss, vaginal changes, and more sagging and wrinkled skin, these women's moods and outlook on life are not really affected. Other women are hit hard, both mentally and physically, after menopause, pregnancy, or reproductive surgeries like hysterectomy or tubal ligation. Hormonal loss then becomes bigger than anything an attitude change can overcome. It's not fair to tell people that are deeply affected from hormonal loss to just cheer up.

Whatever stage of life, it's important to educate yourself on the state of your hormones and to check they are at a level where they can perform the tasks your body requires. Replacing missing hormones can be achieved safely with the use of bioidentical hormones that are exactly the same as your own body makes.

I am not a doctor. I can only share with you what I have learned. I imagine if you are reading this book 10 years from now that there will be a vastly greater amount of knowledge available on this subject, and this chapter might be woefully outdated. But, the word must start trickling out now.

The "Issue of Blood"

Several years ago, my health began to decline rapidly. I asked God so many times to heal me from my uterine problems. I felt a special connection with the woman in the Bible who had *"the issue of blood,"* which she had suffered for too many years. She knew she had to only touch the hem of Jesus' garment to be healed (Matthew 9:20-22).

I also knew God could heal me from my own uterine bleeding condition. However, despite my own desperate prayers, and the prayers of many others, God didn't choose to heal me instantly like He did for the woman in that story. My journey to healing has been slower, longer, but no less miraculous. My healing finally came as I gained knowledge and understanding of hormones and physiology and was able to put that knowledge to practice in my own body. Now I see God's greater plan unfolding in my life. The information I gathered is not supposed to be kept to myself. I have found answers to the many female problems I experienced. Now, rather than simply listening sympathetically while other women tell me about their own struggles, I have solid answers.

It's a Female Thing

Most women have suffered at some time in their life from either migraine headaches, postpartum depression, painful breasts, PMS, heavy periods, irregular cycles, lack of libido, dry vagina, weight gain, water retention, menopause, and post hysterectomy problems—need I go on? This list only makes a small dent in the scroll of ailments women suffer when hormones are out of kilter. These ailments are lumped together under the phrase, "female issues," and are so common we often think they are normal. They are not normal. They're tell-tale signs that our hormones are not quite right, or in some cases, far from right. Our body is telling us something through these symptoms and we need to listen. For too many of us, these problems progress from annoying to debilitating.

If you suffer from common female issues, you can educate yourself now and turn things around before they progress into more serious issues and unnecessary surgery. Like some mothers, I was one of those women who, despite nursing my babies around the clock, would get my period back early. I'd look forward to a nice break so I wouldn't have to worry about getting pregnant right away and then—Oh no, I'd be bleeding again at a few months postpartum. Heavy bleeding crept up slowly over the years, started to be a nuisance, and finally developed into a severe hormone imbalance that resulted in a very thick uterine lining with polyps and fibroids. Finally, the condition made everyday life a misery.

Hindsight is useless, but if I'd known how to start balancing my hormones a decade ago when I began to notice some of these issues emerge, I'm sure I would have avoided a lot of hardship. However, a lot of this information is new and was not even available to us 10 years ago.

In the end, I was faced with hysterectomy. There were times when I hemorrhaged so badly, felt so weak from anemia, and could barely open my eyes from the pain of the migraines that accompanied my bleeding sessions, that I longed to go "get it done." During my darkest moments, ripping my uterus out almost sounded like a relief.

I wrestled with that decision. On one hand, it seemed I did not have much to lose as the location of fibroids and polyps in my uterus had already resulted in a loss of my fertility. But, I didn't want to cut something out of my body just to stop symptoms. There had to be a reason. I was desperate to figure it out, but nobody could tell me. I went from doctor to doctor, seeking solutions. Not one could give me the "why," They all had "how's." Their "how's" to deal with my problems began with birth control pills. If they didn't work (which they didn't), then surgery on my uterus. If that didn't work (which it didn't), then ablation, which means they would burn the lining of my uterus. If that didn't work, hysterectomy.

I wanted to figure out the "why" before I took the drastic measure of having my uterus removed. Uterine fibroids are the number one reason for hysterectomies in the US and I didn't want to be another statistic if there was any possible alternative. At the lowest point of my health problems, I came across a book at a used book store called, *Natural Hormone Balance* by Dr. Uzzi Reiss. This gynecologist offered solutions to female problems that were very different to the ones previously suggested by the doctors I had visited. He had been subscribing bioidentical hormones to women for over two decades. What he had to say in that book made it feel like the pieces were finally being fit into the puzzle. I read his book over and over until I felt I had a good grasp on the material. It soon became apparent to me that although I was not even near menopause in age, I was experiencing hormonal decline. The delicate balance of hormones my body needed was no longer in place. At last, I had hope. If I could get back that balance, perhaps I could heal.

Sure enough, as I learned to safely replace the hormones that had declined in my body, I changed from a weak anemic woman riddled with pain, who had ridiculously short 19-21 day menstrual cycles (spending most of those three week cycles bleeding or spotting), to a strong fit woman who now has regular 27-30 day cycles and normal menstrual loss. It has not been a quick or easy road trying to figure out exactly what hormones I was missing and what doses of bioidentical hormones my particular body responded to and needed. I am still learning little by little, and still have to change the dosages of my hormones now and then. Hormone replacement takes patience, tweaking, education, and a lot of listening to your body.

The following are some common female problems.

Postpartum Depression

I've known women who have suffered terrible postpartum depression after every baby. I wish I could go back in time armed with my new knowledge. They need not have suffered so badly after what should be the joyous occasion of birth. Postpartum depression is often caused by hormonal deficiencies resulting from extreme highs in pregnancy that drop dramatically after birth. For some women, the postpartum weeks are like a sudden menopause. Some women's brains cannot function properly after the hard crash of their hormone levels.

Milder postpartum depression can be alleviated by a more thorough understanding of what is happening to a mama's hormone levels during this time. The highs of estrogen and progesterone plummet after birth and two other hormones take over. These are prolactin and oxytocin. Rather than resist, it is important to flow along with the power of these two postpartum hormones. They are two beautiful hormones, designed to draw us contentedly to our homes. They calm us, relax us, cause us to bond strongly and protectively with our babies, and even become closer to our husbands.

If we feel more introverted during this postpartum time, we shouldn't fight this inclination. These two hormones are rather insistent that we do not go out and about so much during those more precarious weeks when our newborn is most vulnerable to infections.

Taking on too much during the postpartum period goes against nature and can exasperate postpartum blues. If the thought of going to the store in the first weeks after birth seems like a momentous event, almost too hard to endure, blame it on prolactin. It is a force to be reckoned with. God designed it to rule during the postpartum weeks because he knows what is best for you and your baby. Prolactin naturally pulls you toward staying at home with your newborn as much as possible, for both yours and the baby's protection.

Prolactin makes it feel more difficult for you to not only leave home, but even be your usual social, or extroverted self. Prolactin opposes estrogen. They are essentially at war. Estrogen is the hormone that makes you feel outgoing and social and when your body allows it to rise high enough, it brings back your periods. Prolactin, in contrast, draws your personality inward to your nest and your immediate family, and will halt your periods. It is fully in charge in the postpartum period. When some time has passed after birth and your baby grows fatter, stronger, and more resistant to disease, your estrogen levels slowly climb back up. Once they do, your moods, feelings, and personality should come back to a more balanced state.

Just as it is counterproductive to tense and fight the contractions of birth, it is just as harmful to resist the power of prolactin and oxytocin. Oxytocin is released each time you nurse your baby. It wants to soothe you so you can more calmly nurse and give your baby the security and nurturing it needs. Similar to learning the art of childbirth, where we learn to flow with the contractions of birth to relax and open up, so we learn to embrace the flood of different feelings and emotions from prolactin and oxytocin. Fighting their influence causes discord and confusion in the mind and body and gives rise to more postpartum depression.

Since prolactin and estrogen are natural enemies in the body and one will always dominate the other, problems after birth can become more serious when prolactin becomes dominant to the point where estrogen is pushed too low. Some women find it much harder to cope with lower levels of estrogen than they had before and during pregnancy. A too severe drop in estrogen can lower important neurotransmitters necessary for feelings of happiness. A woman cannot just "snap out of it" when this occurs. This is real postpartum depression, not just the "blues."

Women who get to such a low point don't need antidepressants so much as they need to supplement natural estrogen and progesterone to get their levels to a more functional place. I'm not saying antidepressants should never be used but I would first encourage any mother with these severe issues to find a doctor who understands hormones rather than only band-aiding the problem with depression meds. Dr. Reiss has written a wonderful book called, *How to Make a New Mother Happy* which offers more in-depth information about this subject.

PMS (short for Please Make It Stop)!

Let's talk PMS. Are you one who identifies with being a sane, tolerant person in the first half of your cycle and turning into Mrs. Hyde in the second half? It is usually due to one of two reasons, but can sometimes be a combination of each.

Progesterone Takes a Nose Dive

The first cause of PMS to be investigated is insufficient progesterone. Progesterone is supposed to be high in the second half of your cycle. For various reasons, sometimes it just can't climb that ladder and stay on top. You will know this is your problem if you feel a lot of anxiety, agitation, and breast and nipple pain as you head toward your period. You are simply running out of progesterone. Progesterone raises gaba which relaxes and calms you. Therefore, if you feel the exact opposite of relaxed and calm in the week or so before your period, it's a good indication of progesterone shortage. Sometimes a simple over the counter natural progesterone cream will do the trick. Emerita is good because it does not use parabens in its base formula.

Usually younger women are more easily helped with a low dose cream like this since their estrogen levels may still be in a healthy range. Their PMS symptoms of grouchiness and irritability stem only from a mild progesterone shortage as they head toward their period. A daily dab or two of progesterone after day 14 of their cycle until their period can restore a better hormone balance. A cream like this containing USP progesterone, at 20 mg per dose, can help ease anxiety symptoms, mild breast pain, and premenstrual water retention

Older women (those in their thirties and beyond), or those with more severe cases of anxiety and agitation, will need to have hormone levels measured via blood testing. If results show that low progesterone is indeed your problem, ask your doctor for a higher dosed compounded progesterone formula, or a pharmaceutical made capsule like Prometrium. This is simply micronized progesterone in oral form. Do not waste your money on wild yam creams. These do not convert to the real hormone in the body.

If there are uterine problems, along with the PMS like I experienced, this indicates a more chronic imbalance and you will definitely need higher strength progesterone than what is available over the counter. A long term and chronic lack of progesterone can result in conditions such as fibroids, a thickened uterine lining, or a very short luteal phase (the phase from ovulation to menses). These issues will not usually be helped by low dose progesterone.

Severe conditions like these often call for compounded vaginal progesterone creams at higher strengths, or oral progesterone pills. These delivery systems can make a remarkable difference. A 2005 study at *Westminster Hospital* in London evaluated the effects of progesterone cream on the endometrium of women. They concluded that doses of 40 mg (which is twice as strong as the doses from over the counter products) was insufficient "to fully attenuate the mitogenic effect of estrogen on the endometrium." In plain English, this means it wasn't strong enough to stop, or reverse build up in the lining of the uterus caused by estrogen. An Australian study at the *Sydney Menopause Centre* revealed similar findings. They found that using progesterone cream on the skin, even in doses up to 64 mg, was not enough to make any changes in a proliferated endometrium.

In contrast, progesterone cream, especially made for vaginal use where it has a direct route to the uterus, or micronized progesterone in capsule form, either swallowed or used vaginally, can halt and reverse thickening of the endometrium. A study published in the *Journal of the Climacteric and Postmenopause, Maturatis 20,* provides convincing evidence. Seventy eight premenopausal women were given 100 mg of natural progesterone vaginally from day 10–25 of their cycle. This therapy achieved complete regression of endometrial build-up in over 90% of the cases. Similar results on reducing endometrial build-up have been documented using micronized progesterone, 200 mg orally. These capsules are known as Prometrium, or in the generic form are called Microgest. The hormone used is identical to the one your own body makes.

Estrogen Shortage

The next and very common cause of PMS is insufficient estrogen, or what is known as estradiol (E2) on blood tests. Dr. Reiss notices this becoming more common among his patients. If you experience the following symptoms the closer you get to your period, then a lack of estrogen is likely your problem: greater aches and pains including migraine, more depression and feelings of gloom, mood swings, insomnia, memory problems, brain fog, itching skin, and feeling flat and uninspired.

Decreased estrogen before a period can also express itself as symptoms of too much testosterone. If a woman has a healthy amount of testosterone in her body and her estrogen starts to decline too much, the balance between these two hormones is upset. This results in those pesky premenstrual pimples, oily skin, aggressive behavior, impatience, and short temper.

After reading the lists of symptoms, you may be able to identify what type of PMS you have. But, blood tests are also important. In her book, *It's My Ovaries, Stupid* on the topic of PMS, Dr. Elizabeth Vilet advises women to look more at scientific studies, as well as their own body experience for sound information, rather than only listening to the "progesterone gurus." There are a lot of people on the Internet, and even in multi-level marketing businesses, that sell progesterone creams to women for "whatever ails them." This is a one-size-fix-all approach and it doesn't take into account the uniqueness of every woman's hormonal make-up.

Vilet cautions women not to jump straight on the "progesterone fix all" bandwagon. This is a grave pitfall if it is not the missing hormone causing the PMS. Adding progesterone when another sex hormone is too low can make PMS worse. In her particular practice, Dr. Vilet finds there are more women with estrogen deficiencies as the cause of their PMS, than those with progesterone deficiencies. She writes, "It is actually estradiol supplementation in the luteal phase of the menstrual cycle that gives the most impressive symptom relief for PMS . . . progesterone decreases serotonin while estradiol boosts serotonin . . . Since higher serotonin helps lift depression, it isn't surprising women often feel depressed when estradiol is low in relation to progesterone."

She goes on to say, "For a patient with low progesterone levels in the luteal phase and normal estradiol levels, I would use progesterone. And conversely, if there is low estradiol and relatively normal luteal phase progesterone . . . then it only makes sense to boost estradiol back to optimal ranges as a first step."

If your deficiency is either progesterone or estrogen, or even both, it can be determined via blood testing in the second half of your cycle (from day 18-21). Supplementing with the natural form of these missing hormones, starting with small doses, can make a world of difference to you, and the people who have to live with you. (Smile).

Natural or Surgical Decline

What about mamas who have gone through menopause or currently going through it? As your sex hormones leave your body, you may experience hot flashes, brain fog, weight gain around the middle, skin changes, lagging libido, pain during intercourse, deterioration of a healthy cardiovascular system, bladder issues, and many more symptoms. While you should still test your hormone levels to see how much they rise if you intend to start bioidentical hormone theory, there is no doubt they will be low. To find relief, and prevent further accelerated degeneration of your body, you will likely need to bring all three of your sex hormones (estrogen, progesterone, and testosterone) back into healthy ranges.

Those who have been surgically thrown into abrupt menopause through total hysterectomy may have been frightened and confused by the idea of hormone therapy due to the WHI study and are suffering through the side effects of post surgery extreme hormone loss. You can supplement safely with natural hormones and get your life back. More will be discussed later on the difference between synthetic and natural hormones.

Whether from menopause or surgery, without addressing your tanked out hormones, it will be a much greater uphill battle for you to find a healthy weight. In the book, *Why We Get Fat*, the author, Gary Taubes talks about how sex hormones, such as estrogen and testosterone, have positive effects on our fat cells. When sufficient estrogen is circulating in the body an enzyme called lipoprotein lipase (LPL) is suppressed. That's a good thing as LPL attaches itself to fat cells and causes more circulating fat to be drawn into the fat cells to be stored. In an ideal hormonal environment, LPL enzymes will attach themselves more to muscle cells rather than fat cells and draw fat up to be burned as energy, creating a leaner body.

Taubes points to a study on rats that had their ovaries removed. These rats were given the same amount of food and calories as control rats that still had their ovaries. The rats without ovaries grew obese quickly. They infused estrogen back into these obese rats and they promptly lost their weight, became lean again, and began eating and acting like perfectly normal rats. Taubes writes on page 92, "This very likely is what happens to many women who get fat when they have their ovaries removed, or after menopause. They excrete less estrogen and their fat cells express more LPL."

Tubal Ligations and Partial Hysterectomies

There is evidence that even women who have had a tubal ligation, or a partial hysterectomy where the ovaries are not taken, will still have significant hormonal loss. In her book, *It's My Ovaries Stupid!* Dr. Elizabeth Vilet describes a study that looked at 9,514 women who underwent tubal ligation. The study found that women who had tubals were more likely to report persistent cycle irregularities, painful menstrual periods, and decreases in the number of bleeding days and in the amount of bleeding. Vilet talks about how these changes indicate a decrease in hormone levels. Her theory for this hormone loss is that the tubal procedure of cutting, cauterizing, or tying off the fallopian tubes also affects ovarian blood flow which leads to impaired function of the ovary and decreased hormone production.

When Dr. Vilet measures patients' hormone levels in the second half (or luteal phase of the cycle) in women who have had tubal ligations, she consistently finds that estradiol is lower than normal. Vilet says that as time elapses after a tubal, the gradual decline in blood flow causes lower than normal optimal estradiol levels for most of the cycle. This causes menopause-like symptoms in women who are too young to be in menopause. If this is you, or someone you know, blood testing, then supplementing with a natural form of the missing hormone or hormones can re-establish lost health.

While total hysterectomy will throw a woman into menopause immediately because of the abrupt loss of ovaries, many women suffer a more gradual loss of hormones even with partial hysterectomy (removal of uterus only). Although slower, this loss can have huge negative effects on health. A full 30 to 60 percent of women have menopausal levels of estradiol and testosterone as early as two to three years following the removal of the uterus. Again, Vilet explains that it is lack of blood flow to the ovaries, caused by tying off the uterine artery when it is removed. Vilet cautions women that they will likely experience menopausal type symptoms such as depression, fatigue, headaches, loss of sex drive, and other symptoms within three years of a partial hysterectomy. She urges women to get their hormone levels checked and replace what surgery has taken away. This blood flow issue is even more a problem than after a tubal ligation. Once this artery is tied off it means a loss of over 50 percent of the blood flow to the ovary from the artery.

Years Before the Change

Perimenopause, those years (usually in our mid to late forties) before real menopause when the ovaries are puttering out, can be a difficult time for women. During this time many experience anovulatory cycles. These are cycles that occur when an egg is not released. During perimenopausal years eggs are in shorter supply. If an egg is not released the body does not get the message to send out its usual supply of progesterone to support the released egg. Estrogen is left on its own and this has dangerous consequences to the body. It puts the breasts and uterus at higher risk of cancer rates.

Other symptoms of anovulatory cycles are skipped periods, flooding, large clots, and depressive episodes. These perimenopausal years are the time when many women become so tired of their crazy cycles that they almost looking forward to menopause when all the extremes will stop, or so they hope.

If you know you are having anovulatory cycles, it will be wise to create a steadier and safer cycle by supplementing with regular doses of progesterone for at least ten days a month as a protection for your body. You may also be running low on estrogen at times since these are the years when it is petering out before gushing out during menopause. Don't forget to monitor that hormone via symptoms and blood testing also.

For those of us not quite yet in the perimenopause years and yet still have heavy bleeding and long periods, with lots of flooding and large clots or shortened length between cycles, it is usually because of progesterone deficiency. Anovulatory cycles are not the only reason for lack of progesterone. Age can often be the problem. Many women's levels of this hormone speedily decline as they head into their early thirties. Stress speeds up this process, too. I seem to be a textbook case for this scenario as this is about the age when my uterine problems came with fury. Dr. Gordon Reynolds, a renowned obstetrician states, "In fact, 50 percent of women over age 35 are already no longer producing adequate progesterone . . . as soon as progesterone drops out, the rest of her hormones are now imbalanced. This is what is now known as "estrogen dominance."

The Real Truth on Estrogen Dominance

I'm sure you've frequently heard the term "estrogen dominance," but it's important to know what it really means. Many people associate the term "estrogen dominance" with too high estrogen. The phrase is often thrown around as the cause for all female related problems. Estrogen is looked at as the "big baddie," something we should try to rid ourselves of. But, this is not true. Estrogen dominance simply means there is not enough progesterone to balance out estrogen. Drs. Reiss and Vilet both point out in their books that it is rather rare for premenopausal women to make excess estrogen. That usually only happens with very obese women whose fat cells convert testosterone into too much estrogen.

Even some menopausal women can be estrogen dominant with very little estrogen. They simply have less progesterone than they need for a healthy ratio. While estrogen builds up the uterine lining, progesterone combats it by stopping excessive growth. Natural progesterone needs to be added if it has started to decline since we want that wonderful balance that God intricately designed for us females.

Migraines

I have suffered, and know many women who suffer from cycle related migraines. It took me years of trying every remedy I read about before coming to understand that these headaches are often due to fluctuations in estrogen during the menstrual cycle and they become more extreme with age. Those of us who suffer from these migraines simply cannot tolerate the swinging highs and lows of our hormones as well as we did in our youth. These fluctuations become more intense and cause negative changes in brain chemicals as we age. The lows of our hormone dips sink lower and our body begs for more of that great pain reliever called estrogen.

If you are one of these women, you may notice migraines occur routinely with the fall of your estrogen, right before and during menstruation and right before ovulation. We are also the ones who are often afflicted right after childbirth when estrogen drops from the extremely high levels of pregnancy. I always wondered why I experienced severe headaches after each of my births. Now, I know the reason. These extreme estrogen dips result in inflammation in the cells and lower serotonin. That's not a good situation, because serotonin relieves pain in the body. I am not advocating anyone use estrogen therapy straight after birth to relieve this inflammation, but I find it always helps my state of mind to at least understand what is going on in my body. Serene has also suffered from low estrogen headaches after her births. She has recently discovered that incorporating one to two teaspoons of maca root powder each day into her diet directly after birth helps immensely. Maca supports hormone function, and for some women, it helps balance hormones that have bottomed out.

Some unfortunate women never make enough estrogen to sustain a full, pain free cycle, even in their youth, and endure cyclic migraines throughout the entirety of their fertile years.

It may sound contradictory, but even those of us who suffer from problems of estrogen dominance due to declining progesterone, can still dip too low in estrogen as we head toward our period. I struggled with this concept for a long time. How could I have all the problems associated estrogen dominance and be deficient in this hormone at the same time? This happens when both hormones begin declining. My progesterone went downhill first which left me with uterine problems from estrogen dominance. Not too many years later, at various times of my cycle, my estrogen also headed out the door. Hello, migraines.

The good news is that women can learn to offset these extreme estrogen dips during their cycles that increase inflammation and cause neck, head, and face pain, by supplementing with a bioidentical estrogen cream, gel, or patch during the days in their cycle when estrogen is at its lowest. Doing this can have a profound and positive impact on a woman's life if she has been plagued with debilitating headaches.

Some women find that raising their low progesterone levels will help with migraines. We are all different. While supplementing with progesterone helped my bleeding conditions, it did not alleviate my migraines. Estrogen did help in that area. I have found that it is best to start adding a form of bioidentical estrogen before severe pain occurs. Some women who have long and chronic dips in their estrogen will need to use estrogen cream on day 21 and go right through until the end of their bleeding, or even a couple of days beyond that. These are often the same women who need to supplement when estradiol takes a short dip right before ovulation, but this will be a shorter supplementation time as estrogen quickly rises again naturally after ovulation.

Other women will do well by only using estrogen for a few days around menstruation when they are feeling completely horrid due to their low estrogen state. I suggest women who suffer from cyclic migraines make a chart to show the rise and fall of hormones during a female cycle and track their own headache episodes. This makes it easier to predict the most problematic times. You can then show your chart to your doctor and ask him or her to write a script for a compounded cream using both estradiol (E2) and estriol (E3). This is known as Biest cream. Hopefully, your doctor will be open minded to this approach, although it is preferable to find an anti-aging hormone specialist who treats these conditions more naturally than continually passing out drugs. There are plenty of respected studies available online which show estrogen's success at combating cyclic migraines. Print out some of that information, take it to your doctor, and ask to try this alternative.

You will learn in *Foxy Mama*, Chapter 34 that sex helps to relieve pain and will naturally raise estrogen and endorphin levels which help relieve and prevent migraines. More doctors should write, "Have more sex!" on their scripts!

All Dried Up

What about vaginal dryness and discomfort? It's often accompanied with lowered libido as there is not much desire to be sexual when intercourse involves severe pain. I've listened while women describe their lack of libido when breastfeeding. This is often accompanied by vaginal dryness, sometimes so severe it results in vaginal atrophy. The reason this happens in some women is that breastfeeding suppresses normal ovarian production. While that's a God-ordained occurrence to help create natural child spacing, certain women are more vulnerable to vaginal thinning from the subsequent lack of estrogen. We discussed the role of prolactin earlier with regard to postpartum depression. While prolactin is a necessary and beneficial hormone for breastfeeding, it sometimes pushes estrogen too low and results in the dry vagina syndrome.

A similar problem arises for women who have gone through menopause. The ovaries stop producing sex hormones like estrogen which plump and lubricate the vagina. These women could enjoy sex again if they were to measure their hormones, discover what is off balance, and supplement safely and naturally. Bioidentical estriol (E3) or what is known as "the weak estrogen," can be safely used in cream form, even during breast feeding, to restore natural lubrication and tone to the vagina without being harmful to nursing babies.

Natural estriol is the best way to recapture a healthy, juicy vagina. Although it may be weaker than estradiol, your most powerful estrogen, it can have amazing benefits. According to Dr. Reiss, it completely restores the vaginal integrity of the vagina. He says, "When you supplement estriol, you will find that you may not need another lubricant."

Ask your doctor to prescribe a natural, vaginal estriol cream if you have this problem. Make sure it is not combined with a synthetic estrogen. Most gynecologists, and even general practitioners, are happy to do this. If not, there are also low dose over-the-counter vaginal estriol creams that can be purchased in the US, both online, and at some health stores.

Any married woman with a dry, painful vagina should also have more sex. The reasons for this will be discussed further in *Foxy Mama,* Chapter 34.

Chapter 32

Mama's Wise Choices
(Natural versus Synthetic Hormones)

by Pearl Barrett

We live in an imperfect, toxic world. We can't expect our hormones to stay in perfect alignment on their own. You will only do your body a disservice if your hormones become imbalanced or decline and you think, "Well, this is the way things go with age, so I'll just endure it." God equipped mankind with enough creativity to find a way to isolate these bioidentical hormones from yams and soy. They are exactly like the ones He made within us.

I think of it in this way. God left it up to man to figure out how to create fire, but He made sure all the necessary requirements were available. God is a creator by nature and he told us in Genesis 1:26, *"Let us make man in our image."* I believe that as a Father, He is very pleased when His children discover new things. He certainly supplied us with some amazing ingredients when He created the world. I, for one, am thankful for those who have been blessed with scientific minds and who make discoveries to benefit the rest of us.

Therapy using bioidentical hormones is a relatively new science here in the U.S. It's an important one for us to learn, not only for ourselves, but for our daughters as they embark on their own journeys into the different facets of womanhood.

Let's be clear, I am not talking about synthetic hormones. You should avoid synthesized hormones at all costs. I only encourage the use of natural bioidentical hormones when they are needed. Dr. Steven Hotze, a bioidentical hormone specialist and founder of the *Hotze Health and Wellness Center* in Houston, describes synthetic hormone drugs as not hormones at all, but counterfeits. Concerning synthetics, he says in an interview in Suzanne Somer's book, *Breakthrough*, "They are drugs that mimic hormones. Hormones exist in nature and in our human bodies. Those are the only true things that are hormones."

Pregnancy is a good example of the safety of natural hormones. Pregnancy raises hormones in the female body to extreme levels. Two forms of estrogen soar 10 times over their usual amount. The third form of estrogen (estriol) goes up 1,000 times! Progesterone levels increase by 100 to 400 fold. Human growth hormone (HGH) increases by about 20 percent and available testosterone does the same. These intensely elevated hormone levels in pregnancy leave women with a decreased risk of breast cancer with each full term pregnancy.

WHI Study—the Study that Changed Hormone History

In 2002, the conclusions of *The Women's Health Initiative* (WHI) study were published, and this is when female hormone therapy became known as dangerous. The media had a heyday with the study results and fear was ground into the hearts of women. The problem was that the distinction between the synthetic hormones used for the study and natural hormones, identical to what our own body makes, was not clarified by the media. It's important to understand that the study did not look at the results of supplementing with natural estrogen, progesterone, and testosterone (the three main sex hormones your own body makes). Instead, it evaluated the use of premarin (conjugated equine estrogen) and provera (medroxyprogesterone acetate) on women. The first is a horse estrogen; the second is a synthetic hormone not natural to our female body.

The WHI study concluded that "hormone therapy" was associated with a rise in breast cancer and cardiovascular disease. With such a pronouncement, hormone replacement therapy suddenly became the "evil" phrase. Estrogen was now thought to be dangerous. Somehow, natural hormones were lumped into the results of this study when they were never part of it!

The facts are that premarin and provera, the synthetic hormones used in that study, are dangerous to females. Anyone still using one, or both of these, should ask her doctor to switch her to bioidentical replacements. Bioidentical estrogen and progesterone are completely different. In natural doses, they protect you from diseases rather than cause them.

"Natural" Decline

Some women, who have been scared off all hormone replacement by the negative press opt to steer clear from hormone therapy so they can be more "natural" about aging. They often try herbal remedies to help get them through. However, replacing our lost hormones directly with bioidentical ones is far more natural than using herbs. Herbs can help sometimes, but the body has receptors for natural hormones and inherently knows what to do with them. We have no herb receptors in our bodies and the pathways they take cannot always be relied upon. However, the supplement maca is able to nourish your whole endocrine system which is the foundation for hormones. The herb vitex (chaste tree berry) has shown in studies to aid progesterone pathways in females and have a balancing effect on all sex hormones. You can do a self study on these supplements to check if they could benefit you, but they will not restore what menopause or surgery takes away.

Deciding not do anything about hormone loss is like saying, "My eyes are not working as well these days, but I am not going to wear contacts or glasses because that is not natural." Should one not get a hip or knee replacement when it is necessary? This fallen world we live in has sin, sickness, and disease, but that doesn't mean we lay down and give in to it all. In my mind, the idea of not replacing hormones is like not wanting to replace a vitamin or mineral when it is low in our bodies. Vitamin D levels are one of the important nutrients that lower as we age. Should we stay "natural" and not replace them also?

Counterfeit or the Real Thing

Let's compare the differences between synthetic (or counterfeit hormones) and bioidentical hormones.

1. Counterfeit estrogens increase inflammation. Bioidentical estrogen decreases it and decreases C-reactive protein (CRP) which is a general marker for inflammation. Doctors who switch their menopausal women from synthetic estrogens to bioidentical often find they report a reduction in joint pain, which is a good indicator of inflammation.
2. Counterfeit estrogens increase body fat and decrease lean body mass. In contrast, bioidentical estrogen decreases body fat and allows for muscle growth. Refer to the study about the rats in Chapter 31.
3. Counterfeit estrogens raise cardiovascular risk and venous thrombosis (deep vein clots). Bioidentical estrogens protect against heart disease and do not pose a risk for blood clots. Dr. Uzzi Reiss has treated more than 20,000 women with bioidentical estrogen and has not observed a single cardiovascular event associated with estradiol treatment in cream form.
4. Premara, a chemical horse estrogen, increases incontinence (leakage of urine). Bioidentical estrogen significantly helps this problem.
5. Counterfeit progesterone, like provera, increases the risk of breast cancer. Bioidentical progesterone dramatically decreases this risk by protecting your breasts from too much estradiol. There are many progesterone receptors in breast tissue for this purpose, but no provera receptors.

6. Counterfeit progesterone promotes diabetes and bone loss. Bioidentical progesterone helps to build bones. In the right balance, natural progesterone does not raise insulin resistance.
7. Counterfeit progesterone destroys sleep quality. Bioidentical progesterone is the perfect sleep aid as it raises gaba in the brain. It is a calming, restful neurotransmitter.
8. Counterfeit progesterone, like progestins and provera, are harmful to the brain. Bioidentical progesterone has the opposite effect. It has been shown in human studies to generate new brain cell growth. It critically protects the neurological system.
9. Counterfeit progesterone promotes anxiety and feelings of aggression. Bioidentical progesterone naturally soothes and calms.

The Pill—It Sure isn't Natural

The media frenzy on the danger of supplementing hormones is ironic. Often doctors give out prescriptions for birth control pills like they are candy, yet many of them will not prescribe natural hormones, because they think they are "too risky." A doctor who offered me several forms of birth control did not feel comfortable prescribing safe, cancer fighting progesterone, or a compounded estrogen for the times in my cycle when it dipped too low and I felt rotten. Things are upside down. We need to educate ourselves first, and then take the truth to our doctors.

Right this minute, millions of women's bodies are being negatively altered, possibly permanently, by using counterfeit hormones. You guessed it—they're taking the pill. In *Pearl's Story*, Chapter 30, I described how a doctor convinced me to try the birth control pill to see if that would regulate my massive bleeding problem. While bleeding lessened a little, my uterine fibroid condition did not improve. Instead, oral birth control made me depressed. I gained weight (because I no longer had my healthy natural estrogen and testosterone levels), and I also lost most of my libido. Now, I understand the science behind what happened.

Oral birth control shuts down the ovaries so they can no longer make any estrogen and progesterone. Chemical progestins and estrogens are substituted for the body's natural ones; otherwise a menopause state would occur. But, the ovaries also make testosterone which the pill fails to replace. You may think of testosterone only in the terms of it being a male hormone, but it is essential to females also. We make about a tenth of what men make, but that small amount gives us much of our sex drive, vitality, muscle tone, confidence and emotional strength, healthy memory and brain function, clitoral and nipple sensitivity, orgasmic response, and feelings of happiness.

The pill has a devastating effect on testosterone levels in women, decreasing them by about 70 percent. To make matters worse, oral contraceptives dramatically raise SHBG (Sexual Hormone Binding Globulin) which causes whatever testosterone that is left to be bound up and unable to be used. Essentially, any testosterone available to most women on the pill is close to nil. It's even less than a woman who has been through menopause, with the exception of rare women who make ample amounts of testosterone from their adrenal glands. It's no wonder I became an insecure, moping version of myself who wondered if I should have ever become a mother. I needed my testosterone! I was so glad to have "Pearl" back again when I stopped taking the pill.

Although big pharmaceutical companies have been quiet on this topic, studies now back up the fact that taking the pill increases a woman's likelihood of depression. A 2005 study from Australia's Monash University found that the pill increased average depression ratings to 17.6, compared to 9.8 in women not on the pill. None of the women studied had a history of depression before use. It sounds exactly like what happened to me. Like most of these women, I was offered an antidepressant when I mentioned my mood changes to my doctor. Fortunately, I didn't pursue that route. SSRI's like Prozac, Zoloft, and Paxil are most often prescribed for depression, but these only complicate matters more. They can further inhibit libido by raising serotonin to the point where it lowers dopamine. Remember, it is all about balance. Dopamine is a crucial brain chemical for libido and sense of well being. Inhibiting it is a ridiculous idea when a woman's libido is already squelched from the pill.

It is sad to think that young teenage girls are being prescribed oral birth control to help clear up their acne, or regulate their periods, and as a result, they often end up with depression, weight gain, and sometimes a permanently damaged libido. Studies have shown that women who go on the pill for prolonged periods often never fully recover their testosterone production and libido due to the amount of time their HPOA (ovary production) was shut down. What a travesty that these girls may never have the full, delightful, sexual response to their future husbands that God intends them to experience.

Yes, the pill often works to clear up acne, but this is only because it eliminates testosterone which can produce androgenic symptoms like acne when it is not in balance. For girls, or even adult women, who have a major problem with acne, their problem is usually too little estrogen to counteract the dominant expression of testosterone. It is insane to shut off all testosterone to try and help clear up skin. To me, that is about as ridiculous as the blood-letting doctors used to do to try and purge disease. It makes much more sense to safely add some bioidentical estradiol to restore testosterone/estrogen balance. Another option for acne issues is to look into the supplement, Coenzyme A which can have a positive effect on oil glands in the skin.

The Low Dose Pill

What about low dose birth control pills? These are the latest inventions by manufacturers due to the release of such strong data on the danger of synthetic hormones. These "low dose" pills are designed to only deliver a very small amount of chemical estrogen with the theory that this would be a safer approach. Unfortunately, ovary production is still shut down, but now, not only is the woman going to lose her testosterone, she will also plunge into an estrogen deficient state which is highly inflammatory—and a whole new list of symptoms occur.

Remember, God made estrogen to be the "happy hormone" for us females. In the right balance, estrogen is a mild MAO inhibitor which causes us to feel more euphoric and less grouchy. The estrogen amount in these new pills is much lower than what a woman's body naturally makes. Natural hormone doctors, like Uzzi Reiss, are noticing symptoms such as frequent memory loss and declines in cognition, even in young women who take these pills.

Chapter 33

Mama Knows Her Body

(Putting Hormone Therapy to Practice)

by Pearl Barrett

Now you know the "why" about natural hormones. Let's get practical and discuss the "how."

Blood Testing

I recommend you get a full blood test for all necessary hormones, along with a complete blood count (CBC). This will show where your cholesterol and other important telltale levels stand. If your insurance will not cover hormone tests, or if you do not have insurance, The Life Extension Foundation (www.lef.org) has excellent blood tests for very reasonable prices. Another site to order inexpensive blood tests is www.PrivatemdLabs.com and they have year round affordable prices. Neither of these sites requires a doctor script for tests. You can choose your own tests.

LEF has full male and female hormone panels which go on sale each year during the months of April and May. On sale, they cost less than $200 for a full panel of tests. At their regular price, they cost a little more than $200. But this is about a fifth of most blood test costs.

If you need individual tests, for example, an estrogen test only, you can order that too. It costs about $30.

Order your tests over the phone or online. They send you a form which you take to your nearest Lab Corp center. Lab Corps are found all over the country and the process is smooth and easy. Take your test results to the doctor of your choice, or one they recommend in your area. Show the doctor where your results show deficiencies and ask for bioidentical hormone scripts. Of course, it is never a good idea to take hormones unless you have a deficiency.

Another way to obtain inexpensive blood testing is to find a federally funded or nonprofit clinic in your county. They usually have sliding scales, and if you don't have insurance or you have a large family, blood tests can be very inexpensive to obtain. We have a clinic in our rural county that uses Lab Corp and I can get the tests I need for a minimal expenditure. I just have to convince the medical staff that my tests are necessary. Go armed with your list of tests and educated reasons of why you want them.

Take charge of your own health. Keep a file with every progressive blood test and you will be able to track your own progress. Don't solely rely on your doctor to figure out what you need. Instead, try to become partners with him or her in promoting your health.

Many doctors may look at your results and say, "Well, you're in range, so you are fine." This is absolutely untrue in many cases. Ranges are often age adjusted. You must consider any symptoms you have then take into consideration the difference between your test results and where a person in their prime would be. Sure, you may be just in range now, but you were probably a lot higher when you were at your healthiest.

You'll have to become more educated than your doctor about your individual hormone needs. If your doctor has a god-complex and does not want to listen when you respectfully share your new knowledge and the help you require from him or her, find a better doctor. A good way to do this is to locate a compounding pharmacy in your area and ask them for the name of some doctors that prescribe bioidentical hormones. I tried this a few years ago. Even though we live in a rural area with only small surrounding towns, I found a very open minded local doctor who is a strong believer in the healing power of hormones and is proving to be immensely helpful to our family.

I even recommend men and women as young as their late teens and early twenties that are not having any problems, to get their hormones tested. These results will be a great reference point later in life to show what their hormones looked like in optimum doses for their individual bodies. I certainly wish I had numbers from my early twenties when my periods were great, migraines were unknown, and my breasts were full, but not swollen or painful. It would be interesting to see where estrogen, testosterone, and progesterone levels were when my body felt best. This would give a better direction on what to shoot for now.

Test your hormones through serum blood, not saliva, with the exception of cortisol. Saliva can show major elevation in estradiol and progesterone which may not be a true reflection of what's going on. Dr. Reiss has treated women whose doctors had taken them off their hormones because saliva results showed their cells were showing levels hundreds of points higher than their ranges. But, these women still had deficiency symptoms. He tested their serum levels and found they were not high at all and, in some cases, their hormones needed to be increased.

The Big Seven

Below is a list of hormones most important to test and why they are important. I call them the Big Seven. The results will give you a good picture of what's going on inside your body.

If you are still a menstruating woman, it is the best idea to get a hormone panel done between day 18-21 of your cycle. In this way, you will catch the peaks of most of your hormones, especially progesterone. Menopausal women can test any time.

Estradiol

This hormone is known as E2 on blood tests. It's synonymously called estrogen, but it's really only one of the many estrogens we women have in our bodies. We test this one because it is the most potent of the three main estrogens. It gives the most health benefits, but also the most harm when it is not in proper balance. There are no cookie cutter optimum levels for this hormone. Women with smaller breasts often have less of it and function well that way. Curvy women often need more of it but find themselves with problems when it rages out of control.

There are a couple of constants on which you can rely. As long as you do not test during your period (when estrogen takes a nose dive), your numbers should be at or above 100. If they come back any lower, you are probably in estrogen deficiency. Most women approaching menopause begin hot flashes when estradiol dips near 50, but estradiol levels less than 100 will often wreak other types of havoc on women. Their breasts may begin to flatten and sag. They will be less happy. Brain fog is a huge indication. They will have trouble with memory. Their vaginas will become drier. They will notice deeper wrinkles forming. They will not care about their bodies as much, because estrogen gives us that sense of femaleness, that essence that keeps us in tune with the wonder of being a woman.

Many women feel best with estrogen levels around 200. If they are not experiencing symptoms of dominance like water retention, sore breasts, or excessive bleeding at that level, then this is likely where they are supposed to be.

Estrogen, in balanced levels, can be our greatest protector. According to hormone expert, Dr. Shippen, author of *The Testosterone Syndrome*, "Women who take real hormones like estrogen, in a balanced way, have higher levels of good HDL (good cholesterol) and lower levels of unhealthy LDL (bad cholesterol). They have lower levels of fibrinogen and lower levels of homo-cysteine, which is important, because homo-cysteine is an indicator of how much of an inflammatory state the body is in. They have lower levels of insulin and glucose, and they have increased blood flow to all parts of the body, including the brain, heart, muscles and bones."

Optimum levels of estrogen give us greater tolerance to pain. In fact, it decreases all forms of pain by lowering homo-cysteine and inflammation markers. Supplementing estrogen when it is lacking can even be more effective than antidepressants when depression is a problem.

Estrogen may be tested via urine also. This is a good way to detect how your estrogen is converting in your body. Many anti-aging doctors will order a 2/16 ratio test to evaluate the ratio of safe versus harmful estrogens in your body. This test is a good way to be proactive about preventing breast cancer.

If you are experiencing estrogen deficiencies and it is reflected in your blood work, it's time to decide which delivery method will work best for you.

Estrogen Creams and Gels

Trans-dermal creams allow you to top up your hormones as you feel the need. Some women metabolize estrogen much faster than others. While one woman may only need to apply an estrogen cream once a day, another woman may feel better relief from symptoms using smaller doses three times a day. You have a lot of control over how much or how little to use with a cream.

Ask your doctor to write a script for a compounded Biest gel or cream. This is an 80/20 combination of estriol to estradiol. Estriol is the third form of primary estrogen (E3). It protects the breasts and does not cause uterine build up, while estradiol, its big sister, does all the heavy lifting such as restoring peak brain function. The two put together in a cream are a safe, yet powerful combination.

Biest cream is best used at the top of the inner thigh or inner arms and face. It even works wonders on facial skin, plumping it up and fighting wrinkles. If your estradiol levels are already sufficient, a simple estriol (E3) cream can be bought without prescription. It is excellent for the skin on the face and when applied vaginally, it is the best way to restore normal moisture levels. (See *Mama Glows*, Chapter 40 for more information).

Estrogen Pellets

Natural estrogen pellets can be placed under the skin and will deliver a steady stream of this hormone for about four to six months. There is usually more cost involved than with creams and adjusting doses is not as easy but some women like the freedom to not have to worry about daily applications.

Estrogen Pills

Do not use oral estrogen pills. Although you can find bioidentical forms of these and they are very inexpensive, they require breakdown in the liver which raises SHBG (sexual hormone binding globulin) too high in the body. Oral estrogen breaks down into high levels of estrone (E1) which is the estrogen more prone to producing breast cancer. Menopausal women have high levels of estrone which is made in their fat cells once the ovaries shut down. The menopausal age is the time when breast cancer rates begin to soar in women.

If your doctor gives you a blank look if you ask for a compounded estrogen cream and will only prescribe oral pills, usually known as Estrace, you could look into using them in an off label way through your mucosal system. Some women place the pieces of the tablet between the front of their gum and their front bottom teeth and let it dissolve to avoid the problems with oral use where it has to be metabolized by the liver. This is called buccal absorption and is usually a very efficient route. More of the hormone is absorbed buccally, thus only 1/6 to ¼ of the tablet is needed at each dose. This is a very inexpensive way to supplement natural estrogen. Talk to your doctor about this option.

Women who have had their uteruses removed sometimes do a similar thing with Estrace tablets, but rather than using them via buccal absorption, they cut pieces of the tablet and place them in the vagina—another excellent absorption location. It is quite easy to achieve healthy systemic estrogen levels this way. Women who still have an intact uterus may not want to use the tablet pieces in their vagina due to the strong link between the uptake from the vagina to the uterus. There is the risk that it could cause too much proliferation. If your doctor thinks this route would be fine for you, even with an intact uterus, be sure to monitor your uterine thickness via ultrasound.

Estrogen Troches

Some doctors are now prescribing bioidentical hormone troches. These are little dissolvable squares that are used buccally (between front gum and chin). They usually combine concentrations of all three sex hormones, including estrogen, progesterone, and testosterone. Depending on the pharmacy, these troches can be less expensive than creams.

Note: If you are menopausal, and even if you do not have a uterus, do not use estrogen without including a form of progesterone as progesterone is protective for the breasts. Young women with estrogen deficiencies who are still making sufficient progesterone should not have to worry so much about including progesterone. Remember, it's all about only replacing only what's missing.

Progesterone

This is the second most important hormone after estrogen. It is responsible for enabling a woman to get pregnant by maintaining the uterine lining. When we have enough progesterone, estrogen is balanced and cannot cause symptoms of dominance.

One of progesterone's most important roles is to protect you from breast cancer. In his book, *The Natural Superwoman*, Dr. Uzzi Riess points to a study of French women who used bioidentical progesterone cream on their breasts to decrease pain. It was found they enjoyed an overall decrease in the incidence of breast cancer. He cites another French study which revealed that women who used chemical progestins experienced an increase in breast cancer, while women who used bioidentical progesterone experienced a 10 percent decrease.

Progesterone protects the brain, hinders cardiovascular disease, improves immunity, builds bones, improves hearing, decreases allergies, and prevents water retention.

Dr. Uzzi Reiss believes progesterone levels of 18-20, on a range of 5-25, give women the best uterine protection. Many doctors consider any number over five to be sufficient for postmenopausal women who use natural hormones if there are no symptoms of estrogen dominance at that level. Depending on your test results, and the symptoms that accompany them, some supplementation may be in order. If you are still a cycling female and progesterone level comes back at 10 or under, which mine did, you should seriously consider adding this hormone.

Progesterone Creams

Postmenopausal women with an intact uterus need to be discerning when it comes to progesterone formulations. If you are postmenopausal and decide to replace your missing estrogen levels, an over the counter progesterone will not be high enough to balance things out. Dr. Uzzi Reiss believes women get enough uterine protection with a prescribed 10 percent progesterone skin cream, but anything less than that will not be enough balance to counteract more youthful uterine levels. Other doctors believe only oral, buccal, or vaginal dosing of progesterone offers full uterine protection. Women without a uterus will be fine using a regular trans-dermal progesterone cream. Even an over the counter one should be fine since their uterus is no longer at risk for proliferation.

Progesterone Pills

Prometrium is a pill filled with micronized bioidentical progesterone and peanut oil. Many doctors prescribe this due to the ease of simply taking a pill each night. The progesterone molecule is larger; consequently it does not have the negative issues when taken orally as estrogen does.

Younger women with problematic uteruses are often prescribed prometrium or one of its generic equivalents. Raising progesterone in this way helps heavy bleeding from the uterus over time by causing more efficient bleeds. Progesterone makes sure the uterus sloughs the lining more efficiently. It must be mature in order to slough off efficiently and enough progesterone is needed to help the lining mature.

Women with inadequate progesterone levels during pregnancy are often prescribed promethium. It is an effective way to increase their lagging progesterone levels to protect from miscarriage. Doctors sometimes tell their patients with low progesterone pregnancies or problematic uterine conditions to insert these pills vaginally. The pill breaks down in the warm environment of the vagina and is effectively absorbed into the blood stream.

Prometrium is another option for postmenopausal women as part of their complete hormone therapy and often their insurance company will cover it. But some women find they are over-responders to progesterone and become very sluggish due to its relaxing effects. This is more common when swallowing a progesterone capsule than with other methods. Other women with high cortisol levels cannot handle the hormone taken in this oral fashion. They sometimes feel dizzy, and due to highly elevated cortisol, can retain water weight or put on weight around their belly.

Postmenopausal women who find themselves in this position are sometimes advised by their doctors to only use a 12 day course of oral prometrium every three months. This makes sure any build up of their uterine lining is sloughed off. It causes them to bleed for a few days. Many women find this more tolerable than taking a promethium pill every night and feeling constantly draggy and bloated.

Note: Sometimes finding the right individual balance takes time when supplementing with hormones. Don't quit if everything does not feel quite right at first. Keep adjusting. Suzanne Somers says you'll know when you are in optimum balance, because your body feels like it is singing.

Progesterone Troches

This method can be an excellent progesterone delivery system, eliminating some of the side effects some women feel from a progesterone pill. It is also quite inexpensive. It should work well for premenopausal women, but blood work will have to be monitored carefully if it is to be used alongside estrogen therapy in postmenopausal women. You need to make sure enough of the hormone is received to protect the uterus as troches don't always result in high levels.

Testosterone (T)

You should test for both Free T and Total T levels when testing this hormone. Total T can vary greatly from woman to woman, depending upon their body type. According to Dr. Uzzi Reiss, those with little body hair and muscle will usually have natural ranges anywhere from 20-40 on a scale of 20-100. I am in that category, with my natural levels showing at the bottom of the scale in the low 20's.

This is the difference between Serene and me who is much more of a natural testosterone type. We can do the same exercise program and I will have some tone at the end of it, while she will have a six pack and rippling muscles all over her body. Not fair! On the other side of it, I have to shave my legs much less often than her, Ha-ha! I am sure my levels were higher in my early twenties, as testosterone begins declining in women after the age of 25. Women with more body hair and muscle will often have ranges from 50-100.

Free T gives you an idea of how much of your total T the body is able to use. Indicators show that most women need to see their free T higher than 0.6 to have a functioning libido. My free T level came back at 0.5 when I first tested. Strangely, I did have some libido at the time of the blood test, but it dramatically skyrocketed once I supplemented with small doses of testosterone.

Adding small amounts of testosterone cream, as in 1-3 mg a day, can greatly improve a woman's confidence. It also helps protect bones, counteracts sexual dysfunction, battles depression, and is important for women suffering with infertility. It is not advisable for women with problems of acne or facial hair to supplement with testosterone as this is often an indication they have plenty. Some women's adrenal glands are effective testosterone producers. These are the rare women who still have ample amounts of the hormone after menopause, and even while on the birth control pill. Women with PCOS (poly-cystic syndrome) already overproduce testosterone, so they should not supplement either.

Testosterone Creams and Gels

A low strength, compounded T cream or gel can be prescribed by your doctor and may be applied to the inner thigh, vaginally, or the labia where there are a lot of T receptors. As with the case of estrogen and progesterone, a testosterone cream allows adjustments to be easily made to doses. This is extremely important when it comes to testosterone because too much can result in personality and physical changes.

Testosterone Shots

The most cost effective way to supplement testosterone is to inject small doses. One vial that would last a man 4-6 months for less than $100 will last a woman ten times longer (but expiration date must be considered). Doctors used to give women with depleted testosterone levels bigger injections which would spike testosterone very high and this was supposed to last the woman for several weeks. Now, it is more common for a woman to self inject about 10 mg of testosterone cypionate once a week with a little insulin syringe, or make two injections of 5 mg on different days of the week. These shots are relatively painless and do not even have to be injected into muscle.

When it comes to testosterone, I need to add a caution, especially when it comes to testosterone shots. Going too high can be just as bad (or even worse) as being in a low state. Remember, hormone replacement is all about finding that perfect balance for your individual body. Due to the inexpensive cost, injections are how I started my testosterone therapy to try and raise my negligible levels. As I mentioned, I have a low T body type, so even very low dose T shots made massive changes to me.

Testosterone can have a major impact on brain space. I felt great at first with more energy, confidence, and zest for life. It enabled me to work out more efficiently. I didn't run out of steam so easily. I was never a very strong person, but after being on testosterone for a while, I could get down and do at least 30 male style pushups! I felt very powerful and unstoppable.

But, after a few months I noticed my libido rising to the point where it no longer felt natural for me (being honest here). I'm a big believer in being a willing and wanting wife, but this was overboard. It was an odd feeling thinking about sex all the time. Good grief! I had always had a rather healthy libido, but it was more an emotional yearning for sex with my husband. Now I felt like I needed it physically, and often! I found this very distracting. Now I know how a lot of men feel about sex!

My chin broke out with acne. I began snapping more at my children and husband, and had less patience with people in general. My brother, who I'm grateful to say is one of my best friends, commented that I had turned into a . . . well, he called me not a very nice word! But, it was true. I was no longer kind and caring.

I realized I had to reduce my T dosage or my family and friends would soon be sick of me. I simply cannot tolerate much exogenous T at all. I now know that a tiny bit goes a long way for me. Testosterone is the hormone that empowers men to go out into the world and conquer. It creates more ambition and is not the most nurturing of hormones. Please, if you need to add testosterone, listen to your body and be willing to talk to your doctor about lowering your doses if you find yourself being bossy, aggressive, seeking a lot more adventure outside the home, or experiencing hypersexuality.

After a year of testosterone therapy, my injection doses needed to be reduced to such small amounts that I figured it was hardly worth the trouble. I found that taking a daily DHEA tablet was enough to keep my libido in fair enough working order so I stopped T injections altogether.

I can no longer get down and give you 30 excellent pushups and I no longer want to work out with the same gusto, but I'm doing okay. I can still do 20 half hearted pushups—not too shabby. I will keep a good eye on my T levels, and you can bet that once I head into menopause, I will begin supplementing again (under a doctor's care again, of course). I never want to endure the bottomed out T state I was in during the time I used the birth control pill for my uterine problems. Next time around, I will be more likely to use a gel, cream, troche, or whatever they have in the future that will allow me to have more control over dosing.

It can take a little while to figure out how much T your body can handle without turning you into a very different person. What may have been the perfect dose for someone else with a higher T type body was simply too high for me. If your body is low in testosterone, you may want to ask your husband to please bear with you while you try your first doses. While testosterone can be an amazing and necessary addition, there is that "just right" dose for women who need to supplement with it. Be mindful that more is not always better.

Testosterone Troches

Some women can better tolerate a troche that contains testosterone because it has a shorter half life in the body. This means it doesn't linger very long in the blood stream enabling more side effects. It is also quite cost effective and maybe the best way to start out using testosterone. I have a good friend who uses testosterone troches and she swears by them.

Testosterone Pellets

Women who have estrogen pellets implanted can have testosterone included in the pellets so it is steadily released for several months. While this approach is less fuss, I would not recommend any woman include T with her estrogen pellets because of my own hyper reaction to it. Pellet dosages cannot be reduced without going back into the incision and replacing higher dosed ones with lower.

DHEA (dehydroepiandrosterone)

It is important to test DHEA sulphate or DHEA(s). Simply testing DHEA serum will not give you an accurate result of how much your body is able to use.

DHEA is the most prevalent hormone in our body and is called the "master" hormone. This is because, down the line, it converts into other hormones that we need. It is made in the adrenal cortex and unfortunately it usually begins to decline after our mid-twenties. Most of us lose between 80-90 percent of our DHEA between ages 30-90. This proved true with my DHEA results which showed my number of 133 to be okay for my age range. But, don't be fooled by these age adjustments labs make. Progressive anti-aging specialists recommend people try to get their levels to those of healthy men and women in their twenties. I try to shoot for around 200. Youthful levels offer optimum protection.

Declining DHEA levels should be addressed, because even a 10 percent decrease is associated with a 48 percent increase in all causes of mortality. With few exceptions, low or deficient DHEA is found in all illnesses. The exception is PCOS where it is thought the body elevates its own DHEA to try to combat hyper lipid levels. DHEA helps to lower cholesterol levels, lowers insulin levels, and protects against diabetes. It is protective against arteriosclerosis, which in turn lowers risk for Alzheimer's.

Here's the good thing. In women, raising DHEA levels can increase testosterone expression in cells, but it will not usually raise blood levels of this hormone. A higher expression of testosterone in cells can enable a woman to feel the beneficial effects of this hormone. I noticed it had a positive effect on my libido when I started taking it and it has played an important role in finding a balance between my sex hormones. Those who are still premenopausal, but have a lagging libido may, want to give DHEA a try before taking the plunge into supplementing with testosterone. It may help you to become that "wanting wife" we will discuss in *Foxy*

Mama, Chapter 34. Postmenopausal women may not be so fortunate with raising their libido this way and may need testosterone to make a big enough difference.

Studies confirm that supplementing with DHEA decreases the incidence of breast cancer and auto immune diseases. It decreases anxiety and depression, improves memory, builds a smarter immune system, aids in muscular development, and improves bone strength. It is an important aid in balancing levels of cortisol when they are too high and it raises HGH (human growth hormone).

DHEA does wonders for dry skin. I had been suffering from this condition for several years and a health adviser told me it could enhance natural oil production. The transformation in my skin was swift and almost miraculous. Within a month I stopped layering moisturizer all over my face several times a day because my skin always felt so thirsty. Now, I also apply a very inexpensive estriol cream to my face since estriol has been shown in studies to reduce wrinkles, soften skin, and increase collagen. I can't think of a better and cheaper way to have soft, excellent skin that is no longer aging the swift way it was before using these hormones.

DHEA Delivery Methods

Most women who supplement with DHEA use oral capsules or tablets. Thankfully, in the United States we do not need a prescription to purchase DHEA. Just make sure you buy a standardized, micronized product. I use a *Nature's Plus* DHEA tablet with bioperine for added absorption and it gives me good results.

Here's the caution with DHEA. Women cannot take too much without side effects appearing; watch for acne and even male type hair growing on the face. We don't want that! But, these conditions will recede once dosage is bought back in line. Usually, most women cannot tolerate more than 15 mg a day.

I swallow a 10 mg capsule of DHEA a day. Some women will not be able to go over 5 mg a day without causing breakouts in the skin, but you'll find your sweet spot, and even that very small dose will benefit you.

Women under the age of 30 do not usually need to supplement with this hormone and it should not be used while pregnant. Also, women who have very low levels of estrogen may need to address this deficiency via natural estrogen therapy before they can tolerate DHEA. Without enough estrogen, the androgenic side effects of DHEA can express themselves too dominantly in cells producing acne and unwanted hair. Conversely, a few rare women may be able to tolerate 20 mg or more and not notice any unwanted effects.

Take DHEA with food in the morning.

Note: While DHEA taken orally usually converts to a more androgenic pathway in women, often raising libido and energy, it can raise estrogen in men. Males are often better off using a DHEA cream on their skin so it does not have to be metabolized by the liver and possibly convert into estrogen. Male dosages are between 25-100 mg a day.

Thyroid

A lot of general practitioners think testing for TSH (thyroid stimulating hormone) is a sufficient gauge for this hormone. That is not accurate. Make sure you at least test free T3 (Triidothyronine). The following are the optimum thyroid tests and ranges if you can convince your doctor to write a script for them. If not, it may be best to use an online lab and pay out of pocket. If you cannot afford all these thyroid tests, the most important will be TSH and Free T3.

TSH is best between 1-2; anything over 2.5 may indicate hypothyroidism. Any result over four indicates a definite problem.
Total T3 (best in upper ⅓ range)
Free T3 (best in upper ⅓ range)
Free T4 (best in middle of range)
Free T4 (best in middle of range)
ReverseT3 (best in lower half of range)

All organs in the body are affected by thyroid hormones. They regulate temperature and metabolism. Thyroid imbalances will affect every hair on your head (it will start falling out) down to your toenails (they will be brittle with ridges). Watch out for other symptoms of low thyroid:

Unexplained weight gain
Chronic pain
Fatigue and energy loss
Dry skin
High blood pressure
Irregular heartbeat
Missing outer third of eyebrows
Memory loss
Constipation
Cold hands and feet
Increased cholesterol
Cystic breasts or ovaries
Mental and emotional problems

You can see the importance of thyroid balance. If you are not making enough, weight loss will be an uphill battle unless you address the problem. My mother, who has lived on an optimum diet most of her life, started having unexplained weight gain around her middle. We know that lack of estrogen can cause this because it elevates insulin, but thyroid also needs to be checked. Her TSH came back normal. So did T4, but if we had not bothered to test T3, we wouldn't have seen that it was at the bottom of the range and a big cause of the problem. Now, she supplements with the full spectrum of natural hormones that menopause depleted, including thyroid, and is back on the road to a trimmer body and overall better health.

If you are have thyroid problems, it will be even more important for you to make sure you get enough of the hormone while you are pregnant. The state of pregnancy can require larger doses. Thyroid deficiency during pregnancy is a greater risk for birth defects.

Thyroid Delivery Methods

Natural thyroid supplements do not come in creams or pellets. They are swallowed. The best tolerated thyroid tablets are a combination of both T4 and T3 hormones like Armour (USA), or Erfa (Canada). They require a prescription, but thankfully they are inexpensive, and are often tolerated better than thyroid medications like Synthroid which is made up of only the T4 hormone.

It is important to know that the body makes both T3 and T4, but T3 is the hormone our body uses. All T4 must be converted into T3 before we can receive any benefit.

People that have adrenal glands in good working order are much more efficient at converting T4 into T3, so these folk often do fine using T4 only meds like Synthroid. However, it's common for people's adrenal glands to get a real beating through the stresses in life so folks with poorly functioning adrenal glands are certainly not rare. Low ferritin (iron stores) and inadequate B12 levels are other problems which halt the conversion of T4 into the usable T3 hormone. Once those deficits in the body are brought up to par, sometimes people can tolerate thyroid meds like Synthroid much better.

But, even if you do decide to use an Armour type med, you should test your cortisol, because without enough cortisol the thyroid hormone cannot be taken up into the cells. It just sits there, pooling in the body.

Many anti-aging doctors prescribe an adrenal gland supplement to help better cortisol production. Vitamin C is also important for adrenal function. An herb called rhodiola can help with cortisol issues, too, by allowing cortisol to have a longer life in the body. But, since it is an adaptogenic herb, it needs to be cycled so the body doesn't build up a tolerance to it.

If the adrenal glands are in too bad a shape to be helped by these measures, some doctors prescribe small doses of bioidentical cortisol itself, known as Cortef, or generically as hydrocortisone. These doses are usually only 10-30 mg per day, divided into 2-4 doses.

Some cutting edge doctors are now trying to raise their patients' low cortisol by the use of pregnenolone cream. Pregnenolone is the mother hormone in the body. It swims downstream in the body and fills the cortisol bucket naturally. Physicians who are trying this believe it may be a better route to raise cortisol because it does not suppress the body's own feedback loop. Taking oral hydro-cortisone can cause high surges which have the potential to suppress the body's own production of the hormone. One can end up with highs, then lows, rather than a feeling of steady energy. Using pregnenolone cream on the skin lets the pregnenolone release slowly through the fat cells and provides steadier levels for some.

Cortisol

Hormones depend upon each other. We have just discussed how a properly working thyroid depends upon cortisol. It's also important for many other bodily functions. Cortisol enables us to respond to stress and then bounce back to a calm state once the stressful situation is resolved. The average person naturally makes 20-30 mg of cortisol a day. Problems arise when our lives are too full of stress and we require more cortisol than what our bodies can make. The end result of prolonged stress is cortisol depletion.

Lifestyle is very important in regulating cortisol. Trimming a too-full life back to basics can allow your adrenal glands to heal and your cortisol levels to have a chance to return to normal. Most of us take on too much. Raising children, cooking meals and looking after your husband and home is a huge job. Adding too much more than that on your plate can drain the best of us.

If you test your cortisol and it comes back too high, this means that your body is being forced to generate too much of it. It is a warning of worse things to come. Eventually, the adrenal glands will become tired of constantly releasing that much hormone and this will lead to adrenal fatigue and then burnout. This is the dangerous situation where there is not enough cortisol to deal with any stress and heart attack or stroke is often the result.

As we age, our cortisol output declines. Late nights accelerate this, as cortisol responds to light. Levels are supposed to naturally lower at night as the sun goes down and we settle in for rest. In our modern world, many of us are up past midnight with artificial light, so our cortisol hormone does not know how to turn down. Let's give it a break! We need to keep reserves available because healthy amounts of cortisol boost energy levels, improve digestion, ease joint movement, ease inflammation, stimulate the brain and heart, fight certain cancers such as leukemia and lymphomas, and promote a healthy sexual response.

You can get a serum blood test for morning cortisol, but that doesn't show what is happening throughout the rest of the day. If your serum morning cortisol level comes back low, you know you are going to need some help in this area. Even though saliva is a less than optimum testing choice for other hormones, it is the best way to test for cortisol since it can show what is happening throughout the day. Your doctor does not need to write a script for one of these saliva cortisol tests, which tests your saliva four times throughout the day. They can be bought online. I ordered my saliva cortisol test through www.ZRTlabs.com.

Basically, you want your first reading of the day to be at the top of the range and your nighttime reading to be near the bottom. Many people with fatigued adrenal glands have results that come back in the opposite way, low in the morning and high at night. This causes the common issues that many experience of being unable to sleep at night and fatigued in the morning. Taking the supplement phosphatidylserine at night and using pregnenolone or Cortef in the morning can help reverse that situation and create a more natural rhythm.

If your 24 hour saliva test comes back showing low cortisol throughout the day, with no morning spike and two or three of the four measurements low, this is a good indication that some bioidentical supplementation is needed. You were probably over-generating cortisol for years, and at this point, you are essentially running out.

Cortisol Delivery Methods

You can ask your doctor about a pregnenolone cream, or try an over the counter pregnenolone cream as this may help raise your cortisol. Or you could try taking a 25-50 mg over the counter pregnenolone tab. As previously mentioned, pregnenolone is a mother hormone that may help cortisol levels because it fills hormone buckets when they are low. Cortisol is not too far downstream from pregnenolone. Theoretically, if pregnenolone levels come up, some of that should spill over and raise cortisol.

If pregnenolone does not work, your doctor may want to prescribe some bioidentical hydrocortisol or Cortef (they're the same thing, Cortef is the brand name). These tablets can be swallowed in 5 mg doses, usually four times throughout the day.

If you are very low in cortisol, supplementing it back into your body is important. Or, you will need to make extreme lifestyle changes to help your adrenal glands regroup. Without enough cortisol we simply cannot survive. Do not confuse hydrocortisol with the strong steroid prednisone. They are completely different.

Pregnenolone

Although this is the chief mother hormone of the body, I have saved it for last. Dr. Uzzi Reiss notices that most patients he sees have negligible and sometimes undetectable levels. Pregnenolone spreads itself very thinly as we age, trying to fill all the buckets of our declining hormones. Most of us don't have much left after our twenties. Optimum pregnenolone levels should be close to 200. Dr. Reiss sees many people with numbers in the twenties or less.

It's a good idea to test pregnenolone to have a reference point for when you start supplementing the hormone to see how much of an increase occurs.

Pregnenolone is important, not only for enabling healthy cortisol levels, but in order to reduce high cholesterol levels. As the mother hormone, it puts cholesterol to work, causing it to make other hormones rather than just sitting around. It boosts memory and cognitive skills, helps generate new brain cells, and helps arthritis pain. In the fifties pregnenolone used to be doctor's pain relieving choice for their patients with arthritis. They prescribed very high doses for sufferers of arthritis until cortisol was discovered and found to be more effective.

Pregnenolone Delivery Methods

You can purchase an over the counter pregnenolone cream under Life-Flo brand online or in some health stores. Each dose gives 15 mg and this is enough to do the job for many people. Others, however, are fast metabolizers of hormones and need far more. A doctor can prescribe a 10 percent compounded pregnenolone cream to allow for much higher doses if needed.

Pregnenolone tablets can be purchased inexpensively and do not need a prescription. Dr. Uzzi Reiss puts most of his female patients on at least 50 mg per day, best taken in the morning.

Chapter 34

Foxy Mama

by Pearl Barrett

Prelude Dilemma

I have to admit we had much discussion back and forth between our publisher (Hi, Mom!) and Serene and me as to whether we should include this chapter in this book, or make it available separately for purchase. Our main concern wasn't because sex is too delicate a subject, but because we know your teenage daughters may want to read this book and will love trying out the recipes.

We finally came to the conclusion that healthy intimacy with your husband is foundational to being a *Trim Healthy Mama.* We recognize there are various comfort levels in sharing this subject with your daughters, and also the timing of the sharing. This chapter is definitely "girl talk among close friends," so we'll leave it up to you to decide if your older daughters are ready to read this section. Simply ask them to skip the chapter for now if you do not feel the content is age-appropriate for them. Or, paper-clip these pages together.

We Need to Talk

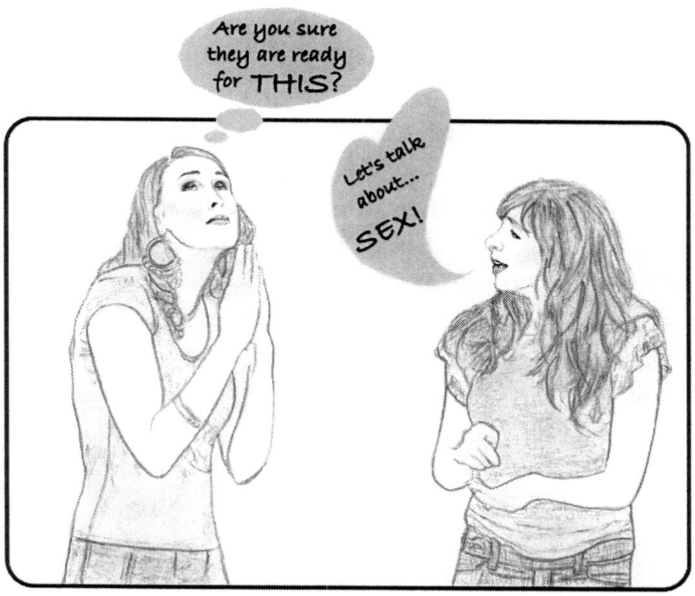

I have noticed that sex is a subject seldom discussed within the circles of Christian women. That's a shame, because as followers of the Scriptures, married couples can have the most exciting and meaningful sex lives of all. We have a God-given guideline explaining how to have long lasting sexual intimacy.

Similar to the way in which Serene and I discovered the simplicity with which the Bible tells us what to eat, we also found it very plainly advises us about married sex.

You'd think there would be a lot of good healthy instruction on the topic of married sex for Christian women. There is more biblically-based information trickling out in recent years, but on the whole, there is still a lot of silence, confusion, stereotyping, and an entrenched sense of taboo about this subject. Also, as with most subjects, the authors and speakers brave enough to broach the topic have vastly different opinions.

Overall, I think the sex subject is frequently avoided because it is not considered a very "spiritual" matter. As a result, many have not yet tapped into the beauty and importance of married sexuality. God designed it and sanctioned it after all. We shouldn't feel embarrassed to bring up sexual issues, challenges, and questions in appropriate company. You're a mama, and so am I. I'd say that makes us appropriate company for well-needed sexual discussion, so it's gonna happen right here. This is not the blatant sex advice you see splashed on women's magazines like Cosmopolitan, but coming back to God's original plan for womanhood.

Shake off the Shackles

The Bible is not a prudish book. God does not dance around the subject in either the Old or New Testaments, and one entire book is completely devoted to His way of sex and intimacy. If the Bible tackles this subject head-on, why shouldn't we?

If you're a little uncomfortable with this chapter at first, it's my hope that by the end of it you will be more relaxed about the subject, possibly have a change of heart (if your heart needs a-changin'), and feel inspired enough to share the good news with others. And, since we know each other better now, I might have a little wiggle room to raise my voice a bit. Got things to yell about!

Whenever my sisters and I speak on this topic at women's seminars, we notice a lot of mouths dropping at the beginning of the session. "You didn't just say that!" Oh, yes we did! However, at the end of the session most of the ladies have become more comfortable. All around, there are smiles, laughter and of course, some tears from challenged hearts. It's really hard to stay uptight when my sister, Evangeline takes the microphone. If you have heard her speak, you are nodding right now.

Gotcha

Regaining your health and your weight is great. Learning new tips and tricks to feed your family is helpful, but if your sex life is left in the dust, we have done you a disservice in our nearly five years of putting this book together. We don't want to get you all revved up in the kitchen to make more healthy foods and consequently be even less revved up in the bedroom.

So read on, Mama. I think you will soon see why we need to brush the cobwebs off this "married sex" topic and shine it up "real nice." As a married woman you'll see 1) why you need it, 2) why you need to give it gladly, and 3) why God wants you to have lots of it.

It's your Attitude that Counts

While we discussed lagging sex hormones in the previous chapters, lack of sexual desire in marriage cannot always be blamed on declining hormones. Yes, we should address our sex hormones if they are lacking so we can be the optimum possible for our husband and ourselves. Hopefully, you'll now have a better direction as to how to go about doing that. At least, if you're over 30, try out DHEA to see if that gives your libido a boost, if boosting is in order. Also, if you have a dry painful vagina, ask your doctor for a natural estriol cream, or seek one out for yourself online.

A healthy libido is a wonderful thing, but people can sometimes have perfectly tuned hormones and still have a selfish attitude toward their married sex life. I know of women who have addressed their lacking hormones, got themselves hormonally tuned up, then poured all their extra energy and gusto into everything else but their intimate relationship with their husband. Many times low sex frequency stems from a wrong mindset and I can't very well discuss sex without touching on this subject

Many women fill their lives with activities. They run around here and there, depleting their energy, and have very little left to give their husband. He's the last on their list. They are often gracious about giving anyone else their time, but think 20 minutes of intimate contact in bed with their husband is too much of a bother.

Honestly, Mama, if you have time to help out at a church function, bake for a family in need, scrapbook, or pursue some other hobby for an hour or so—even brush your own teeth and have a shower—but you don't have the same amount of time for enthusiastic fun in bed with your husband, what's wrong? Your priorities are upside down! Definitely brush your teeth and have a shower, but, you got my point. Forgive my verbal spanking, but I care deeply about your marriage, and as you continue reading I will offer you a way to turn your priorities right side up.

It Starts Today

You're not yet at your ideal weight yet? Don't wait until you think your body is perfect enough to start building a better sex life. It is likely your husband does not have the same perfectionist ideals that you do and is attracted to you just as you are. You're on your way to a healthy sized body now if you're following the principles outlined in this book. The journey toward your healthiest weight will be only benefited by having a greater understanding of married sexuality and living it out.

I don't get it when a wife believes her husband should be okay with being sexually rejected, rationed, avoided, and rebuffed, and yet expect him to still be an affectionate, happy, and helpful guy around the house. Are you kidding? If your husband is often rebuffed sexually and is still Mr. Nice guy, he's a saint! You'd better show him pronto what he means to you for hanging in there and not turning into Mr. Jerk. If he currently is Mr. Jerk, let's see what we can do to help change that.

The Scriptures Say . . .

The Scriptures in 1 Corinthians 7:3-5 discuss married sexuality. We should probably memorize them and take them seriously to heart. They remind married couples that their bodies are not their own, but rather under the authority of their spouse to enjoy whenever desired. Ironically, I grew up a PK (pastor's kid) and heard these Scriptures many times, but their significance did not hit me until years into my own marriage. It was like seeing them for the first time. Here they are for you, just in case you don't believe me . . . *"Let the husband render unto the wife due benevolence: and likewise also the wife unto the husband. The wife hath not power of her own body, but the husband: and likewise also the husband hath not power of his own body, but the wife.*

Defraud ye not one the other, except it be with consent for a time, that ye may give yourselves to fasting and prayer; and come together again, that Satan tempt you not for your incontinency."

According to these Scriptures, your body is essentially your husband's and vice versa. If he desires to make love with you, you are his to enjoy. Of course, if you are sick, he would hopefully be respectful of your situation. I know this may sound rather "cave man" in this modern age, but it's in the Bible, and God has good reason for the admonition. This injunction goes both ways in your marriage. There is no free pass to either gender. The same thing applies to your husband when you desire him physically. You may be thinking, "My husband doesn't need any encouragement in that area, I'd rather not discuss these Scriptures with him." This may be the current dynamic in your relationship, but it is not always the case, nor does it need to remain that way.

Silent Anguish

Although I'm not writing to men as this book is addressed to women, I do need to address an issue concerning husbands before we continue. It is rarely mentioned out loud, but some wives feel alone and ashamed with the secret that their husband does not desire them sexually. The last thing they want to hear is the advice to wear something sexy to bed so their husband will magically find them desirable. They've tried that, and more, to no avail. There is a common stereo type that all husbands constantly want "it" and wives should give in now and then to make their guy happy. Yes, it is true that a husband can tend to have a higher sexual drive, but it is not a rarity for the scale to be tipped the other way. I want to acknowledge that these situations exist and I will not ignore the mamas who live with this pain.

Male hormone loss can be a common cause for low drive and will be addressed in the next chapter, *Don't Forget Your Man.* Hang in there if this is your guy. That chapter also deals with issues like erectile dysfunction, often resulting from the rising epidemic of Type 2 diabetes.

Another reason for infrequent initiation by a husband can be the result of a basic lack of understanding about biblical spousal requirements. This can show up in both men and women as a selfish mindset when it comes to sexuality in marriage. Not all men are wired to constantly want sex, believe it or not. Without a biblical mindset on the subject, these men may not understand the hurt they inflict by holding on to the power of their own body, rather than surrendering it to their wives.

Pornography can be another sex-life robber. Sometimes extreme pornographic addictions result in a man becoming wired to only receive sexual gratification from stimuli other than his wife. Men in this situation may abandon normal sexual function with their wife for visual erotica over the internet. In some cases, the man ends up in a state where normal intercourse is no longer possible, so he avoids it. Past sexual abuse can also be a reason for a damaged healthy sex drive, as can some medications like blood pressure meds and antidepressants.

Men who have low testosterone, a selfish sexual mentality, a serious pornography addiction, or a damaged sex drive from sexual abuse are in need of help. These problems seldom, if ever, clear up on their own. Do not sweep the issue under a rug, due to shame, if this is the case in your marriage. You need to communicate plainly, yet kindly, that things are not okay the way they are and you'll both need to work together to get help. God wants better for both of you.

I would suggest you become extremely proactive about finding help for your husband. Refuse to allow this darkness to continue in your marriage. Don't resign yourself to a sparsely-sexual or non-sexual marriage. Please find a safe and wise counselor, such as an older woman or pastor, to share this burden with so you can begin the road to healing. A turnaround will take a determined "let's get better together" approach. Be prepared for resistance. Men often find this subject very difficult to talk about. They can feel worthless and "less of a man" when they do not feel they can sexually satisfy their wife. Give diligence to avoid contributing to these feelings, yet be firm in your resolve for change. Ask his opinion about where you should both start to a path of healthier intimacy.

Back to you, Mama

Put this anguish that some women live with on the other foot and you've got the situation that many men face day after day, month after month, year after year. While they might not express their emotions in the same way as females, they are still hurting. Many of them think that's just the way it has to be for guys. They may not be faced with outright rejection from their wives (although this is far more frequent than you'd think). Often men are up against their wife's lack of interest or a general reluctance to celebrate their sexual union.

Let's go back to 1 Corinthians 7:3-5 where the Scriptures paint a picture of complete yielding. Giving the "power" of our body over to our husband emulates being completely surrendered, willing, and open before God. It's a type. Just as we give over control of our own lives to God, we mirror this surrender physically with our sexuality in marriage. A person who lives the 1 Corinthians 7 way chooses to think differently about their own body. After all, life is about choices. We can direct our own thinking, and thus the course of our lives, and the contentment and well being of our spouse.

How about adopting one of the following mindsets?

"My spouse is the captain of my body. So when he wants to sail, let's sail!"

Or, *"I am not the gatekeeper of my own sexuality. I place the big old gate key I have been carrying around in the hands of its rightful owner."*

Or nix the metaphors. Perhaps something more practical will resonate with you. *"When my spouse desires me sexually, there is no book that can't be put down, no text or phone call that can't wait until later, no TV show that can't be turned off, no hobby or craft that takes greater importance, no ipad touching or computer game playing that is more important. I am willingly his and he is mine."*

Reading things like this may sound extreme because they are in such stark contrast to our current culture where most married people believe they are in charge of their own body, and their own time. But, this way of thinking is not a burden. It is a joy—and the pathway to freedom! If you hold all the cards in your marriage regarding when you and your husband make love, you are only doing yourself and him a disfavor. Lay down your power! According to God, it is not yours to wield.

Of course, there are certain times when you may need to give your spouse a rain check for a near future time if you're helplessly tied up with something. But hopefully, your rain check will not be past the next day or two.

Let's not get hung up on exceptions. I'm guessing all sorts of scenarios may come to mind right now that seem valid reasons to not have sex. I'm sure you have a considerate enough husband who will understand that once you've got the baby to bed, you'll be ready. And yes, if you've recently given birth, you're not expected to make love to your husband! As in all areas of life, common sense applies. There will naturally be consensual breaks after childbirth and during menstruation. There will be times when your husband will understand if you're absolutely exhausted due to circumstances beyond your control. Hopefully, you can give that same understanding back to him when he offers you a rain check for a not too distant time when he is wiped out. Times of grave illness or mortal disease are a whole different category and are true grounds for consensual sexual abstinence.

This 1 Corinthians 7:4-5 way of life is not about legality. Instead, it encourages a heart attitude adjustment. It's not about clinging to exceptions and a bunch of rules about when, where, and how you will or won't make love to your husband. It simply instructs spouses to willingly surrender to one another. We don't need to complicate it with a long list of "but what ifs."

Who is in Control?

I love how the Scriptures deal so clearly with the problem that many secular books on sexual intimacy grapple to find solutions. If these Scriptures (1 Corinthians 7:3-5) are not practiced in marriage, the lower-drive spouse in the marriage almost always controls the sex life. You can pretty much bank on that.

The spouse who needs more sex plays a constant "waiting game." They wait and wait for their partner to be "in the mood." Sometimes it feels like the stars must line up before their wife or husband concedes that the circumstances are finally right for them to have sex. Rape is wrong of course, even in marriage, so if one spouse doesn't feel like "doing it," there's not too much the other spouse can do about it. They can either continue a life of waiting or get out of the marriage, as many do. Hello, high divorce rate!

Sex therapy books offer wide and varying advice for ways to work around this common problem in marriage. Instead, the Bible cuts to the chase with a novel idea—*your body is not your own*! Give away the power. What a notion! Once again we see the simplicity and common sense of the Bible as amazingly profound.

For couples who do not put themselves under the authority of the Bible, I imagine that sex therapy, sex counseling, or a lot of book reading on the subject would be necessary. All sorts of psychotherapy would be in order because the question of who holds the decision to have or withhold sex can unravel into a complex issue. More challenges usually arise which reveal even more issues to resolve. Thousands of conversations are spent discussing the whys and wherefores of a dismal sex life without a solid resolution. Tail chasing. Vicious circles. No answers.

I don't know about you, but obeying the simplicity of the Scriptures seems like a much smarter and less painful route to sexual equality and satisfaction in marriage, not to mention the effect on the pocketbook!

Does it sound a little scary to give over the power of your body to your husband? What's the worst that can happen? What if he's a real high drive guy and wants sex every night? What if—oh no—he might want it both morning and night? Good for you, if that's as bad, or should I say . . . as good as it's going to get. You will be physically blessed and your health will flourish as a result (you'll learn about this in more detail soon). Typically, most men aren't going to chase their wives all day, every day, even if given the green light. They have work, church, family obligations, and they get tired too. By the end of this chapter, I hope you're doing some chasing of your own.

Desire is Unreliable

Interestingly, 1 Corinthians 7:3-5 does not mention physical desire. The passage doesn't say spouses have authority over each other's bodies, unless one of you is not in the mood. A good married sex life does not rely on physical desire as the only green light for sexual go-ahead. Physical desire is fickle. So many interruptions can squelch it such as a burned supper, a late bill, a trying afternoon with the children, a late night, or an argument. Sometimes you may find yourself yearning for your husband in the afternoon while he's at work. You can hardly wait until he gets home to make love, but by the time you fall into bed later that night, you're beat. Sex is the last thing on your mind, yet he is suddenly in the mood.

These are the times we can draw from a deeper well than the more shallow depths of physical desire. At these times we can be secure in the knowledge that it's a good thing we aren't captain of our own body, otherwise we'd be inclined to mumble, "Goodnight" rather than whisper, "Come a little closer, Honey!" Let your husband know that you are available if he needs you. Obviously, you don't have to make love every night, but if it's been a few days, that's probably not healthy and you need to keep the flame of your love glowing.

Roommates or Lovers?

When you married, you merged into what God calls "one flesh." Couples owe it to each other to practice being "one flesh," whether or not strong physical desire is always present. Without sexual intimacy, you are just roommates. This is not God's plan, nor His picture for marriage. Marriage is a picture of the close intimacy between Christ and his bride. If you're not being intimate with your husband in the way God planned from the beginning, you're not revealing this picture.

I recommend taking time throughout the day to think positive sexual thoughts about your husband. Getting primed up sexually is a decision. Focusing on his faults lowers your desire for him. Concentrate on his good points. He does have some! You may have just forgotten them. Remind yourself daily of his attributes and spend time dwelling on them.

When he's home it's a great idea to make it a priority to not pass your husband in the house without giving him some sort of touch. This conveys love and respect and also keeps your brain and hormones more primed for sexual activity. If fatigue hits you when the opportunity for lovemaking finally arises, you will have a better emotional and physical foundation on which to act.

What's so hard about sex that it should be considered another chore? It's awesome, fun, God-given, clean, pure, and as you'll find out soon, sooooooo good for you. Your husband may know that you are willing, but he also needs to see that you are wanting. Believe me, you can adjust your thinking to turn yourself into a "wanting" wife. You can learn to "pour" on loving sexuality toward your husband, rather than only offer a trickle here and a drop there. Does he deserve a "shower" of love? You bet. He's your husband! He may not be perfect, but he is precious.

Get Out of Those Sweats

Sometimes, it's a matter of getting back in touch with your own sexuality and not being in constant mom mode. Are you constantly wearing "mom" type clothes when he'd like to see you in something sexier now and then? You don't have to show your curves to the rest of the world, but your husband certainly needs to see them. I know myself that when I'm wearing baggy sweat pants and old T shirts, my hair needs washing, and I haven't applied makeup, that I don't usually feel sexually inclined. When I take time to restore my disheveled appearance, my sexual feelings often return. I feel more lovable once I look my best and I feel like I'm more able to give love.

The way you dress and look can really make a difference to how sexually primed you will be for your husband. It's possible your husband may still find you sexually attractive in a disheveled mess (although he deserves better), but you will not find yourself very sexually attractive or eager for a romp in this state. Thinking and acting more like a temptress can be as practical as changing your clothes into something you know inspires appreciation in your husband.

Remember, you are a wife first and you will still be your husband's lover when the children have grown—hopefully (with me yelling in your ear). Learn to be a better lover. Work on these skills. Why not? No man should have to put up with a prude for a wife, nor a wife to have a prude for a husband.

Make Room for your Husband

Maybe it's time to take some extreme measures if you no longer have much desire for your husband. I suggest completely wiping your event calendar if it is preventing you from a healthy sex life. We've talked much about needless carbs in this book. Much of what might be contributing to a too-full plate that barely allows time for sex with your husband can be looked at like macaroni and cheese. You might think you need it because you are used to it, but it's not the best option. It only harms your health. You need to get rid of it and make more room for protein.

I look at married sex as the protein we continually need in order for our marriages to grow and flourish. Protein repairs damage to our cells. In the same way sex helps repair the little distances that grow between husbands and wives. It knits them back together, closer and stronger.

A 2003 report from the *Kinsey Institute for Research in Reproduction, Gender and Sex* located in Bloomington, Indiana brought to light a developing problem in our society. Married women these days are having much less sex than their 1950's counterparts. The report revealed that only one married woman in three now makes love to their husband more than twice a week. How dismal!

Look how far we've come. Every grocery store isle has magazines flashing "sexual how to's" but it sure isn't improving the state of the marriage bed. Oral birth control is now common place so women can have sex without worrying about pregnancy. Surely that would increase sexual frequency! No so! The pill has stripped fertility, along with normal sexual desire, and now there is less sex happening in marriage beds.

Things were simpler for women back in the 50's. It was normal to get married and actually settle down. It was rarer for women to have jobs, or even second cars. Consequently, they didn't cheat themselves or their husbands out of sex nearly as often. Today, women get married, but there's not a lot of settling down. Instead they are busy, busy all the time. I'm not saying we should sell our cars, wipe out all outside activities, or not contribute to family finances in some way, but most women take on too much. It's ironic that the women's movement, with its agenda of liberation, has actually caused a major regression in sexual intimacy in marriage.

Free yourself up as best as you can to focus on your husband and your sex life. A great, HOT, sex life is integral to the health and stability of your family. Everything else stems out from the two of you being secret, crazy lovers. I notice the difference in my own inclination for the wonders of sex with my husband when life is consumed with all the things that need to be done, done, and done. Once my too-full plate is stripped back to manageable levels, I find myself dwelling on and planning for this important part of our relationship again.

You can learn to be better organized, a better homeschooler, a better housekeeper, or a better Sunday school teacher. All those things are good, but insignificant compared to the need for better intimacy with your husband. Sexual intimacy cements and protects your marriage. Look at it as the superglue that keeps your marriage tightly intact. With a tightly glued marriage, your children are far more protected from the heartache they could experience from parental breakup.

Maybe you're thinking, "Well, a great marriage is not all about sex." No, it's not everything, but when you get down to the core of things, it's a huge part of it. It's what separates marriage from all other relationships. No other person can fill your husband's need in this area—it's your job, or should I say, your delightful task. It's time to start taking it seriously. You'll have a lot of fun at the same time if your attitude is in the right place.

What's Love Got to do with it?

The three of us older sisters were discussing the topic of sex one day. (Our youngest sister, Mercy is not yet married, so she wasn't in on this conversation. When she sees our conversations heading toward sexual issues she walks speedily out of the room). My sister, Evangeline mentioned how she had discovered a real gem of truth in Titus 2:4, the familiar Scripture directed to wives, *"That they may teach the young women to be sober, to love their husbands, to love their children . . ."*

This Scripture exhorts older women to teach younger women to love their husbands, and then to love their children. Evangeline noticed that husbands come first. There is nothing happenstance in the Bible. God puts everything in the right order. The word "love" in the Greek is *thilosteeknos*, which means "to be a friend, to spend time with, or as we say these days, "hang out with."

Where does your husband want to hang out with you? As we asked ourselves this question, each of us grinned and agreed. Yes, there's one place most men like best. If I were a betting woman, I'd wager that your husband enjoys your company most of all in bed—and with your clothes off! Yeah, I said it!

This same Scripture goes on to encourage women to be pure and keepers at home. However, those admonitions are further on down the line. After the encouragement to be sober, which means to have sound understanding of God's plan for you as a woman, "love your husband" is at the top of the list. It comes before everything. You cannot love your husband properly without loving him sexually. In marriage, love and sex are intertwined. The two cannot be separated. Your love for your children, friends, and parents can be demonstrated in many ways. Your love for your husband has one huge distinction—married love was designed by our Creator to be sexual at its core. That is what God means by "one flesh."

You may believe you are showing enough love to your husband by speaking kindly, preparing his meals, spending time with him, and asking about his day. They're all great things to do, but he can get those forms of love from anyone else. If they are all in place of "the real thing," I'm sorry, but to put it frankly, you are not *really* loving your husband. Those other ways of showing love are excellent in their own merit, but they are a shoddy replacement for sex itself which is the nucleus of married love.

Actually, how can I be sorry for saying that? We are commanded (not asked) in the Bible to love our husband. Therefore, we'd better include the one thing that separates married love from all other relationships. When you decided to marry, you essentially promised to be a sexual person. You can't change your mind half way through your marriage. You signed up for sexuality when you said "I do." If you do not think of yourself as a sexual person, it's too late to go back and get unmarried, unless there's very real cause. Therefore, lest you be guilty of "defrauding" your spouse (as the Bible states in 1 Corinthians 7:3-5), it's time to make things right.

Now that I am stepping on toes, I may as well keep going. I have to admit it that irks me when I hear some women talk about their Quiet Time with God in the mornings. They're very religious about taking time alone in the morning to have devotions, pray, and keep the intimacy they crave with Christ alive. Sadly, I've often heard such women complain about the intimate time their husbands want with them for sex.

You might guess by now that I don't keep my mouth shut when I hear this. Taking time to minister to your husband sexually is holy. Quiet Times in the mornings to pray and read the Bible are important, but in that same Bible God tells you to love your husband in a "one flesh" relationship. Obedience is God's love language.

Maybe you attend prayer meetings at church, or you're on the worship team. You're witnessing to your neighbors. You're hosting ladies meetings in your home. It's all very Christian-like. However, the Bible says in the famous love chapter, 1 Corinthians 13:1 that if we have not love, all our religious acts are like *"sounding brass and tinkling symbol."* To put it bluntly, we're full of baloney!

Am I pushing over the "comfy" cart? Sisters talk like this to each other, don't they? At least, my sisters and I do! We don't dance around the topic when something needs saying.

Who are you taught to love <u>first</u>? Can I say it again? Your husband. Make him and his needs your top priority and you're doing something God cares about deeply. The rest will naturally follow. You can still reach out to others and show Christian love to them, but don't forget the order in which you do things.

I believe this is why the Apostle Paul mentioned it was better for him to be single. Married folk are required to first meet the needs of their spouse and then the needs of others. This takes time, effort, and cultivation. Paul had a huge job to see to the needs of the early church, to travel far from home for years at a time and to write a whopping 14 books of the New Testament. It's no wonder he was called to a life of singlehood. His life would not have been fair to a wife, nor a stable foundation for intimacy. It's probably fair to say it would have caused a wife anguish and pain. If you are married, your priorities are different from Paul's calling. So, if you don't have a lock on your bedroom door, run (don't walk) to your nearest handyman store and purchase one. You are going to need it very soon.

Grown up Sex = Faith Sex

A good, married sex life doesn't happen by itself. It does at first, when you're in the throes of early love and everything is new and exciting. Remember how easy it was when children weren't waking you up during the night and you had yet to hit the hard bumps of marriage, where life stresses kill natural sexual spontaneity? Things changed, didn't they? Relying on spontaneity, or only having sex when the feeling strikes will eventually take you down the road to a waning sex life and that ultimately leads to a sad and struggling marriage. This is true for both husband and wife. Men get tired, stressed, and overwhelmed with life's cares, too.

There comes a time for all of us, when the art of married sex needs to be relearned. This calls for "grown up sex," or sex with a mature mindset. The urgency for passion between a husband and wife dwindles after a year or two. It's the natural way of things. However, something far greater can take its place. This is not what is portrayed in the movies, on TV, or even in most romantic books. In those instances, it is usually the newness of relationships that is celebrated and romanticized. A certain look between a couple causes sparks to fly and next thing you know . . . clothes are coming off. Mature sexuality no longer relies on feelings that inspired sex at easier times in our lives. Grown up sex is based on unselfish commitment to each other and lots of practice!

Our sex lives need to be protected against laziness and disinterest. They need to be valued for their priceless worth. They need to be fought for tooth and nail when they are threatened. They ought to be constantly watered and fed, so they can grow rather than wilt, and, of course, prayed over very frequently.

Once we step out in faith and behave in a giving and loving sexual manner with our husband, whether we have the specific physical desire or not at that moment, our body will catch on. You'll have a great time— give yourself the opportunity. If you do not feel interested at first, simply open yourself up to getting that way. Please don't act like you'd rather be reading a book, be asleep, or be anywhere rather than being sexual with the man you married.

Having an enthusiastic attitude (and I don't mean you must suddenly jump all over him if you're tired, but that's fine too) means having an open attitude toward your husband when he reaches out to you. Receive his sexual affections with delight, rather than with a "not again" attitude. Science tells us that when we smile, we actually release "feel good" brain chemicals throughout the body. Smiling, even pretend smiling, releases endorphins and serotonin. It works on a positive feedback loop. The more you smile, the more "feel good" chemicals are released.

The same principle applies with "faith sex." You *decide* to be a sexual person. Forget the mindless attitude of "I guess I'd better do this because I should," which can lead to feelings of resentment and backfire on a healthy sex life. Instead, step out in faith, armed with the full knowledge of why cultivating intimacy is so important. Keep the positives in mind. Once you act like a sexual person, your body will start signaling to all its various parts that you *are* a sexual person. Our intricately designed bodies back us up with their amazing feedback loops when we step out in faith. Thankfully, God designed us to receive great rewards from this "faith sex" as you will now find out.

The Health Factor

Since this book is titled *Trim Healthy Mama*, we could not leave out how huge sex can be in creating a healthier mind and body. Nor could we omit sharing about its incredible anti-aging abilities. Not only is a healthy sex life important for the wellbeing and health of your marriage, it is equally as important for the wellbeing and health of you and your husband physically. The health benefits of monogamous sex are astounding. Basically, the more sex you have within the confines of a committed marriage relationship, the better off both you and your husband will be. God made sex to be a fantastic swapping of gifts. In spectacular ways, you and your husband give perfectly designed presents to benefit one another's health.

Semen . . . Gotta Love it!

After doing much study on this subject, I now hold my husband's semen in incredibly high esteem. I know that probably sounds strange. You might think I've fallen off the deep end, but hold on—I have good reason for this belief. Semen is a health tonic like no other, and thanks to God's great design, and my husband—it's free. Why pay ridiculously high dollars for some health elixir at a vitamin store when you have a better, more potent health promoter, and mood brightener at home?

Semen is incredible, not only because it contains life-giving sperm, but it's also a potent fluid, full of all the things God knows a women needs. The vaginal walls are one of the most absorbent areas of your body and your husband's semen gives you a shot of incredible healthy goodies that are absorbed directly into the blood stream, promoting positive changes in your mind and body each time you receive his ejaculation.

Semen contains many necessary minerals and it is loaded with zinc which helps to build your immune system. It has high amounts of vitamin C and B12 which nourish your adrenal glands and promote better energy and ability to fight disease. It contains three major cancer fighting agents. The first two are selenium and glyco proteins. The third is TGR beta (transforming growth factor beta), a molecule that can increase the number and activity of "natural killer" cells in your body. These killer cells recognize and then fight cells that promote tumors. All of these are rapidly absorbed into your bloodstream after sex. Too cool!

A 2002 study at the *State University of New York* suggests that semen acts as an antidepressant for women. The study which was published in the *Archives of Sexual Behavior* showed that women who had sex without condoms had fewer signs of depression than women who used condoms, or abstained from sex.

Youth and Beauty

Semen also has nutrients that plump up your skin and strengthen your hair**.** But, it's not only semen that helps promote a more ravishing appearance. The very act of sex with your husband offers many appearance enhancing benefits on its own. Sex pumps oxygen around the body which boosts circulation and the flow of nutrients to your skin. This gives you a more radiant complexion and smoother skin. Go look at yourself in the mirror after sex and you'll likely see a rosy glow about yourself.

In fact, if you want to take at least six years off your looks, monogamous sex is the way to do it. Dr. Oz, the famous television surgeon, appeared on The Oprah show and announced that having sex 200 times a year (which is about four times a week) can reduce the physiological age for both men and women by an average of six years. He bases this on a study from *Duke University* that surveyed people on the amount and quality of sex that they had over time. Think about it—six years younger! That's not only a regain of younger skin; it also includes regenerated internal organs and a younger mind. Who doesn't want that? Dr. Oz believes it is not only orgasm that is responsible for the reduced physiological age, but he attributes some of the benefits to the spiritual bonding that sex provides between two people in a long term relationship.

Another study headed up by Dr. David Weeks, a renowned Scottish neuropsychologist from the *Royal Edinburgh Hospital,* found even better results for appearance. It revealed that both men and women who reported having sex four times per week on average looked approximately 10 years younger than they really were. This was a large study that spanned 10 years with over 3,500 people, ages 18-102.

HGH (human growth hormone) starts to decline after our early twenties, but every time you have sex with your husband, it triggers the release of small amounts of this hormone. Perhaps it is partly this release of growth hormone that is responsible for the "younger you" that sex provides. HGH helps decrease wrinkles in skin and makes it less prone to sagging. It also increases lean muscle, while decreasing fat.

Burn the Calories

Sex even goes a long way to help your weight control. Cardio wise, sex is the equivalent of going for a brisk mile walk or doing 15 minutes on the treadmill, and it's a lot more fun than those two options. The state of arousal caused by sex raises the heart rate from an average of 70 beats per minute to 150. This is about the same as an athlete putting forth maximum effort. The result? You burn about 200 calories. Awesome!

Female Stress Buster

Oxytocin, a hormone that is released during sex, fights feelings of stress. It is a bonding hormone, the same one that is released when you breastfeed your baby. It contributes to that strong sense of attachment you feel for your baby while you nurse and the ability to relax while your other children are pulling the house down around you. This bonding translates over to your husband during sex and creates the actual "feelings" of love and connection to him and vice versa. It helps to reinforce the reasons you were drawn together in the first place, lest you forget them with the business of life.

Oxytocin brings a sense of calm and fights depression and anxiety. It's God's own female stress buster. Studies looking at the benefits of oxytocin report that it reduces "neurotic tendencies." I know I need that, especially after a hectic day, or maybe before a hectic day. While oxytocin becomes elevated in your husband during sex to a certain degree, you get a much greater five-fold increase. God knows we women need a heftier dose!

A Natural High

Endorphins, which create that feeling of "a high," or extreme happiness, are released in large amounts during sex and orgasm. Endorphins are natural pain relievers, similar in effect to morphine. If you are one who experiences headaches, you are much better off having sex than avoiding it. Try this next time, "Honey, I have a headache, can we get naked?"

Endorphin release is part of the reason researchers believe that arthritis sufferers who have frequent sex have less pain from their condition than low sex arthritis sufferers. I talked to a woman recently who told me sex relieves her terrible fibromyalgia pain. For some time, during and after making love with her husband, she does not suffer so much.

It should be noted that studies reveal that it is primarily married sex where these health benefits are reaped.

Estrogen to the Rescue

What other blessings do you receive by having sex with your husband? It actually increases estrogen in the female body which helps your vaginal tissue stay moist and the PH of your vagina stay in a healthy zone. A series of studies carried out by Dr. Winnifred Cutler at *Penn* and *Statford* universities in the 1990's showed that regular love making could double a woman's estrogen levels.

Estrogen also increases female feelings of flirtiness. This may be why more frequent sex for females actually causes the desire for more frequent sex. This is true in my case. What do you do when you flirt? You smile more, which in itself releases "feel good" chemicals into the body. Smiling at your husband makes him feel loved and more like your hero. When he feels like your hero, it's easier for him to show love right back at ya! Oh yeah, he's going to love it that you read this chapter. I predict his bad moods may significantly decrease.

These surges of estrogen, produced by sex, help to sharpen the mind, strengthen bones, increase skin collagen, and restore emotional wellbeing. Dr. Uzzi Reiss, in *The Natural Superwoman* writes, "In my experience, bioidentical estrogen is the most ideal antidepressant medication available to women." That's a pretty big claim from this renowned doctor, considering that the medical industry makes billions from antidepressants. It seems there is a better way.

Long dry spells without sex can actually lower a woman's sexual desire. Remember this: frequent sex for females causes the desire for more frequent sex. It's an intricate cycle set up by the fascinating interplay of our hormones and neurotransmitters. Science is now only beginning to scratch the surface on how all of this works. The way God designed our bodies keeps blowing me away!

Studies show that menopausal women who have more sex have better natural lubrication and less vaginal pain and discomfort, that's estrogen to the rescue again. The raise in estrogen may also be part of the reason sex makes positive changes to bladder health and fights incontinence, as lack of estrogen causes both those issues. The physical side of sex also helps to alleviate incontinence problems by toning the muscles that are responsible for bladder control. All that tensing on the way to orgasm helps create nicely toned pelvic muscles in females. Did you realize that similar muscle control during sex helps create six pack abdominal muscles for men?

Breast Health

The fact that your husband likely finds your breasts fascinating can really help your health and prevent disease. God made breasts desirable to men for both purpose and pleasure. You might have seen the studies that show breastfeeding significantly reduces cancer risks. Dr. Halid Mahmud, author of *Keeping aBreast: Ways to PREVENT Breast Cancer* has further surprising information on this subject. He suggests that nipple and breast stimulation from your husband is also important in fighting this disease.

In a transcribed interview in Suzanne Somer's book *Breakthrough*, Dr. Mahmud says, "If people would have their breasts stimulated or massaged regularly . . . there is actually scientific evidence that it increases the secretion of oxytocin, which not only helps remove pent up secretions from the breast ducts, but also fights breast cancer in several ways." You don't even need a full orgasm to increase oxytocin. We like those, of course, but even a little breast play from your husband causes your body to make more of this fascinating hormone.

Dr. Mahmud explains that fluid in the breast duct becomes stagnant and the contents break down and release free radicals. The job of these free radicals is to cause DNA damage to the cells. Once DNA damage occurs, the cells become abnormal. He goes on to say, "That is why I stress breast massage and nipple stimulation to keep the fluid moving."

You know your husband has a natural knack to make this happen. It's fantastic if he treats your breasts like his favorite toy. It's not weird or wrong if he wants to have his own turn at your breasts even, while they are lactating. If he likes the taste of your milk, you need not make him feel like a pervert. What on earth is wrong with that? You may be having babies and either pregnant or nursing for a decade, or even two. You don't need to make your breasts off limits to your husband just because they are lactating. Look at Proverbs 5:18-19 which speak beautifully on this subject and hopefully shed some unneeded hang-ups and taboos, *"Let thy fountain be blessed: and rejoice with the wife of your youth. Let her be as the loving hind and pleasant roe; let her breasts satisfy thee at all times; and be thou ravished always with her love."*

According to the Strong's Concordance, the Hebrew meaning for "satisfy" in this Scripture means "slake the thirst or take the fill." It also means "to bathe in, to make drunk, to water, to soak, and to satiate abundantly." Notice the constant emphasis on liquid, thirst, and satisfaction. If your husband wants to take that literally, he's not being unbiblical! I also like the word "fountain" that is used. It underscores the attitude of pouring on sexual love, rather than puttering forth a trickle here and there. Fountains are constantly flowing.

Now, please don't take what I'm saying the wrong way. I'm not advocating some strange, husband breastfeeding cult. I'm sitting here wondering how many horrified letters and emails I'm going to get! Your husband may have a lessened interest in your breasts while they are lactating. All couples are different. I don't want to paint every married couple with the same brush strokes, how boring. I'm just saying, "Shake off the hang ups." You are one flesh after all. Biblical truth is not uptight. It is natural. Allow your marital intimacy to flow in a natural way. Don't be like the Sadducees and Pharisees that made a bunch of laws up themselves and acted as if God made them. Give your marriage bed the beautiful freedom that God ordained.

When Jesus was being questioned by the religious leaders, He answered one of their questions about marriage with, *"Have ye not read, that he which made them at the beginning made them male and female . . ."* (Matthew 19:4).

The word "female" that Jesus used simply means "nipple" or "to give suck." You are essentially a nipple! Of course, a lot more than that, but I like the definition. Big, small, or in between, it doesn't matter, God thinks your breasts are wonderful enough to define you as female.

The word breast is used many times in the Bible and is associated with nurturing and comfort, or it can also refer to the chest area, as on a man. But, in Proverbs 5:19 the meaning alludes to the actual shape of the female breast and has the definition as "the seat of love." I think that is beautiful. I love that God put such thought into molding the shape of the female breast so they could symbolize the "seat of love" for our husband.

Your breasts are an integral part of God's "one flesh" plan. Sharing your breasts with your husband is a natural and bonding part of your relationship that creates protective health benefits for you. However, I shouldn't really say, "your breasts." They're not actually yours, but your husband's also as we learned in 1Corinthians 7:4.

Breasts were designed with purpose. They were not supposed to be left alone. If you are a married woman, they are not supposed to sit hardly moving in your bra all day and under "do not remove" frumpy PJ's all night. Babies keep your breasts healthy by nursing, but so does your husband in his own manly way, even after you are finished with the nursing years. The marriage bed allows nipple stimulation to be a perfect give and take. It's likely your husband enjoys touching your breasts, and for your health's sake, you need him to fondle them a lot.

Healthy Sex Life = Healthier Husband

What about health benefits for your husband? One of the largest studies ever conducted on longevity and sex was carried out in Wales and cited in *The British Medical Journal*. It found that men who had sex less than once a month had double the risk of dying prematurely than those who had sex two times a week. Scientists think one of the reasons for this life extending benefit of sex is that in the male body, the hormone DHEA rises up to three times the regular level just before orgasm. DHEA is a master hormone in the body and has immune building effects. It helps create a blue print in the body for fighting disease and aging so our natural killer cells can be smarter about their attacks on diseases that try to afflict the body. Essentially, DHEA creates a smart battle plan against the ravages of disease rather than just random fighting.

Another decade long study at *Queens University* in Belfast found that men who had sex three times a week were half as likely to die from heart attacks or stroke than men who had less sex. Sex strengthens the heart, helps to regulate blood pressure, and has a positive effect on the tone of all blood vessels. Research from Wilkes University in Pennsylvania found that both men and women who had sex at least once or twice a week contracted fewer colds and flus than people with less frequency. The research showed that the higher frequency folk had

30 percent greater levels of an antibody called immuglobulin A which is known to boost the immune system.

Here's the biggie for your man. Sex protects the prostate from inflammation and cancer. Much like the situation I described with stagnant breast fluid, the prostate can be vulnerable to a buildup of cancer-causing compounds when it gets too stagnant. Sex flushes out the accumulation of these dangerous compounds. Ejaculation for a man is essentially cleaning the pipes, and this is crucial.

A *Harvard University* study showed that men who had 20 monthly ejaculations were one third less likely to develop prostate cancer than men with lower frequencies. Some researchers have theorized that sex releases psychological tension that quiets the nervous system, which when agitated, may contribute to prostate cell division and cancer growth. Now, if you're doing the math like me, this study works out to having sex five times a week! Okay, that's a little difficult to achieve for some of us, especially if you have little sweethearts that like to climb in bed with you. Jobs and other life circumstances don't always allow for such frequency. But, there are ways for the willing and it's certainly not impossible. Some weeks, you might achieve that sort of frequency; others might post numbers even higher than that! Then there are other seasons when life just gets in the way.

The saying goes, "If you shoot for the stars, you'll reach the treetops." Maybe you won't ever manage five times a week, that's okay. However, consensus seems to be that fewer than two ejaculations a week for men can lead to inflammation of the prostate where the seminal fluid can turn into a rancid state and raise the risks of prostate problems.

There are no norms for married couples as to sexual frequency. Some couples are happily loving each other every day, others are very contented with a couple of times a week. However, if one spouse is unhappy with the sexual frequency, it's up to his or her spouse to step it up a notch and help their partner feel less neglected. Did I just say "less neglected?" That's pathetic of me. I should say "fully cared for."

It appears from the vast majority of studies on sex that major health benefits are only truly experienced when it is quite regular, in most cases, at least two times a week. Personally, I think that when sexual frequency is lower than that number, it is not enough. I'm probably the lone voice going out on a limb to say such a thing, but my opinion (for what it's worth), is that healthy sexual frequency starts at two times a week. I base this assumption on the studies I have mentioned and the science that reveals that we are blessed by natural health benefits of monogamous sex when it is highly frequent.

The Challenge

If your frequency is less than two times a week, you owe it to your husband and to yourself to step it up and do your part to protect him from prostate issues. But, more than that is the even greater reason of living out the design God created for marriage. I issue this challenge to my friends, so here it is to you, too. Make it a goal to seduce your husband two times each week!

Please hear my heart. I don't want to encourage you in married sexuality only to place my own heavy law of "You shall have sex two times a week" on your life. This challenge is merely an idea, a proactive way of living out your new understanding. This is your gift to your husband. If he wants to initiate other times, that's great—the more the merrier! It also takes the pressure off him. See if you can race him to initiate. Planning is half the fun! I know that can be harder for women who have husbands with very high drives. He's so busy pursuing you that it's hard to get the chance to pursue him. But, that could be because things have only been the way they have been, and he is yet to experience the love you are capable of giving.

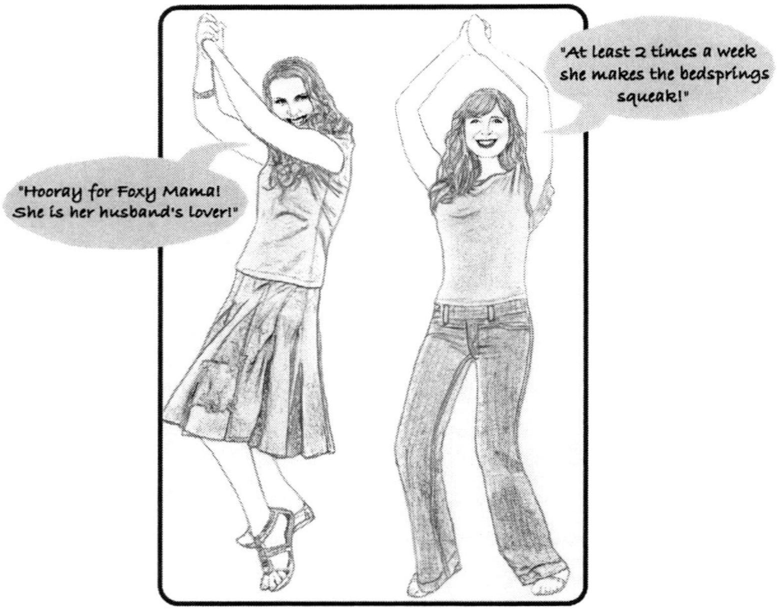

The *Trim Healthy Lifestyle* is all about being practical. Taking measures to ensure you are sexually bonding with your husband at least twice a week is not too ridiculous a goal. It ties in with the doable approach to food and exercise that we promote. If your sex life has been seriously dwindling lately and the idea seems a bit daunting, look at it another way. There could be five days each week when you won't be having sex. Implementing this idea into your life won't leave you constantly between the sheets without time to do anything else. It's only going to add joy, not take it away. It's only going to add health, not take it away. It's certainly only going to add love, not take it away.

My mother constantly confesses, "Things don't just happen; you have to make them happen." You have to also take time to think and plan on how to enrapture your husband. If your husband enjoys lingerie, settings, music, or even dancing, why shouldn't you bless him this way? You might be laughing right now as you picture yourself looking ridiculous, shimmying for your husband in a belly dancing outfit. Would he think it silly, or just you? And even if you both get a good laugh, that's fine. Sex shouldn't have to be so serious all the time, and it's good to laugh at yourself. I've made a fool of myself plenty of times and my husband only loves me the more.

We pour our creativity into our lives, homes, and hobbies. We plan, practice, and hone our skills. Why do some of us cut all this off in the bedroom? Something is wrong! Why not celebrate intimacy? We celebrate food in this book. We encourage seasonings to make food taste even better. Chicken is a great food in its own, but it tastes even better with salt, pepper, and spices. Likewise, spicing up our sex lives is only natural. Why, as people made in the image of our creative Father, would we stifle creatively "seasoning" this area of our lives?

Practice Makes Perfect

The marriage bedroom is where creativity can really shine. Throw away your pride and embarrassment and be "a fool in love" for your man. You'll probably feel like an idiot at first, but remember the smiling phenomenon? Play the part and your body will start to believe it. Think about how to seduce your husband. Try out the role. This doesn't mean you should put on a French accent and wear a "naughty maid" outfit (unless you really want to, of course), but God created you sexually and you only need to tap into it. If it is not natural to you at first, it doesn't mean it won't become natural with time and practice.

Let me tell you, I don't always feel like being a kind, patient mother with my children. I'm far from a perfect mother, but I certainly don't allow myself to act the way I sometimes feel (such as tearing my hair out and yelling for everyone to leave me alone and give me some peace!) I determine to be kind to my children and remind myself to be patient because that is what children deserve from their parents. They don't deserve a mother who doesn't at least try her best to be nurturing and loving, even when she doesn't feel like it. Likewise, just because we don't necessarily feel like a sexy wife, it doesn't mean we should not seek to be sexy to our husband. It is what a husband deserves, simply because he is a husband.

We can all learn, grow, change, stretch ourselves, and emerge into *"new creatures in Christ."* If there's anything in this book we want you to absorb, it is this: just because something does not come naturally to you, it doesn't mean you give up thinking "that's just not me." You can learn with knowledge and practice to manage your weight and health. You can also learn with knowledge and practice to become more of a foxy mama.

Wise Advice

I've been blessed to converse with a woman I consider to be very wise. She and her husband are both in their fifties now. They have wonderful, fulfilling, and very frequent sex. Sounds all rosy and perfect, right? Actually, things were far from perfect for the first 25 years of their marriage.

This woman's husband was a wonderful father to their biological children and also to the special needs children they adopted. He loved his wife and family, did not abuse alcohol, or chase other women. He was kind, pleasant, church attending, and a great guy to be around. But, he had little interest in sex. He could physically have sex, but seldom had the inclination. Every couple of months or so, his body would tell him it was about time, and he would show some interest in his wife, but long, dry spells were more common.

This very attractive lady described to me her agony over decades of not feeling desired by her husband. She would sleep completely naked next to him and not even this would spur any sexual response from him. She tried everything, from trying to endure her situation with patience, grace, and much prayer to crying, demanding more attention, and eventually considering separation. He always promised to do better since he loved her devotedly, but things would revert back to the way they were.

Six years ago, when things were at their bleakest, her husband had his blood tested for a testosterone deficiency and it came back dramatically low. Apparently, he had an injury as a teenager to his testicle area that was never fully investigated by physicians. He probably never made as much of this important hormone as he should have in his adult life. Age had caused what little he had to decline even further.

Once he started testosterone therapy, the complete sexual transformation in her husband was astonishing. He finally felt and acted like a vital, sexual male. He began chasing her around the house! Five years later he is still very amorous toward her and this woman feels she is the luckiest lady on earth.

After his sexual awakening, he mentioned to her that he loved her in heels and that looking at her legs when she wore heels turned him on. This wise woman promptly went out and bought a lot of very comfortable heels and whenever she is around her husband she wears heels—she even does her gardening in them!

Now gardening in heels may sound extreme, but she takes none of her husband's sexuality for granted. It gives her such joy and honor to be the one who turns him on that dressing in whatever manner he finds desirable is never too much trouble. It reminds her of the awesome miracle that occurred between them. She is constantly thankful to God because she knows how bleak her life was when her husband had little sexuality.

Meat and Potatoes

The above mentioned types of stimulation don't matter to some men. It would be silly to force something like erotic dancing or stiletto heels on your guy if he's not into it. Maybe your husband has a more meat and potatoes approach to sex. What will bless his socks off? Ask him, if you've never actually taken the time to find out. You might be surprised what he'd like, or what he doesn't.

If he's not into skimpy lingerie and high heels and he prefers you simply clean and naked, then make sure you get clean and naked for him. Be bathed and clean soap smelling with all the parts shaved, waxed, or permanently lasered that help to make you feel more alluring. I'm sure you have a say in whether or not your husband keeps a beard or is clean shaven. Do you know your husband's preference for your intimate parts? We trim our yards, prune out trees, style our hair, shave our legs—it's human to take care of things. Hopefully, you're equally as caring about the areas only your husband is meant to see. Maybe he doesn't mind either way. That's fine, hair or no hair, or somewhere between the two, it's what makes you feel more sexual and alluring.

Grooming yourself for sexual purposes, rather than only to look "proper" at church, helps reinforce and remind you that you are sexual. It can also increase confidence and is an important part of the "faith sex" mentality. We do these things, not because we are always consumed with desire (it's nice when we are), but mostly out of obedience to being yielded and available to our husband.

Queen Esther literally spent one year preparing herself for her night with the king. You can bet every detail of her body was attended to. She saved a nation by making herself pleasing to her husband. Taking time to enthrall and seduce your husband can make him feel pepped up enough to go out and change the world.

Older women are supposed to teach younger women how to love their husbands. Having just turned 41, I don't feel old, but I do feel compelled to set right the lack of sound information there is on this subject and yell from the rooftops to every wife, "Hey, give your husband great sex!"

It's Doable

Captivating your husband need not always be a big event. We may not always take the Queen Esther approach. Busy seasons in life don't always afford large amounts of time and planning. Please don't throw up your hands and say, "I don't have the time and energy for all that," and overwhelmed, do nothing at all. Let's be honest, it takes five seconds to slip on something sexy before bed. Sometimes a cute outfit and a "come hither" smile are all your husband needs. Or, tell him what you're going to do to him that night—and follow through! Touching your husband frequently throughout the evening can also be another simple, yet wonderful, form of seduction.

Be sure to make things really special on occasion, or as often as you are able, but just keeping a bold, flirtatious, and seductive manner toward your husband is the most important thing. Also, be honest with yourself about your time constraints and keep in mind the check list. Are you taking time to help out with church functions? Are you finding time for reading, hobbies, and time with friends? If you spend more time playing with your iphone rather than "playing" with your husband—then tut, tut. You can think of me waving my finger at you and giving your derriere a friendly boot.

Extra Effort

If you have experienced a miserable and scant sex life in the past years of your marriage you may need to go the extra mile to create a clean slate. My challenge to seduce your husband twice a week is probably not going far enough to reverse the tide of your sex life. I came to know a woman who, due to shame over things she had done in her past life, never really embraced her married sexuality for the 10 years of her marriage. What an amazing change happened in her husband's general demeanor after she changed her attitude and began to live the 1 Corinthians 7:3-5 way of life.

We talked about things she could practically do to remind herself that her marital intimacy was going to move in a whole different direction. Not all of these ideas may work for you, but if you know you need to drastically make changes then adopt some of these ideas.

Buy a Lock

Take ownership of this change by buying that lock I mentioned earlier. Don't rely on your husband to attach it to your door. It's easy enough to do it yourself. This is a sign to him that you are now taking your sex life seriously.

Watch your Privacy

If you have allowed any of your children older than two years to set up permanent residency in your room, it might be time to think about finding them a place of their own to sleep. The "family bed" idea can be taken too far and sometimes children can begin to have control over parents that is not healthy for a marriage. Of course, your door will only be locked during certain times, so little ones can always have access to you when they need you. Remember, according to Titus 2:4, husband first, then children.

Older children in their teens need to be aware that they cannot rule the house late at night, especially if your bedroom is in close proximity to where they like to "hang out." Yes, they like to stay up as they get older, but they need to be taught to give their parents respect and alone time. We have a rule in our house that our older ones need to be in their room and retired by 9.30 pm on week nights. This does not mean they need to be asleep, but it does mean they cannot wander the rest of the house, destroying privacy. This way, you do not have to wait and wait and wait some more until everyone is in bed before you can feel free to make love with your husband. Your teens will not be deprived; it gives them more time to read in their bedrooms and improve their mind.

A New Bedspread

Think about removing and tossing the cover on your bed into the trash if it is where you have avoided and refused your husband. Turn over a new leaf—or cover, so to speak—and buy a new bedspread. Choose a color that speaks of intimacy and passion. You needn't spend a lot of money; think thrift stores or yard sales. This will be a reminder and a symbol of your new goals.

Create a Boudoir

Use your creativity to turn your bedroom into a seductive boudoir. Create a setting that speaks romance and fun. If your room is chaotic, cluttered, too feminine, or too boring, change it up so that it literally feels charged with sexual energy to you, and hopefully, to your husband.

I'm sure Serene won't mind me mentioning her creativity in this area. Just as many of her recipes are exotic, so is her bedroom. She has draped her walls above and around her bed with luxurious fabrics. It looks like a Bedouin tent, fit for a sheik. All over her richly painted walls, she has painted prose and verses that speak of love and romance. The Song of Solomon is quoted in beautifully painted calligraphy on her walls and ceiling. She has incense and candles ready to burn and Middle Eastern music in the stereo ready to be played, to set the final touch to the scene.

I'll admit, my own bedroom is nowhere near that level of creativity, but my husband is the "country boy" type and is not inspired by that style. One thing we do have, which I will encourage, is a noise maker. This is used to block out any noise that you and your husband will hopefully be making when you get together—and the rest of the family does not need to hear. You could also play music, use a high powered fan, or suitable TV station (if you have one in your room).

Surprise Him

Establish a bedroom wardrobe. It needn't be expensive. You'd be surprised at the awesome bedroom wear thrift stores have sometimes. Collect new items your husband has never seen you in before, or if you have the talent, sew some yourself. You can buy a lock box to have beside your bed with intimate lotions, etc., to make sex more pleasurable and sensuous.

Age Factor and Sexual Difficulties

There will often be challenges as we move past our twenties and thirties. Sex is not as physically easy as it once was. But, don't let age slow you or your man down. My husband is 56 now, (15 years older than me) and sex for us has only become better, and on a far more deeply bonding level as the years have passed.

Don't think that my husband and I have not had our share of health, hormonal, and emotional challenges that we have had to help each other through in order to keep this intimate part of our marriage strong. I am not writing this chapter because things have been naturally easier for us than other couples. I don't speak from a lofty soap box. I speak as a woman who has known pain along with joys in my marriage. Both my husband and I have had to dig in our heels and fight to keep this integral bond when faced with challenges and circumstances that would have stolen it from us. Sexual intimacy can grow rather than wane with the passing of years, but an attitude that's proactive toward working through, or around, both physical and emotional issues is necessary.

Do I think things will be perfect from here on out in this aspect of my marriage? No. We had to slay some giants to get to this place of fullness that God wants married couples to enjoy. There will likely be more challenges. But, anything good is worth fighting for.

It's important not to let things slide to a standstill if you are having problems, and merely hope things will turn around on their own. Complacency is a healthy sex life killer. Letting awkward silence fall between you and your husband over sexual problems, due to embarrassment or shame, will only cause the issues to continue or get worse. Be proactive and seek hard for solutions. God will help you find keys if you diligently pursue answers. He wants you to have a great sex life.

While we can stay as fit and trim as possible, our bodies, brains, and faces will be touched by time in various ways. Imprinting our changing selves in our partner's minds and hearts is the key to making great married sex last. Sexual imprints can only occur when sex is highly regular. Our breasts may not be as perky, but they are the ones we constantly give to our husband, so to him they are still highly sexual. Our husband's physique may not be quite what it was when he was young, but if his body is frequently crushing ours in loving passion, then these are the wonderful sexual images to which we respond. A mind that has been hardwired by the fervent love of a spouse, rather than images of porn or fantasy about others, is one like the Scripture in Proverbs 5:19 which is "always captivated."

Shame—Sex Life Killer

Some women I have talked to have the notion that very creative and exciting sex is for the promiscuous. Now that they are "nice Christian" wives, they just lie there and are no longer adventurous. Sex becomes something that simply happens sometimes, a sort of sanctioned meeting of genitals. They may have had pasts, where they did things before marriage that they are not proud of, so now they revert to the opposite extreme and try and remove themselves from who they used to be.

Or, they may have grown up with false religious ideas that sex is "dirty" and the subject was always awkward or taboo in their home. Carrying these burdens of shame into marriage is not fair to the spouse. They should get the best of our sexual creativity and willingness, not the "leftovers." We should not let our past continue to ruin our present and our future. My heart grieves for sexual abuse survivors, but it is still important to get sound Christian help and be proactive toward moving forward for yourself and your husband.

The marriage bed is not a place for shame and guilt. Hebrews 13:4 makes this clear, *"Marriage is honorable in all, and the bed* ***undefiled*** *. . ."*

The Greek word for undefiled is *amiantos*, which means "pure and unsoiled." Interestingly, it is the same word used in Hebrews 7:26 describing Christ, our High Priest, *"For such an high priest became us, who is holy, harmless,* ***undefiled****, separate from sinners and made higher than the heavens."*

The Bible actually uses the same word to describe your marriage bed as the spotless Lamb of God himself. If that doesn't dispel your shame, I don't know what would. It is the place for freedom and great pleasure for both of you. There are no "nasty or dirty" parts to you or your husband. God created every part of the male and female body and called us *"very good"* (Genesis 1:31).

Very Precious

Don't overlook the word "*honorable*" in Hebrews 13:4 either. It is the Greek word *timios*, which means "costly, esteemed, most precious, and accounted of great price." The love and sexual union between a husband and wife is precious in God's sight.

There are always at least two witnesses to Scripture in the Bible. I love the way the Bible always agrees with itself. Hebrews 13:4 is no exception. It simply expounds on what was already laid out clearly in the Old Testament. If we return to Proverbs 5:18-19, where we read of the husband always being satisfied by his wife's breasts, we see that the context of the whole chapter was intent on instructing a young man to steer clear from any woman other than his wife. The chapter shows the contrast between God's blessing on the sexual union in marriage and the curse on any sex outside of this union.

Hebrews 13:4 explains the same thing in the second part of the verse. It separates the undefiled marriage bed from any sexual act outside of marriage by a colon which indicates a different situation. It states, *"But whoremongers and adulterers God will judge."*

God makes it simple. Sex in marriage equals blessing. Sex outside of marriage equals judgment.

Real truths are uncovered by looking at the original Hebrew manuscript. Let's look at the word "ravished" from Proverbs 5:19, *"Be thou ravished always with her love."* Here it is used within the context of God-sanctioned intimacy. The word is used again in verse 20, but in the negative context of adultery or with wayward women, *"And wilt thou my son, be ravished with a strange woman, and embrace the bosom of a stranger?"*

Surprisingly in both cases, the ancient Hebrew word for "ravished" is *shagah*. Its meaning is not what you might expect. It means to "stray or transgress (through the idea of intoxication), to be enraptured in a way that causes one to go astray, to reel as in drunkenness, and it signifies the staggering gait expressing the ecstatic joy of a captive lover." The inference once again is that the sexual union between a man and his wife is sanctioned by God and intoxicating pleasures are the name of the game.

A similar point is established with the word for "breast" that we read earlier in Proverbs 5:19. Remember, it means "the seat of love." Of the four times this particular Hebrew word is mentioned in the Bible, all are sexual in context, but three times the word is associated in a negative context of idolatry and adultery. God is not pleased with the situation and uses the sexual breast to show the whoredom that he hates. But, in Proverbs 5:19 the inverse happens with this word for "breast" as it does with the word "ravish." What God hates in the other three examples of the sexual breast, He smiles upon in the marriage bed.

We don't have to wonder what God thinks about it. It's clear that in marriage sex is blessed, smiled upon, and is the place where you lead your husband to intoxicating pleasure. Hopefully, he leads you right back. Why on earth would we destroy what God thinks is pure by a needless sense of shame or repulse?

I can't resist sharing another beautiful example of how the Bible agrees with itself in both Old and New Testaments. The yielded sexual "power" of spouses of one to another revealed in1 Corinthians 7:3-5 is also clearly and beautifully portrayed in Song of Solomon 2:16, "*My Beloved is mine, and I am his: he feedeth among the lilies*." The word "mine" depicts ownership or control. She owns her beloved. He owns her. How perfect.

Resist the Flesh

While we are taught as Christians to *"put off the flesh,"* this theology should not be transferred to the marriage bed. Sometimes in Christian circles, I hear people talking about "sexual gluttony" in negative tones, even in the context of marriage. Men are made out to be such vulnerable creatures to sexual sin that the wife's job is to temper their appetites. Wives should not even wear sexy outfits to bed and don't allow things to be too thrilling—that could be a slippery slope into depravity. Good grief! Yes, as Christians we must allow Christ to help us overcome laziness, temper, pride, etc., and steer clear of sex outside of God's boundaries. But, this doesn't mean we should dampen our sexuality within marriage and turn it into a non-creative act.

The art of "ravishing" that Proverbs talks about cannot occur when sexuality is tempered and watered down. Is the following thought familiar to you? Several women have verbalized this to me in their own words. "My husband is too sexual. It will be good for him to go without for a little while. He needs to concentrate more on his spiritual life rather than his constant sexual appetite."

We are not our husband's judge and it is our job to creatively celebrate his sexual appetite rather than sneer at it. God put testosterone in men for good reason and they temper it when they keep their sexual advances and desires toward you only and not other women. How excellent if your husband brings all his sexuality to you and heeds the warnings in the Bible against adultery. How could that be a bother when he is doing as God asks? Surely, it wouldn't be preferable if he were a eunuch?

Take Action

Think about a young baby. He or she needs lots of touch, kisses, hugs, and almost constant skin to skin contact to flourish and develop normally. Who would want to deny a baby of such natural, physical love? That would be a form of abuse. The needs for affection and sexual intimacy in marriage are also God-given. Why would we want to harm our spouse's natural growth and maturity by denying, defrauding, and tempering what is only natural and essential?

Are you enrapturing your husband with your love as expressed in Proverbs 5:18-19? Do you notice that it is the wife's love that is the action in these Scriptures? The husband is "ravished" by his wife! I told you the Bible is a pro-sexual book, and it becomes more evident as we understand the real "jewels" of the Hebrew. It inspires the wife to not only give a responsive sexual love and willingly yield to her husband's advances, but to actively captivate him and make him drunk with love. She is to bathe him in her love. She can lead him astray from the problems and burdens of the day as she transports him to a place of delight.

The Common English Bible translation of Proverbs 5:19 says, *"Let her breasts intoxicate you all the time; always be drunk on her love."* Do you have an intoxicated husband?

Here's one more picture from God's point of view in case you are not yet convinced. Song of Solomon 4:9 says, *"Thou hast ravished my heart my sister, my spouse, thou hast ravished my heart with one of thy eyes."* Who is doing the ravishing? Again, it is the bride. The Hebrew word for "ravished" in this Scripture is *lavav* and means "to take away or transport the heart with love." The same word is also used "to be wise and intelligent." It is the wise wife, seeking to build her marriage and home, who takes time to enrapture and ravish her husband with delights.

That is why I suggest the idea of seducing your husband a couple of times a week. It's a practical baby step toward this greater understanding of the healing power of a wife's love. As hearers and doers of Titus 2:4 where we are commissioned to first love our husband, we see that "love" in this Scripture is a verb. Proverbs 5:19 also gives a glimpse into the nature of that verb. It is pouring on infatuating love to completely "ravish" the husband. Can you imagine the changes in marriages that would occur if this was commonly taught to Christian women?

Your husband will feel like the most blessed man in the world when he sees you delight, desire, kiss, and caress him. He'll feel sorry for all other men and won't even be able to tell them why. It will be his joyous secret. You are the only person who can make him feel the luckiest man alive! To put it candidly, a woman who brings this joy to her husband is a better picture of a "nice Christian wife" than the one who looks and acts so piously in church services, but gives her husband the cold shoulder in bed.

Begin to initiate more communication with your husband on this subject. You'll likely have to be the one to do this, as many men are not as verbal (another stereo-type, I admit, but it holds water for a great majority of men). Generally, men are doers rather than talkers. If you need information, it may not be the best approach to ask 100 demanding questions—that could be a turn off. Gently find out what he loves and desires, even if it feels awkward at first to discuss these things. If you find it difficult to talk about these things, adopt an attitude of trial and error. Try new outfits, positions, and scenarios. Try not to be offended if he doesn't appreciate some of them. Logically assess his reactions and store your information in "this works" versus "this doesn't" department of your brain.

Let your husband know what you love and need sexually in return. Please don't criticize him if he doesn't do things exactly as you want, but you can kindly lead him to understand what makes you purr. Your husband may have a vague idea about what you like, but maybe you need to open up to him about what really works. It's okay to be a little bold. Your husband wants to send you over the moon with pleasure. He needs to be your sexual hero and you have to let him know how to do that.

It's time to wear something that will delight your husband, give him some prostate protection, and cure yourself of being neurotic in the process! Go for it!

Chapter 35

Don't Forget Your Man

by Pearl Barrett

If your husband is young and still full of vigor, this chapter may not apply to him so much. However, you may have a father who will benefit from some of this information. Regardless, it's good practice to be armed with knowledge so you can be better prepared to help your husband as he ages.

While menopause for women is a lot more obvious, men go through similar changes only they occur at a slower rate. Testosterone levels begin to decline steadily in men after age 30. Anti-aging doctor, Jonathan V. Wright has authored several books on hormones. In the book, *Stay Young and Sexy with Bioidentical Hormone Replacement*, he writes about the male hormone decline called andropause, versus female decline, "By contrast, andropause is a much more gradual, almost imperceptible process, usually beginning during men's 40's and following the slow but steady decline in testosterone secretion by the testes. Each man follows his own unique pattern, of course, but sooner or later, the results are pretty much the same for all."

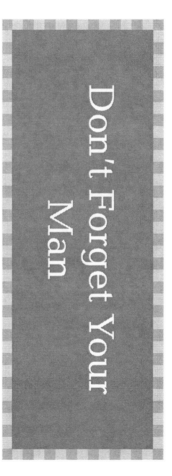

The Check List

If your husband, or father, is over 40 and showing signs of lack of interest in things that used to give him joy, it is a warning sign his sex hormones might be in steady decline. If he has a few or more of the following conditions, then low T could be the culprit—depression, muscle wasting, increasing abdominal fat, sloping shoulders, couch potato syndrome, lack of drive or vitality, decline in libido, erectile dysfunction, fatigue, and irritation at things that he could let slide in the past. Or, if you sense that the man he was is fading away, encourage him to get a hormone panel taken. That might mean making the appointment for him.

Tests

Here's a very basic list of the main hormones that should be tested for a male. It's important to test both total T and free T levels.

Total T (Testosterone)
Free T or bio-available T (Testosterone)
DHEA (Dehydroepiandrosterone)
Estradiol (E2) (Estrogen)
LH (Luteinizing Hormone)
FSH (Follicle-stimulating Hormone)

Do not let a doctor tell your husband or father that because his levels come back within range that everything is fine. The ranges set for total testosterone encompass men from 18-80, usually ranging from 250-900. Let's say your guy is showing many low T symptoms, yet his tested levels come in between 300-400. While that may be in range, it is more likely the average of a 70 year old man, with all the problems 70 year old men complain about. Most of the averages taken as given ranges for these labs are from men who were already exhibiting negative symptoms.

The Bottom Line

Any total T result less than 450 could signal a real decline and your man may have a lot of trouble tackling life properly at these levels. But like us females, male bodies are unique. While one man may function okay between 400-500, another man may have severe low T symptoms at that level. He might be functional with that number if all he had to do was lie on a hammock on an island all day, but I don't know any guy who has that option.

When testosterone levels decline, cholesterol levels usually go up, coronary artery dilation diminishes, insulin levels rise causing greater abdominal fat, both strength and energy decrease, and the heart is at much higher risk for disease. My several years of study on this subject suggests that functional total T levels start at around 500 for most guys and many men require quite a bit higher than that to regain their free T into healthy levels.

Dr. Eugene Shippen, a doctor who specializes in male hormone therapy and author of the book, *The Testosterone Syndrome*, explains that very few men have testosterone levels that stay at or near youthful heights right into old age. Dr. Shippen says, "I have never seen an older male in excellent mental and physical health whose testosterone levels were not well within the normal range. And the healthiest, most vital individuals are always in the high normal ranges."

If a male is to have an optimum quality of life, he usually needs to be closer to the top third of the range for total testosterone and free testosterone. This will be much closer to 600-900 for total levels. Healthy T levels will go a long way to help restore lost drive and give him back a great deal of his youthful gusto. The need for diabetic medicine is often cut in half or completely eliminated when testosterone is restored. Cholesterol levels drop and LDL (lousy cholesterol) often declines as much or more than 30 points.

Human growth hormone and testosterone are the only two hormones that construct repairs in a man's body. When a man's T declines, he cannot heal as fast or recover from daily wear and tear. Simply put, he weakens. That is why restoring this hormone helps to prevent age related diseases. A man with higher T levels is much better equipped to fight them.

He Doesn't have to be Superman

If your husband is not showing low T symptoms, he should not seek to elevate his levels in order to achieve a "superman" state. Some body builders, who push their T levels to extreme highs through the use of steroids, pay dearly when their endocrine systems crash and sometimes cannot be restarted. Natural hormone therapy is about finding a healthy balance for both males and females and only restoring what has been lost over time.

Do not confuse testosterone therapy and steroid use. Putting these two in the same category only fuels unfounded fears. The "roid rage," which you have likely heard the media associate with steroid users is not applicable to testosterone therapy. Most men who regain their missing T levels find their moods and happiness improve, leading to less anger, not more.

While oral, synthetic testosterone has been associated with liver problems, this is definitely not the case with bioidentical testosterone. As with female natural hormones, it is exactly the same as the hormone the body makes and in no way negatively affects the liver.

The Prostate Myth

Natural testosterone therapy can reveal a prostate cancer that is already there, but testosterone will not cause it. Surprisingly, the latest studies on testosterone and prostate cancer show a positive effect on active prostate cancer and testosterone therapy. Men in their late teens and early twenties have the highest levels of testosterone and prostate cancer is almost unheard of in this age bracket.

Prostate cancers rise when men begin to lose more and more of their testosterone. Sometimes during this latter season of male life, estrogen levels also climb. This is thought to be one of the imbalances that causes prostate troubles. Keeping a man's testosterone levels healthfully elevated, and his estrogen levels in check, is one of the best ways to avoid prostate cancer. That is, along with lots of married sex as we've already discussed in the previous chapter. Couldn't resist that dig!

Before any man starts TRT (Testosterone replacement therapy), he should have his PSA (Prostate Specific Antigen) levels tested and have a digital rectal exam to rule out prostate cancer. Most doctors will not prescribe testosterone for men with active prostate cancer, but there are some more progressive doctors who are realizing that T supplementation has been shown to improve mortality rates in prostate cancer patients and has no impact on making the cancer any worse.

One of the latest studies on testosterone and prostate cancer was released in the *Journal of Endocrinology* in 2011. It followed 13 men with untreated prostate cancer who also had deficient testosterone levels. These men were started on Testosterone and monitored for a median of 2.5 years, with many follow up tests and biopsies. The results were startling. There was no local prostate cancer progression or distant disease in any of the men in the study. But, here's the huge piece of news, which is turning the urology world on its head. There was no cancer found in 54 percent of the follow-up biopsies. The cancers had disappeared!

Dr. Morgentaler, of Men's Health in Boston, writes of the study, "These men were rigorously followed. The cancers in these men were typical of the prostate cancers for which men have undergone invasive treatment with surgery or radiation for 25 years. Clearly, the traditional belief that higher testosterone necessarily leads to rapid prostate cancer growth is incorrect."

Different Testosterone Therapies

All men are unique in their response to various testosterone treatments. There are now several safe ways of delivering this hormone into the male body. Personality can play a big part in what treatment will work best for a man. Some forms, like pellets, may cost a little more, but after the brief procedure of a small incision in the skin, a man can take a more "fix it and forget it" approach. Gels need to be applied every day, but provide the most natural rise and fall of the hormone. Injections are by far the cheapest route. Let's take a more in depth look at some of these methods.

Gels and Creams

Trans-dermal methods work well to restore libido and give a good sense of well being and energy. Dr. Crisler, anti-aging specialist and founder of the All Things Male Center in Lansing, Michigan, advises his patients to try a trans-dermal testosterone product first, as this application is more similar to the rise and fall of a young man's testosterone throughout a 24 hour period.

Androgel and Testim are commonly prescribed testosterone gels that are often covered by insurance for men with low T. Both these gels come in 1% strength while more recently Androgel is available in a slightly higher delivery strength.

Most doctors will start a man out at four pumps of Androgel (five grams), but men often need double that dose to feel right. Blood should be tested again at the four week mark to see if levels have risen sufficiently. Both symptoms and blood levels need to be considered as every male will have a different response.

If lack of insurance is an issue, a doctor can write a script for a compounded 10% testosterone cream. The Life Extension Foundation pharmacy will compound such creams which costs about $20 per month if you send in your doctor's script. Put this in contrast with the large pharmaceutical company-made products like Androgel that cost between $300-500 per month without insurance. There are sure to be local compounding pharmacies in your area if you do not want to send in your script to a larger compounding pharmacy like LEF. Local compounding pharmacies usually charge about $30-$40 for a one month supply of trans-dermal testosterone.

Men with young families need to be mindful when applying gels or creams to keep the application areas to unexposed areas of their body. If a man has young children in the house, or a pregnant wife, he should not expose his family to freshly applied skin. Shoulders and upper arms are the most common applications sites and a simple T shirt covering these areas will prevent unwanted transfer. Also, most gels and creams are completely absorbed within four hours, so if a man applies his gel in the morning, goes to work for the day, then climbs into bed shirtless with his wife some twelve or so hours later, transfer is not an issue.

Some other downsides to gels and creams are that some men do not absorb them well, especially if they have thyroid issues as that tends to cause thickened skin. Exfoliating the treated areas beforehand with a loofah may help make the skin more absorbent enabling more of the hormone to enter the blood stream. If, after raising gel dosages, along with exfoliating applications, T levels still do not respond, then another form of testosterone will be needed.

Pellets

This delivery system is growing more popular among men because they do not have to worry about daily applications of gels or transferring the hormone to their wives or children. Upsides to pellets are that they are usually highly effective in raising T levels to young, healthy levels. They are also less likely than other modes of delivery to raise estrogen levels. This is important for some men who have estrogen spikes when their T levels rise. The two hormones need to have a wide ratio in males for T therapy to be effective.

However, a minor medical procedure is required and the pellets will need to be replaced every four to six months. If the dose is too high or too low, more pellets will have to be taken out or added through the small incision. The procedure itself usually costs about $250 each time so that's not exactly cheap. However, men who like not having to worry about implementing their own T therapy on a daily basis often think the money is well worth it. I personally know quite a few men who say they are very happy with their testosterone pellets.

Shots

Testosterone shots are certainly the cheapest way to go when administering testosterone. A vial of testosterone should cost less than $100 and last a good five to six months. Doctors used to give men big injections in their office which were supposed to last from two weeks to a month. That caused highly elevated levels for a few days and then huge drop offs where men would feel extremely depleted before their next injection. Now, most open-minded hormone doctors let men do their own injections at home. Most men should do at least one injection per week, but many need two smaller injections per week to keep up steady levels. Some even do much smaller injections, every other day, to achieve greater stability but that is usually not necessary. Huge needles are not needed. Insulin syringes are usually quite sufficient with small gauges, like 29. Usually, the injections are painless and can either be done into the muscle or sub Q (into the fat layers).

The down side to shots is they can elevate estrogen more easily than pellets and gels for some men. The testosterone/estrogen balance is delicate and when thrown off can take away the benefits of T therapy.

The Trouble with Estrogen

Most anti-aging doctors or hormone specialists will keep a keen eye on estrogen levels in their male patients' estrogen levels. However, some general practitioners need to be informed about the changes in this hormone that may occur once T therapy is started. Males should fight hard to get estradiol tested, especially if they feel their T therapy is not working as they hoped.

Estrogen levels that spike too high after the administration of testosterone can mask much of the good progress that testosterone gives a male. If using Lab Corp for blood testing, it is important that men ask for the sensitive estradiol test, not the standard test which is for women. The sensitive test has a range for males from 3-70 and its code no is 140244. The standard test may give elevated estrogen results that don't really reflect a man's true level. If levels are elevated much above 30 on this sensitive test, it may be indicative that estrogen is becoming a problem.

Sometimes, lowering the dose of testosterone will help bring estrogen back into range. Unnaturally high levels of testosterone are more likely to cause elevated estrogen. If lowering doses does not help, an estrogen blocker will be needed. Some doctors prescribe very small doses of the drug Arimidex to stop testosterone from aromatizing into estrogen. Other doctors may try to combat estrogen problems through the use of pregnenolone or progesterone. A lack of these two hormones may naturally cause estrogen to be elevated since they have a naturally balancing effect on estrogen in the body, just as they do in females. Once pregnenolone and progesterone are bought into better range, some men find elevated estrogen is no longer a problem. However, balancing all these naturally is not for the faint of heart.

Zinc is a supplement that can help keep estrogen in line. But, regardless of estrogen, zinc is an important supplement for all aging males, especially while on testosterone therapy. The usual suggested daily dose for men is 50 mg of zinc along with 2 mg of copper. Zinc not only helps inhibit too high estrogen, it is also protective and nourishing to the prostate. Another way that it is helpful is that it naturally chelates iron in the body. Testosterone causes better generation of red blood cells which can elevate iron and hemoglobin in some older men.

Keep an Eye on Hemoglobin

Hemoglobin (red blood cell count) always needs to be tested after a man begins testosterone therapy. If hemoglobin goes too high (much higher than 17 on a range of 14-18), it is important for men to give blood to keep this level down. Giving blood every 56 days to the Red Cross is an excellent idea for most men over 40 since many studies show males in this age group who donate blood are less likely to have a stroke and heart attack. And, of course, giving blood saves lives.

A study of 2,682 men in Finland, reported in the *Journal of Epidemiology* showed that men who donated blood at least once a year had an 88 percent lower risk of heart attacks than non-donors. Another study published in the August, 1997 issue of *Heart* found that men who donated blood were less likely than non-donors to show signs of cardiovascular disease.

I make appointments for my husband to give blood at the Red Cross every 56 days and they appreciate his donation. I appreciate the results of his lowered red blood cell count and I love that he can help others in need.

Pregnancy and Testosterone Therapy

Any couple considering testosterone replacement for the husband should know that in order for it to work properly, it shuts down a man's own production of this hormone and replaces it with the exogenous source. This can result in the testicles shrinking somewhat since they are not busy constantly producing the hormone. Sleeping testicles can cause infertility in men while they are using the therapy.

Most men using T therapy are older (past the age of 45). These men have hormonal loss from mere age or it is bought on by diseases like Type 2 diabetes. Often their wives are past the child bearing years so it doesn't matter as much that they lose sperm production while using testosterone.

However, some younger men require testosterone therapy because they have what is known as "primary hypogonadism." This is when their pituitary gland cannot properly signal for the testes to make testosterone. These men lead miserable lives with low T levels so they need to use testosterone. However, this can interfere with their ability to father children as it can take several months after stopping testosterone to restore sperm production back to normal.

Some males use the substance HCG as part of their testosterone protocol to prevent this testicle shrinkage from occurring. It is thought to also allow a much quicker response to restoring sperm production again. Some men, (although this is more rare), can even make their wives pregnant while using HCG, thus experiencing no loss of fertility. As always, there can be a down side. Using HCG can further increase estrogen levels in some men and they may need an estrogen blocker.

Other men in this situation, who do not want to bother with the use of HCG, but desire their wife to be pregnant, can come off therapy for a while and use a medication called Clomid which helps increase sperm production more speedily. Once their wife is pregnant, they can return to T therapy so they are once again able to enjoy life to the fullest.

The Turn Around

Don't expect abrupt changes in your husband as soon as he starts T therapy. Not all men will respond quite as dramatically as the husband in the story I told in *Foxy Mama*, Chapter 34. But, there will be improvements over time. His malaise will not likely disappear within 24 hours. He may not (probably not) start chasing you around the house after his first application of gel or injection. Hormone receptors in cells take a while to become re-saturated after long droughts. The brain also has some rewiring to do, but it will rewire after testosterone has flooded the body for a while. The body and mind will shape up after they realize there is a new Sherriff in town and its name is "More T."

Things should progress to a better overall picture slowly and surely with the deepest changes occurring from three months to one year. Energy should return, interest and ambition will likely come back, depression will often lift, and healthy sexuality should become a more natural part of life.

Testosterone therapy works best when it is combined with diet improvements and resistance exercise. Although returning T levels to healthy ranges can halt the muscle wasting that occurs when T is low, it won't create a younger buffer physique without a man helping it out through his own efforts. Most men are more inclined to start exercising, or at least become more active, once they have higher T levels in their system. A low T state is often the reason why men are loathe to exercise as they don't have the energy. However, T therapy, along with our **S** and **E** plan, and some muscle resistant workouts is a recipe for big rewards.

Cold Hard Facts

T therapy can go a long way to help men who suffer from erectile dysfunction, but it's not always a cure all. Erectile dysfunction (ED), can cause some real insecurities, sometimes so much so that a man would rather not perform at all rather than try and fail.

Maybe it seems strange to talk about issues like ED in this book since we are writing it specifically to mamas, but Type 2 diabetes is now a rampant disease and growing in numbers. It not only negatively affects the person with the disease, but it also greatly affects their spouse. If your husband has been diagnosed with Type 2, or you suspect he has it, you will be walking a challenging journey with him.

What's diabetes got to do with T therapy and ED? Men that are diagnosed with this condition are 300 percent more likely to experience ED. Sometimes it is the first sign of adult diabetes. Constant elevated blood sugar damages penile tissue by destroying nerves, blood vessels, and muscle function. If a man complains of an ED issue at a doctor's visit, the first protocol for the attending physician is to immediately order a blood test for diabetic conditions.

I'm going to share some statistics with you. Some of them are hard to hear, but it will make you understand my deep concern over this diabetic trend and its far-reaching and devastating impact. As of this year (2012), around 12 percent of all American males over 20 have already been officially diagnosed with the condition. That is not counting the millions more that are thought to already have the disease, but have not yet received blood tests for confirmation.

The 12 percent figure jumps up in dramatic bumps with each 10 year age gap. Of men that have Type 2 diabetes in the up to 20 age bracket, nine percent of them already have ED. That's still a high statistic for a man in his prime—almost one in 10 of those men! But, if a man reaches the age of 70 with Type 2 diabetes, his probability of having ED is 95 percent! The longer a man has the disease, the more the certainty he will suffer with ED. Within 10 years of diagnosis, a full half of Type 2 diabetic men will already suffer with serious erectile problems. It's really a matter of "when," not "if."

These figures are staggering. Think about it. Younger and younger people are now succumbing to diabetes, thanks to our modern high starch/sugar diet. A full third of adults in this nation are thought to have the disease. And to be clear, there's no confusion on what's to blame. Diet is the evil culprit of this epidemic. Even young children are now succumbing to this condition. Never before in history has this occurred. This is unchartered territory for humankind.

Will these young boys who are freshly diagnosed with Type 2 Diabetes even be able to experience normal sexual relations once they are adults or will it be over for them before it even starts? Will they be able to marry and fully consummate that marriage? Father children? The negative effects of diabetes on penile tissue are often permanent. I hate to think about the futures for some of these children and young people.

Clear the sugar and needless starches out of your home, Mama, and not just because sugar causes tooth decay. It may contribute to the decline of our species! Pardon my drama, but if anything calls for being dramatic, this does!

Shroud of Silence

It's a huge blow to men to lose their sexual function. It results in a feeling of inadequacy which can bruise the core of a marriage. Men tend to withdraw emotionally when they can no longer respond physically. Wives feel the pain just as deeply. Many couples silently deal with this trauma because it's considered an embarrassing and shameful subject. Making things worse is the continuing stereo typing that depicts all men constantly wanting sex. It's rampant in church circles, pulpits, Christian books, and is humorously interwoven in conversations. But, it only makes these couples feel worse.

There is a desperate need for answers, but a shroud of silence prevents healthy discussion about this issue. Wives don't want to embarrass their husbands by sharing his problem and who would they go to for help? Most pastors are not equipped with information to deal with this.

I'm crazy enough to ignore polite social etiquette when it comes to this subject. Secretly, many are thirsting for real help. I want to pull back the shutters of shame and offer any and all information I can share. No more closing our eyes to this growing problem, pretending it doesn't really exist, and that many church attending married couples aren't deeply suffering.

Men that have Type 2 diabetes also have significantly lower testosterone levels than men without the condition. It's a bit of a "chicken or the egg" pickle. No one really knows if diabetes leads to low T or if low T leads to diabetes, but the negative end result speaks for itself. Thankfully, as I mentioned earlier, many diabetic men who start T therapy can often lessen, or stop, their diabetic medicine. This is due to the extremely positive effect testosterone has on muscle cells. Muscles are more able to accept and burn blood sugar with higher T levels.

More Help Required

While T therapy can have a positive impact on erectile function, the psychological aspects of it may linger. The worry of not being able to perform becomes a self-fulfilling prophecy for some men who've suffered from ED for a while. Anxiety ends up destroying the natural response.

In other cases, there is damage to penile blood vessels from Type 2 diabetes. High blood pressure, and years of undiagnosed low testosterone which often means years of impaired blood flow to the penis can also damage penile tissue. A higher T state won't always be able to mend this sort of damage. Men who have had prostate surgery may also suffer from ED due to damaged blood vessels from the surgery. These are the cases (along with psychological anxiety) where more help may be needed, along with testosterone therapy, to restore a healthy sex life between husband and wife.

It is a great idea for men who have suffered from ED to ask their doctor for 5 mg daily Cialis to go along with their testosterone therapy, especially at the beginning of therapy. Cialis is in a class of medications called PDE5 inhibitors. It is a remarkable drug which widens blood vessels and allows better blood flow, not only to the penis but to all areas of the body. Recently, in 2011, a similar PDE5 medication kept a baby alive after undergoing three heart surgeries. The impotence medicine kept her stable by radically improving her circulation. It helped her combat daily cyanotic spells which had previously turned her blue as her body struggled to circulate blood. The medical community is finding more and more great uses for Cialis and similar drugs. It has recently been approved for pulmonary hypertension. Some doctors are now prescribing it to help keep men's hearts healthy, thanks to its promotion of better blood circulation.

Due to the positive influence on blood vessels, Cialis can also help combat high blood pressure and there is some evidence that it has a protective effect on the prostate. It protects penile tissue from atrophy that comes with age and helps maintain those spontaneous nocturnal and morning erections which are a great indicator of both penile and general health. Most need not be concerned about any long term side effects with the medication but rarely it may induce some lower back ache and even more rarely vision disturbances.

Note: Males who use nitrates for heart issues should never use Cialis or Viagra. The combination of these type of meds can cause an unsafe drop in blood pressure.

Unlike Viagra, which has a small time window, Cialis can be taken like a vitamin once a day. It has a 24-36 hour time window to work so lovemaking can be a natural occurrence. Adding in a med like this can help unload the pressures and fears that are more the psychological aspects of ED, but it can also help overcome the physical challenges of ED too. A husband is then more able to relax during intimacy with his wife, knowing he has his bases covered.

Unfortunately, Cialis is not cheap. Some insurance plans cover the daily dose, but due to rampant recreational use of this drug in recent years by males who don't have a real need for it, some insurance companies have stopped covering it. Generic Cialis is known as tadalafil. The patent for Cialis runs out in 2016 so it's very likely other companies will start manufacturing tadalafil and prices will be much more reasonable.

What could your husband do if he has a need for this med? Four years away for cheaper versions sounds a long time for couples in need. Many doctors will give out free samples regularly so remind him to ask his doctor about this. If his doctor does not have samples of the daily 5 mg dose, he may have samples of the 20 mg tablet. Some men cut the tablet into quarters for daily use.

Men who have had surgery on their prostate are often encouraged by their doctors to use daily Viagra or Cialis after surgery for several months to help them get back their sexual function. This enhances the chance for full sexual post surgical recovery. Some of these prostate cancer survivors cannot afford the cost of all of this medication so they end up ordering tadalafil from overseas pharmacies. These men report that this is their only effective solution.

Please remember, I am not speaking as a doctor or lawyer, and regarding imported forms of this medication, I am only relaying information I have acquired on prostate cancer forums on the internet. Men turn to these forums desperate for answers. Officially, it is illegal to import prescription medications from overseas pharmacies, but apparently the law is a little muddy on the subject. Prostate cancer survivers who use this imported med say there is a clause in the law that says as long as the medication is for personal use, is not for more than three month's worth, was purchased with a script from a licensed doctor, and is not for resale, then it is allowable. Make sure to look up the laws in your state as importation laws for prescription medications vary.

If your husband is having some erection issues, but is reluctant to try or does not have access to a med like Cialis, he could try taking the amino acid l-arginine. This supplement may also offer improvements for erection difficulty, but the doses need to be high, 5000-10,000 mg per day. For some men l-arginine in these doses results in significant erectile improvement, but it doesn't work for all men.

Don't Focus on Performance

I want to say clearly that the married sexual union does not have to break down even when there are extreme challenges and genitals no longer work they way they are supposed to. Men with chronic diabetic or prostate surgery induced ED can resort to pumps, penile injections, and sometimes even penile implants if nothing else works. In the end, "one flesh" in marriage is not only about perfectly working parts; it's about sharing ourselves physically with our spouse, giving and serving each other sexually, whether all appendages are in working order or not.

Putting too much emphasis on performance, function and orgasm can cause anxiety in both partners. Patience, understanding, and making sure expectations aren't unrealistic is of utmost importance. Some of these solutions I've mentioned simply give men more confidence, which in turn makes them less likely to withdraw from the sexual union. As I encourage women to take measures to remedy the "dry, painful vagina" syndrome, men can seek and find answers for their sexual challenges as they age (maybe with a little help from their wife).

Bullet in the Foot

It's quite common for men and women to unknowingly shoot themselves in the foot by the medications they take. Some antidepressants, and many blood pressure medications, result in a lessening of sexual function.

Antidepressants like Zoloft and Paxil have a dampening effect on the prosexual neuro transmitter dopamine. They can hinder sexual desire in both women and men, but with a further complication of delaying ejaculation in males. That may not be a problem for younger men, but it is certainly a more common concern for aging males.

Raising testosterone alone may help alleviate depression, but if more help is needed, some doctors will prescribe Wellbutrin. This antidepressant does not have the negative sexual side effects more commonly associated with SSRIs. It works on relieving depression via dopamine pathways.

In *Mama's Secret Weapons*, Chapter 41, I talk about a natural supplement called Mukta Vati that works well to lower blood pressure. Some men are skeptical about using an herbal formulation for any of their physical problems. They only want to take what their doctor prescribes them. If this is true for your husband, you can be the little birdie who tweets the reminder in your husband's ear to ask his doctor about some other alternatives. There are options for blood pressure meds that don't have these negative effects.

The most popular BP medications prescribed for hypertension are water pills (diuretics) and beta blockers. Both of these can cause unwanted sexual side effects. Diuretics can decrease forceful blood flow to the penis, making it difficult for men to achieve an erection. They can also deplete the body of zinc which is necessary to make testosterone. Beta blockers can affect the nervous system reaction that causes an erection. They can also make it difficult for the arteries in the penis to widen to let in enough blood flow for healthy male function.

A class of blood pressure medications, known as ACE inhibitors (Angiotensin Converting Enzyme inhibitors), are a little less hard on a man's sex life, but are known to cause ED for a small percentage of men. They are also responsible for causing a dry cough that won't go away.

There are newer BP drugs now available called ARBs (Angiotensin 11 Receptor Blockers). These work through a different mechanism than ACE's which simply inhibit the activity of the ACE enzyme that causes blood vessels to constrict. ARBs block the binding of the ACE enzyme, rather than inhibit it. They relax the blood vessels and, here's the good thing, they do not cause erectile dysfunction. In fact, one study showed that ARBs actually improved erectile function for men.

Hence, if your husband is having negative sexual side effects with other BP meds, he can ask his doctor about a medication like Cozaar which is in the family of ARBs. Cozaar is much less likely to cause a dry cough also.

If water retention is still a problem, the BP drug Lasix can work to reduce edema and further lower blood pressure without causing sexual problems like most other water pills. Lasix is known as a "loop diuretic" rather than a water pill. It inhibits the body's ability to reabsorb sodium. In higher doses, it causes its own share of adverse effects. However, a very small dose of Lasix, along with a drug like Cozaar, can be a good combination for men who aren't willing to try a natural supplement, but who also do not want to experience sexual side effects. If Lasix is used, a potassium supplement should also be used to prevent an imbalance of electrolytes in the body.

Hopefully, your husband will be willing to join you on the **S** and **E** plan and his high blood pressure may well take care of itself as he loses excess weight. A carbohydrate conscious diet like our plan helps bring down high blood sugar which in itself may prevent both an accelerated low T state and the often permanent damage that Type 2 diabetes causes to many vital parts of the body.

Chapter 36

Get Movin', Mama

by Serene Allison

If you are content with low energy levels, waning sex drive, and a body losing muscle mass by the year, the next four chapters are not for you.

We hear about the benefits of exercise and we sure know we need it. But, the need for exercise is as simple as "If you don't use it, you will lose it."

Life in the 21st century is filled with motorized contraptions for almost every duty. We can press a button for nearly everything and we have built larger contraptions to carry our sedentary bodies around from place to place. Most of us do not exert the physical intensity we were created for in our everyday jobs or home life. Think of the primitive hunter tribes, or even the pioneers of the new world. With all of our modern technologies, we are one, two, or maybe thousands of steps behind them—I'm talking literal steps.

As a society, we are more advanced in many areas. We don't need to take that for granted, but we have become overweight and sedentary. The average westerner doesn't have to walk an hour to work in the morning, or wash her clothes by hand in the river. Our push button lifestyle, on top of a trashy diet, has made it a common sight to see the wonderful human body severely distorted. Huge distended bellies and out of proportion backsides are not a rare sight these days. God's wonderful design was created for use, not neglectful abuse. The human form is always beautiful, no matter what body type you may have, once it is allowed to reveal its true genetics.

Due to modern lifestyle changes, we now have to slot in a little time for training our bodies, building our muscles, and strengthening our bones. I said "little," so don't quit reading this chapter, thinking I am going to suggest hours every day. Hey, I'm not Jillian from the Biggest Loser. I'm a mother of nine, and who has time for the hours that show prescribes (can't say I'm not a fan of the show, though). However, we need to devote some time to maintain our natural shape and turn over the engine regularly so our vehicle does not rust into a dumpy heap of broken down parts.

Get up and Go

Many people say they are too tired for exercise with everything else they have to get done in life. The truth is, exercise increases energy levels and floods our bodies with endorphins (euphoria producing chemicals, the same ones Pearl mentioned that increase during sex). These make us feel on top of the world and ready to accomplish anything that comes our way. Exercise is our key for giving us the "get up and go" we need for our busy modern lives.

Exercise has been proven to be one of the most effective methods for reducing stress and treating mild depression. It stimulates the production of alpha brain waves which keep us feeling calm and relaxed. Serotonin, the happy hormone, is released. It brings feelings of joy, well being, personal security, self esteem, and the ability to concentrate.

I feel invigorated and almost on a "natural high" after a good workout. Many people get addicted to the healthy, happy, energetic feeling that exercise brings. Marilyn Demartini, a national sports and fitness journalist says, "When at the top of your physical game, you'll be at the top of your mental game . . . Feeling fatigued, unattractive, sleep deprived and achy, the overweight and under-exercised majority may tell us that it is the reality of aging . . . Science and experience show how to arm our bodies for the war against aging . . . Kick your body into full gear and tap your own fountain of youth. It's not in a bottle, it's in your veins."

Murdering Epidemic

Obesity in America is rampant and continuing its bulging rise at alarming rates. In 1987, not one U.S. state had an obesity rate above 15 percent, according to a report by the centers for Disease Control. Years later, while Americans have fallen into the trap of being sedentary and eating carby junk, six states in less than 10 years had reached this level. By 2001 the national obesity rate had skyrocketed to 22 percent! This has sadly resulted in 61 percent of adults being overweight. The majority of Americans are sick and deteriorating, the best part of their lives being choked away by fat. Statistics indicate that the second most common cause of actual death, right behind tobacco use, is poor diet and exercise of which 400,000 die a year.

More than 900,000 adults were studied for 16 years. The researchers involved estimated that over 90,000 cancer fatalities annually could be avoided if every American maintained a healthy weight. This study also revealed that overweight men have a 52 percent higher risk of dying of cancer than for men of normal weight. This risk is 62 percent higher for women.

The correlation between being overweight and diabetes is staggering. Pearl spoke about this epidemic but let me add a couple of statistics. Because someone has not been diagnosed with diabetes does not mean it is not forming in their bodies. In his book, *Ready, Set, Go! Synergy Fitness,* Phil Campbell writes, "Eight million Americans have undiagnosed diabetes and 650,000 Americans will learn they have diabetes this year."

As you have already learned in this book, there are simple yet powerful dietary steps you can take to prevent and treat this murdering epidemic. The balanced approach to prevention is always more thorough. A one sided battle attack is not as well strategized as an assault from two angles. Diet and exercise together are the ultimate weapon to wage war against killers like diabetes and other degenerate diseases. Why use only one arrow when you can have two at your disposal?

No Longer Optional

I don't want be another voice telling you to start an exercise program. I know, you've already done that. You've put it on your New Year's resolution list more than once—and broken it. They say March is the best time to purchase cheap exercise equipment on Craigslist or eBay. Only three months after New Year and most people are done with all that! Somehow, it needs to sink in that healthy habits of diet and exercise are our key to survival. It is now a matter of life and death. But, I'm not talking about long arduous workouts to add misery to your life. You'll soon learn that we have a quick fix approach.

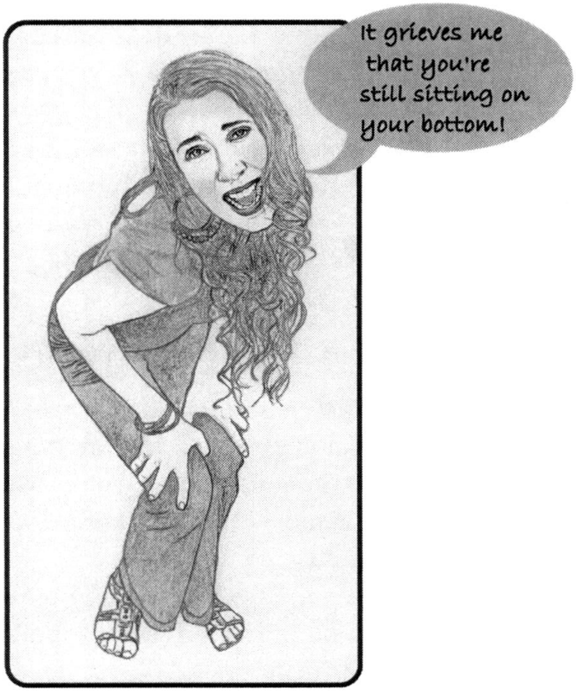
It grieves me that you're still sitting on your bottom!

It's not an optional decision anymore. Do you want to be free of disease and around for your children, and maybe grandchildren? When I say "around," I don't mean surviving on 50 different medications like a zombie. If so, you have to make physical movement part of your life. After all, the fascinating human physique was created for action.

Better than Pills and Potions

As I bring your focus back towards the natural and the fundamental movement of your body, I want to inspire you with a few more facts. Sam Varner (former strength and conditioning coach of the US Olympic team) says, "The pills, potions, and cosmetics in our billion-dollar health industry are evidence of our society's continued fixation on everlasting youth and beauty. But, if you could rank all the proven methods known to retard the aging process and enrich our health, exercise would be at the top of the list. It truly is the fountain of youth!"

In his book, *Slimmer, Younger, Stronger*, Varner talks about a recent study that showed regular exercisers who smoke cigarettes had fewer health risks than sedentary individuals who did not smoke. He talked about smoking being horrendous for your health, but lack of exercise is a similar killer.

Below are three studies results mentioned in his book that I found astounding.

1. Sedentary individuals are 80 percent more likely to develop coronary heart disease than more physically active individuals.
2. Scientists in Finland tracked the health and physical activity of 16,000 twins for 19 years and found that the twin who exercised at least 30 minutes, six times a month, was on average 56 percent more likely to have outlived his or her sedentary twin.
3. One in two men and one in three women are in harm's way of cancer's ravaging claws. There are many contributing factors to its growth, but the initial introduction is due to a lack of available oxygen to cells. Some oxygen starved cells become abnormal and can mutate into deadly cancer cells.

Oxygenate, Cleanse, and Hydrate

Exercise bathes your cells in precious life supporting oxygen. It is this abundant circulation of oxygen that plays a vital role in the prevention of cancer. Those who exercise regularly have 30,000 to 60,000 more miles of capillary blood vessels that are created throughout the body than those who would rather commune with the couch. This means an expanded highway system for oxygen delivery.

If all this wasn't enough, exercise pumps out the lymphatic system by stimulating the circulation of lymph fluid. In a properly working lymphatic system, cellular waste is removed. A sluggish clogged lymph system produces trapped cellular waste, toxicity, and disease. A normal lymph flow is 125 miles per hour, but moderate physical activity pushes this to 1800 per hour.

Exercise makes you feel the need to intake detoxifying liquids. You sweat out the toxins and create a giant thirst to rehydrate your body with life-giving water. We all know we need to drink more water, but sometimes it is difficult to get it down. During, and after a vigorous exercise session, suddenly pure water becomes the only thing you desire and you get to chug the good stuff with a passion.

More Happy, Less Hungry

Exercise dulls sugar cravings, and contrary to what you might think, lowers your appetite. It is hard to believe, but reclining in the Lazy Boy and zoning out to TV makes you hungrier than a heart-pumping work-out. Increased blood flow from exercise releases more nutrients and oxygen to circulate and nourish your cells. The liver also excretes extra glucose which can naturally stabilize lowering blood-sugar.

This balanced blood sugar controls the urge for a sugary snack. Exercise also elevates brain serotonin levels, which not only makes you feel happy, but controls your hunger and does a good job suppressing sugary carbohydrate and alcohol cravings.

There are still more benefits, to boot. Consistent exercise increases your insulin sensitivity. This is a good thing, because, as you've already read earlier, insulin resistance is where your body becomes almost numb to this hormone. Your body then requires larger and larger amounts of insulin to stabilize a blood sugar spike. Remember, insulin is our fat storage hormone and large secretions of insulin mean large fat deposits.

I could enjoy preaching on for hours about the benefits of exercise to your body. Unfortunately, Pearl will label me with OCD (obsessive compulsive disorder) and I dislike that. She's been telling me to calm down a little, but I reminded her how fervent she became in her own chapters (especially the one on sex) and she is now sheepishly backing off my case.

This does it for my pep talk. Are you convinced? Good. The "why" is only the beginning. I will also show you the "how."

Chapter 37

Quick Fix

by Serene Allison

Is there a form of exercise that gives you more bang for your buck?

Definitely. There is a way that is not only better for you, not only gives you faster results in a shorter time, not only gives a greater surge of all the benefits we have talked about, but will give you a complete metamorphosis, if you need it.

Intense

Yes, you read right, INTENSE. I am not talking about busting your body for long periods of time. This is the beauty of this kind of exercise. Everyone has time for it. No more need for 45 minute sessions on the treadmill at a methodically boring pace. An hour of exercise is out! A hike through the woods is different, that's simply not being sedentary.

No More Long Workouts

In his book, *Perfect Weight, America*, Jordan Reuben writes, "Long duration exercise downsizes the heart's capacity to rapidly provide you with big bursts of energy when you need them, increases LDL cholesterol and triglycerides, elevates clotting and inflammation factors and creates loss of bone density."

After 45 minutes to an hour of exercise, cortisol turns on, which is your stress hormone and breaks down the body. Super long bouts of exercise become catabolic (breaking down the body) instead of anabolic (building up the body) and it is the anabolic state we want our bodies to be in during exercise.

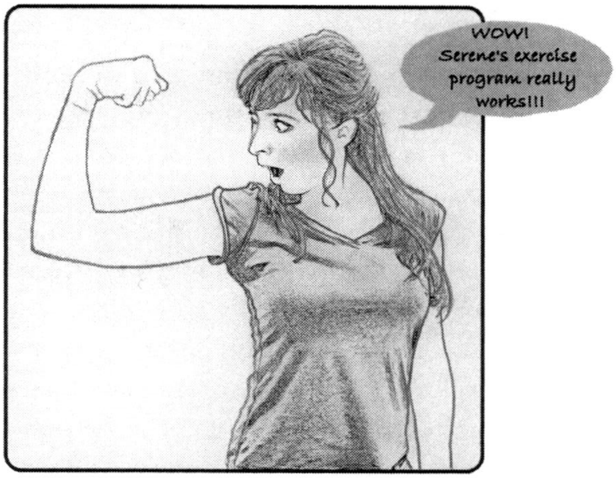
WOW! Serene's exercise program really works!!!

Short Bursts are Best

We want to build up our muscles and build up our bone density. Short bursts of intense movement, followed by brief periods of rest are all you need. Exercise done like this need only take 10-20 minutes of your time, a mere pittance. Of course, if you want more, go for it. Just don't go over 45 minutes to an hour. That is destructive.

If you have ever watched the Olympic Games, you have seen both the catabolic and anabolic state right before your eyes. The skinny, wasted, wizened up bodies of the marathon runners are perfect examples of catabolism in action. The beautifully strong, sleek, muscular, robust physiques of the track and field sprinters are the pictures of health that anabolism provides.

Over Exercising is Detrimental

Sam Varner, US Olympian team coach, says that one of the main problems he notes in athletes on a professional level is over training. He calls this the "more is better syndrome." He goes on to explain it as, "The biggest detriment to a client's physical progress. When you work out too much and too often, you set yourself up for increased fatigue, decreased motivation, increased chance of injury, heightened exposure to illness, needless muscular soreness, and stagnating progress."

I told you how lack of exercising is destroying our nation, but now you can see that over exercising has its pitfalls as well. Just like the balance we encourage in our **S** and **E** plan, we must also find this balance for exercise. The thought of having to spend so much time in exercise is such a major deterrent, especially for busy mothers, but finding 15 minutes is easy and lifts the rest of the day.

Got Five Minutes?

Sam Varner encourages keeping your workout length shorter than an hour. Don't put off exercise, if you can't even find 20 minutes. Just do five minutes if that's all you've got. Once you are five minutes in, you start to get motivated, feel your blood start to pump and you are more inclined to squeeze in another five or ten.

If you can't squeeze in any additional time, do a series of five minute bursts, spread throughout your day. By nightfall, you may have calculated a full twenty minutes in all. Quoting from Sam Varner again, "Personally speaking, my lifting routine used to last one and a half to two hours a day, three to five days a week. However, by reducing the amount of workout time to LESS THAN 35 minutes, just four days a week, I noticed greater intensity, improved strength, lower body fat, sharper mental concentration and a more invigorating workout. To this day I find it is much easier and much more productive to consistently follow a shorter, more intense exercise routine, rather than a longer, more drawn out one. And isn't that the key?"

There are many scientific reasons supporting shorter, more intense forms of exercise. I would need a whole book to do any of them proper justice, but I need to mention the Human growth hormone. Research has shown that blood levels of this youthful hormone peak after 35-45 minutes of intense exercise. This hormone subsides after 60 minutes and from a hormone standpoint, any exercise done beyond 60 minutes is counterproductive. The cortisol that starts to pump at this time, tends to not only break down your body, but rearrange your body fat all towards your middle and lock it there. It's that stubborn tummy fat again.

Short and Intense is More Natural

Exercising in short intense bursts is not foreign or unnatural. In fact, it is moving at the same speed for extended periods that is unnatural. If you watch children at play, you will see the most natural way of exercising. They get an impulse of energy and chase each other around the yard for a bit. Then they slump to the grass panting, giggling, and out of breath. They rest for a couple of minutes before eyeing a ball and playing a wild toss and catch, followed by a run inside for a drink of water and a loll on the couch. They won't lay there long. Somebody decides to jump on the trampoline and they race outside to see who can get there first. Jumping energetically and taking turns resting on the side will go on for a while before another bright, energetic idea comes along.

This is considered fun for children. At one time in our lives, we thought it was enjoyable too. Then we grew up and thought that exercise had to be serious, boring, and long.

Children have very high amounts of human growth hormone and they instinctively move and play in a way that maximizes this hormone. If we start to move in fast, intense, but brief spurts, followed by little rests, we can maximize the human growth hormone as well. If you want your body to produce more of the most powerful fat burning, muscle toning, anti-aging substance known in science, then move like a child again.

Make Your Own

The benefits and clock rewinding power of human growth hormone has an estimated 500,000 adults injecting this substance and hundreds of thousands more using supplements that promise to raise it.

Human growth hormone injections have been proven to reverse the ravages of aging to the equivalent of 10-20 years. Bioidentical HGH can be prescribed for people with a deficiency, but it is very expensive and also has a bad rap due to body builders who overuse and abuse it beyond natural levels. You don't have to inject yourself to increase more of your own.

The picture of youth and vitality is not available without HGH. Children and young people naturally pulsing large amounts. Phil Campbell writes in *Ready, Set, Go! Synergy Fitness,* "On average, growth hormone can pull off 28 pounds of body fat from a 200 pound adult and it can add eight percent lean mass. We're talking about a powerful substance."

In his book, Phil Campbell goes on to discuss the benefits of exercise induced HGH without having to use expensive injections that many doctors will not prescribe anyway. Research has shown it can be produced naturally within our own body by intense short periods of exercise (like sex with your husband as Pearl already mentioned), adequate deep sleep, or as an affordable nutrient, namely two grams of L-Glutamine. A significant increase of this powerful hormone has been observed by taking these simple steps.

Exercise induced growth hormone blasts body fat like a targeted missile for two hours after working out. I will share with you how you can keep it pulsing for the entire time and not cut it short from common mistakes.

Skin Deep

Who'd have thought that the type of exercise I'm promoting would help your skin more than expensive creams. There is a link between strength training, anaerobic exercise, and beautiful skin. Dr. Perricone, a leading dermatologist writes in his book, *The Perricone Prescription*, "Resistance training releases growth hormone while increasing muscle mass. It also lowers stress, resulting in lower levels of catabolic, destructive cortisol. For the skin, this means increased cell growth and repaired and restored collagen fibers."

Burn Calories While You Rest

Anaerobic exercise beats aerobic exercise in regards to the percentage of calories and fat burned. Anaerobic far exceeds aerobic exercise in raising your metabolic rate, which enables you to burn off even more calories while you are at rest.

During an hour session of aerobic exercise you burn 210 calories compared with 650 calories for an anaerobic session of the same time. Two hours after your aerobics session 25 calories are being burned, but 150 calories are being burned two hours after your anaerobic session. This is the clincher: three to 15 hours after aerobic exercise no additional calories are being burned. Yes, that is a zero. But, 15 hours after anaerobic training, 260 calories are still burning into smithereens. Yee Ha Grandma! Remember, we don't want you to do a full hour, but the point is made.

Don't Adapt

In the eighties, the cardio craze was all the rave. This decade flew the "cardio burns fat" flag and this was promised on every magazine and exercise book. The facts are that during the steady state workout, where you maintain a constant pace, your body does burn a higher percentage of calories from fat. This misguiding fact is why cardio has been so worshiped. On the surface it sounds promising, but there are two huge problems which cause the dominoes to fall. Aerobic activity allows your body to adapt. Once this happens (and it will happen), your body will burn fewer and fewer total calories. Your body has been programmed to do this. Just as we change up our **E** meals that burn glucose and our **S** meals that burn fat for fuel, we need to do the same when it comes to exercise. Short bursts of intensity keep your body in guess mode.

The second problem is that because of the adaptation process that occurs in the so-called "fat burning zone," your body will actually start to store fat. This is your body's preservation mechanism. Our bodies are incredibly equipped to survive and storage is one form of survival to help us through the lean times.

Miserably Ineffective

A well known fitness trainer and author, Rachel Cosgrove has shaped her body to be sleek, strong, and beautiful using anaerobic, intense intervals, and weight training. As a life goal, and also to prove a point of cardio's inferior ability to actually burn fat, she trained seven months for an iron man competition. She watched every calorie and calculated that she exercised for a total of 374 cardio hours, coming in at an average of 13 hours per week.

In an article entitled, *The Final Nail In the Cardio Coffin,* she says, "If I burned just ten calories in a minute, it adds up to 224,400 calories. Doing the math (at 3500 calories per pound) 224,400 calories should equal 64 pounds weight lost. Needless to say, I did not lose 64 pounds. Over those seven months, training an average of 13-14 hours a week, I lost all of five pounds. That was it."

She tells how she already knew that steady state aerobics was not effective for fat loss. Rachel says, "But still . . . I thought it would have been more effective than this. A lousy five pounds after doing 374 hours of training, while keeping tabs on what I'm eating! It's enough to make a girl give up in the gym and take refuge in a box of Krispy Kremes." Even though Cosgrove only lost five pounds of fat during her aerobic training months, she also lost much of her muscle tone, and for the first time, had no six pack to show. She said she actually became rather "flabby."

Get it Back with Short Bursts

The exciting and fortunate news for Rachel, as well as for you, is that short duration intensity is the answer to "gettin' it back." Rachel was able to undo the seven month aerobic damage in eight weeks. She did it by eliminating all steady state endurance exercise, which meant no long sessions of running, biking, swimming or the like. She implemented workouts for short bursts of high intensity, either with weights or metabolic interval sessions. She lifted three days a week and did short interval sessions on the other two. She would crank her heart rate up for two minutes, then recover. In only eight weeks, she dropped 15 pounds of fat and her abs came back. She was once again lean and sculpted and no longer had the wasted but flabby look of an endurance athlete.

Target Fast Twitch Muscle Fibers

The intense anaerobic exercises are more effective for the many reasons we have already discussed, but another reason is that they target more of your muscle. Cardio exercise uses mostly slow twitch muscle fibers and not enough fast twitch muscle fibers. It's the fast twitch fibers that give you firm muscles and quick results.

Younger in a Week

Training these fast twitch muscle fibers reverses the aging process, because these muscles are the first to deteriorate as we age. This is due to the fact that neurons stop communicating with them. Lucky for us, we can greatly increase firing rates after only one week of anaerobic training.

Studies and data back this up. It's sad how many people are slogging it out at the gym on their treadmills and bicycles when they could be taking much less time and getting better results by doing intense short burst training.

In December, 2006 Canadian researchers found that only two weeks of interval training boosted women's ability to burn fat during exercise by 36 percent.

A 12 week *Skidmore College* study found that exercisers who added high intensity total body resistance routines lost more than twice as much body fat, in particular, more than four times as much belly fat than other groups of exercisers.

In January, 2007 a six month study was published, showing that adding aerobic exercise had no additional benefit on body composition over diet alone.

Another study released in June, 2007 that ran for twelve months, monitored subjects doing six hours of aerobic exercise per week, training six days a week for a year. The average weight loss was only three pounds for that one year period.

But hey, if you love to run, sprint! Seriously, if you really love a nice run, by all means go ahead. Do it for the love of it and because you are not a couch potato. Just know there are better, more effective ways to make your body its best.

Examples of anaerobic exercise:

Jumping rope or rebounding
Sprint intervals using either running, swimming, walking or cycling
Body resistance/strength training including weights, kettlebells, and bands
Poly-metrics (our eight minute Spew session)

Off my Tuft

I had been writing this chapter and sitting on my tuft for a few hours but have come back refreshed from a five minute, intense exercise burst. I feel so much better and have a clear head again. This is an example of how a busy mother, with the additional project of a book deadline, can still fit in exercise. Now, where was I?

Set the Right Conditions

Intense bursts of movement are considered anaerobic and this is what we shoot for. There are certain factors that need to come into play to ensure the release of HGH.

Out of breath
Muscle burn
Increased body temperature
Adrenal response (slightly painful)

These benchmarks are telltale signs that your body has the right conditions to release HGH. I urge you to use common sense. Even a well-trained athlete that is not accustomed to anaerobic training needs to work up to their goal slowly. In other words, don't go all out the first day of training and regret it with an injury, but get a little bit more intense with your workout each session.

By out of breath, I mean nicely winded, where you find it hard to talk (like at the end of a sprint race). I do not mean hyperventilating. The muscle burn is the deep burning sensation you feel while performing exercise. You need to raise your body temperature by one degree for HGH to release. This is attainable in the first two minutes of intense workout.

A research team from the University of Virginia found "adrenal hormone release function" plays a central role in HGH release. The release of epinephrine (adrenaline), which supports your body in stressful situations, as well as norepinephrine (which maintains normal blood circulation), are both major triggers of HGH release. Phil Campbell describes how, "Exercise must achieve the out of breath, slightly painful level of intensity that produces an epinephrine response before HGH is released."

Twenty minutes is our target goal for exercise, but less will still do you good. By the time 20 minutes of high intensity training is up, the body will have released a significant amount of HGH. This surge continues its rise until it hits a peak around the one hour mark into recovery. It takes around two hours, and some studies say even three, to return to its pre-exercise level.

It is super important to take advantage of this amazing two hour opportunity to turn your body into a fat burning furnace.

Here are some things you should not forget if you want HGH to surge.

Fuel It

If you haven't eaten for a while and you want to exercise, you'll need a little fuel because you'll need some energy to get you through the intense bursts. That is why I suggest eating an **E** snack right before, or an **E** meal about an hour before exercising. That should offer your muscle cells some glycogen so the right intensity can be achieved. But, what if you're doing a full **S** day and starchy carbs are out? Coconut oil is a great fuel and source of energy in place of carbs. Professional athletes often take advantage of this secret. If you don't want to spoon it down, you could enjoy some *Skinny Chocolate* (*Snacks,* Chapter 24), or enjoy one of our whey protein smoothies that contains coconut oil. This is not a hard and fast rule.

Another idea I incorporate is to have my daily one cup of coffee half an hour before my workout begins. There is much evidence that coffee fuels stronger intensity during workouts. However, I don't believe in constant medicating with coffee. If you are truly tired in the afternoon, take a nap (if you can). It will be better for your body rather than propping yourself up with coffee. Some days your body will tell you to take a rest from training as it signals, "too tired." Please don't stomp on this signal with coffee boosts.

Supplement It

Take two grams of L-glutamine in plain water, or even better, in sparkling (carbonated) water. Carbonated water causes greater absorption of this powerful supplement. L-glutamine is a cheap supplement that is powerful in stimulating HGH release if taken right before exercise. It is naturally used up in your body by almost 50 percent when exercising with high intensity. It is good to supplement L-glutamine to keep a healthy level of this nutrient in your body, regardless of its HGH benefits. It is also used for anti-aging purposes and raises immune function. If that isn't enough, it is also incredibly healing for the bowel wall and can reduce sugar and starch cravings.

Guzzle It

Drink plenty of pure water during exercise. HGH research teams have found that not enough water during training will greatly reduce your HGH response during training.

Protein It

It is a must to support your muscle growth and repair by taking 25 grams of protein within a 45 minute window after training. I do it within five minutes, but some cannot stomach the thought right after exercising. If you do not apply these principles, your body will eat its own protein and cannibalize muscle, which stops progress, strength, and the physical changes you desire. If you are trying to build a high peachy derriere instead of a flat drooping backside, please eat your protein.

Supplementing with whey protein makes this easy, especially if your appetite is dulled straight after working out. Just mix it with water and shove it down the hatch! In *Foundation Foods*, Chapter 17 we talk about whey's benefits and the best brands available. One scoop is usually around 25 grams of protein. If you don't have the money for a good whey source, the following food sources provide 25 grams of protein:

Four ounces of chicken, fish, or beef
6 oz. water packed tuna
Three eggs
1 measuring cup of cottage cheese
1 measuring cup of Greek yogurt (regular yogurt contains less protein)

Don't Ruin it

For the two hour window following your workout, it is best to eat an **S** meal for the following reasons. We never want to eat high-carbs after exercise as this stops HGH in its tracks. Although **E** meals on our program are never excessively high in carbs, sticking with **S** meals has other advantages. The healthy fats will support your hormone production which is imperative at this time. Also, besides the HGH fat burning benefits, eating mainly fats and proteins will help slip your body into a fat burning mode. Carbs will not be available for energy so the fat you eat, as well as any excess on your body, will be used.

Aside from inhibiting growth hormone release and spiking your insulin, carbing out post exercise has other pitfalls. You will still find exercise gurus saying that eating carbohydrates post exercise is essential for success. They believe your muscles must be refilled with glycogen energy stores straight afterward because they want to take advantage of the insulin that results from eating high-carbs as an anabolic hormone. But, let's look at the science. A study in September, 2007 from the *AMJ Physiol Endochinol Metab* showed that the inclusion of carbohydrates in post workout nutrition does not increase protein synthesis. In other words, it does not help in rebuilding muscle tissue.

In fact, high-carbs post workout raises insulin levels. The spike of insulin that always comes after a spike in sugar from carbohydrates causes the release of high levels of muscle eating catabolic hormones like cortisol. Straight after a rigorous training session, when you want results, who wants to tear it down with too high levels of the fat storage hormone, insulin, or the muscle eating hormone, cortisol?

Having said all this, there are people like me who tend to get skinny when training hard. We're the ones who should think about adding some carbs to our after-training meal so our body does not burn only fat. Be careful not to make the carb level too high as that will prevent a HGH surge. A **Crossover** snack or meal would be perfect.

Chapter 38

Jump Right In, Mama

by Serene Allison

The simple key to anaerobic success is intense bursts followed by rest periods that are only long enough for your heart to stop pounding through your chest. Repeat these bursts for a 20 minute goal.

If your effort is very concentrated as in "The Spew" described below, your overall time can be reduced even further.

At the end of this chapter I will supply you with a list of DVD resources that incorporate ideas for intense short exercise.

However, the following are a few HGH promoting workout ideas you can do today—and you don't even have to purchase anything! They are only suggestions. Please have fun with your own creativity.

The Spew

20 squats
20 lunges (switching legs each time)
20 jump lunges (same thing as simple lunges, but add a jump to propel you into the next rep)

20 jump squats (same thing as regular squats, but jump as high as you can between each one)

Do this routine with the best form you can muster. Hands should stay clasped behind your head so you do not support yourself by leaning on your thighs.

Do these motions as fast as you can, but not so fast that your form suffers.

To squat: keep feet at shoulder width apart and sit your bottom back until your thighs are parallel to the floor as though you were sitting down on a chair. Think about all your weight centering on your heels, not on the balls of your feet. Keep your back erect and eyes focused straight ahead, not on the floor.

To lunge: take a good step forward and lower yourself until the front thigh is parallel and the back knee almost touches the ground. Again, keep back erect and think of sinking down, rather than leaning forward.

Do the entire sequence and then rest for double the time it took you to perform it. Repeat sequence. Now you're done, and it probably took you less than 10 minutes, including your rest time. How's that for time efficiency?

This is a very demanding workout. Even when I am in top physical condition it whips my behind. Don't beat yourself up if you can't do the entire sequence straight through at first. It took me a few weeks to work up to completing it without cheat breaks. But, I am very tall, so it may be a tad harder for us tall folk. Well, that's my excuse.

My husband named this routine "The Spew." He wondered why I was finishing my exercise in under eight minutes and calling myself done for the day. He thought I was being a wimp and wanted to prove his macho manhood by doing it all the way through the first time, with height and gusto. By the way, he's 6' 5". The floors were shaking. By the end he was yelling, "I want to spew" and lay on the floor to recover. Luckily, he managed to avoid vomiting, but the name stuck. Hey, have fun! Maybe it could be part of a date night. Ha-ha.

Seriously though, if you have a bunch of children, it is fun to do this in the evening with daddy included. It's a real laugh and the children love it. Of course, it's easy for them as they are much lighter and probably do this type of thing naturally in their play.

Sprint Intervals

I like to do this one running up our field at home. If you have a "70 yard" dash area, you might like to try it. Some people do this up their suburban street or go to a park. Basically, you want to work up to eight to 12 second, all-out sprints (not necessarily running, but it may be).

Depending on your natural abilities, this sprint could involve running all out, or it could be an extremely fast speed walk. Postpartum mothers should not attempt to run these sprints before three months, at least. The same goes for those who are very unfit. Sprint walks of about one minute, followed by two minutes of pleasure walking is a great option. You can also swim sprint intervals in a pool, or sprint on a stationary bike.

If you have a treadmill, or a stationary bike machine, you can sprint on these machines. However, because you can't go all out on the treadmill, due to safety and because the bike supports some of your weight, equipment based sprints need to be longer. Sprint for 30 seconds.

You need to complete eight intervals. You will increase your pace slowly with the first four with a goal of an all out sprint for the last four. To begin, walk to your starting spot and begin your first lap (we like to call it a hit) of about 70 yards with a slow jog. Walk back. Jog slightly faster for the second hit. Walk back, then make the third hit a run, and the fourth a fast run. The next four are all out "bustin' gut" dashes.

It is important to know that if you sprint all out the first day you try this, you will likely injure yourself and halt your exercise progress. I speak from personal experience. Even for the last four sprints, you should hold back to 80 percent exertion during the first month. Your muscles need to slowly become accustomed to the exercise.

This workout should be completed in less than 20 minutes. It is meant to be quick and effective. It's a great idea to invite the children to join you in this one. If training with competition makes you, or them, feel discouraged or tense, have everybody start at opposite ends of the field, street, pool, or stagger your start times so nobody is aware of who comes second, third, or last.

Jumping Intervals

Jump rope as fast as you can for 300 counts as a goal. When first starting, you may want to only jump 100 counts.

Now your rest period. You can jump on a mini trampoline (rebounder), doing only a relaxing light bounce by keeping toes touching the tramp. Or, you could walk around your living room in circles until rested, but not in relaxed mode for longer than two minutes.

Now, get that rope moving again and repeat the hits and the rests until you feel like you've had a good workout—about 15 minutes.

Mixed Intervals

Here's one to stop you from getting bored.

Do the 300 count skip as in Jumping Intervals. Rest as described.

Do 20 squats, followed by 20 jump squats. Rest.

Do 20 lunges, followed by 20 jump lunges. Rest.

If time is an issue today, you are finished. If not, you can repeat this sequence for a full 15-20 minute workout.

Body Resistance Max

The goal is 90 seconds per exercise although only do what you can. A stopwatch makes this easier, but you can watch the second hand on any clock. Don't give up too early. You can always do a few seconds more than you think.

Plank: Keep body in a straight position from heels to head.

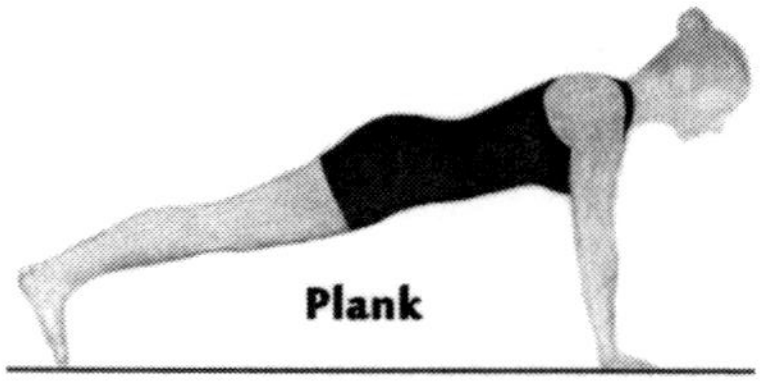

Body Hang: For this exercise you need to purchase a cheap pull up bar which you can insert between your door. You can get one for less than $10.00 from Walmart. However, I said you shouldn't have to buy anything, so leave out this exercise if you're penny pinched.

Grip the bar with your fingers facing toward you and raise your knees at a 45 degree angle. Keep tummy tight like a corset. Try and lift your body a quarter of an inch and hold for a goal of 90 seconds. This lift is only imaginary, but it helps with form and initiates the right muscle action. You may only be able to hold for 15-30 seconds in the beginning.

I have to do mind games to keep holding on for 90 seconds. I imagine I am holding my child from falling off a cliff. There's nothing that would make me let go. Or, you could imagine crocodiles below you, whatever works for you.

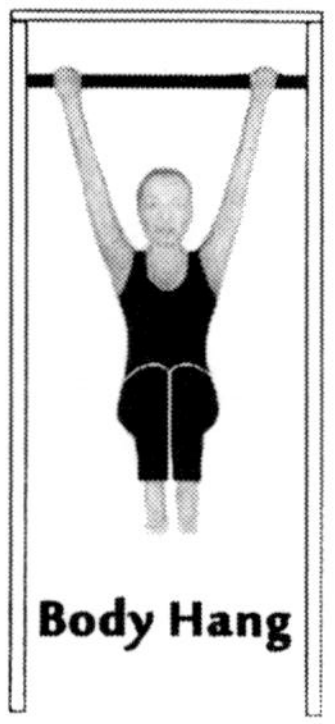

Superman: Lay on the floor on your tummy. Raise your legs and arms at the same time, reaching in opposite directions. If your buttock muscles are not shaking after a minute, you may not be lifting your legs high enough.

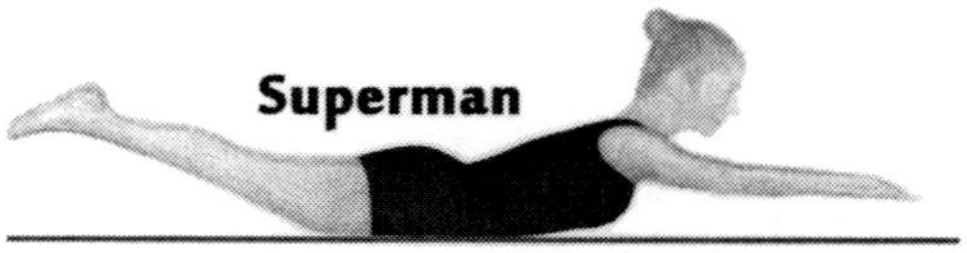

Pushup Elevator: Ultimately, this exercise is performed as a male-style pushup. If that is not possible for you at first, use a higher incline like a bench, table top, or a set of stairs, going down a step as you become stronger.

When I first started anaerobic exercise, I could not do one male-style pushup without collapsing in the middle. Now I easily push out a set of 20 or more.

Start at the top of a male-style pushup or plank position, supported by hands. Hold for 5-10 seconds, depending on strength.

Lower two inches and hold again for 5-10 seconds.

Lower two inches and hold again for required time.

Lower now to bottom pushup position and hold again.

Rise in intervals of two inches at a time with 5-10 second holds.

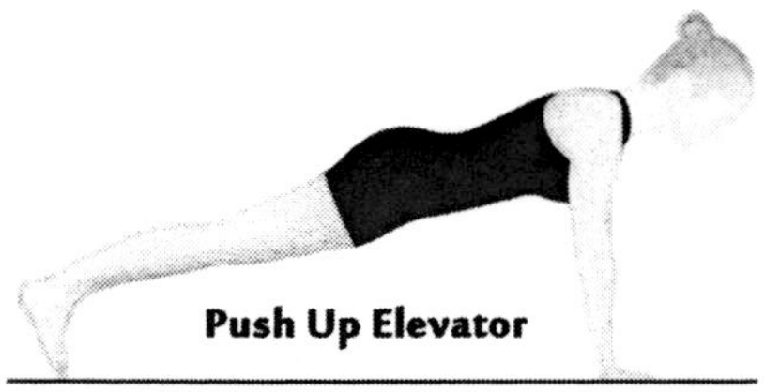

Wall Sit: Take a seated position with your back against the wall as if you are seated on an imaginary chair, hands on head, not on thighs for support. Sit for 90 seconds.

You might have to yell a bit to get through this one like a Romanian Olympian doing a shot put. For advanced athletes (not me yet), get your toddler to sit on your lap while doing this.

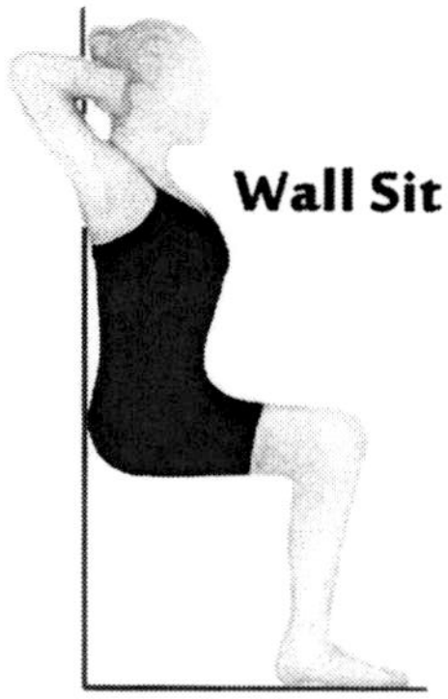

You have now finished this workout, but if you don't want to stop, there is another optional exercise to throw in for good measure.

Balance Ball Core Challenge: The goal of this exercise is to hold for only 60 seconds as it is so intense.

Start on knees with elbows supported on stability ball. Now rise onto your toes. Keep tummy tucked deep into your spine and keep your chest high, not caving towards the ball. Try to keep your form perfectly straight and balance for a goal of 60 seconds.

This workout is a complete intense training session, targeting all major muscle groups in a functional format. No expensive machines and still under 20 minutes. You could do this in your PJs. Oh Yeah! Actually, it only involves less than 10 minutes of exercise with a lot of panting in between.

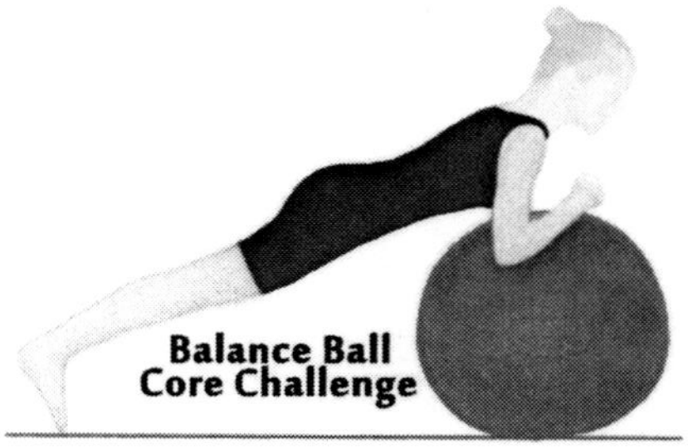

From Door to Floor

Reach up with your arm and touch the highest place on your door frame that you can, then get down and do a pushup. Depending on your strength level, use a male-style pushup on floor, or on higher inclines such as bench, stairs, or coffee table. If you cannot achieve that I'll close my eyes and you can do female-style pushup reps on your knees.

Now reach up and touch the door frame again, then get down and do two pushups.

Reach up, then down again for three pushups. Each time you will add a pushup.

Continue to do this until you are at complete muscle failure. This is a great routine that involves both aerobic and anaerobic movements. You need very little space. It is great for motel rooms and travel times.

Kettlebells

Do you want a quick explosive workout that gives superior results in a short amount of time? The kettlebell is one of the speediest methods for fat loss through its ability to incorporate resistance training with heart pounding intervals.

The kettlebell can be the best friend of any woman who wants to take back control of a sagging rear and flabby hamstrings, the muscles that run down the back of the thigh. No woman wants jelly hammies. It is also one of the top exercises for strengthening the core. When Mike Mahler, a fitness training expert, author, coach, and lecturer on physical strength and hormone optimization was asked if woman should train with kettlebells, he replied, "Yes . . . only the smart ones."

The great thing about kettlebells is you don't need a lot of space. I discovered this when my husband's job took us to apartment living for several months. I was desperate to exercise, but our tiny apartment was situated above an Italian restaurant and I couldn't jump around without complaints from the fine diners below. Kettlebells were my answer. There is no jumping around and you only need a 5x5 space to get a quick workout like no other.

If you have small children, confine your kettlebell workout to a room where you can shut the door, or a time when your little ones are napping or outdoors. You will be swinging a hunk of iron and do not want to injure anybody.

I have now become addicted to kettlebells. They are fun. I don't know if it's the swingin' thing or the many different freestyle movements that make you feel so alive and like a child again. As far as targeting all the ideals desired for intense short burst exercise, it has them all. It's the main exercise I do now! The more you learn, the more you advance and achieve more spectacular results. I feel like a child who found a favorite play thing, instead of a busy mother grudgingly fitting in her miserable workout.

Resources for Kettlebells

KETTLEBELL DVDs:

Workout DVD's are a great idea because when you press "play" you no longer have to rely on your own motivation. Below is a list of workout DVDs that are quick and also utilize our intense "change it up" approach.

It's a good idea to gather a collection of these DVDs, as finance allows, so you won't get bored and your body will have frequent new challenges. Some of these websites offer quality bells, but you can always purchase a bell from Walmart for much less, if you're strapped for money.

Visit www.busywomansworkout.com where you can order *The Busy Woman's Workout* series with Maureen Martone. I enjoy the following two DVDs from this series: *Kettlebells 6-Minute Routine for Women* and *Kettlebell Interval Training for Women*. The *Interval Training* DVD allows you to choose your workouts between 4, 8, and 12 minutes long. The exercises are randomly shuffled which yield infinite workout possibilities.

Maureen Martone and her husband, Jeff Martone are a Christian couple who are highly skilled trainers. My husband owns a couple of Jeff's kettlebell DVDs and is hooked. Their motto is "MAXIMUM RESULTS IN MINIMUM TIME." If you visit the website www.tacticalathlete.com you can order his DVDs for your husband also.

Visit www.Dragondoor.com to purchase the DVD, *Kettlebell Goddess Workout* with Andrea Du Cane. I truly value this DVD because it has many workouts on the one disk to mix everything up.

Visit www.socaltrainer.com by Lauren Brooks. This lady is a mama of little ones and carries excellent kettlebell DVDs, including a safe pregnancy workout DVD called *Baby Bells*. Don't think the *Baby Bells* workout is only for pregnant women. I do it with my younger sister, Mercy, and it kicks her behind.

Visit www.nofearfitness.com which is a website devoted to kettlebells from a woman's perspective by Lisa Shaffer.

Books:

From Russia with Tough Love by Pavell is a great kettlebell book that taught me correct form which is important for kettlebells. I downloaded it onto my kindle for quarter the price to purchase it hardcover.

Strength by Sara is an e-book by Sara Cheatham. This can be ordered as a pair with *Baby Bells* at Lauren Brook's website, www.socaltrainer.com. Or, google the title and order it from her personal blog. This book is designed for pregnant women with every safety precaution, modification, and encouragement you will need through your entire pregnancy. I used this e-book right through to the day I delivered with my most recent pregnancy. I have never experienced such a comfortable and fit third trimester.

DVD Resources utilizing other quick intense methods:

Visit www.suzannebowenfitness.com to order her *Gorgeous Core* DVD of which Pearl and I are big fans. The workouts on this DVD are 12 minutes or less. They utilize mostly body resistance, but you can use some weights with them, too. We love to do her "Metabolism Bootcamp" workout. It takes about 12 minutes and you can add weights as you get better to make it even more intense. The title of the routine sounds wild but Suzanne has a graceful approach to exercise that is not overwhelming. Pearl really enjoys doing this routine. Suzanne has another five minute workout on her DVD called *Total Core Fast Blast*. We like to layer these two together, if we have time, for a very well rounded workout set or do them individually on busy days.

Suzanne Bowen is married to our cousin, Levi Bowen and she is a world-renowned female trainer. She also has a prenatal DVD called *Long and Lean Prenatal Workout*. It's one of my favorites and has kept me in great pregnancy shape until delivery in my last two pregnancies.

Visit www.fityummymummy.com by Holly Rigsby. This site is another great source of anaerobic training for busy moms and she includes lots of kettlebell work. Her website is a must see. All her workouts are 15 minutes only and she recommends no more than 90 minutes total workout time per week. Her exercise DVDs fit with our lifestyle and eating plan perfectly. They will guide you step by step from post-baby belly bulge to a fit yummy-mummy. This is an excellent site for women who are overwhelmed and not sure where, or even how, to begin on an exercise journey. Check out her site even if you are an extreme fitness expert. Her workouts, while quick, also advance to the toughest levels.

Visit www.beachbody.com for a workout series called *Ten Minute Trainer.* These are great ten minute, very intense workouts that WORK! Out of the five workouts in the series, we only do the *Total Body* and *Lower Body* workouts as we find them the most effective 10 minute sessions. You could do the others if you want to, of course. Once you get to know the workouts, you might want to lower the volume as his training style may be offensive to some.

Visit www.jillianmichaels.com to order *30 Day Shred*. These 20 minute workouts are extremely intense, so take your time moving up to the next level. Her DVD is found in many stores, even Walmart, if you don't want to order online.

Visit www.mytrainerbob.com to order his *Inside Out Method.* This DVD has two workouts. We only do the 20 minute *Butt and Balance* workout which we love. The other workout is the cardio but it is too long. This DVD is worth getting for the *Butt and Balance* workout alone. Pearl and I have one copy of this DVD which we share (I mean fight over constantly). To make things worse, our younger sister, Mercy, who is also an avid exerciser loves it too and steals it whenever we are not looking. We never know who has it and have to call each other to say, "Get that thing over here now! I want Bob!" Sometimes we all do the workout together and that is fun. This DVD is also available at most stores like Walmart or Target.

Visit www.walmart.com for an excellent 20 minute mini trampoline workout DVD. The DVD is called *Gold's Gym Mini Trampoline Workout*. It is so much fun bouncing in all the different ways and the trainer Mia Finneagan is both gentle and encouraging. You can buy the DVD at any Walmart store if you don't want to get it online.

Tips and Tricks

The ideas and resources I have been talking about so far are good for using as entire routines. But there are also some little tips and tricks you can use to fire up your metabolism on days you are not exercising, or if you find yourself sitting down a lot during the day.

Give Me Ten

What about the plain old pushup? Get down and give me ten, or maybe you're up to twenty. This is one of the best full body exercises you can do. It tightens your core, lifts your pecs, and strengthens your arms and shoulders.

Perhaps you've been replying to emails for a while, sitting at the table helping your child with school work, or flattening your behind writing a book all day like us. Adding in some pushups can make you feel great about yourself. Sometimes, on the weekend when I take days off from exercising, or I've sat down and watched a movie with the children, a set of pushups peps me up again by releasing good blood flow.

Just Squat

What about the simple squat? I'm not a great television watcher but if I watch an occasional show, I sometimes do squats (and many times my children join me) during the ads. We try not to stop until the show resumes.

Sam Varner, in his book, *Slimmer, Younger, Stronger* explains that the squatting motion is considered the best and most effective movement. This incredibly simple squat movement involves over 65 percent of all the muscles in your body. It is super effective and efficient for those with little time on their hands.

It stimulates human growth hormone more than other weight bearing movements. This is because it is a compound movement which means it involves two or more compound joints. A compound movement gives you "more bang for your buck" in the words of Sam Varner.

Research has also found that it tones the muscles and reduces fat in the upper as well as the lower body. Basically, it gives you a full body workout with one movement. In one study, the barbell squat was performed three times a week for six weeks. No other exercise was added. The results were inspiring— a surprising reduction in the waist, gained muscle, including such areas as biceps and shoulders, and a decrease in body fat.

Let's hear it for the squat! Cheers!

Join the Jumpers

Here's another idea to keep that metabolism kicking. Take a lesson from your children. If you've been sitting inside for too long and you notice your children having fun on the trampoline, why not join them? Although, maybe you'll want to skip the back flips. You may be surprised how winded jumping on the trampoline can make you feel.

The rebounder (mini trampoline) is another great metabolism booster and you don't have to do 20 minutes at a time. Use it for a few minutes right before you cook dinner, during the ads of your favorite family TV show, or you and the children can put on a CD and each one can take a turn for one song each on the rebounder, including you.

Cell Exerciser:

The rebounder, sometimes known as the "cellucizer," stimulates every cell in your body through the forces of acceleration, deceleration, and gravity. This G force has such a full body effect that it even causes facial exercise to occur and prevents and reverses drooping facial muscles and skin. Your cells are gently squeezed at the bottom of the bounce, detoxifying the cells and forcing them to become stronger. Amazingly, rebounding has been shown to dramatically increase the mitochondria count in each cell. This is important news since the mitochondria is the nucleus in the cell which is responsible for all our energy.

As far as regular cardio exercise is concerned, rebounding trumps all as far as time efficiency. Rebounding is 68 percent more effective than regular cardio exercise. That's good news for mothers like us because we are all about getting more results in less time. A study by NASA, in the *Journal of Applied Physiology* concluded, "For similar levels of heart rate and oxygen consumption, the magnitude of the biochemical stimuli is greater with jumping on a trampoline than with running on a treadmill."

Lymphatic Pump:

Rebounding cleanses the body through the lymphatic system. It stimulates the lymphatic system more than any other exercise. Studies have shown that even moderate rebounding, for just a few minutes a day, can significantly increase the effectiveness of the lymph system, resulting in less toxins in the body.

From NASA to Garage Sales:

Like any piece of exercise equipment, high end models are expensive such as the Needac designed by NASA. But, in our experience, you can usually find a great rebounder at a yard sale for about $5.00 that will do the job. If you can't be bothered going to the trouble to seek one out, they are less than $20.00 at Walmart and come with a motivating DVD workout. It takes around 20 minutes and is a lot of fun.

Keep it Around:

Don't put the rebounder away, out of sight. It needs to be part of the furniture in your living room. The children love it and having it in sight, in fact, having it in the way where you actually have to step over it to get somewhere else, helps you get on it more. Remember, quick bursts are what we advise. You can do a one or two minute sprint or five minutes of a more basic bounce whenever you remember throughout the day.

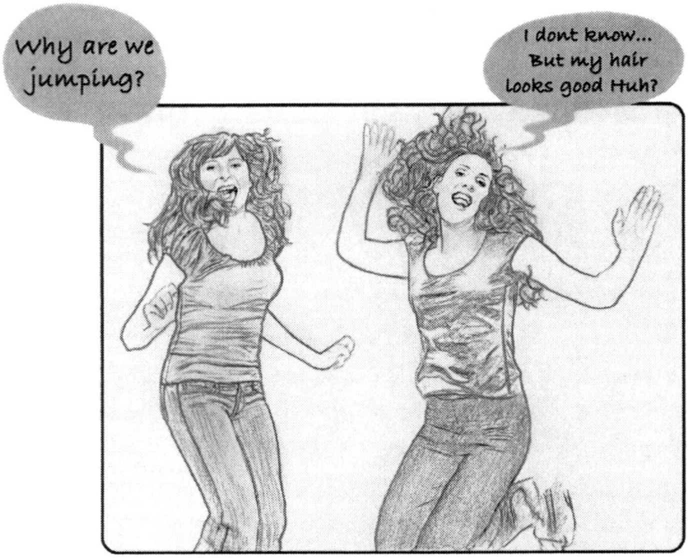

Ball Time

Sometimes, sitting inside for long periods cannot be helped. To make it better for your body, you can use a stability ball for your seat at the computer, folding laundry, or watching a movie etc. Your core is activated in this position and every time you slightly move, it has to contract tightly to re-stabilize you. Strong abs anyone? These balls are inexpensive (about $10.00) and are readily available at most stores like Walmart and Target. During school hours at our home and whenever I'm at the table helping my children, I sit on my ball.

Give it a Rest

Don't train every day of the week! Three to five days of intense routines are sufficient for each week, depending on your goals. You need at least two non-training days to allow for muscle growth. You will actually inhibit strength gains by training every day. Remember, your training days are designed to break down your muscles and your rest days are to repair and rebuild.

Take a week's rest every month or two and take some walks and do some stretches instead of your usual anaerobic training. (You could research muscle foam rolling, the cheapest, deep muscle massage you'll ever get). Resting allows for proper hormone balance, prevents overtraining, and keeps you less susceptible to injuries. Plus, you can look forward to these reward weeks. Some women like to take this time off during their periods. Just make sure you start up again. If you need motivation get back to exercising, re-read THE MURDERING EPIDEMIC paragraphs a few pages back.

What's the Deal?

If you are still not serious about committing to the priority of exercise in your life, imagine me in your face right now. Imagine that I have just done my morning resistance workout, swinging kettlebells. I am sweaty and revved up and will not take any lame, pathetic excuses. So tell me, what's holding you back? No time? Sorry, we have covered that. You have five minutes here and there throughout the day. If you give enough importance to brushing your teeth, but don't give at least that same amount of time to strengthening your body, what's the problem? Hopefully, after reading Pearl's *Foxy Mama*, Chapter 34 you realize you eliminate other things to make time for sex. Exercise is only going to give you more energy for sex and make it better in every way. The two go hand in hand. Sex is great exercise, but adding additional small spurts of exercise into your day will give you better energy for sex, and help to increase your libido.

Feelings Don't Factor

You don't ask yourself, "Should I brush my teeth today?" You always brush them, whether you feel like it or not. If you don't, you'll have horrible breath and your teeth will rot. You don't have to feel like exercising to do it. Feelings don't factor with most priorities in life. You don't feel like getting up when your baby cries at night, but of course you do. You know you have to. The word is commitment. The same principle applies to making your body move.

Is the thought of starting too overwhelming? Do you feel like you are already too far gone to even begin? Rubbish! If you are still breathing, you can start. Do not believe those lies. Maybe you've never been the exercising type. Well, I'm telling you, you are. But, you are just going to baby step your way there. Seek for little improvements every week. You owe it to yourself, your husband, and your children.

Not Vanity, but Responsibility

I look at it like this. At the altar on our wedding day, my husband made an investment in me for his future. Looking after my body, and consequently my health, is looking after his investment. I want the best, not only for me, but for him. Should I let the value of his stocks fall? Aren't I supposed to be his helpmeet and look after the things that matter to him? Exercise is not vanity; it is responsibility. It is respect for yourself and your husband.

There is no choice. God made our bodies to move. Get up and get moving.

Chapter 39

Movin' with the Belly

by Serene Allison

Pregnancy is not the time for the kind of intense exercise that reaches the benchmarks for HGH release. You don't have to worry about this, as pregnancy raises HGH on its own by 10 percent. Science declares infallibly that pregnancy is a super state for health and well being. It floods a woman's body with youthful, anti-aging, and healing hormones. Enjoy this time of glowing skin, rounding breasts, and even the remission of many pre-pregnancy sicknesses. It can be a time of renewed youth and super abundant health.

It is not such a fragile state that you should limit yourself to a sedentary lifestyle. It is not an illness and it is not a handicap. There is no reason you cannot stay active. In fact, not only is it safe to continue to exercise during pregnancy, it is one of the healthiest things you can do for you, as well as your baby. Exercising regularly throughout your pregnancy improves the supply of glucose and oxygen for the baby. It also enlarges the life support organ for the baby which is the placenta.

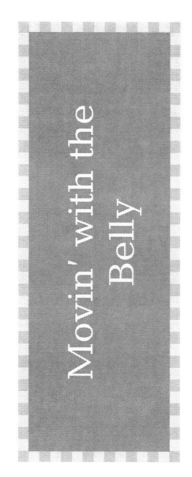

The Careful Way

It's important to make a caution here that there are exceptions to the majority of low risk, healthy pregnancies. There are conditions during some pregnancies that may call for extreme careful measures, i.e., incompetent cervix, impending miscarriage, pre-term labor, or major illness.

We must take a "common sense" approach to pregnancy which is to have, above all, concern and respect for your growing baby within. Keep an awareness at all times of the way your body, as well as your baby, is responding to a particular exercise. There should be a beautiful harmony between a good vigorous workout, the comfort of all reproductive supporting ligaments, and a thriving baby.

1. No exercise should be continued if you feel a pulling or "twining" sensation in the area of the abdomen.
2. No exercise should be continued that leaves you exhausted for several hours afterward.
3. No exercise should be continued that initiates early contractions that do not slow down during the rest period post workout.
4. No exercise should be an all out "gut bust" i.e., no sprints or Spew routine.
5. No exercise should be fueled through caffeine to make you push harder. You need to be aware of your true energy levels. Small amounts of coffee may be fine during pregnancy, but don't use coffee as an intensifier for a workout during this time.
6. No exercise should be initiated without a well-nourished and hydrated body. It's very important not to start your workout in a fasted state. This means you should not be three hours past your last meal or exercising first thing in the morning before eating. A small snack is all that's required. Also, don't forget your protein after your workout. It is even more important to remember to eat protein during pregnancy where your macronutrient requirement is higher, regardless of exercise.

Always make sure you get plenty of rest in a balanced measure to your exercise. If you have completed a workout, been to the grocery store, and have been outside chasing your toddler, you'll need to rest and recuperate to get the forces of gravity off your cervix for a while.

The Vigorous Way

After all these precautions, I'm sure you understand that you don't have to march in place or lift only one pound dumbbells. I am not into only doing a leisurely walk around the park and a few light stretches either. While there's nothing wrong with that, it will not sustain muscle tone and will not be enough to strengthen the pregnancy supportive muscles of the lower back and girdle muscles. Birth is an athletic event, similar to running a marathon. It truly is labor and requires excellent blood pressure, endurance ability, and a strong heart. A meander around the park, while much better than nothing, doesn't give you all that.

Back in your Jeans

If your aim is a rapid return to your favorite jeans, your ticket to success will be some sort of body resistance or the use of tools like kettlebells. My desire is to enjoy the "baby moon" after the birth of my little one, without the creeping depression of 30 pounds plus to lose. If you are shooting for that too, you need to do more than walk around the block with a pregnant friend. But, don't cut that out altogether. It's tradition, right?

Pregnancy is a time where a woman becomes more insulin resistance so there is a higher chance of body fat gain. The body tries to reserve sugar stores for the baby's brain and high progesterone helps us do this. Our own muscle cells will say "No more" to the sugar they are offered. They do this to spare it for the baby. Isn't that a beautiful sacrifice? You don't even know you are doing it when you are pregnant, but you're already sacrificing for the baby.

To ensure this doesn't result in too much weight gain, exercise helps increase your metabolic capacity, insulin sensitivity, muscle mass, and the use of fat stores to supply energy requirements. Of course, *Trim Healthy Mama-ing* will go a long way to stop excess sugar floating around wildly in your body and looking for a home in your fat cells. Let's flourish the baby, not the backside. The bump should stay in front!

Fears Relieved

If you're worried that anything more than a walk in the park may bring on pre-term labor, I've been in this situation. I've had two pre-term impending labors, one in which my baby arrived two months early and had to be in the NICU for three weeks. However, in both of these pregnancies, I mostly walked for exercise. Plus, I was faced with a lot of excess stress (not just dishes in the sink stress). In succeeding pregnancies, I carefully added body resistance and free weight workouts. My workouts were a lot more intense, yet I went overdue! Studies run by Dr. James F. Clapp III MD, an OB and author of the book, *Exercising Through Your Pregnancy* reveal that even vigorous exercise does not increase the incidence of either membrane rupture or pre-term labor.

This is only my personal theory, but I think my rich protein diet, along with exercises that supported muscle gains and strength, helped ward off my prior issue with early dilation. Entering my last two pregnancies I felt stronger all over, and I believe my core and pelvic floor were also at a new level of strength. The *Trim Healthy Mama* lifestyle, with its significant focus on protein and resistant exercise, restored the fragile weak state of my body. Many years of veganism, along with muscle wasting and long hours of steady state endurance exercise (with no change of pace), could have been one of the causes of this pre-term issue that I was able to overcome.

My Favorites

I am pregnant again now (the second time around during the writing of this book) and I love the *Baby Bells* DVD. This workout is longer than the more intense non-pregnant protocols where we usually keep things under 20 minutes. Since you shouldn't shoot for that kind of intensity while pregnant, it's okay to go a little longer. *Baby Bells* is 35 minutes because it keeps the heart rate from jumping too high. But, it seems to go fast, because it layers three different fun circuits, including the warm up and cool down stretching sessions which are very relaxing. I do it two times a week because I have other DVDs that keep things fresh for me. I hate to get bored.

Suzanne Bowen's *Long and Lean Prenatal Workout* is like the meat in my sandwich. I can't do without it while pregnant. It's an intense 40 minute workout, but in a deep massage kind of way, not the boot camp kind. After talking with her personally, she suggested breaking it up into two 20 minute sessions. You can do the "standing work" one day and the "floor work" another day.

While pregnant, I think it's good to aim for some resistance exercise for at least three to four days a week. The other days can be for meandering walks.

The Gentle Way

I try to exercise right through to the delivery day when possible. However, I make sure I take things nice and slow post birth.

For the first couple of days, I mostly stay in bed and allow my body to contract back as much as possible. On day three, I start kegels (contractions of the perineum and vaginal muscles—google for directions) and belly breathing. These are tummy exercises that are described in the book, *Maternal Fitness*, by Julie Tupler. It is a foundational read for any pregnant woman. If you purchase only one book while pregnant, that might be it. At this two to three day mark, I also start some light stretching on my bed.

The entire first week I try to take it completely easy. The less gravity on my body the better. Every day I do a little more kegels, belly breaths, and light stretching. I don't do any walks or formal exercise. I spend my time kissing and caressing my baby and resting so my milk comes in rich and creamy.

Week two is when I may start what I call "granny walks." These are even more relaxing than the meanders most pregnant women take around the mall. They are short, lazy strolls. Of course, I continue my routine of kegels, belly breaths, and stretching. These are the most important for getting the post partum corset laced up tight again.

After week three, if I am feeling great and have mostly stopped bleeding, I may begin Suzanne Bowen's *Long and Lean* routine, only one session at a time for 20 minutes, tops. On the same DVD, she also has a 10 minute postnatal ab toning session. That's a good one to add in around the three week mark.

From four weeks onwards, I listen to my body and allow a little more exercise intensity as my body gains strength. Labor and birth, as well as the plummeting of hormones after pregnancy, requires this time of recuperation. Bones, joints, and ligaments separate for birth and all need to slowly move back into place. Some people say you should be able to bounce right back and return to whatever exercise you were doing pre-pregnancy. I believe a slower approach is much safer and better for your long term maternal health.

I am one of those crazy folk who actually love exercise. It's hard for me to hold myself back, but I don't want to end up with a prolapsed uterus or fractured bones. Also, my focus is on my newborn in those first few weeks. Regular, vigorous exercise during my entire pregnancy helps make me feel deserving of this special break.

By the twelve week mark, you should easily be able to start back into your more intense DVDs and short burst approach. However, don't do sprint intervals on the first day back to full exercise. Ramp up slowly and carefully.

Chapter 40

Mama Glows
(Your Skin Care)

Your skin is like a sponge. Think about it. Nicotine patches, birth control patches, and hormonal replacement creams are all actual medications that are absorbed through the skin and make huge impacts in the body.

Our skin is also our largest detox organ. It is meant to be a place where toxins come out, not go in. Therefore skin creams, even if they say "all natural," can be a dangerous onslaught of chemical cocktails.

You need to watch out for the following harmful ingredients in most hair and skin products:

Parabens
Phthalates
EDTA
Propylene glycol
Synthetic colorings
Ureas
Vegetable oils

It takes years for some of these chemicals to break down when absorbed through your skin.

Another thing for you and your teenage sons and daughters to consider is to avoid antiperspirants that contain aluminum. Your under arm is right next to your lymph system and there is much concern that the absorption of aluminum may lead to greater risk of breast cancer. There have been many conflicting studies on this subject, some finding cause for concern, others finding no increased risk. We think it's better to err on the side of caution. Find effective alternatives at your health food store. There are also highly effective homemade recipes using baking soda which you can google online.

The best thing you can do for your skin is to stay on a low gylcemic way of life. This is far more important than any expensive cream you purchase. Dr. Perricone, the world renowned dermatologist, talks about how inflammation is the destroyer of skin. Sugar and high glycemic carbohydrates such as excessive amounts of sweet fruit or starchy vegetables (like white potatoes), cause rapid inflammation at a cellular level. These elevated blood sugar levels cause chemical reactions that create free radicals and attack the lipid bi-layer membranes of our cells. The result is premature aging in our skin.

Dr. Perricone writes in *The Perricone Prescription*, "Even a healthy body is damaged by sugar in a phenomenon known as glycation. When foods rapidly convert to sugar in the blood stream, as high glycemic carbohydrates do, they cause browning, or glycating of a protein in your tissues . . . Glycation can occur in skin as well, creating detrimental age-related changes to collagen and that means deep wrinkles . . . Glycation causes irreversible cross links between adjoining collagen molecules. This extensive cross-linking of collagen causes the loss of skin elasticity."

Perricone goes on to describe how that when a young person smiles or frowns, creating lines on the face, the skin returns easily to an unlined state. But, the skin of a person who has eaten a high-carb diet for years and cross-linked their collagen will not snap back and smooth out. He also says, "These deep grooves remain because that is where the sugar molecules have attached to collagen, making the fibers stiff and inflexible."

Beware of using harsh scrubs or derm-abrasion products. Don't get caught up in the alpha hydroxy craze. These peel off the protective outer layers of skin and destroy a natural pH balance. These creams destroy the natural rhythm of skin growth and shedding. This leads to overly dry skin that is more prone to wrinkles. Support your skin, do not turbo sand it.

So, what should we use on our skin? For those older than 30, we suggest considering estriol. We stumbled upon using an estriol cream (a bioidentical form of the estrogen secreted during pregnancy) as the most amazing skin restorer. We both use pea-sized amounts of estriol cream from the brand Life-flo. It is called Estriol-Care and we order it from www.swansonvitamins.com. It costs around $10.00 for a 2 oz. bottle which lasts a couple of months.

We use it on our face and neck every morning and evening. Estriol is a safe hormone that increases collagen, moisture, and elasticity in the skin. It restores youthful plumping and hydration. In the small doses we use Estriol-Care it does not contribute to estrogen dominance and can even be used while nursing. We love the fact that it also has no parabens. If we stop using this cream, we notice the dry parched feeling came back to our skin; it keeps a soft and toned look to the face. When we run out, we race over to each other's home to borrow until we get more.

We look at estriol cream as underwear for our skin. But, we also need to dress, right? Here's what we use to dress our skin each day:

Kit Naturals (Kath's Intensive Treatments—All Natural creams, Salves, Lotions, and Balms). Available from www.kitnaturals.com.

You'll love us for introducing you to these products. And, we love the gal who has created this incredible and inexpensive line of skin food.

We did say "food." You can literally eat every ingredient in this product line, not that we're recommending that. Kath has children with severe allergies and has created these creams to be free of the eight major allergens (milk, tree nuts, shellfish, fish, eggs, peanuts, wheat, and soy).

Her products have zero carcinogens and zero parabens. They are made with the medicinal properties of fresh herbs and pure oils. Kath uses a process that is very rare in the skin care business today. She infuses the oils with the herbs in small batch creations. This results in creams that are antioxidant rich, naturally antiseptic and antifungal, while deeply nourishing the skin.

We have longed to use creams like Kit Naturals before, but could never afford the ones that had only organic and edible ingredients. Other organic skin creams, not even as pure as Kath's, which sell as "all pure and edible" run at exorbitant prices. It's hard to find facial creams like these without spending at least $50 for a one month supply. Since Kath runs this as a family business, with older homeschooling children, she is able to keep costs way down, yet still delivers exceptional quality.

Kath's *Orange Silk Hydrating Cream* which we are crazy about for our face and body, is only $14 for 2 oz. Can you believe it? The jar lasts us much longer than a month's worth, even using it on our body as well as our face.

Kit Naturals products are made with both coconut and olive oil as their base. Olive oil protects against free radicals, slows the signs of aging and fine lines, offers vitamins A and E, and helps maintain elasticity, while coconut oil keeps connective tissue in the skin strong and supple. It prevents age spots, repairs, heals, penetrates into the layers of skin, and naturally combats infections with its antibacterial and antifungal properties.

Aloe Vera is another superstar in Kit Naturals. It forms a natural barrier that shields skin from toxins. It moisturizes, keeps skin flexible, increases strength and synthesis of skin tissue, lightens dark spots, treats acne, and improves the ability of the skin to hydrate itself. Aloe Vera is an excellent "carrier." It enables the healing properties of the herbs in to be drawn more effectively into the skin layers where they can work their magic.

Calendula is Kath's chief herb in all of her products. It has been called the "mad skin plant." It is anti-inflammatory, antibacterial, promotes fast healing and regeneration of skin, promotes youthful glow, treats acne and scars, and is full of antioxidants which protect against the damages of time and exposure.

We love these creams, not only because of what they do, but how they smell. Ah, the aroma of orange essential oil. It's full of vitamin C, one of the most anti-aging components for skin regeneration. Along with being a natural antibiotic, orange oil is nature's antidepressant with its ability to promote happy feelings, stimulates cell activity, and growth in the skin.

Two other important ingredients in these creams should be mentioned. Beeswax is also anti-inflammatory, antibacterial, antiviral and acts as an emollient and a humectant, drawing moisture to the skin and sealing it in. Vitamin E plays a key role too. It reduces the appearance of fine lines and wrinkles and is another strong antioxidant. It treats scars, prevents water loss, and helps retain moisture.

Now you can understand why we're nuts about these products and their price.

Pearl chats: My husband experienced severe dry skin on his hands every winter without fail. His hands got so dry that they cracked and bled, sometimes even getting infected from the open wounds. I tried every possible lotion and balm throughout the years to help, but nothing alleviated the problem.

This past winter someone gave me a jar of Kit Naturals cream as a gift. I'd never seen or heard of it before, but it smelled great and I was excited about its purity. I loved the results on my face, so I started applying it to my husband's hands. I didn't really expect any dramatic results since his condition was so acute and all my other attempts had failed. His hands were already dried out because we were in the month of December. Within one week of using the cream, the dryness subsided. The cracks disappeared after another week and his hands completely healed to smooth skin. He was astonished and so was I. Once they were healed, I made sure to rub some of the cream into his hands every few days and that was enough to ensure that none of the dryness returned. It was a little miracle.

Serene chats: Finding Kit Naturals was like stumbling over a treasure chest for me. After reading this book, you may have figured out that I am a complete purist, sometimes to the point of being ridiculous. Nothing I could afford was ever pure enough for me. I would end up putting straight oils on my face that always looked greasy, felt heavy, and didn't absorb properly. I even put pure red palm oil on my face. Some people thought I had a liver disease with my orange face.

In comes Kit Naturals to save the day. Here was something that finally met my strict and psycho standards. The icing on the cake is that Kit Naturals is not only incredibly effective, but affordable. I now feel not only like an "all naturaaaaal" girl, but I no longer look strange and greasy.

I have always obsessed about wrinkles. Even when I was too young to have them, I was still concerned about them. I once taped my face (at 13 years), when I went to sleep at night in case I rolled over, squished my face in the pillow, and created lines and furrows. After all the pain of ripping tape off the red raw screaming skin, I never tried that again! Now, in my mid thirties, when most women begin worrying, I am at perfect peace with Kath's creams babying my skin.

This chat has been a confessional of some of my absurd behaviors and since I have come clean on some, I will throw in another one for good measure. You'll really believe I am a little nuts after this, but hey, there may be someone as nutty as me who may like this idea. Every morning and night, I spray a little fresh milk onto the palm of my hand and dab it all over my face and neck. You might be asking, "What fresh milk, and how does one spray it? Is this a new aerosol product? Well, not exactly, but . . . well . . . um . . . it's my own breast milk, when in season!

Now, before you think I am a completely loony, science backs me up. Breast-milk is incredibly rich in anti-fungal, antiseptic, antibacterial, and soothing middle chain fatty acids. It is an incredible therapy for rashes, eczema, burns, acne, bites, and infections of the skin. It can also be used for ear infections and sore throats. My aim may not be so good for spraying for these purposes, but a little expressed milk put in an eye dropper does the trick. I have only skimmed the surface about the amazing healing properties of breast milk with its immunoglobulins and other goodies.

I think most mamas will want to stick with Kit Naturals, but I had the itch to share my latest craze. I mean, we feel like family now after writing to you in this book for over four long years.

Another great source for affordable yet pure skin care lotions and other products is http://www.frontierfamilyfarms.com/. They are another family business that focuses on full body organic soaps and lotions. Thankfully, like Kit Naturals they won't break your bank and their soaps and lotions smell and feel amazing.

Chapter 41

Mama's Secret Weapons
(Supplements)

It would be nice to say that a whole foods diet can give you all the vitamins and minerals you need, but this is the real world. Let's face it, we need a few extras to keep our bodies protected and running at optimum.

We could lament that our soil is not as good as it used to be and even organic produce is not near the quality of what our forefathers ate. Depressing. On the brighter side, there is a trade off in this technological age. Science has discovered many potent, anti-aging healing substances that are now available to us in a carefully concentrated state. Great-great Uncle Joe didn't have access to the vast array of supplements now widely available to us.

Okay, we know what you are thinking . . . $$$. You don't have enough, right? We want to give you a bare bones affordable supplement list. Hey, there may be times you cannot even afford these basic supplements, but don't beat yourself up. You will at least be eating the most optimum way on the **S** and **E** plan, and that is the best you can do.

For those who can stretch their budget a little more, we have included a basic, and a more thorough list of important supplements. If you can afford all those, more power to you! We're jealous.

Bare Bones

Cod Liver Oil

This is nature's richest source of vitamins A and D. It provides essential omega-3 acids, EPA, and DHA for crucial brain health and growth. Cod liver oil plays an important role in supporting cardiovascular health. It also contributes to calcium metabolism and bone health.

This oil is essential for children's brain and nervous system development and crucial for women in their reproductive years. It helps to relieve depression and menstrual disorders while it also aids metabolism and weight loss.

Try to purchase a bottle which has been molecularly distilled so any toxic heavy metals have been removed. You can choose lemon, mint, or orange flavored oils which disguise the fishy taste. For those who get fishy burps, which we have never noticed, enteric coated capsules are available.

One of the best brands is BLUE ICE Fermented Cod Liver Oil—Arctic Mint, available from www.greenpasture.org. This is a very good oil, but not affordable for those on bare bones. A cheaper one we approve is Swanson's Pristine Norwegian, available from www.swansonvitamins.com.

Vitamin D3

Most of us are deficient in this nutrient which is more like a hormone than a vitamin. Fortunately, it is inexpensive and readily available.

Spending time in the sun enables your body to make vitamin D, which is why it is called the sunshine vitamin, but this is not always effective. As we age, our ability to absorb it from the sun wanes. Plus, in later years, we are more prone to avoid the sun to preserve our skin. Many cold climates are not appropriate for attaining healthy levels of vitamin D as less time is spent outdoors and less sunlight is available.

Half an hour in the middle hours of a summer day, with arms and legs bare to the sun, will give you about 10,000 iu (international unit, which measures biological activity, or effect of a substance). That's a nice healthy dose. The problem is, once you have developed a decent tan, absorption is not as great.

One of the best things you can do to prevent cancer is to increase your vitamin D levels. Low levels are associated with all forms of cancer and immune diseases. Vitamin D increases the fighting power of your immune system which is so important with new viruses creating worldwide epidemics. Most people know it is important for strong bones and teeth, but it is less commonly known that Vitamin D is essential for cardiovascular health. A recent *Harvard* study, tracking 18,000 men, showed that the men with the highest blood levels of vitamin D were the least likely to have heart attacks, while the men with the lowest D levels had the highest risk. According to several studies, and one more recent 2011 study published in *Archives of*

Internal Medicine, vitamin D deficiency increases the risk of premature death from all causes by 26 percent.

The lack of vitamin D is a big cause of asthma in children. It is a good idea to get the whole family tested for vitamin D. While cod liver oil provides you with a dietary source, it is not enough to increase levels if they are lacking. Even without testing, it is safe for children to take 400 iu of vitamin D a day. Adults can safely take 1000-2000 iu a day. More is often needed once levels have been verified by a 25-hydroxy vitamin D test. Oil soft gels are the best form.

While taking vitamin D, it is a good idea to keep cod liver oil in your diet. D supplementation in high doses can have a lowering effect on vitamin A levels in the body. Taking cod liver oil helps to ensure a good balance between the two vitamins.

Pearl chats: I read about vitamin D deficiencies a few years back and started to take 2000 iu of vitamin D a day. I have avoided direct sunlight for many years as I have fair skin and tend to freckle. I figured I'd probably be rather low in this vitamin. I took this dose for three months and then had my levels tested. I guessed I'd probably come back in the high range since I considered 2000 iu a hefty dose. To my surprise, my level only came in at 33 (with a range of 32-100). I must have been very low to begin with (scary). Simply being in range does not mean you are covered. According to most cutting-edge, anti-aging doctors, D levels should be between 60-90. Interestingly enough, I had chronic asthma as a child, another sign of low vitamin D, so I have probably been deficient most of my life. Now, I dose 5000-8000 iu a day.

My father tested his levels and they came back at only 13. That is dangerous for a man of his age. He started on a high dose of 8000 iu a day. After three months, his levels only climbed to low thirties. Strangely enough, he gets a lot of sun and has a deep tan. After 10,000 iu for six months, his levels only reached the mid fifties. This is a good example of how it often takes a lot more for elderly people to get their levels up into protective numbers.

Serene chats: To be on the safe side, if you want to supplement more than 4000 iu a day, you should do a test to see how your body reacts. I took on average 4000 iu a day for six months before I ever tested. My levels came back at 76.3. That's great. I don't need more, because optimum is between 60-90. But, I do get a lot more sunshine than Pearl.

Green Supplement

The cheapest ways to get more supplemental greens are via alfalfa tablets or liquid chlorophyll concentrated drops. Greens build the blood. For those of us in our reproductive years, this is extra important. Greens are powerful cleansers. They detox the body and build the immune system. They help to eliminate odors from the body so those of us who use chlorophyll will stink less. Yay!

Serene chats: Superfood green powders are superb, but they have not been affordable for me. What I love about concentrated chlorophyll drops is that you have the option of purchasing mint flavor. I love adding green minty drops to my chocolate smoothies. It's like a York Pattie in a drink and much easier than choking down gummy green powders that stick to the roof of your mouth and teeth.

Pearl chats: I buy a large organic jar of alfalfa tablets from swansonvitamins.com where I purchase most of my vitamins at very low prices. I get 360 organic tablets for just under $10.00 and take from four to eight per day.

There is evidence that alfalfa improves the cholesterol panel, creating a better ratio between HDL and LDL. The fiber content of alfalfa sticks to cholesterol so it doesn't stay in the blood and cannot be deposited on blood vessel walls. Alfalfa helps us assimilate other foods since it contains all eight essential enzymes needed to aid digestion for all four classes of food—proteins, fats, starches, and sugars.

Alfalfa helps to heal problems with the intestinal tract. It is used in treatment for ulcers and colitis. It is incredibly high in protein, at 18.9 percent! It is also high in iron and can help increase red blood cell count in a beneficial way. It promotes lactation and increases milk supply. It is rich in vitamin K which helps blood to clot after an injury. It helps postpartum women shorten duration of bleeding and may benefit females with excessive and long periods.

Note: If you take aspirin to thin the blood, you may not want to use alfalfa since it may interfere with anti-clotting medication. Alfalfa should also not be taken by anyone who has lupus as it can aggravate this condition.

Vitamin C

No bare bones list should be complete without this one. Why? Not only does it support the immune system, but vitamin C is vital for the adrenal glands to work properly. Our adrenals regulate energy and the ability to cope with stress. Take enough vitamin C per day to tolerance; whatever you can stand without getting diarrhea.

Magnesium

This mineral calms the body, soothes the nerves, and helps relax the muscles and arteries. But, here's the really great thing. It makes certain you "go" in the morning. You know what we mean, right? It won't leave you constipated.

There is plenty of fiber in the nutritional guidelines we advise, but magnesium gives you the daily guarantee that you will not feel bloated with stuck poop when you wear your jeans. Yes, we did just say that. We ask for grace. As sisters, we have "poopy" conversations probably far too often.

Magnesium is cheap. In citrate form, it is a little pricier, but it is still under $8.00 for two month's supply. It is better absorbed by the body so you get the added health benefits for the nervous system. Take at night on an empty stomach to ensure bowel evacuation the next morning. Usually two to five tablets will do the trick. Any more than that may cause diarrhea, but everyone is different and some people may need more.

Note: Those who have IBS type conditions which result in bouts of diarrhea would not want to use this on their bare bones list.

Pearl chats: I purchase Nature Made brand magnesium oxide tablets from Walmart for only a couple of dollars. They are not absorbed well by the body in oxide form so I'm probably getting less of the other benefits of magnesium, but it is inexpensive this way and a great help to my regularity. I take three to five 250 mg tablets every night and am the most regular woman you could find. It really helps when I have to travel with time differences and when sitting for long periods (such as writing this book) that would usually affect my regularity. When I have a little extra money, I take magnesium in citrate form as well. This enables me to absorb more and to have greater positive effects on my nervous and muscular systems.

Extra Supplements

If you have some extra cash, you could add the following:

Curcumin

You can either purchase the supplement or use a lot of turmeric in your cooking. Curcumin is a potent anti-inflammatory. Remember, inflammation triggers the formation of disease and Curcumin is a powerful anti-cancer weapon.

Selenium

Again, an excellent cancer fighting tool. Many of us have heavy metals in our body. Selenium will not pull them out, but does neutralize the heavy metals from poisoning us. It helps convert the inactive thyroid hormone T4 into the active thyroid hormone T3. This is essential for an optimum metabolism. Up to 200 mcg (micrograms) a day is fine. More than that can be toxic. If you'd rather not buy selenium in supplement form, eating five Brazil nuts a day will give you 200 mcg.

Tart Cherry Extract

This supplement is almost worthy to go on the bare bones list because it is relatively inexpensive, yet the punches it packs are powerful. Tart cherries are natural pain relievers. In some studies, they have shown tart cherry to be 10 times more powerful at lowering inflammation than aspirin. Those who suffer from headaches and pain from arthritis or fibromyalgia can receive great relief from tart cherries. It has a similar effect on pain as ibuprofen or naproxen.

Tart cherries have two natural anti-cancer flavonoids called isoquercritrin and quercetin. But, cherries have another secret weapon that fights cancer called perillyl alcohol or POH. This has been called nature's own chemotherapy agent because of the way it targets cancer. POH shuts down the growth of cancer cells by depriving them of the proteins they need to grow.

Research at the *University of Iowa* has shown that tart cherries are extremely powerful in reducing the incidence of all kinds of cancer. POH has shown significant results in the treatment of advanced carcinomas of the breast, prostate, and ovaries. In animal studies, it has shown to induce the regression of 81percent of small breast cancers and up to 75 percent of advanced breast cancers. Studies also show that tart cherries significantly inhibit the growth of colon cancer tumors.

A study at the *University of Michigan* in 2007 found that tart cherries lowered blood sugar, fat storage in the liver, and oxidative stress. This means that tart cherries may be a handy tool to reduce the likelihood of Type 2 diabetes and the metabolic syndromes of our current western lifestyle.

Tart cherries are chock full of anthocyanins. These are potent antioxidants that are the sought after power weapon in berries and are what create the bright color of cherries and berries. Anthocyanins are able to make many positive changes in the body. This is the reason tart cherries protect against heart attack and stroke, protect the brain and neuromuscular system, support the immune system, help lower LDL cholesterol, and naturally lower blood pressure.

Tart cherry juice is available as a common remedy for pain relief, but we recommend buying the extract in capsules to avoid the sugars in the juice. The least expensive place to purchase these capsules is at www.swansonvitamins.com. They often have a two for one sale.

Resveratrol

You've probably heard some news reports on the benefits of resveratrol as a "life extender." This is because it contains a mechanism for eliminating free radicals and activates a longevity gene. The only other mechanism known to turn this longevity gene on in the human body is calorie deprivation, and that's not a fun way to live. In studies done on worms, rats, yeast, and flies, resveratrol extended life by a whopping 70 percent. When humans take resveratrol, it simply "turns on" the genes that protect us from disease even if we are not practicing calorie restriction.

Resveratrol fights mutated and malignant cancer cells by suppressing the action of the key protein that feeds them. This is known as Nuclear Factor-kappa B, or NF-KB for short. Since resveratrol comes from the skin of red grapes, some studies show that three to four glasses of red wine per week can supply us with enough of this substance to suppress NR-KB.

As a supplement, it is not yet known how much is too much. To be on the safe side, it is recommended to take one to two 250 mg capsules per day.

Multivitamin

We only endorse food-based multivitamins, not synthetics. In our opinion, the best are New Chapter brand where the food-based potent extracts have been fermented for much better absorption. Vitamin Code from Garden of Life is another excellent multi. Both of those are pricey, though. *Now* brand has a cheaper whole food-based multi called Multi-Food Complex which should cover all bases.

Be careful about using a multi with iron if you are a menopausal women or an older man. Women who have stopped menstruating can easily get elevated iron as they are no longer losing red blood cells during menses every 28 days. Too much iron in the body is not healthy. It can cause free radical damage in the body which is thought to be one of the contributors to cancer. Getting a complete blood count to check for iron, hemoglobin, and hematocrit is a good idea before taking any iron supplements if you are not in child-bearing years.

Cholesterol Supplements

If you have a less than perfect cholesterol profiles we need to talk about what not to use first. Statins are widely overused since they are a billion dollar industry promoted by drug companies. The important thing to look for with your cholesterol profile is your ratio. This ratio is obtained by dividing the HDL cholesterol into the total cholesterol. The goal is to keep the ratio below 5:1, with ideal being less than 3.5:1.

Statins, which are often handed out like candy to keep LDL below 100, should be carefully considered before use. They inhibit CoQ10, which is a very important and essential nutrient. It is responsible for the production of energy, especially in the heart and liver. Statins affect the mitochondria of the cell and can cause muscle dysfunction and wasting. Statins bring about conditions in groups of nerves that cause pain. They can lower sexual desire and function because cholesterol is synthesized into our sex hormones. They can alter immune systems, cause inflammation of the muscles, lead to breakdowns in muscle fiber, and even cause brain damage through inhibiting cholesterol to the brain.

Please, if you are on any kind of statin, be sure to take a CoQ10 supplement to prevent this depletion. Statins may keep your cholesterol low, but with a lowered CoQ10 level, your heart is at risk for even more severe damage than high cholesterol. The reason is that each cell has mitochondria, but the heart muscle has more mitochondria than any other place in the body.

We have all been told that HDL is the "goody" and LDL is the "baddy" when it comes to the good and evils of cholesterol. While there is truth to that, it is the size of the particles that matters most. According to Dr. Arthur Agatston, author of South Beach Diet Heart Program, "Not all HDL is good enough to do its job efficiently. Some types of HDL are simply too small. Like shuttle buses with too few seats, small HDL particles, even if you have a lot of them, cannot transport enough cholesterol out of your artery walls."

We want big particles of both kinds of cholesterol. The carbohydrate-conscious way of eating we outline in this book should help to make your cholesterol particles bigger and fluffier. It is the smaller, more densely packed particles that move through the inner cell lining of the artery walls and create more plaque.

You can look at your triglyceride levels if you want to get a good guess at how big or small your cholesterol particles are. Triglycerides over 100 are a warning sign. High-carb diets are the biggest culprit with regard to high triglyceride levels. Most people, once on a reduced carb diet for several months will notice their triglycerides drop to well below 100 and their cholesterol particle sizes increase.

Even the dreaded LDL is not always the ogre it is made out to be. In the book, *Eat Fat, Lose Fat: The Healthy Alternative to Trans Fats* and *Nourishing Traditions* by Mary Enig and Sally Fallon, the authors point to the famous Framingham, Massachusetts town. Residents have been studied for 50 years for major risk factors associated with heart disease, stroke, and other diseases. One of the many scientific papers from the studies found that women in Framingham over the age of 70 years had a greater risk of heart disease if their LDL was low.

Sometimes, highly elevated LDL cholesterol is simply a sign that there is a lack of certain hormones in the body. Essentially, there is a breakdown somewhere in the synthesis of cholesterol into hormones. Often optimizing thyroid and pregnenolone levels will remarkably reduce LDL levels without adding statin type drugs or altering diet. It is important to get a hormonal panel done if you have any cholesterol concerns. Men with low testosterone often find that when they replace more youthful levels of T back into their body, their LDL levels naturally reduce to safer levels.

As was explained in *Mama's Wise Choices*, Chapter 32, most adults are low in pregnenolone. Because it is our mother hormone, it gets stretched very thin with all the work it must do as we age. If your LDL cholesterol is too high, you could try using an over the counter pregnenolone cream such as Life-Flo brand. Try a pump or two a day, depending on how it makes you feel. Three months later, check your cholesterol to see if it makes a positive impact on your levels.

Niacin

For people who have cholesterol ratios that don't look too great, niacin can come to the rescue. It is also called nicotinic acid, but it is simply vitamin B3. You can think of it as "the little vitamin that could."

Here are some of the ways niacin can improve your blood lipids:

1. It enlarges small dense cholesterol particles so they are less able to move into arterial walls and become plaque.
2. It has been proven to raise HDL levels from 15-24 percent.
3. It can lower triglycerides by 20-50 percent.
4. It can reduce LDL levels by 5-25 percent.
5. It is the only medication that effectively lowers the level of lipoprotein(a) or Lp(a). This particle is often known as the "widow maker," because it is so closely linked with heart attack and stroke. A normal Lp(a) is 30mg/dl or less. Any greater level than this can dangerously increase the risk for heart disease, even in young people. Statins, diet, and exercise will not lower this protein—only niacin and a good hormone profile.

Before you run out to your local health food store to load up on niacin, you need to know it has a strong side effect. It causes flushing. Flushing is not dangerous, but it can be a scary feeling if you are not prepared. Niacin opens all your tiny little blood vessels and this causes a warm, even hot, and sometimes, strong prickling feeling over the body. This is actually very healthy, but can feel rather uncomfortable. It's likely your face and ears will turn red for several minutes. The flushing gets less as your body becomes more used to the niacin dose, but every time you increase your dose substantially, you will notice more flushing. Many experts suggest jumping up doses in very small increments to help avoid this strong side effect.

Taking niacin in doses below 1000 mg will have a positive impact on HDL levels. It helps raise them in these smaller doses, but one usually has to take between 1-2000 mg to see a significant drop in LDL levels.

It is best to start slowly to get the body used to the flush. Start at 100 mg. After a few days you'll notice the flush will be more tolerable. Jump up to the next dose that you can handle, maybe another 100 mg. Keep increasing slowly, until after a couple of months, you are taking between 1-2000 mg. Taking your dose with a meal will significantly reduce the flush, as will taking a baby aspirin beforehand. If you take too much too soon, and feel like you are on fire, drink lots of water and this will help reduce the longevity of the flush. There is no need to rush to the emergency room because you think you are burning up! It will pass.

Some people do not have the patience to ramp up slowly. They may want to consider asking their doctor to script Niaspan for them which is slow release niacin. A very similar formulation can be purchased at most drug stores without a prescription. It is called Slo-niacin. The flush with slow release niacin is not usually noticeable to people, so larger doses can be taken.

It is important to monitor liver enzymes when taking over 1000 mg of niacin. While rare, some people may get an elevated liver enzyme count, so their dose will need to be reduced.

There are many "non flush niacin" supplements available. There is no evidence that they have the positive and significant effects on cholesterol, triglycerides, and the all important lipoprotein (a), as does regular or slow release niacin.

Red Yeast Rice

You may have heard of this supplement. It will lower cholesterol that is too high, but it is simply a statin in a natural form. Be careful if you decide to use this supplement as it also lowers CoQ10 levels in the body. However, it is more "natural" than a pharmaceutical drug if that is the route you decide to take.

Blood Pressure Supplements

Pearl chats: My husband discovered he had blood pressure problems at the age of 50, about six years ago. We tried many different supplements, all to no avail. He went on medication for a while, but even on medication he could not get his blood pressure into an optimum range. He felt sleepy and drained. I hated the idea of him having to take meds for the rest of his life.

I wasted a lot of money trying many supplements advertised to lower blood pressure. We tried garlic, hawthorn berries, and several formulations with a combination of various other BP lowering herbs, some of them promising to drop BP by 20 points! Nothing really made a dent in his BP readings. Once he lost over 30 pounds by eating **S** and **E,** his BP dropped quite a bit, but not perfect enough for my peace of mind.

My husband does not love to exercise. I feel his BP could have reduced all the way to normal with more exercise, but hey, he started to eat so well, I didn't want to nag. Well, I did every now and then. "Sorry, Honey!" I should add that he is much better about including exercise now that he has better energy levels on his T therapy, so I nag way less. That is good for both of us!

I finally read about an ayurvedic formula called Mukta Vati. I didn't hold out much hope, but decided to purchase it and see if anything positive happened. Smart decision if I say so myself. Mukta Vati lowered my husband's BP back to perfectly normal range. That was a big victory! When we run out, it goes back to borderline levels, so we have to order more online. Purchase from eBay or google for Ivy's brand.

Mukta Vati can cause a stuffy nosed feeling in the first couple of weeks. It also takes a couple of weeks to see any results. Hang in there for the first couple of weeks, even if you feel like giving up, because the stuffy nose usually passes. It may be used alongside BP medication, so BP monitoring will be necessary after commencing to see if meds need to be reduced or eliminated.

Chapter 42

Frequently Asked Questions

Why don't we count carbs and calories for meals on this plan?

Because this concept leads to the assumption that lower is always better. Our plan is about changing up fats, carbs, and calories, not diminishing them to a constant low state. Each day on plan will be naturally different from others.

While we have the basic threshold of 45 carbs for an **E** meal, it is only grains and fruit we estimate. We don't bother counting non-starchy vegetables even though they do have some carbs.

Remember, we are a carbohydrate conscious lifestyle, not a low-carb lifestyle. Constantly counting carbs is a waste of time. We have designed **S** and **E** so that when you feel lower in energy some days, or desire a starchier meal, an **E** meal is the ticket. If you had two or three **E** meals in one day, the total carb amount for that day will be a lot higher than a day when you only included one **E** snack. Why even keep track? Calorie and carb change ups will happen naturally. We would hate to urge you to keep carbs under a certain amount each day. That would take away your freedom to enjoy food. We want you to immerse yourself in the health benefits of all food groups and listen to your body, rather than count obsessively.

It's a similar issue with counting calories as it is to carbs. Constantly limiting calories to a set number will lower your metabolism and adversely affect your leptin and ghorenelin hormones. Those are crucial to a healthy bodily cycle of eating.

We believe in superfood fats like coconut oil, fish oils, olive oils, avocadoes, grass fed butters, and even good old cream. These are higher calorie foods, yet they make up the core of our **S** plan. They nourish our endocrine system and deter cravings so satiety kicks in. This allows high calorie foods to not be considered "the enemy," but rather extremely healthy options.

Be mindful that <u>constantly</u> eating high calorie fats may be too much if you have challenging pounds to lose. Sometimes, you can ladle the butter and cheese on without a lot of reserve in your **S** meal. Other times, enjoy your **S** meal, but don't make your fats so abundant. Remember, even slight calorie change ups, even in your **S** meals, are a good idea to stimulate your metabolism and ward off weight loss plateaus.

To avoid continuous calorie abuse, don't have several coffees with cream per day. We generally stick to one or two coffees per day. They may include cream if they coincide with an **S** meal. But, we don't pour half, or even quarter of a cup of cream in each time. That's a waste of calories. This doesn't mean you can't have a coffee with cream and then extra whipped cream on top as a treat after meals sometimes. But, don't do that every time you have coffee. It's great to be indulgent, but not at every meal. Food is to be celebrated, but not to the point where we feel the liberty to take calories for granted and think they have absolutely nothing at all to do with weight control. They play a role even though they are not solely in charge.

Sometimes you can do what we call (between ourselves) a pulled back **S**. Instead of eating a three cheese, sausage, and bacon quiche, you could have a lightly sautéed fillet of salmon with a large salad drizzled with just the perfect amount of medium-fat vinaigrette. Do you see the calorie change up even within an **S** category? Sometimes we bathe our body with two or three superfood fats per meal and, at other times, enjoy a more conservative portion of one. Sometimes, you can eat a rich fatty dessert, but it's also wise to eat more calorie conservative desserts like *Choco Pudding* a little more often. Remember to include some **Fuel Pull** snacks and meals so you force your body to juggle that third, much lower calorie ball we talked about earlier in the book.

If I have an E snack, like an apple with peanut butter, can I have an S meal an hour later?

Not if you want to stay in weight loss mode. To make sure the blood sugar rise produced by eating carbs does not get mixed up with the digestion of heavy fats, you need to wait at least two and a half hours, better yet, three hours between switches. It is easy to keep meals and snacks two to three hours apart from each other because eating closer than that is needless, unless you are breastfeeding a hungry baby.

The only likely reason you would feel hungry an hour after a meal or snack, is if it was not protein-centered and you overdid the carbs. Remember, overdoing carbs causes excessive hunger. If you are really craving that apple but know you want to eat an **S** meal soon after, eat half of it and add a little more protein to your snack. That way, you wouldn't be officially entering **E** territory, but making it more of an **S Helper** or neutral snack. You'd be fine to enjoy your **S** meal after that.

If you got busy and forgot your mid-afternoon snack, resulting in a small lapse of time between snack and meal, think ahead to coordinate them—**S** snack followed by **S** meal, or **E** snack followed by **E** meal. Or, simply have a **Fuel Pull** snack which makes things less complicated so you don't need to think at all.

What do you think about eating late at night?

The later you stay up at night, the more likely you will want to eat again. That is one of the reasons we suggest getting to bed by 10.00 pm or close after. This is often when the nighttime munchie monster rears its ugly head. Metabolism slows down in the evenings and you don't want to consume heavy calories at this time of the day.

But, there are times when you are genuinely hungry. It is okay to have a bed-time snack if you do it right. We actually recommend this for pregnant women and breastfeeding mothers. You may also need a snack if you have had a very physically demanding day.

The best snack for you to eat late at night is our *Choco Pudding* or *Lemon Mousse* (*Desserts*, Chapter 23). Why? Both these options are super low in calories, yet creamy and satisfying, thanks to the zero calorie superfood glucomannan. You could eat a full cup of one of these dessert/snacks for a pittance of calories and feel full enough to retire to bed without the rumbly tumblies.

We suggest keeping bed time snacks small so digestion issues will not disrupt sleep. We both have a few different suggestions.

Pearl chats: I usually have a nice hot cup of peppermint tea before bed. Sometimes, I may think I'm hungry, but it is really the desire for hand to mouth satisfaction. Holding a cup of tea in my hands is often enough to quell this feeling. If I am still really hungry, I'll have a few bites of *Choco Pudding*. If I'm not in the mood for sweet food, I'll have a small handful of almonds, or maybe a couple of pieces of cheese.

My digestive system has always been overly sensitive at night. I have learned my lesson to only eat a small snack, or gas pains for me!

Serene chats: Like Pearl, I like to test my true hunger with a nice hot drink first. It could be a soothing chai with a little raw cream, or a Swiss water decaf coffee with cream also. I use these more filling drinks when I know a clear herbal tea will not cut it. At other times, a simple peppermint or chamomile fits perfectly.

A freshly squeezed lemon or two over ice water and stevia gives great satisfaction on a hot summer night. Chewing on the ice also satisfies like I am eating something (although they say that it is not good for your teeth).

I often have a glass of *Earth Milk* (Chapter 27) as this satisfies, but does not tax my digestive system.

When food is the only thing that will fill the gap, I opt for low-carbs and have a little protein snack. This ensures I don't trigger my hunger further and is also an anti-aging tool. Research reveals that purposely eating a small protein snack before retiring will turn on more of your human growth hormone that naturally starts to pulse in the first few hours of sleep. It doesn't turn on with a late night bedtime! I eat a little Greek strained yogurt with a tad of almond butter swirled in, or one egg—hard boiled or lightly sautéed.

On the weekends (hey, I gotta be honest here) my late night snack is sometimes a glass of dry red wine and a couple of squares of Lindt very dark chocolate, 85-90%. My husband and I enjoy this ritual together after all the squabbles have been resolved, the snotty noses wiped, the diapers are on, and all the children are tucked in. Ahhhhh!

I've never liked salmon. Can I do this program without it?

Yes, you can. Use other fish, or keep to chicken and good sources of beef. But, before you stick to your notion, open your mind for a minute. We can relate to your aversion. Neither of us were big salmon eaters. Remember, Serene had not eaten any meat for almost two decades. Most of our likes and dislikes are simply mindsets that can be changed. If you tell yourself about all the benefits with its superfood qualities, and learn to prepare it in a yummy way, the mindset will fall away as it did for us. Try different ways to cook it and find your favorites. If you are worried about a fishy taste, season well and pour the juice of a whole lemon on top. That will take care of that. Serene is rearing to say more.

Serene chats: When I first began eating meat, I began with salmon and had an interesting journey. In the beginning, even one fillet on my plate was too overwhelming. I would have to flake it in small pieces and sauté it with yummy veggies like eggplant and onions. I also learned to enjoy it flaked in soups. Salmon burgers are also good for a beginner.

If you don't like it baked, try it broiled. Still not happy? Try it lightly fried to a crisp. This can be made even crispier by making a "breading" out of sesame seeds or crushed nuts and spices. If this does not hit the spot, try it sautéed in dry red wine and lots of butter. I like nutritional yeast, black pepper, and Celtic salt sprinkled on both sides and lightly fried in coconut oil. My new favorite is simply poached in a tasty broth.

I hate to eat salmon cold, it gives me the willies. But, if there are any leftovers, they can be reheated in the pan with a little butter or oil, and this is divine. After all the ways I learned to prepare salmon in order to get it down my throat, it has now become my favorite food "anytime, anywhere, anyway."

My husband says he is not interested in changing the way he eats, yet his weight is not healthy. I want to follow S and E all the way. What should I do about him?

Start with yourself. He'll eventually notice all the good results you are gaining. Even without going completely on this program, he'll receive benefits for himself by eating the low glycemic family meals you now prepare. These delicious "male food" type meals should not meet his resistance.

Offer to make him scrumptious breakfasts before he leaves for work. If he is the type of guy who has developed a sweet tooth, why not serve him *Basic Cheesecake* in the morning? Or, try out the *Cookie Bowl Oatmeal* on him. It's extremely hard for someone to not like a sweet breakfast recipe.

What man would turn away a sliced steak omelet for breakfast? He won't miss the white toast. You could even add a warm buttered *Oopsie Roll* or one of our *Country Biscuits* (*Muffins, Breads, and Pizza Crusts*, Chapter 19). If he goes to work very early, you can leave some *Savory Protein Muffins* (*Morning Meals*, Chapter 18) in the fridge for him. He can easily heat them before he leaves, or they're great to eat cold, too.

By starting the day off healthfully and ending it with one of your night time **S** or **E's**, he will be on the road to change and not even know it. Don't nag him as this will only make him dig in his toes even more. Let him know you want to steer the nutritional direction of the household in a healthier, more low glycemic direction, and would love and appreciate his support.

He may have some bad habits, like chocolate chip cookies, Fritos, or potato chips that he likes to snack on when he's home. You know the time he usually reaches for these. Get clever and offer him one of your new exciting creations to taste test before his snack time, perhaps some spicy crispy nuts, one of our cracker recipes, or cheese crisps. Who knows, even though they are green, he might enjoy *Kale Chips* (most women love them, but some guys can get on board with them, too). Maybe he'll love our *Chunky Cream Pops* if he gets a hankering for something cold and creamy, or our peanut butter flavored *Tummy Tucking Ice Cream* (both found in *Deserts*, Chapter 23). We have yet to meet one person who doesn't enjoy those.

The goal is to fill him up on your food so he needs to eat less of his. Anticipate his needs. Ask him what he is in the mood for. Be creative enough to put your healthy spin on his cravings, using our principles. Don't expect him to want to read our book and understand that he shouldn't mix **S** and **E** foods, although if he wants to that's great. Pearl's husband has been doing the plan for over four years and still doesn't know what's **S** and what's **E**! He just loves all the food he's given.

If all these tips still don't work, a happy marriage is better than a hen-pecked man who would rather be somewhere other than home.

I thought bananas were healthy. This is the first time I've been told to not eat them. What about other fruits like watermelon, pineapple, and mangoes?

Yes, bananas are healthy. God made them for a purpose. They are excellent for growing children and for people who struggle to keep on weight. The reason for this is that they are much higher in sugars than the other fruits we suggest. Tropical fruits on a whole have less fiber and more sugar.

This doesn't mean you should totally exclude them from your diet. You can have small amounts of these with **E** meals, e.g., mango in some salsa, pineapple in some cottage cheese, small piece of watermelon, or half a banana. Personally, we stay away from bananas, but we had addictions to them in the past. Three in one sitting was not beyond us, so they are trigger foods for us.

God created such a variety of fruits in order to satisfy different tastes and different cultures. The starchier, sweeter varieties are great for children who run around all day and burn lots of energy. Fruits like berries, grapefruit, and green apples are perfect for adults who have stopped growing and need to keep control of their weight. There are also middling fruits like oranges and pears. They can be a regular part of your diet, but they need to take second place to lower glycemic fruits like berries.

We call bananas and other high glycemic fruits healthy since God made them, but only for those whose blood sugar can handle them. If something is chock full of vitamins and minerals and yet causes your waistline to expand and spike your blood sugar levels, which is aging and inflammatory, it is not healthy for you.

I love dried fruits. I always thought they were like healthy candy. You mean I shouldn't eat them?

Again, these are fine for children. However, caution must be taken even when feeding your children a lot of dried fruits as they can damage teeth with their extremely high sugar potency.

Fruit, in its natural state, usually has high water content. This helps dilute the sugar content and helps to eliminate the severe bloat for which dried fruit is famous. Drying fruit, by removing the water, simply leaves sugar balls. Yes, all the vitamins, minerals, and antioxidants are left, but the high doses of sugar spike your insulin just like the white sugar you buy at your grocery store. Sure, dried fruits are not empty calories, but for your waistline and the health of your pancreas, the results can be similar to a Snickers bar.

If you are at your ideal weight or you have a high metabolism, small amounts of dried fruit, mixed with nuts to temper the rush of sugar, is a healthier **Crossover** choice.

> *Serene chats:* I lived on organic dried fruit and thought it was an integral part of my superfood raw diet, but I suffered with terrible yeast problems. When I was pregnant on that sort of diet, I could not eradicate this constant issue. I had a colon cleanse (colonic irrigation) and was told that my intestines were full of froth and bubble, as if I had consumed a lot of alcohol. I told the irrigationist that I had never touched a drop to my lips. She replied that I must be eating something that was very high in sugar because it was fermenting in my intestines and turning into alcohol. Yuk! And to think I was so proud about never letting even one white grain of sugar into my body!
>
> Since living on a low glycemic diet, I never suffer with yeast. I am six months pregnant right now and haven't felt one annoying itch. I even had to go on antibiotics (rare occurrence for me) for an ear infection I picked up swimming in the creek and I still did not get a yeast infection after I took the full course. This is truly a miracle for me!

I have a child who is a picky eater. She won't eat much more than mac n cheese, cereal, and chicken nuggets. Help!

We know peace is easier than a battle, but this is serious. You are going to have to wage war against your child's vulnerability to diabetes and other diseases that could develop later in life. You must ask yourself the following questions.

- Is it okay for my child to develop a weight problem on my watch?
- If it's not an issue already, is it okay with you if she develops insulin resistance (prediabetic state) and has a weight problem when she is older?

- It is likely that weight will become an issue, but even if it doesn't, is it still okay with you that your child becomes depleted of vitamins, minerals, amino acid, and antioxidants that are essential for good health?
- Are you fine with the fact that these inflammatory promoting foods are a breeding ground for degenerate disease?

We're sure you're not okay with any of the above—but that is the big picture. You know the saying, "You have to be cruel to be kind." Her regular foods will have to be removed to make room for healthy ones. They could be used for treats now and then.

Pearl chats: Two of my five children are rather picky. They would be much worse, but I have not allowed it. One of my sons cannot stand fruit and does not like salad. For a while, I didn't like all the complaining and the confrontation and so I gave in to him and hoped he would change as he got older. This caused me to make different meals for him. Some of my other children got on the bandwagon and I found myself having to "make something extra here and leave off something there." It was exhausting and ridiculous and I was not doing my children any favors.

Now, the rule in our house is that they eat what is on their plates, or else! They are not allowed to complain. They can only compliment. They know I try to make meals tasty, but I let them know their health is Mommy's priority and educate them on the benefits of healthy foods. It was hard at first, but now my children are used to it. They know they have to eat what is put in front of them and be happy. They also know I rotate their favorite meals so some nights they'll be eating exactly what they want. They have to man or woman up the other nights and eat without complaints.

I'll admit my children do get some regular treats. Now and then, they are allowed store-bought ice cream and they get to eat chocolate chip cookies made with natural ingredients, but the majority of their diet is whole food.

Serene chats: I do not bring junk food into our kitchen cupboards so the temptations are not available for my children. Of course, this does not mean that they don't ask for them when we go shopping. I just say No, and they know that my No is No. Having unhealthy food choices in the home may be an issue if your husband likes you to buy treats for him. This is where you have to use extra firmness with your children. You have the opportunity to mold their eating habits, but you can't force a change in your spouse.

I like to make healthy *decadent* chocolates or little peanut butter balls for the children so treats *are always* on hand. My children love the *Secret Agent Brownie Cake* (*Desserts*, Chapter 23) made with honey. When it comes to eating something they *don't* like, it is as simple as *eat or go hungry*, and when you are ready to eat again, it will be the same thing you refused. This sounds tough, but I don't want this to continue into their adulthood. It limits their ability to establish their health, promote stable weight, and prevent disease. Besides, a picky child who turns into a picky adult is no fun to cook for and can create unneeded marriage problems.

I am worried about bowel regularity if I eat the way you promote. It doesn't seem like there would be enough whole grains to keep the bowels moving.

S and **E** are so rich with non-starchy vegetables, which are the highest in fiber and water content, that we don't see how this could be a problem. It is true, however, that whenever you change your diet drastically, the digestive system isn't used to the new foods and often needs a week or so to adjust.

Although we have mentioned this before, here's a little more detail about the benefits of supplementing magnesium. Constipation can be easily alleviated by taking magnesium citrate or oxide (or a combination of both) as a supplement before bed at night. This is extremely healthy as magnesium is depleted from modern soils and is essential for nerve and brain health. It is also a natural relaxant and loosens the bowels without causing addiction to laxatives.

We have found that even though the citrate form is better absorbed by the body if your major reason for taking it is bowel regularity forget the more expensive citrate form. We buy inexpensive magnesium oxide from Walmart, two bottles for less than $5.00. Two to four tablets before bed, on a reasonably empty stomach, should do the trick. Pull back if you get diarrhea. If you take an iron supplement, you might need to increase the dose. Iron in oral form leads to constipation, but enough magnesium can remedy that.

Don't get us wrong. We go fine even without magnesium, but we love the extra assurance. Therefore, we continue magnesium supplementation just for the health of it, and consequently, bowel issues are never a problem.

If you are really concerned, here are some other good tips to try.

- Eat two stalks of celery a day.
- Make sure you get some sort of exercise.
- Drink a fresh lemon squeezed into warm water upon rising in the morning.
- Eat fermented vegetables.
- Glucomannan puddings will help you, too.

- Add chia and flax seed to smoothies or breakfast oatmeal. Make sure to drink enough water if adding these seeds.

What if you really have a stubborn bowel? We have counseled people with these ill-behaved bowels and here's a protocol that should be a sure-fire solution when all else fails.

1. Take magnesium oxide at night on an empty stomach.
2. Before you eat anything in the morning, drink a strong organic coffee with a little cream to help stimulate your bile. Sip slowly. Don't gulp it down and try not to dwell on whether you will have success in the bathroom. Just relax as a tense bowel will not perform on demand.
3. Wait 20 minutes. If you still haven't gone to the bathroom, fry up two to three eggs in a good amount of butter or coconut oil. This fatty, protein rich breakfast really stimulates your bile which is paramount for bowel evacuation. Fiber usually gets the limelight while bile doesn't get enough recognition. This under-praised digestive aid is the real superstar. Coffee on an empty stomach is highly stimulating to your bowel. Topping it off with a good dose of bile excretion should send you to the "loo" as we say Downunder.
4. Still having issues? Surely not, but if so, jump gently on a mini trampoline (rebounder) for a few minutes. Intense exercise at this moment won't work to help you go. Stay relaxed as you bounce and let the poop descend with the gentle pull of gravity as you bounce. You can tell we are entirely too comfortable talking about this! It's a sister thing! Time to move on before we get worse. Oh wait, mooooove on. Yea, that's hilarious, to us at least!

I don't have a lot of time for making healthy treats for myself. Is there any chocolate I could buy that is approved for this plan?

Yes, you can visit www.netrition.com and purchase Lucienne's sugar-free chocolate which is sweetened with the healthy sweeteners we recommend, but it is too pricey for some of us. Your good old regular grocery store should have 85% dark chocolate. Don't make a habit of eating store purchased chocolate any less percentage than 85%.

Very dark chocolate like this does have some sugar content, but it's usually so low that, per serving the carbs are about six grams or less. That's within **S** limits. Keep this chocolate to **S** settings as it has ample fat. We both enjoy 85% dark chocolate sometimes with brands such as Green and Black, or Lindt. They are smooth and not as bitter as you might think. Don't go overboard with portions and you'll avoid a blood sugar spike and the consequent fat gain. Stick to a serving as indicated on the chocolate packet.

I'm pregnant and I don't think this is a good time to go on a diet. Can I still do the S and E plan?

Emphatically yes! It is very important to stabilize sugar while you are pregnant. High levels of progesterone during pregnancy cause our cells to naturally be in a more insulin resistant state and this is the reason why many women suffer gestational diabetes on regular western food.

We are not doctors, but between us, we have had 12 biological babies. We think any weight gain over 30 pounds is not necessary for a healthy baby and makes recovery much harder. Neither do we think a woman should gain less than 20 pounds unless she is obese to start with. However, some women may gain 40 pounds no matter what. As long as they are not overdoing carbohydrates, they can rest assured that this is natural for them. The weight that is accumulated from natural change in hormones and normal gestational growth will come off easily. The stubborn pounds are the ones accumulated from sugar spikes.

Post pregnancy hips will slowly come back in as the bones move back after separating for birth. Loose skin will tighten again and if your stomach muscles separate, they will return to normal. The soft pillow where the baby was growing may poke out for awhile, but this is not fat. As the stomach muscles regain their strength, it will flatten again. Any extra tire of fat that is noticeable when you stand up cannot be blamed on the pregnancy. This is from overdoing carby foods.

What about breastfeeding?

Breastfeeding, on its own, is usually enough to lose extra weight after birth. If you have gained more than 30 pounds stick to the **S** and **E** program more purely (without adding a lot of **Crossovers** or **S Helpers**) and this will melt the rest away. **S** and **E** have enough nutrients and balance of food groups to support an abundant milk supply. Eat frequent **E** meals that contain quinoa as this will help stimulate your milk supply and is so nourishing for both you and the baby.

You will be hungry more often when you are breastfeeding so don't forget your snacks. Eating frequent small meals does not cause weight gain. It actually helps you to lose. Also, remember to drink enough liquids which is majorly of important for a healthy milk supply.

There are some breastfeeding women who lose baby weight very quickly. These women will need to incorporate **Crossovers** to ensure a healthy strong body.

Do you have any quick lifestyle tips for us?

We will both give you 10 tips each. Some of these will be recap, but we would like to hit them home.

Serene's Tips:

1. I drink a glass of pure water with something green in it every morning before I even know I am awake and realize how gross it tastes. I can't afford Barley Green or Perfect Food (green food supplements), but I use straight wheat grass powder or chlorophyll drops which are the cheapest and they last for months.
2. I exercise in the first half of the day and make this babysitting time for my older children, even if that means a little recess from homeschool. If I leave it until later, I never do it. Most days I only do 20 minutes and I usually take the weekends off. I like to read to my children and also sit a lot while I school them. I hate to feel my bottom is joining in with the sofa. Therefore, I like to get my circulation moving and keep my metabolism warmed. I do this every hour or so by doing a few star jumps, running on the spot with my children, or doing a set of 10 pushups. This sporadic form of exercise is actually the most beneficial to metabolism.
3. I do five minutes of relaxing stretches before I get in bed at night.
4. I make sure to drink lots of fresh water, green tea, and herbal drinks throughout the day. This not only keeps my body hydrated, but makes for a nice relaxing break when I sit down to a warm tea.
5. I try to incorporate lots of raw berries and a nice green salad every day, as well as raw fermented dairy. I also eat 1 Tbs. of cultured veggies when I eat a cooked meal. Snacking on raw nuts and seeds with a little raw cheese is also a practice of mine. This supports my enzyme levels.
6. I never eat after I feel satisfied, and if I am not sure, I opt for a warming tea—creamy chai or Swiss water decaf with some cream after an **S** meal. I tell myself that even though my taste buds want more, my body doesn't need more. Giving my body what it doesn't need and can't process easily is like using it as a trash can and throwing in useless waste. (I don't follow this rule at Thanksgiving and Christmas).
7. Another helper I use is little mints (brand name SPRY called Supermints) that are made from pure mint extract and xylitol. Xylitol is a low glycemic sweetener that is excellent for preventing bacteria in your mouth and gums. I use them when I want to eat because I am bored or at nighttime when I want to eat but I don't need to. I go to bed with a delicious mint breath for my husband and don't have to feel yucky because I gave in and ate a couple of pieces of toast before bed.

8. I try to get to bed by 9.00 p.m. and this way I am usually in bed by 9:30 p.m. Sleep is so important for health and anti-aging as well as proper weight control.
9. I try not to be a stressed out, harried person. This doesn't always work and I am often stressed out and completely frazzled. I try to give my worries to God and rest in the fact that He alone is the One in control of my life and my children's lives, and take a deep breath and relax.
10. If I am running out of the house on errands, going to church, or spending a day at a friend's house, I always pack some healthy snacks for the children and me. This way, I am never stuck being hungry with no healthy options. I also keep my metabolism revved and don't arrive at home or a restaurant absolutely famished and ready to eat anything that comes my way.

Pearl's Tips:

1. I could not do without my supplement list that I have attached to the side of my fridge for my husband and myself. It lists the supplements I should take each morning and night. If I don't check my list, I forget some, or don't take them at all, or forget to lay them out for my husband.
2. I never eat leftovers from my children's plates. If they can't quite manage to eat their whole meal, it's not my job to be the vacuum cleaner. Some people have the notion that it is terrible to waste food. However, I think if certain foods are not going to benefit your body, they are better in the trash or put back in the fridge for your child the next day, than in your stomach.
3. I do the salad rip trick a lot in order to eat more raw food and fill up. I rip up some organic lettuce, put it on my plate, pour on some dressing, and then add my protein of meat or eggs—it's done!
4. I always try to get to bed by 10.00 to 10:30 on week nights. I stay up much later on the weekends, because after all, life is for living.
5. I make sure to exercise in the morning (sometimes in the afternoon if mornings are crazy) about four times a week. Believe me, I never feel like it. Vigorous exercise doesn't come naturally to my personality. In fact, it is usually so hard to work up the motivation that I have to call Serene and ask her why I need to exercise. Sitting and watching the birds outside my kitchen window and drinking a coffee or green tea sounds much more sane. But, I have gained so many benefits from exercise that I make sure to call and get my pep talk when I need it. She's always ready to preach to me and I end up revved and convinced! If you are like me, I suggest you find someone who you can call and who will give you a motivation speech, or buy an exercise DVD that helps

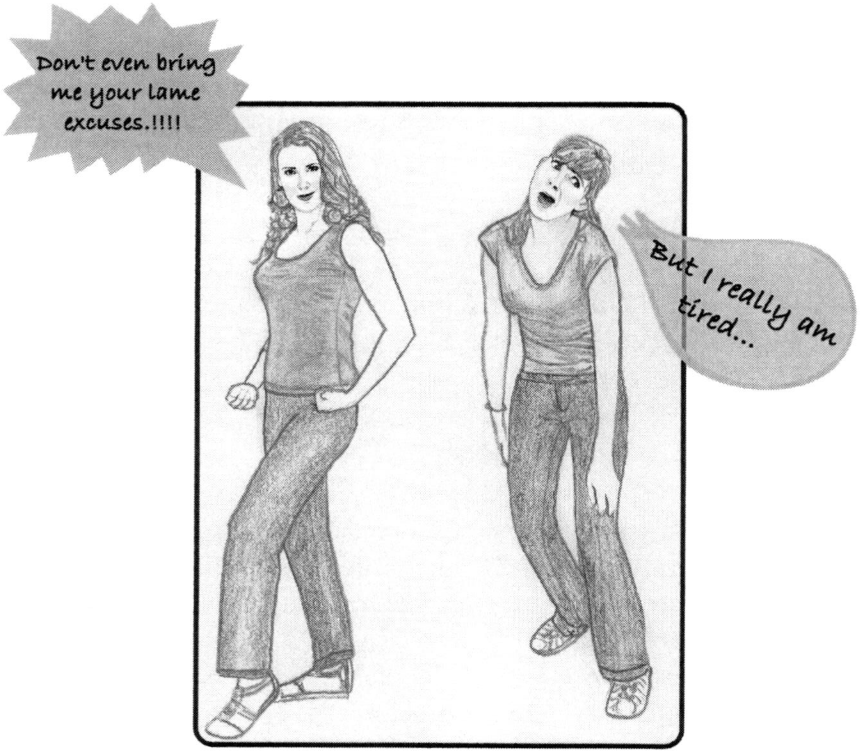

motivate you. Some of us don't have those inner voices telling us why we should get out of breath and feel muscle pain. We need somebody else who is more wired that way to remind us.

6. In the early evening or late afternoon, when it is warm enough, I like to take a stroll. This is not for exercise, but to enjoy nature, decompress, think about the things I am grateful for and thank God for them.

   Recently, I read an incredible book about being thankful called *A Thousand Gifts*. The author, Ann Voskamp makes a challenge to herself to practice thankfulness in the little things of daily life. It's a lesson in contentment like no other and she weaves it through vivid scenes of her own personal struggles inside her home and community.

   These walks are when I try to really focus on the things in life for which I am thankful. It's time to count my blessings. Ann Voskamp writes a list with pen and paper. I walk and list in my head, but it works for me. My "grateful walks" always refresh me and walking helps digestion to boot. I need no motivational talks from Serene to do this.

7. I make every effort to not go to bed with my makeup on. I always notice my skin is negatively affected the next morning if I do. Also, making sure to take my makeup off keeps me in the routine of moisturizing with all the goodness of Kit Naturals before bed.
8. I have such a long list of books I want to read and find it hard to get through them all. I am usually reading three or four study and research books at the same time. I now bring my books to the table with my children while they homeschool so I am right there if they have any questions. (Math hour is out since I'm always trouble shooting, but some other subjects allow time for this). This way, they see that Mom is an avid reader and we continue to learn our whole lives through. Also, this way, I get two things done at once.
9. I have given up fussing about the house all day. We get on with our lives and let it go. We all have one big clean up after lunch and then another one after supper. If you come to my house in between those times, I feel sorry for you. Picture perfect it is not! At least this way, we wake up to a clean house and have a while to relax in the afternoon when it is not in shambles.
10. I try to change my clothes and put a little makeup on before my husband comes home at night to help keep that romantic spark alive. He didn't fall in love with a grubby woman in sweats with a frown on her face. He fell for a woman who made the best of herself and smiled a lot, so I remind myself to do that for him. I slip up now and then.

    If your husband is not a makeup liking sort of guy, do something to yourself that he will notice and like. Maybe it's brushing your teeth and applying lip balm. That helps. Acknowledge that you are glad he is home when he walks in the door. That is huge! Don't gauge your actions on whether you think he deserves it. It's too easy to keep a record of little wrongs. Let them go! Do it because he's the man you chose to marry and that means he deserves your best.

Chapter 43

Time for Goodbye

That's it, Mama! We've pictured you in our minds all throughout the writing of this book. We imagine you reading little snippets of it when your children are in bed, when you get a few minute's break in the afternoon, or maybe even when you're using the bathroom! Hey, we know what it's like.

You are in our hearts and we want to hear from you as you start toddling on your way toward nutritional freedom. We want to hear about your first joy-filled running steps once you learn to eat, love, and live to the fullest.

Support will be your key. You can visit our website, www.trimhealthymama.com. We'll pop in there as we are able (we may not always be able!). There'll be a place for you to post recipes of your own that fit the plan and can bless others. We know some of you will surpass us in culinary ideas and skills.

It may be a great idea to start up or attend a *Trim Healthy Mama* group in your area. Getting together with other mamas to encourage one another, support each other through challenges, and discuss the principles of this lifestyle will go a long way to help keep you on track.

We have our own natural support group of friends that have similar nutrition and life goals as we do. It benefits us all to get together now and then. A great idea is to make the gathering a lunch time at someone's home. Decide if the lunch will be **S** or **E** and have everybody bring a dish to match. **S** might be the best way to start.

One mama can bring the greens for a salad, another could bring a quiche or tasty meat item, another the delicious dressing and spicy nuts for the salad, and someone else can bring the scrumptious dessert. You can enjoy one another, have fun, share recipes, encourage each other to exercise the smart way (maybe even do a short workout DVD together before lunch—what a laugh!) and of course, exhort one another to love your husband with the full knowledge of that meaning!

We hope to meet up with you again in our next book, *Trim Healthy Mama Rides Again.* Like the name? Or maybe we should title it, *Get Slim Eating Puddings, Ice cream, Shakes, and Cakes*! Isn't that the crazy truth? Now that title might be a real seller. We'll need to think about that.

Hopefully it won't take us another five years to write the next one. We promise to do better on our time management next time around.

Love you, Mama. The ride begins now!

Serene and Pearl
www.trimhealthymama.com
Facebook: Trim Healthy Mama

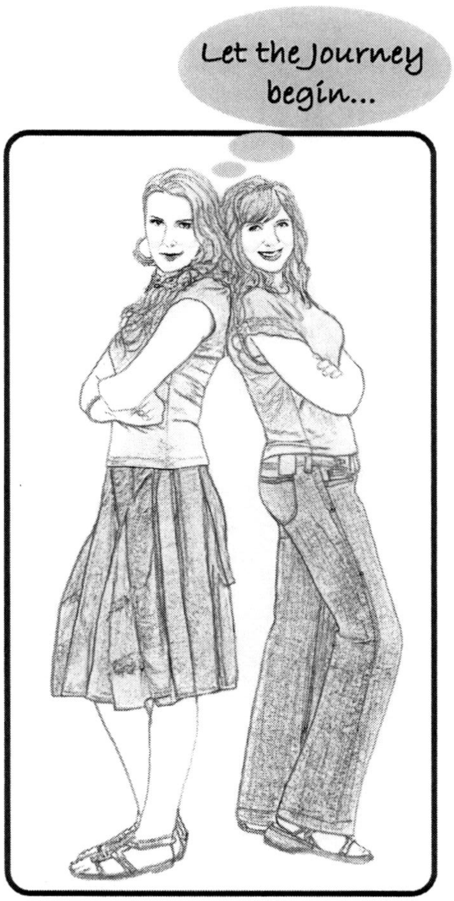

RECIPE INDEX

D

E

F

G

H

I

J

K

L

M

N

O

P

Q

R

S

T

V

W

Z

SUBJECT INDEX

A

B

C

G

H

I

J

K

L

M

T

V

W

X

Y

Notes

Notes

Notes

Notes

Notes

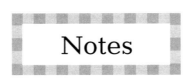

Notes

Notes

Notes

Notes

CPSIA information can be obtained at www.ICGtesting.com
Printed in the USA
BVOW062204060613

322686BV00002B/15/P

9 780988 775114